Study Guide for

Medical-Surgical Nursing: Assessment and Management of Clinical Problems

Eighth Edition

Prepared by:

Judy L. Maltas, RN, MSN, CCRN
Assistant Professor/Clinical
Department of Acute Nursing Care
School of Nursing
University of Texas Health Science Center at San Antonio
San Antonio, Texas

Sharon L. Lewis, RN, PhD, FAAN
Shannon Ruff Dirksen, RN, PhD
Margaret McLean Heitkemper, RN, PhD, FAAN
Linda Bucher, RN, PhD, CEN

Reviewed by:

Susan A. Sandstrom, RNC, MSN, CNE
Auditor, Department of Quality
Omaha Veterans Administration Hospital
Omaha, Nebraska

ELSEVIER
MOSBY

ELSEVIER
MOSBY

3251 Riverport Lane
St. Louis, Missouri 63043

STUDY GUIDE FOR MEDICAL-SURGICAL NURSING:
ASSESSMENT AND MANAGEMENT OF CLINICAL PROBLEMS

ISBN: 978-0-323-06654-9

Notices

Previous editions copyrighted 2007, 2004, 2000, 1996, 1992

ISBN: 978-0-323-06654-9

Senior Acquisitions Editor: Kristin Geen
Senior Developmental Editor: Jamie Horn
Publishing Services Manager: Jeff Patterson
Project Manager: Megan Isenberg
Design Direction: Teresa McBryan
Cover Designer: Teresa McBryan

Printed in the United States of America

Last digit is the print number: 9 8 7 6 5 4 3 2

Contents

CHAPTER 1

Contemporary Nursing Practice

1. Using the American Nurses Association's definition of nursing, identify which of the following activities are within the domain of nursing (select all that apply):
   _____ a. Writing an order for intake and output for a patient who is vomiting
   _____ b. Establishing and implementing a stress-reduction program for family caregivers of patients with Alzheimer's disease
   _____ c. Explaining the risks associated with the planned surgical procedure when a preoperative patient inquires about risks
   _____ d. Developing and performing a study to compare the health status of older patients who live alone with the status of older patients who live with family members
   _____ e. Identifying the effect of an investigational drug on patients' hemoglobin levels
   _____ f. Using a biofeedback machine to teach a patient with cancer how to manage chronic pain
   _____ g. Preventing pneumonia in an immobile patient by ordering frequent turning, coughing, and deep breathing
   _____ h. Determining and administering fluid-replacement therapy needed for a patient with serious burns
   _____ i. Testifying to legislative bodies regarding the effect of health policies on culturally, socially, and economically diverse populations

2. Choose two or three areas of specialization in nursing that are of interest to you. Using the website of the American Nurses Credentialing Center (www.nursecredentialing.org), determine the educational preparation required for certification in those areas of interest and any other requirements identified.

3. A nurse who has worked on an orthopedic unit for several years is encouraged by the nurse manager to become certified in orthopedic nursing. The nurse recognizes that certification in nursing (select all that apply)
   a. requires a certain amount of clinical experience.
   b. requires successful completion of an examination.
   c. is professional recognition of expertise in a specialty area.
   d. will require membership in specialty nursing organizations.
   e. is an advanced practice role that requires graduate education.

4. Which of the following statements best describes the role of the clinical nurse leader (CNL)?
   a. CNL role focuses on performing nursing research.
   b. CNL role is a generalist clinician with a master's degree.
   c. CNL education provides a terminal degree in nursing practice.
   d. CNL role offers an opportunity for a nurse to specialize at an advanced education level.

5. Identify whether the following statements are true (*T*) or false (*F*). If a statement is false, correct the bold word(s) to make the statement true.
   a. The **simplicity** of the health care environment is affected by rapidly changing technology and expanding knowledge.
   b. Nurses are caring for an **aging population**, which will affect future nursing practice.
   c. Future nursing practice will require critical thinking to make sound clinical judgments. Critical thinking is a **learned** skill.
   d. National Patient Safety Goals (NPSG), such as "improve the effectiveness of communication among caregivers," are set for health care providers by the **Institute of Medicine**.

6. What are the six competencies from the project Quality and Safety Education for Nurses (QSEN) that are expected of new nursing graduates?

   a.

   b.

   c.

   d.

   e.

   f.

7. Place the steps of the evidence-based practice (EBP) process in order (1 being the first step; 5 being the last step).
   _____ Make recommendations for practice or generate data.
   _____ Ask a clinical question.
   _____ Critically analyze the evidence.
   _____ Find and collect the evidence.
   _____ Evaluate the outcomes in the clinical setting.

8. The format for asking a clinical question follows the PICOT format. What do each of the letters in this acronym signify?

   P _____

   I _____

   C _____

   O _____

   T _____

9. Two nurses are establishing a smoking-cessation program to assist patients with chronic lung disease to stop smoking. To offer the most effective program with the best outcomes, the nurses should
   a. search for an article that describes nursing interventions that are effective for smoking cessation.
   b. develop a clinical question that will allow them to compare different cessation methods during the program.
   c. keep comprehensive records that detail each patient's progress and ultimate outcomes from participation in the program.
   d. use evidence-based clinical practice guidelines developed from reviews of randomized controlled trials of smoking cessation methods.

10. Identify the three nursing terminologies that specifically relate to the steps of the nursing process.

    a.

    b.

    c.

11. The nurse working in a health care facility where uniform electronic health records are used explains to the patient that the primary purpose of such a record is to
    a. reduce the cost of health care by eliminating paper records.
    b. prevent medical errors associated with traditional paper records and handwritten orders and prescriptions.
    c. force the use of standardized medical vocabularies and nursing terminologies so that outcomes of patient care can be measured.
    d. provide a single record where all aspects of a patient's medical information is readily available to any health care provider involved in the patient's care.

12. A nurse who studies the structure and processing of nursing information and who builds systems that support that processing is called a
    a. nurse educator.
    b. nurse informatist.
    c. unit nurse manager.
    d. clinical nurse leader.

13. Match the phases of the nursing process with the descriptions (answers may be used more than once).

    _____ a. Analysis of data   1. Assessment
    _____ b. Priority setting   2. Diagnosis
    _____ c. Nursing interventions   3. Planning
    _____ d. Data collection   4. Implementation
    _____ e. Identifying patient strengths   5. Evaluation
    _____ f. Measuring patient achievement of goals
    _____ g. Setting goals
    _____ h. Identifying health problems
    _____ i. Modifying the plan of care
    _____ j. Documenting care provided

14. A 62-year-old patient hospitalized with heart failure has been receiving large doses of diuretics. The nurse notes that the patient has increasing weakness, flabby muscles, increased irritability, and a weak, rapid pulse. The nurse notifies the health care provider of these findings and asks whether the patient's potassium level should be checked. The health care provider orders a laboratory test to evaluate the patient's serum electrolyte levels. The results indicate hypokalemia, and the nurse reports the results to the health care provider. The health care provider orders potassium supplements, daily serum electrolyte levels, and a high-potassium diet. The nurse administers the medication and discusses the dietary order and the patient's status with the dietitian. The dietitian performs initial patient teaching regarding dietary intake of potassium. The nurse helps the patient choose high-potassium foods from the daily menu and evaluates the patient's ability to make correct choices. The nurse also monitors the patient's response to the potassium supplements with daily laboratory results and physical assessment findings.

    What are the independent, collaborative, and dependent functions that the nurse performed in this situation?

    a. Independent

    b. Collaborative

    c. Dependent

15. For the following problems, write "ND" in front of those that are nursing diagnoses and "CP" in front of those that are collaborative problems.

    _____ a. Infection related to immunosuppression
    _____ b. Ineffective airway clearance related to excessive mucus
    _____ c. Constipation related to irregular defecation habits
    _____ d. Deficient fluid volume related to NPO status
    _____ e. Fatigue related to sleep deprivation
    _____ f. Excess fluid volume related to high sodium intake
    _____ g. Imbalanced nutrition: less than body requirements related to anorexia
    _____ h. Risk for cardiac dysrhythmias related to potassium deficiency
    _____ i. Stress urinary incontinence related to weak pelvic-floor muscles
    _____ j. Hypoxia related to chronic obstructive pulmonary disease

16. Read all the data for the case history below, and write a three-part nursing diagnosis statement that clearly describes the problem.

    A 52-year-old man was on prolonged bed rest after fracturing his pelvis. When he begins ambulation, he develops the following signs and symptoms: shortness of breath on exertion; a reported inability to perform usual activities of daily living (ADLs) because of weakness and fatigue; pulse remains elevated after activity for more than 5 minutes.

17. Identify the basis for setting priorities for interventions for nursing diagnoses.
    a.

    b.

    c.

    d.

18. Describe how planned nursing interventions would differ between these two nursing diagnoses: (a) imbalanced nutrition: less than body requirements related to anorexia; and (b) imbalanced nutrition: less than body requirements related to difficulty in swallowing.

19. For the specific written outcome statements below, identify those that are correctly (C) written, and identify what criteria are not met in those outcomes that are incorrectly (I) written.
    _____ a. The patient will recognize the importance of taking the medications as prescribed.
    _____ b. The patient lists the supplies needed to change the dressing by discharge.
    _____ c. The patient maintains a low-sodium diet.
    _____ d. The patient's activity tolerance will be increased by discharge.
    _____ e. The patient will ambulate with a walker from the room to the nurse's station three times a day without assistance.

20. For the nursing diagnoses and written patient outcomes listed below, identify a specific nursing intervention indicated to help the patient reach the outcome.
    a. Nursing diagnosis: Risk for impaired skin integrity related to immobility
       Patient outcome: Patient will demonstrate skin integrity free of pressure ulcers.

    b. Nursing diagnosis: Constipation related to inadequate fluid and fiber intake
       Patient outcome: Patient will have daily soft bowel movements in 1 week.

21. A patient with a seizure disorder is admitted to the hospital after a sustained seizure. When she tells the nurse that she has not taken her medication regularly, the nurse makes a nursing diagnosis of ineffective self health management related to lack of knowledge regarding medication regimen and identifies the NOC outcome of "Compliance behavior, with the indicator 'Performs treatment regimen as prescribed, at a target rate of 3 (sometimes demonstrated).'" When the nurse tries to teach the patient about the medication regimen, the patient tells the nurse that she knows about the medications but she does not always have the money to refill the prescriptions.
    a. Where was the mistake made in the nursing process with this patient?

    b. How would the nurse revise the care plan based on this evaluation?

22. Identify the five rights of delegation.
    a.

    b.

    c.

    d.

    e.

23. Delegation is a process used by the RN to provide safe and effective care in an efficient manner. Which of the following nursing interventions should not be delegated to nursing assistive personnel (NAP), but should be performed by the RN? (select all that apply)
    a. administering patient medications
    b. ambulating stable patients
    c. performing patient assessment
    d. evaluating the effectiveness of patient care
    e. feeding patients at mealtime
    f. performing sterile procedures
    g. providing patient teaching
    h. obtaining vital signs on a stable patient
    i. assisting with patient bathing

24. Match the following care planning tools to the description statement(s). There may be more than one statement per tool and some statements may be used more than once.

    Tools
    1. Nursing Care Plan
    2. Concept Maps
    3. Clinical Pathway

    Statements
    _____ a plan that directs an entire health care team
    _____ used as guides for routine nursing care
    _____ used in nursing education to teach the nursing process and care planning
    _____ a description of patient care required at specific times during treatment
    _____ should be personalized and specific to each patient
    _____ a visual diagram representing relationships between patient problems, interventions, and data
    _____ used for high-volume and highly predictable case types

CHAPTER 2

Health Disparities and Culturally Competent Care

1. A 62-year-old African American man has been diagnosed with lung cancer and has been scheduled for surgery. The nurse recognizes that the major determinant of this patient's health is most likely the fact that
   a. he is African American.
   b. he chose to smoke all of his adult life.
   c. his father died of lung cancer at about the same age.
   d. he has a limited ability to understand and act on health information.

2. A 73-year-old white woman is brought to the emergency department by a neighbor who found the woman experiencing severe abdominal and lower back pain for 2 days and nausea and vomiting for the last 24 hours. She has always refused medical care of any kind and lives by herself "up the mountain" off a dirt road in rural West Virginia. She had two children with the help of a midwife, but they both left for the West Coast years ago, and she rarely sees them. She was not married to the father of her children, and she has not seen him in years. She has eked out a living with piece sewing for a doll company and receives a small amount of public assistance. As ill as she is, she is insisting that she will return home after she sees the doctor.

   List at least four factors in this situation that contribute to health disparities.
   a.

   b.

   c.

   d.

3. Match the factors and conditions that lead to health disparities with the examples provided.

   Factors and Conditions
   _____ a. Race, culture, ethnicity
   _____ b. Geographic location
   _____ c. Income, education, occupation
   _____ d. Health literacy
   _____ e. Gender
   _____ f. Age
   _____ g. Health care provider attitudes

   Examples
   1. Inability to read and understand medication labels
   2. Chronic illness rates higher in minorities
   3. Women are less likely to receive intervention for heart disease
   4. Assumption that immigrants cannot understand modern health care
   5. Inability to access quality health services with high patient-to-provider ratios
   6. Limited screening and less aggressive treatment of disorders offered
   7. Underinsured or uninsured individuals who forego health care treatment

4. Match the following terms with their descriptions.

_____ a. Culture
_____ b. Values
_____ c. Transcultural nursing
_____ d. Acculturation
_____ e. Assimilation
_____ f. Ethnicity
_____ g. Race
_____ h. Ethnocentricity
_____ i. Cultural imposition
_____ j. Stereotyping
_____ k. Biculturalism

1. Identification with a group whose members share a common social and cultural heritage passed through generations
2. Modification of one's culture as a result of contact with another culture
3. Forcing one's own cultural beliefs and practices on others without regard for their culture
4. Principles and standards that serve as bases for beliefs, attitudes, and behaviors
5. The knowledge, values, beliefs, laws, and customs of members of a society
6. Divisions of humankind sharing common ancestry and physical characteristics
7. An individual exposed to two or more cultures
8. The assumption that all members of a culture or ethnic group share the same values and beliefs
9. Loss of one's cultural identity in the process of adaptation to the dominant culture
10. The belief that one's own values, beliefs, and behaviors are the only right and natural way
11. Goal is the discovery of culturally relevant facts to guide care that is culturally appropriate

5. List the four basic characteristics of culture.
   a.

   b.

   c.

   d.

6. Identify the specific components of acquiring cultural competence reflected in the following examples.
   a. Asking the patient what caused the illness and what treatment would be appropriate. _____

   b. Identifying one's own biases toward people of another culture. _____

   c. Working directly with persons from different cultures over time. _____

   d. Creating a safe environment in which collection of relevant cultural data can be obtained during the health history and physical examination. _____

7. Identify one example of how each of the following cultural factors may affect the nursing care of a patient of a different culture.
   a. Time orientation
   b. Economic factors
   c. Nutrition
   d. Personal space
   e. Beliefs and practices

8. When admitting a woman experiencing a spontaneous abortion at the ambulatory care center, the nurse notes that the admission form identifies the patient's religion as Jehovah's Witness. The nurse understands that the patient
   a. should not receive any pork-derived medications.
   b. may ask to have only female nurses and doctors care for her.
   c. may experience some degree of spiritual distress and conflict.
   d. will not be able to receive blood or blood products if an emergency develops during the procedure.

9. A hospitalized Native American patient tells the nurse that later in the day a shaman from his tribe is coming to perform a healing ceremony to return his world to balance. The nurse recognizes that
   a. the patient does not adhere to an organized, formal religion.
   b. the patient's spiritual needs may be met by traditional rituals.
   c. the patient may be putting his health in jeopardy by relying on rituals.
   d. Native American medicine cannot alter the progression of the patient's physical illness.

10. When the nurse takes a surgical consent form to an Asian woman for a signature after the surgeon has provided the information about the recommended surgery, the patient refuses to sign the consent form. The best response by the nurse is,
    a. "Didn't you understand what the doctor told you about the surgery?"
    b. "Are there others whom you want to talk with before making this decision?"
    c. "Why won't you sign this form? Don't you want to do what the doctor recommended?"
    d. "I'll have to call the surgeon and have your surgery cancelled until you can make a decision."

11. A male nurse would be providing culturally competent care by requesting that a female nurse provide the care for a(n)
    a. Arab male.
    b. Arab female.
    c. Latino male.
    d. African American female.

12. Identify at least five classes of drugs that are known to respond differently in other ethnic groups compared with the usual response of whites of European descent.
    a.

    b.

    c.

    d.

    e.

13. In a Latino patient who claims to have empacho, the nurse would expect assessment findings to include
    a. abdominal pain and cramping.
    b. anxiety, insomnia, anorexia, and social isolation.
    c. nightmares, weakness, and a sense of suffocation.
    d. headaches, stomach problems, and loss of consciousness.

14. To communicate with a patient who does not speak the dominant language, the nurse should (select all that apply)
    a. speak slowly and enunciate clearly in a slightly louder voice.
    b. use gestures and pantomime words while verbalizing specific words.
    c. use family members as interpreters rather than strangers to increase the patient's feeling of comfort.
    d. use a dictionary or phrase books that translate from both the nurse's language and the patient's language.
    e. avoid the use of any words known in the patient's language because the grammar and pronunciation may be incorrect.

15. Identify whether the following statements are true (*T*) or false (*F*). If the statement is false, correct the bold word(s) to make the statement true.
    _____ a. The use of standardized, evidence-based care guidelines will **reduce** health care disparities.
    _____ b. Encouraging individuals from **underrepresented** populations to enter a health care profession will help reduce health care disparities.

Health History and Physical Examination

1. A newly admitted patient has a medical history in his record file. Is it necessary for the nurse to complete a nursing history of the patient? Why or why not?

2. While being admitted to the nursing unit from the emergency department, a patient tells the nurse she is short of breath and has pain in her chest when she breathes. Her respiratory rate is 28/min, and she is coughing up yellow sputum. Her skin is hot and moist, and her temperature is 102.2° F (39° C). She says that coughing makes her head hurt and she aches all over. Identify the subjective and objective assessment findings in this patient.

Subjective   **Objective**

3. Give an example of a sensitive way to ask a patient the following questions.
   a. Is the patient on antihypertensive medication having a side effect of impotence?

   b. Has the patient with a history of alcoholism had recent alcohol intake?

   c. Who are the sexual contacts of a patient with gonorrhea?

   d. Does the patient skip taking medications because they cost too much?

4. The nurse prepares to interview a patient for a nursing history but finds the patient in obvious pain. The best action by the nurse at this time is to
   a. delay the interview until the patient is pain-free.
   b. administer pain medication before initiating the interview.
   c. gather as much information as quickly as possible by using closed questions that require brief answers.
   d. ask only those questions pertinent to the specific problem and complete the interview when the patient is more comfortable.

5. While the nurse is obtaining a health history, the patient tells the nurse, "I am so tired I can hardly function." The nurse's best action at this time is to
   a. stop the interview and leave the patient alone to be able to rest.
   b. arrange another time with the patient to complete the interview.
   c. question the patient further about the characteristics of the symptoms.
   d. reassure the patient that the symptoms will improve when treatment has time to be effective.

6. Rewrite each question asked by the nurse so that it is an open-ended question designed to gather information about the patient's functional health patterns.
   a. Are you having any pain?

   b. Do you have a good relationship with your spouse?

   c. How long have you been ill?

   d. Do you exercise regularly?

7. A patient has come to the health clinic with diarrhea of 3 days' duration. He notes that on the third day, he developed abdominal pain and cramping that was not present the first 2 days. He says the stools occur five or six times a day and are very watery. Every time he eats or drinks something, he has an urgent diarrhea stool. He denies being out of the country but did attend a large family reunion held at a campground in the mountains about a week ago. Identify the information in this situation that address specific areas of symptom investigation. Also identify the areas of symptom investigation that have not been addressed that would provide additional important information.
   a. Areas addressed

   b. Areas not addressed

8. The following data are obtained from a patient during a nursing history. Organize these data according to Gordon's functional health patterns. Patterns may be used more than once, and some data may apply to more than one pattern.

   _____ a. 78-year-old woman
   _____ b. Married, three grown children who all live out of town
   _____ c. Cares for invalid husband in home with help of daily homemaker
   _____ d. Vision corrected with glasses; hearing normal
   _____ e. Height 5 ft 10 in; weight 172 lb
   _____ f. Vital signs: T 99.2; HR 82; RR 32; BP 142/88
   _____ g. 5-year history of adult-onset asthma; smokes two or three cigarettes a day
   _____ h. Coughing, wheezing, with stated shortness of breath
   _____ i. Moderate light-yellow sputum
   _____ j. Says she now has no energy to care for husband
   _____ k. Awakens three or four times a night and has to use a bronchodilator inhaler
   _____ l. Uses a laxative twice a week for bowel function; no urinary problems
   _____ m. Feels her health is good for her age
   _____ n. Allergic to codeine and aspirin
   _____ o. Has esophageal reflux and eats bland foods
   _____ p. Can usually handle the stress of caring for her husband, but if she becomes overwhelmed, asthma worsens
   _____ q. Has been menopausal for 26 years; no sexual activity
   _____ r. Takes medications for asthma, hypertension, and hypothyroidism and uses diazepam (Valium) PRN for anxiety
   _____ s. Goes out to lunch with friends weekly
   _____ t. Says she misses going to church with her husband but watches religious services with him on TV

   1. Demographic data
   2. Important health information
   3. Health-perception–health-management pattern
   4. Nutrition-metabolic pattern
   5. Elimination pattern
   6. Activity-exercise pattern
   7. Sleep-rest pattern
   8. Cognitive-perceptual pattern
   9. Self-perception–self-concept pattern
   10. Role-relationship pattern
   11. Sexuality-reproductive pattern
   12. Coping–stress tolerance pattern
   13. Value-belief pattern

9. An example of a pertinent negative finding during a physical examination is
   a. chest pain that does not radiate to the arm.
   b. elevated blood pressure in a patient with hypertension.
   c. pupils that are equal and react to light and accommodation.
   d. clear and full lung sounds in a patient with chronic bronchitis.

10. Match the following data with the assessment technique used to obtain the information.
    _____ a. Normal blood flow through arteries   1. Inspection
    _____ b. Abnormal blood flow in carotid artery   2. Palpation
    _____ c. Tympany of the abdomen   3. Percussion
    _____ d. Pitting edema   4. Auscultation
    _____ e. Cyanosis of the lips
    _____ f. Hyperactive peristalsis
    _____ g. Bruising of the lateral left thigh
    _____ h. Cool, clammy skin

11. The sequence of examination techniques that should be used when assessing the patient's abdomen is
    a. inspection, palpation, auscultation, percussion.
    b. auscultation, inspection, percussion, palpation.
    c. palpation, percussion, auscultation, inspection.
    d. inspection, auscultation, percussion, palpation.

12. When performing a physical examination, it is most important that the nurse
    a. uses a head-to-toe approach to avoid missing an important area.
    b. uses the same systematic, efficient sequence for all examinations.
    c. follows a sequence that is least revealing and embarrassing for the patient.
    d. allows time to collect the nursing history data while performing the examination.

13. The nurse is performing a physical examination on a 90-year-old male patient who has been bedridden the past year. Identify an adaptation for performing the examination that would be easier on the patient.

14. A comprehensive assessment would be performed in which of these situations? (select all that apply)
    a. when a patient complains of chest pain.
    b. when a patient is initially admitted to the telemetry unit.
    c. when a patient is found lying on the floor unresponsive.
    d. when a patient arrives in the surgery holding area of the operating room.
    e. when a patient is being initially evaluated by the home health nurse.

15. Word search. Find the words that are described by the clues given below. The words may be located horizontally, vertically, or diagonally and may be reversed.

E	O	N	T	E	D	L	N	O	R	C	E	S
N	A	O	F	B	I	U	Q	A	R	Q	P	E
N	O	I	T	A	T	L	U	C	S	U	A	T
O	N	T	I	L	C	F	O	C	U	S	E	D
I	G	A	N	P	I	O	N	U	B	H	O	L
T	O	C	E	V	I	T	C	E	J	B	O	N
A	F	O	T	O	S	C	O	P	E	T	M	E
P	I	L	N	O	I	S	S	U	C	R	E	P
L	O	A	O	N	M	T	I	Q	T	E	N	A
A	D	I	N	S	P	E	C	T	I	O	N	S
P	A	J	A	L	O	D	M	O	V	I	A	T
L	O	A	P	T	R	O	O	N	E	N	Y	O

Clues

a. Assessment technique involving touch
b. Data the patient must explain
c. Assessment technique involving visual examination
d. Instrument to examine the ears
e. An examination that is a more detailed assessment of a body system
f. Assessment technique that requires listening to sounds
g. Data that can be observed and measured
h. Assessment technique that produces sound
i. An area that is assessed in symptom investigation.

CHAPTER 4

Patient and Caregiver Teaching

1. In each of the nursing situations described below, identify the goal of patient education.
   a. Teaching a new mother about the recommended infant immunization schedule

   b. Discussing recommended lifestyle changes with a patient with newly diagnosed heart disease

   c. Counseling a patient with a breast biopsy that is positive for cancer

   d. Demonstrating the proper condom application to sexually active teenagers

2. What is meant by this statement?
   "Every interaction with a patient or caregiver is potentially a teachable moment."

3. Which of these statements are true regarding the Teaching-Learning process? Select all that apply.
   a. Learning can occur without teaching.
   b. Teaching uses a variety of methods to influence knowledge and behavior.
   c. Teaching must be well planned to be effective.
   d. Learning has not occurred when there is no change in behavior.
   e. Teaching may make learning more efficient.

4. From the following list of principles of adult education, identify which one(s) is (are) used in the examples of patient teaching.

   _____ a. The nurse explains why it is important for a patient with Parkinson's disease to walk with wide placement of the feet.

   _____ b. The nurse asks a patient what is most important to her to learn about managing a new colostomy.

   _____ c. The nurse teaches a patient how to reduce the risks for stroke after the patient has had a transient ischemic attack, warning of carotid artery disease.

   _____ d. The nurse provides a variety of printed materials and Internet resources for a patient with impaired kidney function to use to learn about the disorder.

   _____ e. When caring for a patient with newly diagnosed asthma, the nurse explains that asthma is a disorder the patient can control and allows the patient to decide when teaching should be done and who else should be included.

   _____ f. The nurse arranges for a patient diagnosed with diabetes mellitus to perform self-monitoring of blood glucose and insulin administration in the nurse's presence.

   _____ g. During preoperative teaching of a patient scheduled for a total hip replacement, the nurse compares the postoperative care with that of the patient's prior back surgery.

   1. Adults are independent learners.
   2. Readiness to learn arises from life's changes.
   3. Past experiences are resources for learning.
   4. Adults learn best when the topic is of immediate value.
   5. Adults approach learning as problem solving.
   6. Adults see themselves as doers.
   7. Adults resist learning when conditions are incongruent with their self-concepts.

5. When a patient with diabetes tells the nurse that he cannot see any reason to change his eating habits because he is not overweight, the nurse determines that the most appropriate action at this stage of the Transtheoretical Model of Behavior Change is to
    a. help the patient set priorities for managing his diabetes.
    b. arrange for the dietitian to describe what dietary changes are needed.
    c. explain that dietary changes can help prevent long-term complications of diabetes.
    d. emphasize that he must change behaviors if he is going to control his blood glucose levels.

6. Translate the following medical terms or diagnoses into phrases that a patient with little or no medical knowledge would be able to understand.
    a. Acute myocardial infarction

    b. Intravenous pyelogram

    c. Diabetic retinopathy

7. An empathetic approach to patient teaching is demonstrated when the nurse
    a. assesses the patient's needs before developing the teaching plan.
    b. provides positive nonverbal messages that promote communication.
    c. reads and reviews educational materials before distributing them to patients and families.
    d. can overcome the personal frustration felt when patients are discharged before teaching is complete.

8. Describe one strategy that could be used to overcome the common barriers to teaching patients and caregivers.

9. To promote the patient's self-efficacy during the teaching-learning process, the nurse should
    a. emphasize the relevancy of the teaching to the patient's life.
    b. begin with concepts and tasks that are easily learned to promote success.
    c. provide stimulating learning activities that encourage motivation to learn.
    d. encourage the patient to learn independently without instruction from others.

10. Identify what teaching interventions are indicated when the following characteristics are found during assessment of a patient for the purposes of developing a teaching plan.
    a. Impaired hearing

    b. Patient refuses to see a need for a change in health behaviors

    c. Drowsiness caused by use of sedatives

    d. Presence of pain

    e. Reading ability at national average

    f. Visual learning style

    g. Primary language is not English

11. On assessment of a patient's learning needs, the nurse determines that a patient taking potassium-wasting diuretics does not know what foods are high in potassium. An appropriate nursing diagnosis for this patient is
    a. risk for cardiac dysrhythmias related to low potassium intake.
    b. deficient knowledge related to lack of recall of high-potassium foods.
    c. imbalanced nutrition: less than body requirements related to lack of intake of potassium-rich foods.
    d. deficient knowledge related to lack of interest regarding dietary requirements when taking diuretics.

12. Write a learning goal for the patient taking potassium-wasting diuretics who does not know what foods are high in potassium.

13. Match the following descriptions or characteristics with the appropriate teaching strategy (answers may be used more than once).

    _____ a. May require the patient to practice between teaching sessions
    _____ b. Used to rehearse behaviors or feelings
    _____ c. Useful to provide participants with basic information.
    _____ d. Non-threatening strategy
    _____ e. Useful when patients have previous experience with subject
    _____ f. Allows for questions and exchange of ideas
    _____ g. Should be supplementary to the nurse's planned teaching sessions
    _____ h. Useful when it is difficult to reach desired goals of the session
    _____ i. Access may vary/information may be inaccurate
    _____ j. Best strategy for teaching motor skills or procedures
    _____ k. Requires maturity and confidence of participants
    _____ l. May be used in combination with almost any other teaching strategy
    _____ m. Offers extensive sources of information

    1. Lecture/discussion
    2. Discussion
    3. Demonstration/return demonstration
    4. Role play
    5. Internet
    6. Printed materials
    7. Videos/CDs

14. When selecting audiovisual and written materials as teaching strategies, it is important for the nurse to
    a. provide the patient with these materials before the planned learning experience.
    b. ensure that the materials include all the information the patient will need to learn.
    c. review the materials before use for accuracy and appropriateness to learning needs/goals.
    d. assess the patient's auditory and visual ability because these functions are necessary for these strategies to be effective.

15. A drug handbook provides the following information about the drug atorvastatin (Lipitor).
    • Action: Inhibits HMG-CoA reductase enzyme, which reduces cholesterol synthesis
    • Uses: As an adjunct in primary hypercholesterolemia (types Ia, Ib)
    • Side effects: Liver dysfunction, dyspepsia, flatus, pancreatitis, rash, pruritus, alopecia, lens opacities, myalgia, and headache
    • Precautions: Past liver disease, alcoholism, hypotension, severe acute infections, uncontrolled seizure disorders, severe metabolic disorders, trauma, and electrolyte imbalances
    • Interactions: Increased effects of warfarin, digoxin, oral contraceptives; increased myalgia with cyclosporine, gemfibrozil, niacin, erythromycin; decreased effects of atorvastatin with colestipol, antacids, bile acid sequestrants, propranolol; increased effects of atorvastatin with erythromycin, itraconazole

    Rewrite the above information as teaching material for an adult patient with an average reading level.

16. A patient with a breast biopsy positive for cancer tells the nurse that she has been using information from the Internet to try to make a decision about her treatment choices. In counseling the patient, the nurse knows that (select all that apply)
    a. the patient should be taught how to identify reliable and accurate information available online.
    b. all sites used by the patient should be evaluated by the nurse for accuracy and appropriateness of the information.
    c. most information from the Internet is incomplete and inaccurate and should not be used to make important decisions regarding treatment.
    d. the Internet is an excellent source of health information, and online education programs can provide patients with better instruction than is available at clinics.
    e. the patient should be encouraged to use sites established by universities, the government, or reputable health organizations such as the American Cancer Society to access reliable information.

17. Identify what short-term evaluation technique is appropriate to evaluate whether the patient has met the following learning goals.
    a. The patient will demonstrate to the nurse the preparation and administration of a subcutaneous insulin injection to himself with correct technique.

    b. The patient will identify five serious side effects of Coumadin that should be reported to the doctor.

    c. The patient will select the foods highest in potassium for each meal from the hospital menu with 80% accuracy.

    d. The patient will ambulate unassisted with the walker 100 feet three times a day.

18. The best example of documentation of patient teaching regarding wound care is
    a. "The patient was instructed about care of wound and dressing changes."
    b. "The patient demonstrated correct technique of wound care following instruction."
    c. "The patient and caregiver verbalize that they understand the purposes of wound care."
    d. "Written instructions regarding wound care and dressing changes were given to the patient."

19. Use of games or a game system would be an effective teaching strategy for a patient from which of the following generations?
    a. Baby Boomers (1945-1960)
    b. Generation X (1961-1980)
    c. Millennials (1981-2000)
    d. Veterans (prior to 1945)

Chronic Illness and Older Adults

1. Identify characteristics of chronic illness from the list below. Select all that apply.
   a. Self-limiting
   b. Residual disability
   c. Return to previous functioning expected
   d. Need for long-term management
   e. Nonreversible pathologic changes
   f. Infrequent complications
   g. Permanent impairments

2. Seven tasks required for daily living with chronic illness have been identified. From Table 5-4, select at least one of these tasks that would specifically apply to the following common chronic conditions present in the older adult.
   a. Diabetes mellitus
   b. Visual impairment
   c. Heart disease
   d. Hearing impairment
   e. Alzheimer's disease
   f. Arthritis
   g. Orthopedic impairment

3. Fill in the blanks.
   a. Actions aimed at early detection of disease and interventions to prevent progression of disease are considered _____ prevention.
   b. Following a proper diet, getting appropriate exercise and receiving immunizations against specific diseases is considered _____ prevention.

4. Crossword Puzzle: Chronic Disease Trajectory and Impact

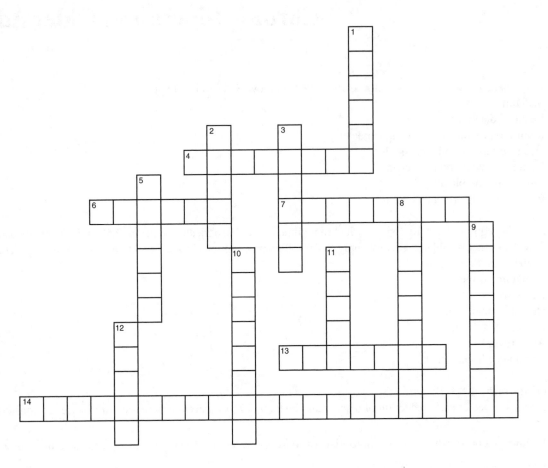

Across
4. Lose control over symptoms/disease course
6. Third leading cause of death in the U.S.
7. Gradual return to acceptable way of life
13. Major contributor to other health problems
14. First leading cause of death in the U.S.

Down
1. Person maintains everyday activities
2. Signs and symptoms are present
3. Second leading cause of death in U.S.
5. Life-threatening situation
8. Over 40% are limited in activities
9. Greater than 6 million Americans do not know they have this disease
10. Increasing disability and symptoms
11. Hospitalization required for management
12. Relinquish everyday life interests, let go

5. Identify two common social conceptions or myths about aging or the aged that illustrate the concept of ageism.
   a.

   b.

6. For each of the nursing diagnoses listed, identify at least two normal expected physiologic changes related to aging that could be etiologic factors of the diagnosis. Changes related to aging are found in the chapters identified in Table 5-7.
   a. Imbalanced nutrition: less than body requirements (see Table 39-5, p. 908)
      Change:

      Change:

   b. Activity intolerance (see Table 62-1, p. 1575)
      Change:

      Change:

   c. Risk for injury (see Table 56-4, p. 1416)
      Change:

      Change:

   d. Urge urinary incontinence (see Table 45-2, p. 1111)
      Change:

      Change:

   e. Ineffective airway clearance (see Table 26-4, p. 504)
      Change:

      Change:

   f. Risk for impaired skin integrity (see Table 23-1, p. 439)
      Change:

      Change:

   g. Ineffective tissue perfusion: peripheral (see Table 32-1, p. 720)
      Change:

      Change:

   h. Constipation (see Table 39-5, p. 908)
      Change:

      Change:

7. The nurse identifies the presence of age-associated memory impairment in the older adult who says,
   a. "I just can't seem to remember the name of my new granddaughter."
   b. "I make out lists to help me remember what I need to do, but I can't seem to use them."
   c. "I forget movie stars' names more often now, but I can remember them later after the conversation is over."
   d. "I forgot that I went to the grocery store this morning and didn't realize it until I went again this afternoon."

8. Indicate what the acronym SCALES stands for in assessment of nutrition indicators in frail older adults.
   a. S
   b. C
   c. A
   d. L
   e. E
   f. S

9. When working with older patients who identify with a specific ethnic group, the nurse recognizes that health care problems may occur because these patients often
   a. live with extended families who isolate the patient.
   b. live in rural areas where services are not readily available.
   c. eat ethnic foods that do not provide all the essential nutrients.
   d. have less income to spend for medications and health care services.

10. An 83-year-old woman is being discharged from the hospital following stabilization of her INR levels (lab to assess effectiveness of warfarin therapy). She has chronic atrial fibrillation and has been on warfarin (Coumadin) for several years. Discharge instructions include returning to the clinical weekly for INR testing. Which of the following statements by the patient indicate she may be unable to have the testing done?
    a. "I will need to ask my son to bring me into town every week for the test."
    b. "Should I just keep taking the same pill every day until I can get a ride to town?"
    c. "It is very important to have this test every week. I have several church friends who can bring me."

11. The old-old population (85 years and older) have an increased risk for frailty. However, old age is just one element of frailty. Identify at least three other assessment findings that contribute to frailty.
    a.

    b.

    c.

12. An 80-year-old woman is brought to the emergency department by her daughter, who says her mother has refused to eat for 6 days. The mother says she stays in her room all of the time because the family is mean to her when she eats or watches TV with them. She says her daughter only brings her one meal a day and that meal is cold leftovers from the family's meals days before.
    a. What types of elder mistreatment may be present in this situation?
    b. How would the nurse assess the situation to determine whether abuse is present?

    The daughter says her mother is too demanding, and she just cannot cope with caring for her 24 hours a day.
    c. What might be an appropriate nursing diagnosis for the daughter?
    d. What resources can the nurse suggest to the daughter?

13. An 82-year-old patient with multiple health problems is hospitalized with a fractured hip.
    a. What Medicare coverage will apply to treatment of the fractured hip?

    b. What criteria must be met for the patient to receive Medicare benefits for hospitalization?

    c. The patient is transferred to a skilled nursing facility for rehabilitation. Will Medicare continue to cover the expense of the skilled facility?

    d. The patient is too frail to complete rehabilitation and it is discontinued. Custodial care is indicated. If the patient is placed in a long-term care facility or taken home to be cared for, what Medicare coverage is available for expenses?

    e. The patient is taken to a daughter's home for custodial care. The daughter and son-in-law are both employed. What community-based service might be appropriate to allow the family members to continue employment?

14. What are three common factors known to precipitate placement in a long-term care facility?
    a.

    b.

    c.

15. An 88-year-old woman is brought to the health clinic for the first time by her 64-year-old daughter. During the initial comprehensive nursing assessment of the patient, the nurse should
    a. ask the daughter whether the patient has any urgent needs or problems.
    b. obtain a health history using a functional health pattern and assess activities of daily living (ADLs) and mental status.
    c. interview the patient and daughter together so that pertinent information can be confirmed.
    d. refer the patient for an interdisciplinary comprehensive geriatric assessment because, at her age, she will have multiple needs.

16. A mental-status assessment of the older adult is especially important in determining
    a. potential for independent living.
    b. eligibility for federal health programs.
    c. whether the person should be classified as frail.
    d. service and placement needs of the individual.

17. An important nursing measure in the rehabilitation of the geriatric patient to prevent loss of function from inactivity and immobility is
    a. performance of active and passive range-of-motion (ROM) exercises.
    b. using assistive devices such as walkers and canes.
    c. teaching good nutrition to prevent loss of muscle mass.
    d. performance of risk appraisals and assessments related to immobility.

18. An older adult patient has hypertension and heart failure and is treated with enalapril (Vasotec) and digoxin (Lanoxin). The pharmacodynamic and pharmacokinetic properties of these drugs include the following:

	Enalapril	**Digoxin**
Dynamics	Blocks conversion of angiotensin I to active angiotensin II, causing systemic vasodilation	Increases intramedullary calcium, increasing cardiac muscle contraction Vagomimetic action and baroreceptor sensitization lead to positive inotropic action and reduced sympathetic response
Kinetics Absorption Distribution Metabolism Excretion Half-life	Oral absorption 60% 20%-30% plasma protein bound 60% converted by liver to active enalapril 60% excreted by kidneys, rest by feces 11 hr	Oral absorption 60%-80% 20%-30% plasma protein bound Small percent metabolized by liver and gastrointestinal flora Most excreted unchanged by kidneys 36 hr

a. What physiologic changes in the older adult affect the absorption, metabolism, and excretion of enalapril?

b. Describe the additional effect digoxin may have on the older adult also taking enalapril.

c. What nursing interventions should the nurse plan to monitor for the potential side effects related to administration of these drugs?

19. In view of the fact that most older adults take at least six prescription drugs, what are four nursing interventions that can specifically help prevent problems caused by multiple drug use in older patients?
   a.

   b.

   c.

   d.

20. Which of the nursing actions below would demonstrate the nurse's understanding of the concept of providing safe care without using restraints? (select all that apply)
   a. making hourly rounds on patients to assess for pain and toileting needs.
   b. placing a disruptive patient near the nurses' station in a chair with a seat belt.
   c. asking simple yes-or-no questions to clarify patient needs.
   d. placing patients with fall risk in low beds.
   e. applying a jacket vest loosely so the patient can turn but can't climb out of bed.

CHAPTER

6

Community-Based Nursing and Home Care

1. The difference between community-based nursing and community-oriented nursing is that in community-based nursing, the nurse
   a. focuses on a population rather than an individual.
   b. provides primary prevention rather than tertiary care.
   c. helps individuals and families manage acute or chronic health problems in the community and home setting.
   d. does not provide direct patient care, but instead coordinates the care provided by other health care professionals.

2. Prospective payment systems for health care services
   a. require that health care is provided by preapproved health professionals.
   b. provide payment for health care based on flat predetermined rates regardless of actual cost.
   c. reimburse the expenses of health care only when costs are approved by the system before treatment.
   d. arrange to pay only those health care providers who contract with the system to provide the lowest-priced services.

3. Identify five factors that have influenced the shift of acute and long-term chronic care to community-based settings and the home.
   a.

   b.

   c.

   d.

   e.

4. A case manager is responsible for
   a. determining when a patient needs to be hospitalized.
   b. setting limits on the financial expenditures of a patient's illness episode.
   c. coordinating patient care during an entire episode of illness in all care settings.
   d. providing home health care to patients following hospitalization for acute illnesses.

5. Using the following list of health care settings, identify the setting that would be most appropriate in each of the described patient situations. Settings may be used more than once.

a. An ambulatory patient with Alzheimer's disease needs a segregated, low-stimulus environment and activity programming.

   _____

b. A diabetic patient with a wound infection at an above-the-knee amputation site has exhausted the DRG days and still requires IV antibiotics and frequent complex dressing changes for a short time.

   _____

c. A stable, comatose patient following a head injury requires tube feedings, IV medications, and continuous nursing support.

   _____

d. A patient with an acute eye infection requires a one-time encounter with health professionals for treatment.

   _____

e. A patient requires assistance in activities of daily living and medication supervision but is ambulatory and cares for self with direction.

   _____

f. A patient is stable following a stroke but has left-sided paralysis with a potential for return of function.

   _____

g. A patient requires IV antibiotics and wound care daily and has family members to provide care.

   _____

h. An alert, middle-aged patient with multiple sclerosis has no immediate family and needs a permanent home in addition to around-the-clock personal care assistance.

   _____

i. A patient has been on a ventilator for 35 days following a diving accident resulting in a cervical fracture and requires extensive medical and nursing intervention.

   _____

Settings
1. acute rehabilitation
2. ambulatory care center
3. home health care
4. intermediate care facility
5. long-term acute care
6. residential care facility
7. skilled nursing facility
8. subacute care unit

6. The patient care setting in which nurses most often perform telephone follow-up with patients is _____.

7. The patient care setting in which nurses are most likely to be required to adapt to a variety of circumstances and make independent decisions is _____.

8. Indicate whether the following statements are true (*T*) or false (*F*).
   _____ a. Medicare reimbursement is not available for health care that is delivered in the home.
   _____ b. Equipment used in home care is restricted to the use of that necessary for mobilization of the patient (e.g., walkers, canes, wheelchairs).
   _____ c. The nurse is more likely to encounter the use of alternative and complementary therapies during care of the patient in the home than during care in an institution.
   _____ d. A licensed nurse is the only one who is allowed to administer parenteral medications to the patient in the home.

9. The primary role of the professional nurse in home health care is to
   a. perform all health and personal care delivered in the home.
   b. coordinate and case-manage all aspects of care in the home.
   c. teach family members to assume all care for the patient eventually.
   d. visit the home at least once a week to evaluate the status of the patient.

10. A 58-year-old man who has had two strokes is cared for by his wife and daughter in his home. The patient is becoming weaker and is almost bedridden. The wife and daughter are both becoming exhausted from the care he requires, they express concern that they aren't doing the right things because he isn't getting better, and the daughter misses spending time with her friends. The patient insists that he remain in his home with family care. What are two nursing diagnoses that might relate to these family caregivers?
    a.

    b.

11. For each of the nursing diagnoses identified in Question 10, describe the nursing interventions that would be appropriate.

Complementary and Alternative Therapies

1. Match each description in the left column with its National Center for Complementary and Alternative Medicine (NCCAM) classification (in the right column) and with its specific type of therapy (also in the right column).

Description

_____ a. Use of hands to realign energy flow

_____ b. Communication with the Creator or the Sacred

_____ c. Manipulation of energy channels with fine needles

_____ d. Use of vitamin and mineral supplements

_____ e. Considers disease as an imbalance of life force and basic metabolic condition

_____ f. A method of learned control of physiologic responses of the body

_____ g. Soft tissue manipulation to relax, stimulate the immune system, and increase flexibility

_____ h. Uses the principle of "like cures like" with small doses of prepared extracts

_____ i. Spinal manipulation and realignment to promote health and well-being

_____ j. Self-directed practice of focusing, centering, and relaxing

_____ k. Use of unrefined plants or plant parts for specific effects

_____ l. Use of finger and hand pressure at energy meridians to improve energy flow

_____ m. Part of Ayurveda practices that include mental and physical exercises

NCCAM Classification

1. Whole medical systems
2. Mind-body medicine
3. Biologic-based practices
4. Manipulative and body-based practices
5. Energy therapies

Specific Therapies

6. Acupressure
7. Prayer
8. Dietary supplements
9. Yoga
10. Ayurveda
11. Healing touch
12. Biofeedback
13. Massage therapy
14. Acupuncture
15. Homeopathy
16. Chiropractic therapy
17. Herbal therapy
18. Meditation

2. Indicate whether the following statements are true (*T*) or false (*F*).

_____ a. The increase in the use of CAM therapies is due, in part, to an increase in chronic disease and stress-related disorders.

_____ b. Research and education in CAM therapies are supported by the National Center for Complementary and Alternative Medicine of the National Institutes of Health.

_____ c. Practices that are considered complementary and alternative in one culture or time might be considered conventional in another place or time.

3. Complementary and alternative therapies are advocated by many nurses because these therapies
   a. promote self-care and self-determination by patients.
   b. are congruent with a view of humans as holistic beings.
   c. are less expensive for patients than conventional therapies.
   d. cause few adverse effects while achieving positive outcomes.

4. Traditional Chinese medicine holds that disease occurs when
   a. yin and yang become imbalanced, altering the flow of Qi.
   b. acupoints in Qi channels become obstructed, preventing the release of Qi.
   c. the body's natural healing abilities are impaired by obstruction of fluid channels.
   d. the individual is out of harmony with nature and requires spiritualism and mysticism to reestablish balance.

5. Acupuncture is used to
   a. relieve pain by causing counterirritation in another area of the body.
   b. reestablish the flow of Qi through meridians to simulate the body's self-healing mechanism.
   c. create an inflammatory response at an acupoint, increasing blood circulation and healing energy.
   d. stimulate the electrical activity of the central nervous system, promoting movement of vital energy through the body.

6. When the members of a postoperative patient's family leave after a visit, the patient tells the nurse that his family gave him a headache by fussing over him so much. An appropriate intervention by the nurse would be to
   a. administer the PRN analgesic prescribed for his postoperative pain.
   b. reassure the patient that his headache will subside now that his family has gone.
   c. ask the patient's permission to use acupressure to ease his headache.
   d. teach the patient biofeedback methods to relieve his headaches by controlling cerebral blood flow.

7. A bedridden patient tells the nurse she has low back pain and asks if the area could be massaged. The best action by the nurse is to
   a. ask the patient if she has ever tried acupuncture for back pain.
   b. position the patient to expose the area and massage the back with effleurage and petrissage strokes.
   c. explain to the patient that massage may only be done by a licensed therapist and offer a PRN analgesic instead.
   d. call the physical therapy department to request that a physical therapist see the patient to provide a therapeutic massage.

8. A complementary and alternative therapy shown to be effective in treatment of a patient with chemotherapy-related nausea and vomiting is
   a. Reiki.
   b. acupuncture.
   c. aromatherapy.
   d. magnetic therapy.

9. When discussing herbal therapy with a patient, the nurse should advise the patient that
   a. preparations should be purchased only from reputable manufacturers.
   b. herbs rarely cause harm or side effects because they are natural plants.
   c. there are no known contraindications or conditions for which herbal therapy cannot be used.
   d. most herbal preparations have been clinically tested for safety and efficacy before marketing.

10. While the nurse is obtaining a health history for a patient, the patient tells the nurse that he uses a number of herbs to maintain his health. The most important thing the nurse can do to address the patient's use of these products is to
    a. ask the patient what effects the various products have.
    b. have a working knowledge of commonly used herbs and dietary supplements.
    c. reassure the patient that the products can continue to be used with conventional therapies.
    d. warn the patient that there is limited research concerning the therapeutic and harmful effects of herbal products.

11. A patient newly diagnosed with type 2 diabetes has been given a prescription to start on an oral hypoglycemic. The patient tells the nurse she would rather control her blood sugar with herbal therapy. Which action should the nurse take?
    a. Advise the patient to discuss using herbal therapy with her physician.
    b. Advise the patient that herbal therapy is not safe and should not be used.
    c. Advise her to give the prescriptive medication time to work before using herbal therapy.
    d. Advise her that if she takes herbal therapy, she will have to monitor her blood sugar more often.

12. The role of the professional nurse related to complementary and alternative therapies should include (select all that apply):
    a. seeking further education on CAT.
    b. evaluating the evidence regarding these therapies.
    c. collecting data on the use of these therapies as part of the nursing assessment.
    d. suggesting specific herbs the patient should take to help with his/her condition.
    e. provide patients information on various therapies so they can make informed decisions.
    f. investigate which of these therapies fall within the nursing domain in your practice state.

13. Crossword Puzzle: Have You Met Herb?

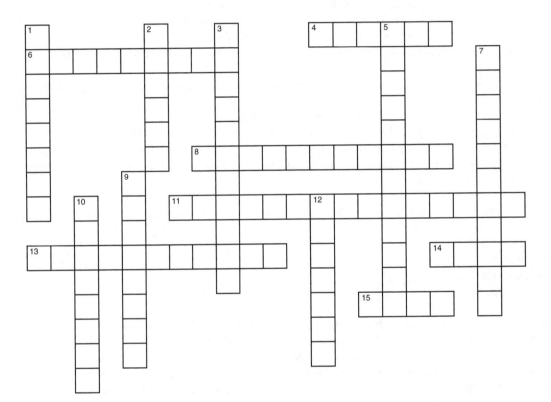

Across
   4. A spice used to treat nausea and vomiting of a variety of causes
   6. Frequently used to prevent and treat upper respiratory infections
   8. Often used to relieve menopausal symptoms by perimenopausal women
  11. Used to relieve skin irritation, eczema
  13. May interfere with liver enzyme system to treat viral hepatitis
  14. An effective laxative that is also used for skin lesions
  15. Strong evidence for its use for anxiety but can cause hepatotoxicity and bleeding

Down
   1. Most commonly used for prevention of migraine headaches
   2. Most frequently recommended to lower serum lipid levels but also used to lower blood pressure
   3. Slows prostate cell multiplication; used for benign prostatic hyperplasia
   5. Has strong evidence for its use in treatment of dementia and peripheral vascular disease
   7. Usual use is treatment of mild to moderate depression and anxiety
   9. Evidence for use in heart failure and coronary artery disease
  10. Frequently used for insomnia and anxiety
  12. May help to control blood glucose levels in type 2 diabetes mellitus

CHAPTER 8

Stress and Stress Management

1. When a patient at the clinic is informed that testing indicates the presence of gonorrhea, the patient sighs and says, "That, I can handle." The nurse understands that the patient in this situation probably
   a. is in denial about the possible complications of gonorrhea.
   b. does not perceive the gonorrhea infection as a threatening stressor.
   c. does not have other current stressors that require adaptation or coping mechanisms.
   d. knows how to cope with gonorrhea from dealing with previous gonorrhea infections.

2. The stage of the general adaptation syndrome (GAS) in which the nurse would expect to observe the fewest physical signs and symptoms is the _____.

3. A patient who is critically ill briefly shows an increase in pulse, respirations, and blood pressure and becomes more alert, followed by a return of previous vital signs and level of consciousness. The nurse identifies the patient as being in which stage of GAS? _____

4. Identify four personal characteristics that promote adaptation to stressors.
   a.

   b.

   c.

   d.

5. Using the word and phrase list below, fill in the boxes below with the numbers of the words or phrases that illustrate the physiologic response to stress.

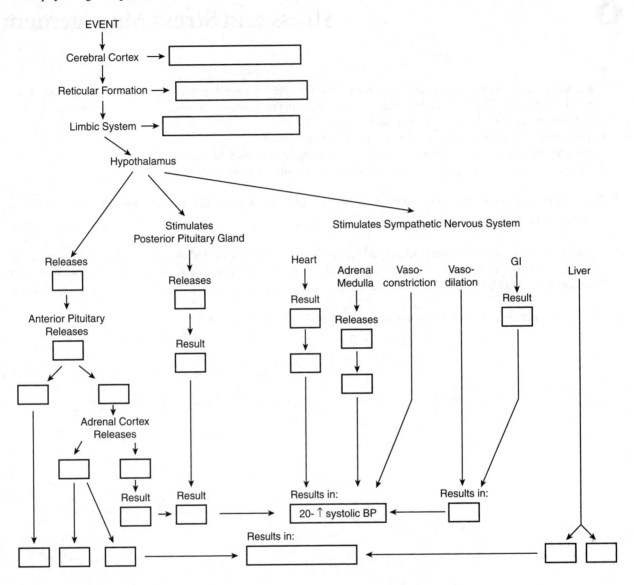

Word and Phrase List

1. interpretation of event
2. ↑ ADH (antidiuretic hormone)
3. cortisol
4. ↑ blood volume
5. ↑ HR and stroke volume
6. ↑ water retention
7. wakefulness and alertness
8. ↑ sympathetic response
9. β-endorphin
10. self-preservation behaviors
11. ↑ cardiac output
12. corticotropin-releasing hormone
13. aldosterone

14. ACTH (adrenocorticotropic hormone)
15. blunted pain perception
16. ↑ gluconeogenesis
17. ↑ epinephrine and norepinephrine
18. ↓ digestion
19. pro-opiomelanocortin (POMC) release
20. ↑ systolic blood pressure
21. ↓ inflammatory response
22. glycogenolysis
23. ↑ blood to vital organs and large muscles
24. ↑ blood glucose
25. ↑ Na and H_2O reabsorption

6. From the diagram on p. 30 and the physiologic responses that are noted, identify eight objective clinical or laboratory manifestations that the nurse might expect and three or four subjective findings.

Objective	**Subjective**
a.	a.
b.	b.
c.	c.
d.	d.
e.	
f.	
g.	
h.	

7. While caring for a patient with Alzheimer's disease and her caregiver husband, the nurse finds that the patient's husband is experiencing increasing memory impairment. The nurse recognizes that one explanation for this finding is that
   a. progressive, nonpathologic memory loss occurs in all people as they age.
   b. chronic and intense stress can cause hippocampal damage, impairing memory.
   c. the husband adequately copes with his wife's condition by unconsciously forgetting events related to the current situation.
   d. the husband is probably also developing Alzheimer's disease because he shares the same environment and exposures as his wife.

8. Identify the behaviors listed below as either positive coping (P) or negative coping (N) strategies.
   _____ a. Starting an exercise program
   _____ b. Smoking cigarettes
   _____ c. Increasing time spent with friends
   _____ d. Ignoring the situation
   _____ e. Joining a support group

9. A patient has recently had a myocardial infarction. Identify two specific problem-focused coping efforts and two specific emotion-focused coping efforts the nurse could encourage him to use to adapt to the physical and emotional stress of his illness.

Problem-Focused	**Emotion-Focused**
a.	a.
b.	b.

10. While teaching relaxation therapy to a patient with fibromyalgia, the nurse recognizes that it is most important to incorporate
   a. relaxation breathing.
   b. soft background music.
   c. progressive muscle relaxation.
   d. concentration on a single focus.

11. After receiving the assigned patients for the day, the nurse determines that stress-relieving interventions are a priority for the patient
   a. with peptic ulcer disease.
   b. newly admitted with cholecystitis.
   c. with a bacterial exacerbation of chronic bronchitis.
   d. who is 1 day postoperative for knee replacement.

12. A 42-year-old patient with rheumatoid arthritis is withdrawn, pulls the covers over her head, and does not initiate conversation with her husband or other visitors. Upon questioning, the patient tells the nurse that she must either withdraw or cry all the time and that she cannot cope with the chronic nature of the disease. An appropriate nursing diagnosis for the patient is
   a. ineffective denial related to inability to cope.
   b. ineffective coping related to disruption of emotional bonds.
   c. ineffective coping related to inadequate psychologic resources.
   d. impaired adjustment related to unwillingness to modify lifestyle to accommodate chronic illness.

13. A 32-year-old man is admitted to the hospital with an acute exacerbation of Crohn's disease. Coping strategies that might be suggested by the nurse during his hospitalization include (select all that apply)
   a. humor.
   b. exercise.
   c. journaling.
   d. relaxation therapy.

CASE STUDY

Stress

Patient Profile

M.J., a 26-year-old unmarried secretary, is admitted to the hospital with right lower-quadrant pain rated as 9 on a scale of 0-10; 10 to 12 watery, blood-streaked stools in the past 24 hours; and a low-grade fever. She has a 7-year history of inflammatory bowel disease.

Subjective Data

Patient relates the following.
- She has been hospitalized four times in the past year.
- She is not currently working because of the illness and has no income.
- She has no insurance.
- Her boyfriend has lived with her for 2 years.
- She does not want her boyfriend to visit because she thinks he has enough problems of his own.
- She has been in bed the past week because of weakness, nausea, and malaise and has been crying and depressed.

Objective Data

- Height: 5 ft 6 in (168 cm)
- Weight: 104 lb (47.3 kg)
- Hemoglobin: 10.5 g/dL (105 g/L)
- Hematocrit: 30%
- Temperature: 100° F (37.8° C)

Clinical Decision-Making Questions

Using a separate sheet of paper, answer the following questions.

1. What physiologic and psychologic stressors can be identified or anticipated in M.J.'s situation? Describe the possible effects of these stressors on the course of her illness.
2. What factors identified in M.J.'s nursing assessment could affect her current adaptation to stress?
3. What physiologic changes would be expected in M.J. as she begins to respond to prescribed treatment?
4. Describe an approach that the nurse could use to assess M.J.'s perception of her situation. Include several specific questions to be asked by the nurse.
5. *Priority Decision:* What are the priority nursing interventions that can be implemented with M.J. to enhance her adaptation to stress?
6. *Priority Decision:* Based on the assessment data provided, what are the priority nursing diagnoses? Are there any collaborative problems?
7. *Priority Decision:* What is the priority nursing diagnosis/intervention for M.J. on admission?

Sleep and Sleep Disorders

1. Indicate whether the statement is true (*T*) or false (*F*). If a statement is false, correct the bold word(s) to make the statement true.

_____ a. During sleep, an individual is **not consciously** aware of his/her environment.

_____ b. Adults generally require at least **5 hours** of sleep every 24 hours.

_____ c. Sleep is **necessary** for normal functioning and survival.

_____ d. **Less than 10% of adults** report day time sleepiness severe enough to interfere with work or social functioning.

2. Crossword Puzzle: Everyone Needs Plenty of Sleep!

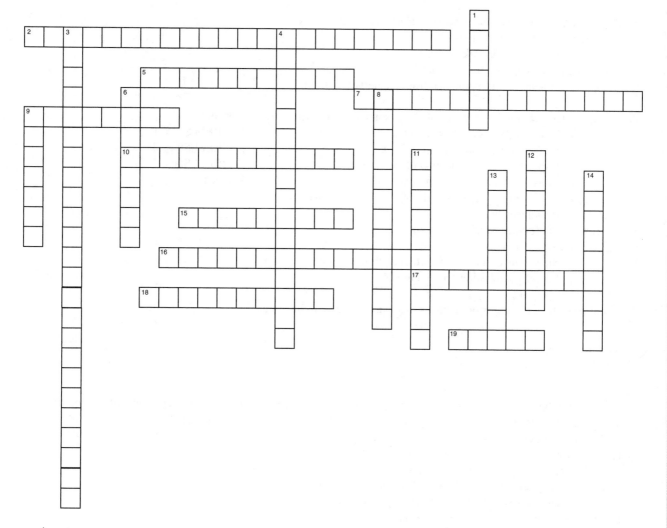

Across

2. Sleepiness following a meal
5. Unusual and undesirable behaviors that occur with sleep are _____.
7. Biologic rhythm of behavior and physiology during 24 hours
9. Condition characterized by shallow respirations
10. Transition from wake to sleep over 10-20 minutes is sleep _____.
15. Brief and sudden loss of skeletal muscle tone

16. Feeling unrefreshed on awakening is _____ sleep.
17. Disorder from brain's inability to regulate sleep-wake cycles
18. Time asleep as compared with time in bed is sleep _____.
19. Cessation of spontaneous respirations lasting longer than 10 seconds

Down
1. Stimulates wake behavior through activating the RAS
3. Abnormal respiratory patterns associated with sleep
4. Difficulty falling asleep
6. Most common sleep disorder
8. Less sleep than one needs to be fully awake and alert is _____ sleep.
9. Practices that are important to have a normal, quality sleep are sleep _____.
11. Frequent awakenings that interrupt sleep is _____ sleep.
12. A condition that results in poor sleep quality is a sleep _____.
13. Endogenous hormone released more in the evening as it gets dark
14. Temporary paralysis of skeletal muscles

3. The cyclic changes between waking and sleep are controlled by
   a. fluctuating levels of melatonin.
   b. the environmental light-dark cycles.
   c. key nuclei in the brainstem, hypothalamus, and thalamus.
   d. a variety of neuropeptides released from the nervous system.

4. Match the descriptions to the stages of sleep (some may be used more than once).
   _____ a. Brain waves resemble wakefulness
   _____ b. Deepest sleep lasting 20-40 minutes
   _____ c. Important for consolidation of memory
   _____ d. Most vivid dreaming occurs
   _____ e. Occurs four to five times during 7-8 hours of sleep
   _____ f. Person easily awakened
   _____ g. Short duration of 1-7 minutes
   _____ h. Slow eye movements
   _____ i. Slowed heart rate; decreased body temperature
   _____ j. Sound sleep lasting 10-25 minutes

   1. NREM Stage 1
   2. NREM Stage 2
   3. NREM Stage 3
   4. REM

5. List at least three behaviors or practices that can contribute to insomnia.
   a.

   b.

   c.

6. A clinical polysomnography (PSG) may be performed on a patient with signs and symptoms of a sleep disorder. This study includes which of the following measures and observations? (select all that apply)
   a. Actigraph watch worn on the wrist to monitor motor activity
   b. Airflow measured at the nose and mouth
   c. Blood pressure monitoring (noninvasive)
   d. Brain activity recorded by electroencephalogram (EEG)
   e. Eye movements recorded by electro-oculogram (EOG)
   f. Gross body movements monitored via audio and visual recordings
   g. Heart rate monitoring
   h. Muscle tone measured by electromyogram (EMG)
   i. Noninvasive oxygen saturation (SpO_2)
   j. Respiratory effort around the chest and abdomen
   k. Surface body temperature fluctuations

7. First line therapy for insomnia is
   a. complementary therapy such as melatonin.
   b. cognitive-behavioral therapies such as relaxation therapy.
   c. benzodiazepine-receptor-like agents (e.g., zolpidem [Ambien]).
   d. over-the-counter medication such as diphenhydramine (Benadryl).

8. The nurse knows that a patient taught sleep hygiene practices needs further instruction when he says,
   a. "Once I go to bed, I should get up if I am not asleep after 20 minutes."
   b. "It's okay to have my usual two glasses of wine in the evening before bed."
   c. "A couple of crackers with cheese and a glass of milk may help to relax before bed."
   d. "I should go to the gym earlier in the day so that I'm done at least 6 hours before bedtime."

9. Which of the following foods or beverages has the highest caffeine content?
   a. Hershey bar
   b. 12 oz diet Coke
   c. 8 oz of brewed tea (nonherbal)
   d. 1 c Ben & Jerry nonfat coffee fudge frozen yogurt

10. Which of the following foods or beverages has the least caffeine content?
    a. 12 oz 7-Up
    b. 8 oz hot chocolate
    c. 8 oz decaffeinated coffee
    d. 8 oz Dannon coffee yogurt

11. A nurse caring for a patient in the intensive care unit implements strategies to create an environment conducive to sleep. Which of these strategies would be most effective?
    a. Turning the lights out in the room during the night.
    b. Having the television on at all times for background noise.
    c. Silencing the alarms on the bedside monitor and infusion pumps.
    d. Administering ordered analgesics around the clock even if the patient denies pain.

12. Which of the following medications is a nonamphetamine wake-promotion drug?
    a. modafinil (Provigil)
    b. protriptyline (Vavactil)
    c. desipramine (Norpramin)
    d. methylphenidate (Concerta)

13. The nurse in a clinic is talking with a patient who will be traveling from the Midwest time zone to Moscow to attend a 4-day conference. The patient asks the nurse how he can minimize the effects of jet lag. Identify at least two recommendations the nurse could give to the patient.

14. Place the events below in the order they occur in the patient with obstructive sleep apnea (beginning with 1).
    _____ a. apnea lasting 10-90 seconds
    _____ b. brief arousal and airway opened
    _____ c. generalized startle response, snorting, or gasping
    _____ d. hypoxemia and hypercapnia
    _____ e. narrowing of air passages or tongue and soft palate obstruct pharynx
    _____ f. risk factors: obesity, large neck circumference, craniofacial abnormalities, acromegaly, smoking
    _____ g. occurs 200-400 times during 6-8 hours of sleep
    _____ h. relaxation of muscle tone during sleep

15. The physician has ordered CPAP for a patient with serious obstructive sleep apnea. CPAP will
    a. prevent airway occlusion by bringing the tongue forward.
    b. be easily tolerated by both the patient and the patient's bed partner.
    c. provide enough positive pressure in the airways to prevent airway collapse.
    d. deliver a high inspiratory pressure and a low expiratory pressure to prevent airway collapse.

16. While caring for a patient following an uvulopalatopharyngoplasty (UPPP), the nurse monitors the patient for which complications in the immediate postoperative period?
    a. Snoring and foul-smelling breath
    b. Infection and electrolyte imbalance
    c. Loss of voice and severe sore throat
    d. Airway obstruction and hemorrhage

17. An elderly patient asks the nurse why she has so much trouble sleeping. An appropriate response by the nurse would be,
    a. "Disturbed sleep is a normal result of aging."
    b. "Have you tried any over-the-counter medications to help you sleep?"
    c. "Don't worry. You don't need as much sleep as you did when you were younger."
    d. "Tell me more about the trouble you are having. There may be some things we can do to help."

18. Nurses who rotate shifts or work nights are at risk for developing circadian rhythm shift work disorder characterized by insomnia, sleepiness, and fatigue. Identify at least three negative implications for the nurse.
    a.

    b.

    c.

19. What strategies could decrease the distress of rotating shifts for nurses? (select all that apply)
    a. Take brief on-site naps
    b. Use sleep hygiene practices
    c. Sleep just before going to work
    d. Maintain consistent sleep-wake schedules even on days off (if possible)
    e. Negotiate to control work schedule rather than having someone else impose the schedule

1. Pain has been defined as "whatever the person experiencing the pain says it is, existing whenever the patient says it does." The definition is problematic when caring for a patient who has
   a. been placed on a ventilator.
   b. a history of opioid addiction.
   c. decreased cognitive function.
   d. pain resulting from severe trauma.

2. On the first postoperative day following a bowel resection, the patient complains of abdominal and incisional pain rated 7 on a scale of 0 to 10. Postoperative orders include morphine, 4 to 10 mg IV q2-4hr. The nurse determines that it has been 3½ hours since the last dose and plans to administer 4 mg of morphine. Routine administration of the smallest prescribed dose of an opioid analgesic when a range of doses is prescribed
   a. protects the patient from addiction and toxic effects of the drug.
   b. prevents hastening or causing a patient's death from respiratory dysfunction.
   c. contributes to unnecessary suffering and physical and psychosocial dysfunction.
   d. indicates that the nurse understands the adage of "start low and go slow" in administering analgesics.

3. List and briefly describe the five dimensions of pain.
   a.

   b.

   c.

   d.

   e.

4. Once generated, what may block the transmission of an action potential along a peripheral nerve fiber to the dorsal root of the spinal cord?
   a. The transmission may be interrupted by drugs such as local anesthetics.
   b. Nothing can stop the action potential along an intact nerve until it reaches the spinal cord.
   c. The fiber produces neurotransmitters that may activate nearby nerve fibers to transmit pain impulses.
   d. The action potential must cross several synapses, points at which the impulse may be blocked by drugs.

5. A patient comes to the clinic with a complaint of a dull pain in the anterior and posterior neck. On examination, the nurse notes that the patient has full ROM of the neck and no throat redness or enlarged head or neck lymph nodes. The next appropriate assessment indicated by the patient's findings is
   a. palpation of the liver.
   b. auscultation of bowel sounds.
   c. inspection of the patient's ears.
   d. palpation for the presence of left flank pain.

6. While caring for an unconscious patient, the nurse discovers a stage 2 pressure ulcer on the patient's heel. During care of the ulcer, the nurse
   a. knows that the patient will have a behavioral response if pain is perceived.
   b. should treat the area as a painful lesion, using gentle cleansing and dressing.
   c. can thoroughly scrub the area because the patient is not able to perceive pain.
   d. understands that all nociceptive stimuli that are transmitted to the brain result in the perception of pain.

7. List in order the nociceptive processes that occur to communicate tissue damage to the CNS. No. 1 would be the first process and No. 4 the last process.
_____ a. Modulation
_____ b. Transmission
_____ c. Transduction
_____ d. Perception

8. Match the following types of pain in the left column with the category of pain in the upper right column and an example of the source of the pain from the lower right column.

Types of Pain
_____ a. pain arising from skin/subcutaneous tissue; well localized
_____ b. pain arising from muscles/bones; localized or diffuse and radiating
_____ c. pain caused by dysfunction in the CNS
_____ d. pain felt along the distribution of peripheral nerve(s) from nerve damage
_____ e. pain from loss of afferent input
_____ f. pain persisting from SNS activity
_____ g. pain arising from visceral organs; well or poorly localized; referred cutaneously

Categories of Pain
1. Nociceptive pain
2. Neuropathic pain

Sources of Pain
3. Sunburn
4. Osteoarthritis
5. Pancreatitis
6. Poststroke pain
7. Trigeminal neuralgia
8. Phantom limb pain
9. Postmastectomy pain

9. Amitriptyline (Elavil) is prescribed for a patient with chronic pain from fibromyalgia. When the nurse explains that this drug is an antidepressant, the patient states that she is in pain, not depressed. The nurse's best response to the patient is that
a. antidepressants will improve the patient's attitude and prevent a negative emotional response to the pain.
b. chronic pain almost always leads to depression, and the use of this drug will prevent depression from occurring.
c. some antidepressant drugs relieve pain by releasing neurotransmitters that prevent pain impulses from reaching the brain.
d. certain antidepressant drugs are metabolized in the liver to substances that numb the ends of nerve fibers, preventing the onset of pain.

10. A patient with trigeminal neuralgia has moderate to severe burning and shooting pain. In helping the patient manage the pain, the nurse recognizes that this type of pain
a. is chronic in nature and will require long-term treatment.
b. involves treatment that includes the use of adjuvant analgesics.
c. responds to small to moderate around-the-clock doses of oral opioids.
d. can be well controlled with salicylates or nonsteroidal antiinflammatory drugs (NSAIDs).

11. In the following scenario, identify the pain characteristics that are present.

T.B., a 62-year-old mail carrier, is admitted to the medical unit from the emergency department. Upon arrival he is trembling and nearly doubled over with severe, cramping abdominal pain. T.B. indicates that he has severe right upper-quadrant pain that radiates to his back, and he is more comfortable walking bent forward than lying in bed. He notes that he has had several similar bouts of abdominal pain in the last month but "not as bad as this. This is the worst pain I can imagine." The other episodes only lasted about 2 hours. Today he experienced an acute onset of pain and nausea after eating fish and chips at a fast-food restaurant about 4 hours ago.
a.
b.
c.
d.
e.
f.
g.

12. List the nine basic principles that should guide the treatment of all pain.
    a.

    b.

    c.

    d.

    e.

    f.

    g.

    h.

    i.

13. A patient with colorectal cancer has continuous, poorly localized abdominal pain at an intensity of 5 on a scale of 0 to 10. The nurse teaches the patient to use pain medications
    a. on an around-the-clock schedule.
    b. as often as necessary to keep the pain controlled.
    c. by alternating two different types of drugs to prevent tolerance.
    d. when the pain cannot be controlled with distraction or relaxation.

14. A patient who has been taking ibuprofen (Motrin) and imipramine (Tofranil) for control of cancer pain is having increased pain. The nurse recommends that an appropriate change in the medication plan would be to
    a. add PO oxycodone (OxyContin) to the other medications.
    b. substitute PO propoxyphene (Darvon), a mild opioid, for the ketoprofen.
    c. add transdermal fentanyl (Duragesic) to the use of the other medications.
    d. substitute PO hydrocodone with acetaminophen (Lortab, Vicodin) for the other medications.

15. A patient with chronic cancer-related pain has started using MS Contin for pain control and has developed common side effects of the drug. The nurse reassures the patient that tolerance will develop to most of these effects but that continued treatment will most likely be required for the
    a. pruritus.
    b. dizziness.
    c. constipation.
    d. nausea and vomiting.

16. The use of a continuous infusion of an analgesic (called a basal rate) with patient-controlled analgesia (PCA) for postoperative pain is not recommended. Why?

17. Match each step of the physiologic pain process (in the right column) with the measures or drugs (in the left column) that may be effective in controlling pain during that step. Some drugs may have actions in more than one step.
    _____ a. NMDA (*N*-methyl-D-aspartate) antagonist drugs   1. Transduction
    _____ b. NSAIDs (nonsteroidal antiinflammatory drugs)   2. Transmission
    _____ c. Local anesthetics   3. Perception
    _____ d. Distraction   4. Modulation
    _____ e. Tricyclic antidepressants
    _____ f. Corticosteroids
    _____ g. Epidural opioids
    _____ h. Antiseizure medications
    _____ i. Relaxation therapies

18. A patient is receiving a continuous infusion of morphine via an epidural catheter following major abdominal surgery. The nurse should include which of these actions in the plan of care? (select all that apply)
    a. Assess the patient's pain relief frequently.
    b. Monitor patient vital signs (BP, HR, respirations).
    c. Ensure that only preservative-free morphine is being administered.
    d. Label the catheter as an epidural access.
    e. Use sterile technique when caring for the catheter.
    f. Assess the motor and sensory function of the patient's lower extremities
    g. Monitor the patient's level of consciousness (LOC).
    h. Check correct placement by aspirating cerebral spinal fluid (CSF) every 4 hours.

19. A patient with multiple injuries resulting from an automobile accident tells the nurse that he has "bad" pain but that he can "tough it out" and does not require pain medication. To gain the patient's participation in pain management, the nurse explains that
    a. patients have a responsibility to keep the nurse informed about their pain.
    b. unrelieved pain has many harmful effects on the body that can impair recovery.
    c. using pain medications rarely leads to addiction when they are used for actual pain.
    d. nonpharmacologic therapies can be used to relieve his pain if he is afraid to use pain medications.

CASE STUDY
Pain

Patient Profile

R.D., a 62-year-old postal worker, is being evaluated for a change in his pain therapy for chronic malignant pain from metastatic cancer.

Subjective Data

- Patient desires zero pain but will accept pain level 3-4 on a 0 to 10 scale.
- He has been taking two Percocet tablets q4hr while awake, but his pain is now usually at 4-5 with the medication.
- Patient reports that pain varies over 24 hours from 5-10.
- He always awakens in the morning with pain at 10 with nervousness, nausea, and a runny nose.
- When pain becomes severe, he stays in bed and concentrates on blocking the pain by emptying his mind.
- He is worried that increased pain means his disease is worsening.
- He is afraid to take additional doses or other opioids because he fears addiction.

Objective Data

- Height: 6 ft 0 in (183 cm); weight: 150 lb (68 kg)
- Rigid posturing, slow gait

Clinical Decision-Making Questions

Using a separate sheet of paper, answer the following questions.

1. What additional assessment data should the nurse obtain from R.D. before making any decisions about his problem?
2. What data from the nursing assessment are characteristic of the affective, behavioral, and cognitive dimensions of the pain experience?
3. Based on R.D.'s lack of pain control with his current dosage of opioid and his symptoms on arising in the morning, what changes are indicated in his medication regimen?
4. *Priority Decision:* What are the priority teaching needs that should be included in a teaching plan for R.D. to titrate his analgesic dose effectively?
5. How could the nurse best help R.D. overcome his fear of addiction to opioid drugs?
6. What additional pain therapies could the nurse plan to help R.D. manage his pain?
7. *Priority Decision:* Based on the assessment data provided, what are the priority nursing diagnoses? Are there any collaborative problems?

CHAPTER 11

Palliative Care at End of Life

1. According to the World Health Organization, palliative care is an approach that improves quality of life for patients and their families who face problems associated with life-threatening illnesses. Identify the specific goals of palliative care from the list below (select all that apply).
   a. Minimize the financial burden on the family.
   b. Provide relief from symptoms including pain.
   c. Offer support to family during patient's illness and their own bereavement.
   d. Prolong the patient's life with aggressive new therapies.
   e. Regard dying as a normal process.
   f. Support holistic patient care and enhance quality of life.
   g. Offer support to patients to live as actively as possible until death.
   h. Assist the patient and family to identify and access pastoral care services.
   i. Affirm life and neither hasten nor postpone death.

2. The husband and daughter of a Hispanic woman dying from pancreatic cancer refuse to consider using hospice care. The nurse should
   a. clarify their understanding of what hospice care services are.
   b. talk directly to the patient to see if she could change their minds.
   c. ask them how they will care for the patient without hospice care.
   d. accept their decision since they are Hispanic and prefer to care for their own.

3. List the two criteria for admission to a hospice program.

4. For each of the following systems, identify three physical manifestations the nurse would expect to see in a patient approaching death.

   Respiratory
   a.

   b.

   c.

   Skin
   a.

   b.

   c.

   Gastrointestinal
   a.

   b.

   c.

   Musculoskeletal
   a.

   b.

   c.

5. A terminally ill patient is unresponsive and has Cheyne-Stokes respiration. The patient's husband and two grown children are arguing at the bedside about where the patient's funeral should be held. The nurse should
   a. ask the family members to leave the room if they are going to argue.
   b. take the family members aside and explain that the patient may be able to hear them.
   c. tell the family members that this decision is premature because the patient has not yet died.
   d. remind the family that this should be the patient's decision and to ask her if she regains consciousness.

6. A 20-year-old patient with a massive head injury is on life support, including a ventilator to maintain respirations. What three criteria for brain death are necessary to discontinue life support?
   a.

   b.

   c.

7. A patient with end-stage liver failure tells the nurse, "If I can just live to see my first grandchild who is expected in 5 months, then I can die happy." The nurse recognizes that the patient is demonstrating
   a. Rando's phase of avoidance.
   b. Kübler-Ross's stage of bargaining.
   c. Martocchio's stage of shock and disbelief.
   d. Martocchio's stage of reorganization and restoration.

8. A terminally ill man tells the nurse, "I have never believed there is a God or an afterlife, but now it is too terrible to imagine that I will not exist. Why was I here in the first place?" The nurse recognizes that the patient
   a. is experiencing spiritual distress.
   b. most likely will not have a peaceful death.
   c. needs to be reassured that his feelings are normal.
   d. should be referred to a clergyman for a discussion of his beliefs.

9. Identify the legal document or other term described by each of the following.
   a. A lay term for statements that give instructions about future treatment if a patient is unable to do so for himself or herself:

   _____

   b. A term used to describe a document designating the person or persons who should make health care decisions if a patient cannot make informed decisions for himself or herself:

   _____

   c. A written document to a health care provider stating the patient's wish to be allowed to die without heroic or extraordinary measures:

   _____

   d. Specific state laws that include a variety of directives related to an individual's wishes regarding medical treatment and prolongation of life:

   _____

   e. The federal law specifying that institutions participating in Medicare must provide written information to patients concerning their rights to accept or refuse treatment:

   _____

   f. A general term used to describe all documents that give instructions about future medical care and treatments:

   _____

   g. A signed written physician's order instructing health care personnel not to attempt CPR:

   _____

10. A patient is receiving care to manage symptoms of a terminal illness when the disease no longer responds to treatment. This type of care is known as
    a. terminal care.
    b. palliative care.
    c. supportive care.
    d. maintenance care.

11. A patient in the last stages of life is experiencing shortness of breath and air hunger. Based on practice guidelines, the most appropriate action by the nurse is to
    a. administer oxygen.
    b. administer bronchodilators.
    c. administer antianxiety agents.
    d. use any methods that make the patient more comfortable.

12. End-of-life palliative nursing care involves
    a. constant assessment for changes in physiologic functioning.
    b. administering large doses of analgesics to keep the patient sedated.
    c. providing as little physical care as possible to prevent disturbing the patient.
    d. encouraging the patient and family members to verbalize their feelings of sadness, loss, and forgiveness.

13. Fill in the blanks.
    a. _____ is the term used when a patient wants to avoid the use of cardiopulmonary resuscitation (CPR) if cardiopulmonary arrest occurs.
    b. Complete and total heroic measures including CPR, drug administration, and mechanical ventilation are known as a _____ .
    c. Allowing only drug administration in the event of an arrest is called _____.
    d. _____ or _____ are the newest terms being used to signify providing all comfort measures to relieve pain and symptoms while allowing a patient's natural progression to death without delay or interruption.

CASE STUDY
End-of-Life Palliative Care
Patient Profile

S.J., a 42-year-old housewife, had unsuccessful treatment for breast cancer 1 year ago and now has metastasis to the lung and vertebrae. She lives at home with her husband, a 15-year-old daughter, and a 12-year-old son. She has been referred to hospice because of her deteriorating condition and increasing pain. Her husband is an accountant and tries to do as much of his work at home as possible so that he can help care for his wife. Their children have become withdrawn, choosing to spend as much time as possible at their friends' homes and in outside activities.

Subjective Data

- S.J. reports that she stays in bed most of the time because it is too painful to stand and sit.
- She reports her pain as an 8 on a 10-point scale while taking oral MS Contin q12hr.
- She reports shortness of breath with almost any activity, such as getting up to go to the bathroom.
- S.J. says she knows she is dying, but her greatest suffering results from her children not caring about her.
- She and her husband have not talked about her dying with the children.
- Her husband reports that he does not know how to help his wife anymore and that he feels guilty sometimes when he just wishes it were all over.

Objective Data

- Height: 5 ft 2 in (157 cm); weight: 97 lb (44 kg)
- Skin intact
- Vital signs: T 99° F (37.2° C); HR 92; RR 30; BP 102/60

Clinical Decision-Making Questions

Using a separate sheet of paper, answer the following questions.

1. What additional assessment data should the nurse obtain from Mr. and Mrs. J. before making any decisions about care of the family?
2. What types of grieving appear to be occurring in the family?
3. *Priority Decision*: What physical care should the nurse include in a plan for S.J. at this time?
4. What is the best way to facilitate healthy grieving in this family?
5. What resources of a hospice team are available to assist this patient and her family?
6. *Priority Decision*: Based on the assessment data provided, what are the priority nursing diagnoses?

<h1 style="text-align:right">Addictive Behaviors</h1>

1. Match the following terms with their definitions.

_____ a. Addiction	1. Absence of a substance will cause withdrawal symptoms
_____ b. Abuse	2. Responses occurring after abrupt cessation of a substance
_____ c. Craving	3. Return to drug use after a period of abstinence
_____ d. Physical dependence	4. Drug use for purposes other than that intended
_____ e. Tolerance	5. Compulsive need to experience pleasure
_____ f. Withdrawal	6. Overuse and dependence on substance that negatively affects functioning
_____ g. Abstinence	7. Refraining from substance use
_____ h. Relapse	8. Decreased effect of substance following repeated exposure
_____ i. Misuse	9. Overwhelming desire for substance after decreased use
_____ j. Psychologic dependence	10. Compulsive use of substances for physical and psychologic effects

2. As a health care professional, nurses have the responsibility to help reduce the use of tobacco. List the "five As" recommended as brief clinical interventions.

   a.

   b

   c.

   d.

   e.

3. On admission to the hospital for a knee replacement, a patient who has smoked for 20 years expresses an interest in quitting. What is the best response from the nurse?
   a. "Good for you! You should talk to your doctor about that."
   b. "Since you won't be able to smoke while you are in the hospital, just don't start again when you are discharged."
   c. "Great! I'll help you make a plan and work with your doctor to get you what you need to start while you are here."
   d. "Why did you ever start in the first place? It's so hard to quit."

4. List two major health problems commonly seen in the acute care setting related to the abuse of the following substances.

   Nicotine
   a.

   b.

   Alcohol
   a.

   b.

   Cocaine and amphetamines
   a.

   b.

   Opioids
   a.

   b.

   Cannabis
   a.

   b.

5. Match the following commonly abused substances with the physiologic effects associated with their use (answers may be used more than once).

_____ a. Increase in appetite
_____ b. Sexual arousal
_____ c. Depersonalization
_____ d. Tachycardia with hypertension
_____ e. Reddened eyes
_____ f. Constricted pupils
_____ g. Nasal damage
_____ h. Decreased respirations
_____ i. Altered perception
_____ j. Euphoria and drowsiness
_____ k. Decrease in appetite

1. Cocaine/amphetamines
2. Opioids
3. Cannabis
4. Hallucinogens
5. Nicotine

6. Use the terms below to fill in the blanks in the following statements.

sedative-hypnotic(s)   stimulant(s)
opioid(s)   hallucinogen(s)

a. Seizures may be a symptom of toxicity in _____ addiction and a symptom of withdrawal in _____ addiction.

b. Assessment findings of tremors, chills and sweating, and nausea and cramps are most likely to be found in the patient with _____ withdrawal.

c. The patient who abuses _____ is least likely to have withdrawal symptoms.

d. Suicidal thoughts and proneness to violence should be assessed in patients during withdrawal from

_____.

e. The safest and most effective method to withdraw the patient from large doses of _____ is with hospitalization and gradual reduction of the drug.

f. A patient with severe central nervous system depression with slow and shallow breathing and coma will respond to treatment with naloxone (Narcan) in acute _____ toxicity, but not in acute _____ toxicity.

7. When the nurse is encouraging a woman who smokes 1½ packs of cigarettes a day to quit with the use of nicotine replacement therapy, the woman asks how the nicotine in a patch or gum differs from the nicotine she gets from cigarettes. The nurse explains that nicotine replacements
   a. include a substance that eventually creates an aversion to nicotine.
   b. provide a noncarcinogenic nicotine, unlike the nicotine in cigarettes.
   c. prevent the weight gain that is of concern to women who stop smoking.
   d. eliminate the thousands of toxic chemicals that are inhaled with smoking.

8. Match the following drugs used for treatment of cocaine toxicity with their specific uses (answers may be used more than once).

_____ a. haloperidol (Haldol)
_____ b. IV lidocaine
_____ c. IV diazepam (Valium)
_____ d. propranolol (Inderal)
_____ e. bretylium (Bretylol)
_____ f. IV lorazepam (Ativan)
_____ g. procainamide (Pronestyl)

1. Tachycardia
2. Hallucinations
3. Dysrhythmias
4. Seizures

9. A patient who is a heavy caffeine user has been NPO all day in preparation for a late afternoon surgery. The nurse monitors the patient for
   a. a headache.
   b. nervousness.
   c. mild tremors.
   d. shortness of breath.

10. The third day after an alcohol-dependent patient was admitted to the hospital for pancreatitis, the nurse determines that the patient is experiencing alcohol withdrawal. Identify four major signs of withdrawal on which the nurse bases this judgment.

    a.

    b.

    c.

    d.

11. The best approach by the nurse to assess a newly admitted patient's use of addictive drugs is to ask the patient,
    a. "How do you relieve your stress?"
    b. "You don't use any illegal drugs, do you?"
    c. "What alcohol or recreational drugs do you use?"
    d. "Do you have any addictions we should know about to prevent complications?"

12. A patient who abuses a variety of depressants and opioids minimizes the amount and frequency of substances used, as well as the specific agents taken, and tells the nurse that a recent overdose episode was a result of experimentation. An appropriate nursing diagnosis for the patient is
    a. defensive coping.
    b. ineffective denial.
    c. ineffective coping.
    d. ineffective health maintenance.

13. To stop the behavior that leads to the most preventable cause of death in the United States, the nurse should support programs that
    a. prohibit alcohol use in public places.
    b. prevent tobacco use in children and adolescents.
    c. motivate individuals to enter addiction treatment.
    d. recognize addictions as illnesses rather than crimes.

14. A young woman is brought to the emergency department by police who found her lying on a downtown sidewalk. Initial assessment finds that she is unresponsive; has a weak pulse of 112; shallow respirations of 8/min; and cold, clammy skin. Identify the two drugs that would most likely be given immediately to this patient, and explain why.
    a.

    b.

15. A patient with a history of alcohol abuse is admitted to the hospital following an automobile accident. To plan care for the patient, it is most important for the nurse to assess
    a. when the patient last had alcohol intake.
    b. how much alcohol has recently been used.
    c. what type of alcohol has recently been ingested.
    d. the patient's current blood alcohol concentration.

16. A patient in alcohol withdrawal has a nursing diagnosis of ineffective protection related to sensorimotor deficits, seizure activity, and confusion. An appropriate nursing intervention for the patient is to
    a. provide a darkened, quiet environment free from external stimuli.
    b. force fluids to assist in diluting the alcohol concentration in the blood.
    c. monitor vital signs frequently to detect an extreme autonomic nervous system response.
    d. use restraints as necessary to prevent the patient from reacting violently to hallucinations.

17. What are four precautions indicated for the alcoholic patient who is alcohol intoxicated and is undergoing emergency surgery?

    a.

    b.

    c.

    d.

18. During admission to the emergency department, a patient with chronic alcoholism is intoxicated and very disoriented and confused. Which of the following ordered drugs will the nurse administer first?
    a. IV thiamine
    b. D_5 in ½ normal saline at 100 mL/hr
    c. IV benzodiazepines
    d. IV haloperidol (Haldol)

19. The nurse uses motivational interviewing with a patient who is dependent on alcohol and hospitalized for gastritis. When the patient says she does not think her use of alcohol is a problem because she can control her drinking when she wants to do so, it would be most appropriate for the nurse to
    a. help the patient consider the positive and negative factors of drinking.
    b. refrain from talking about her alcohol use while the patient is in denial.
    c. explain that the gastritis is evidence that alcohol is affecting her health.
    d. reassure the patient that she can quit drinking when she finally decides she wants to.

20. When assessing an older patient for substance abuse, the nurse specifically asks the patient about the use of alcohol and
    a. opioids.
    b. sedative-hypnotics.
    c. central nervous system stimulants.
    d. prescription and over-the-counter medications.

CASE STUDY
Cocaine Toxicity
Family Profile

N.C. is a 34-year-old man who was admitted to the emergency department with chest pain, tachycardia, dizziness, nausea, and severe migraine-like headache.

Subjective Data

- The patient is extremely nervous and irritable.
- He thinks he is having a heart attack.
- Patient admits he was at a party earlier in the evening drinking alcohol, smoking pot, and snorting cocaine.
- He noted a change in personality, including irritability and restlessness.
- He experienced an increased need for cocaine in the past few months.

Objective Data

Physical examination
- Appears pale and diaphoretic
- Has tremors
- BP: 210/110, HR: 100, RR: 30

Clinical Decision-Making Questions

Using a separate sheet of paper, answer the following questions.

1. What other information is needed to assess N.C.'s condition?
2. How should questions regarding these areas be addressed?
3. What other clues should the nurse be alert for in assessing N.C.'s drug use?
4. What emergency conditions must be carefully monitored?
5. *Priority Decision:* What are the priority nursing interventions?
6. What is the best way to approach N.C. to engage him in a treatment program?
7. *Priority Decision:* Based on the assessment data presented, what are the priority nursing diagnoses? Are there any collaborative problems?

Inflammation and Wound Healing

1. A patient with an inflammatory disease has the following symptoms. Identify the primary chemical mediators involved in producing the symptom and the physiologic change that causes the symptoms.

	Chemical Mediators	Physiologic Change
a. Fever		
b. Redness		
c. Edema		
d. Leukocytosis		

2. In a patient with leukocytosis with a shift to the left, the nurse recognizes that
   a. the complement system has been activated to enhance phagocytosis.
   b. monocytes are released into the blood in larger-than-normal amounts.
   c. the response to cellular injury is not adequate to remove damaged tissue and promote healing.
   d. the demand for neutrophils causes the release of immature neutrophils from the bone marrow.

3. Chemotaxis is a mechanism that
   a. causes the transformation of monocytes into macrophages.
   b. involves a pathway of chemical processes resulting in cellular lysis.
   c. attracts the accumulation of neutrophils and monocytes to an area of injury.
   d. slows the blood flow in a damaged area, allowing migration of leukocytes into tissue.

4. The action of the complement system in inflammation has the effect of
   a. modifying the inflammatory response to prevent stimulation of pain.
   b. increasing body temperature, resulting in destruction of microorganisms.
   c. producing prostaglandins and leukotrienes that increase blood flow, edema, and pain.
   d. increasing inflammatory responses of vascular permeability, chemotaxis, and phagocytosis.

5. Key interventions for treating soft tissue injury and resulting inflammation are remembered using the acronym RICE. State what each letter stands for and describe the mechanism of action.

	Meaning	Mechanism of Action
R		
I		
C		
E		

6. During the healing phase of inflammation, regeneration of cells would be most likely to occur in
   a. neurons.
   b. lymph glands.
   c. cardiac muscle.
   d. skeletal muscle.

7. Place the following events that occur during healing by primary intention in sequential order from 1 to 10.
   _____ a. Contraction of healing area by movement of myofibroblasts
   _____ b. Fibrin clot that serves as meshwork for capillary growth and epithelial cell migration
   _____ c. Accumulation of inflammatory debris
   _____ d. Epithelial cells migrate across wound surface
   _____ e. Fibroblasts migrate to site and secrete collagen
   _____ f. Blood clots form
   _____ g. Enzymes from neutrophils digest fibrin
   _____ h. Avascular, pale, mature scar present
   _____ i. Budding capillaries result in pink, vascular friable wound
   _____ j. Macrophages ingest and digest cellular debris and red blood cells

8. The primary difference between healing by primary intention and healing by secondary intention is that
   a. secondary healing requires surgical debridement for healing to occur.
   b. primary healing involves suturing two layers of granulation tissue together.
   c. the presence of more granulation tissue in secondary healing results in more scarring.
   d. healing by secondary intention takes longer because more steps in the healing process are necessary.

9. Match the following characteristics with the related complications of wound healing. Not all terms will be used.
   _____ a. Bands of scar tissue between or around organs
   _____ b. Risk increased in undernourished or immunosuppressed patients
   _____ c. Abnormal passage between organs or between hollow organ and skin
   _____ d. Large protrusion of scar tissue extending beyond wound edges; may form tumor-like masses of scar tissue
   _____ e. Separation of joined wound edges; healing site bursts open

   1. Keloid formation
   2. Infection
   3. Dehiscence
   4. Hypertrophic scar
   5. Adhesion
   6. Evisceration
   7. Fistula formation

10. Indicate the role of the following nutrients in wound healing.
    a. proteins _____
    b. carbohydrates _____
    c. fats _____
    d. vitamin C _____
    e. B-complex vitamins _____
    f. vitamin A _____

11. Match the characteristics and management techniques of wounds with their types (answers may be used more than once).
    _____ a. Serosanguineous drainage
    _____ b. Adherent gray necrotic tissue
    _____ c. Spray films
    _____ d. Creamy ivory to yellow-green exudate
    _____ e. Autolytic debridement
    _____ f. Dry, sterile dressing
    _____ g. Soft necrotic slough
    _____ h. Clean, moist granulating tissue
    _____ i. Negative pressure wound therapy

    1. Closed wound
    2. Red wound
    3. Yellow wound
    4. Black wound

12. During care of patients, the most important precaution for preventing transmission of infections is
    a. wearing face and eye protection during routine daily care of the patient.
    b. wearing a gown to protect the skin and clothing during patient-care activities likely to soil clothing.
    c. wearing nonsterile gloves when in contact with body fluids, excretions, and contaminated items.
    d. hand washing after touching fluids and secretions and removing gloves, as well as between patient contacts.

13. The patient who is at greatest risk for developing pressure ulcers is
   a. a 42-year-old obese woman with type 2 diabetes.
   b. a 78-year-old man who is confused and malnourished.
   c. a 65-year-old woman who has urge and stress incontinence.
   d. a 30-year-old man who is comatose following a head injury.

14. The most important nursing intervention for the prevention and treatment of pressure ulcers is
   a. using pressure-reduction devices.
   b. massaging pressure areas with lotion.
   c. repositioning the patient a minimum of every 2 hours.
   d. using lift sheets and trapeze bars to facilitate patient movement.

15. Match the stages of pressure ulcers with their characteristics.
   _____ a. Necrosis of subcutaneous tissue to fascia   1. Stage I
   _____ b. Skin loss with damage to muscle or bone   2. Stage II
   _____ c. Loss of epidermis or dermis   3. Stage III
   _____ d. Closed, nonblanchable erythema   4. Stage IV

16. A patient's documentation indicates he has a stage III pressure ulcer on his right hip. Which of the following should the nurse expect to find on assessment of the patient's right hip?
   a. An abrasion, blister or shallow crater
   b. Persistent redness (or bluish color in darker skin tones)
   c. Exposed bone, tendon, or muscle
   d. Deep crater through subcutaneous tissue to fascia

17. *Delegation Decision:* Which of the following nursing interventions for a patient with a Stage IV sacral pressure ulcer is most appropriate to assign/delegate to an LPN?
   a. Teach the patient pressure ulcer risk factors.
   b. Choose the type of dressing to apply to the ulcer.
   c. Measure the size (width, length, depth) of the ulcer.
   d. Assist the patient to change positions at frequent intervals.

CASE STUDY

Inflammation

Patient Profile

L.G., a 28-year-old diabetic, is admitted to the hospital with a cellulitis of her left lower leg. She had been applying heating pads to the leg for the last 48 hours, but the leg has become more painful and she has developed chilling.

Subjective Data

- Complains of pain and heaviness in her leg
- States she cannot bear weight on her leg and has been in bed for 3 days
- Lives alone and has not had anyone to help her with meals

Objective Data

Physical examination
- Round, yellow-red, 2-cm diameter, 1-cm deep, open wound above the left medial malleolus with moderate amount of thick yellow drainage
- Left leg red from knee to ankle
- Calf measurement on left 3 inches larger than right
- Temperature: 102° F (38.9° C)
- Height: 5 ft 4 in (160 cm); weight: 184 lb (83.7 kg)

Laboratory test results
- White blood cell (WBC): 18,300/μL (18.3 × 10^9/L; 80% neutrophils, 12% bands)
- Wound culture: *Staphylococcus aureus*

Clinical Decision-Making Questions

Using a separate sheet of paper, answer the following questions.

1. What clinical manifestations of inflammation are present in L.G.?
2. What type of exudate is draining from the open wound?
3. What is the significance of L.G.'s WBC count and differential?
4. What factors are present in this situation that could delay wound healing?
5. L.G.'s health care provider orders aspirin to be given PRN for a temperature above 102°F (38.9°C). How does the aspirin act to interfere with the fever mechanism? Why is the aspirin to be given only if the temperature is above 102°F? To prevent cycling of chills and diaphoresis, how should the nurse administer the aspirin?
6. What type of wound dressing would promote healing of the open wound?
7. *Priority Decision:* What are the priority precautions to prevent transmission of infection in the care of L.G.'s wound?
8. *Priority Decision:* Based on the assessment data provided, what are the priority nursing diagnoses? Are there any collaborative problems?

14 Genetics, Altered Immune Responses, and Transplantation

1. Crossword Puzzle

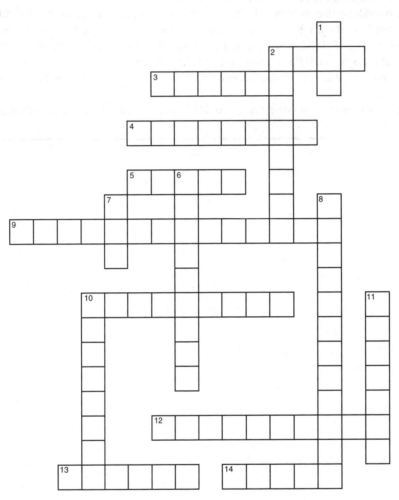

Across
   2. Basic unit of heredity; arranged on chromosome
   3. One of two or more alternative forms of a gene on a particular locus
   4. Permanent change in the sequence of DNA
   5. Physical characteristics that one inherits
   9. Gene expressed in the phenotype of a heterozygous individual
   10. Genetic physical traits expressed by an individual
   12. Structure in cell nucleus that carries genes
   13. Complete genetic information in a complete set of chromosomes
   14. Position of a gene on a chromosome

Down
   1. Double-stranded molecule-forming gene; stores genetic information
   2. Actual genetic makeup of an individual
   6. The 22 homologous pairs of chromosomes
   7. Single-stranded nucleic acid that transfers genetic information for protein synthesis
   8. Having two different alleles for one given gene
   10. Family tree containing genetic characteristics and disorders of that family
   11. Individual who carries a copy of a mutated gene for a recessive disorder

2. The new parents of an infant born with Down syndrome ask the nurse what happened to cause the chromosomal abnormality. The best response by the nurse is
   a. "A mutation in one of the chromosomes created an autosomal-recessive gene that is expressed as Down syndrome."
   b. "An abnormal gene on one of the two chromosomes was transferred to the fetus, causing an abnormal chromosome."
   c. "During cell division the two chromosomes did not completely separate, causing an abnormal number of chromosomes."
   d. "A process of 'crossing over' caused the exchange of genetic material between the two chromosomes in the cell resulting in abnormal chromosomes."

3. When a father has Huntington's disease with a heterozygous genotype, the nurse uses Punnett squares to illustrate the inheritance patterns and the probability of transmission of the autosomal-dominant disease. Complete the Punnett squares below to illustrate this inheritance pattern, using "H" as the normal gene, and "h" as the gene for Huntington's chorea.

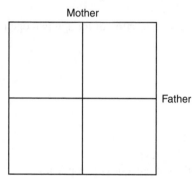

Mother

Father

There is a _____ % chance that offspring will be unaffected.

There is a _____ % chance that offspring will be affected.

4. Identify whether the following statements are true (*T*) or false (*F*). If a statement is false, correct the bold word(s) to make the statement true.
   _____ a. An example of genetic testing that is required by all states is **premarital testing of women for the hemophilia gene**.
   _____ b. An ethical issue that is raised with genetic testing is **protection of privacy to prevent discrimination**.
   _____ c. Genetic testing for **BRCA-1 and BRCA-2 mutations** can identify women who may choose to have mastectomies to prevent breast cancer.
   _____ d. Stem cells from **placenta blood** are different than adult stem cells because they can differentiate into any cell type they are stimulated to become.
   _____ e. The hope for **gene therapy** is that new tissue may be regenerated to replace lost or damaged tissue.

5. Match the descriptions of acquired specific immunity with their types of immunity (answers may be used more than once).
   _____ a. Maternal immunoglobulins in neonate   1. Active natural immunity
   _____ b. Contact with antigen through infection   2. Active artificial immunity
   _____ c. Immediate, lasting several weeks   3. Passive natural immunity
   _____ d. Longest-lasting immunity   4. Passive artificial immunity
   _____ e. Immunization with antigen
   _____ f. Temporary for several months
   _____ g. Boosters may be needed for extended protection
   _____ h. Pooled gamma globulin

6. Complete the following statements.
   a. The central organs of the lymphoid system are the _____ and the _____.
   b. The primary cells involved in the immune response are _____, _____, and _____.
   c. The lymphoid organ primarily responsible for filtering foreign substances from the blood is the _____.
   d. Lymphocytes that differentiate into B lymphocytes are processed in the _____; T lymphocytes are differentiated in the _____.

7. To stimulate an immune response, an antigen must be
   a. captured, processed, and presented to a lymphocyte by a macrophage.
   b. a foreign protein that has antigenic determinants different from those of the body.
   c. circulated in the blood, where it comes in contact with circulating lymphocytes.
   d. combined with larger molecules that are capable of stimulating production of antibodies.

8. T lymphocytes that are involved in direct attack and destruction of foreign pathogens are
   a. dendritic cells.
   b. natural killer cells.
   c. T-helper (CD4$^+$) cells.
   d. T-cytotoxic (CD8$^+$) cells.

9. Interferon is a cytokine that
   a. directly attacks and destroys virus-infected cells.
   b. augments the immune response by activating phagocytes.
   c. induces production of antiviral proteins in cells that prevent viral replication.
   d. is produced by viral infected cells and prevents the transmission of the virus to adjacent cells.

10. The humoral immune response involves
    a. surveillance for malignant cell changes.
    b. production of antigen-specific immunoglobulins.
    c. direct attack of antigens by activated B lymphocytes.
    d. releasing cytokines responsible for destruction of antigens.

11. Activated B lymphocytes differentiate primarily into
    a. plasma cells that secrete immunoglobulins.
    b. natural killer cells that destroy infected cells.
    c. memory B cells that retain a memory of the antigen.
    d. helper cells that in turn activate additional B lymphocytes.

12. Match the characteristics of the immunoglobulins with their types (answers may be used more than once).
    _____ a. Crosses placenta for fetal protection
    _____ b. Predominant in primary immune response
    _____ c. Predominant in secondary immune response
    _____ d. Responsible for allergic reactions
    _____ e. Assists in B-lymphocyte differentiation
    _____ f. Protects body surfaces and mucous membranes
    _____ g. Antibodies against ABO blood antigens
    _____ h. Passed to neonate in colostrum
    _____ i. Assists in parasitic infections

    1. IgA
    2. IgD
    3. IgE
    4. IgG
    5. IgM

13. Identify five important functions of cell-mediated immunity.

a.

b.

c.

d.

e.

14. A 69-year-old woman asks the nurse whether it is possible to "catch" cancer because many of her friends her age have been diagnosed with different kinds of cancer. In responding to the woman, the nurse understands that the increased incidence of tumors in advancing age results from
a. an increase in autoantibodies.
b. decreased activity of the bone marrow.
c. decreased differentiation of T lymphocytes.
d. decreased size and activity of the thymus gland.

15. Identify the types of hypersensitivity reactions from the following characteristics.
_____ a. Cellular lysis or phagocytosis through complement activation following antigen-antibody binding on cell surfaces
_____ b. Antigen links with specific IgE antibodies bound to mast cells or basophils releasing chemical mediators
_____ c. T lymphocyte attack of antigens or release of lymphokines attract macrophages that cause tissue damage
_____ d. Antigens combined with IgG and IgM too small to be removed by mononuclear phagocytic system deposit in tissue and cause fixation of complement

1. Type I: IgE-mediated reactions
2. Type II: Cytotoxic
3. Type III: Immune-complex mediated
4. Type IV: Delayed hypersensitivity

16. Match the following examples of hypersensitivity to their types (answers may be used more than once).
_____ a. Transfusion reactions
_____ b. Asthma
_____ c. Angioedema
_____ d. Transplant rejection
_____ e. Rheumatoid arthritis
_____ f. Allergic rhinitis
_____ g. Tubercular caseous necrosis
_____ h. Goodpasture's syndrome
_____ i. Atopic dermatitis
_____ j. Acute glomerular nephritis
_____ k. Anaphylactic shock
_____ l. Urticaria
_____ m. Contact dermatitis

1. Type I: IgE-mediated reactions
2. Type II: Cytotoxic
3. Type III: Immune-complex mediated
4. Type IV: Delayed hypersensitivity

17. A patient was given an IM injection of penicillin in the gluteus maximus and developed dyspnea and weakness within minutes following the injection.
    a. What are four additional assessment findings that would indicate that the patient is having an anaphylactoid reaction?
        1.
        2.
        3.
        4.

    b. Identify five nursing interventions to be taken to treat the patient's problem.
        1.
        2.
        3.
        4.
        5.

18. The rationale for treatment of atopic allergies with immunotherapy is that this therapy
    a. decreases the levels of allergen-specific T-helper cells.
    b. decreases the level of IgE so that it does not react as readily with an allergen.
    c. stimulates increased IgG to bind with allergen-reactive sites, preventing mast cell–bound IgE reactions.
    d. gradually increases the amount of allergen in the body until it is no longer recognized as foreign and does not elicit an antibody reaction.

19. When administering immunotherapy to a patient, the nurse must
    a. give the injections at the same site each time.
    b. give the injection in the upper arm near the shoulder.
    c. observe the patient for 1 hour following the injection.
    d. have emergency equipment and drugs available for immediate use.

20. A nurse who develops a contact dermatitis from wearing latex gloves
    a. is demonstrating an allergy to natural latex proteins.
    b. can use powder-free latex gloves to prevent the development of symptoms.
    c. should use an oil-based hand cream when wearing gloves to prevent latex allergy.
    d. has a type IV allergic reaction to chemicals used in the manufacture of latex gloves.

21. Although the cause of autoimmune disorders is unknown, the two factors believed to be present in most conditions are _____ and _____.

22. Plasmapheresis is indicated in autoimmune disorders to
    a. obtain plasma for analysis and evaluation of specific autoantibodies.
    b. decrease high lymphocyte levels in the blood to prevent immune responses.
    c. remove autoantibodies, antigen-antibody complexes, and inflammatory mediators of immune reactions.
    d. add monocytes to the blood to promote removal of immune complexes by the mononuclear phagocyte system.

23. Currently, histocompatibility leukocyte antigen (HLA) typing can be used to
    a. determine paternity and predict risk for certain diseases.
    b. match tissue types for transplantation and determine paternity.
    c. establish racial background and predict risk for certain diseases.
    d. predict risk for certain diseases and match tissue types for transplantation.

24. The most common cause of secondary immunodeficiency disorders is _____ .

25. The disorder in which viable T lymphocytes infused into an immunodeficient patient destroy vulnerable host cells is _____ .

26. Match the types of transplant rejection with their characteristics (answers may be used more than once).
    _____ a. Most commonly occurs with kidney transplant
    _____ b. Organ must be removed when it occurs
    _____ c. Infiltration of the organ with B and T lymphocytes
    _____ d. Treatment is supportive
    _____ e. The recipient's T-cytotoxic lymphocytes attack the foreign organ
    _____ f. Usually reversible with additional or increased immunosuppressant therapy
    _____ g. Occurs when recipient has antibodies against donor's histocompatibility leukocyte antigens (HLAs)
    _____ h. Long-term use of immunosuppressants necessary to combat the rejection
    _____ i. Irreversible, immune-mediated injury to transplanted organ

    1. Hyperacute
    2. Acute
    3. Chronic

27. A common combination of immunosuppressive agents used to prevent rejection of transplanted organs is
    a. cyclosporine, sirolimus, and muromonab-CD3.
    b. everolimus, mycophenolate mofetil, and sirolimus.
    c. tacrolimus, prednisone, and mycophenolate mofetil.
    d. prednisone, polyclonal antibodies, and cyclosporine.

CASE STUDY

Allergy

Patient Profile

M.W., age 54, has been diagnosed as having perennial allergic rhinitis. He is to undergo skin testing to identify specific allergens. His health care provider has prescribed oral antihistamines for control of his symptoms.

Subjective Data

- Itching of eyes, nose, and throat
- Stuffy nose, head congestion

Objective Data

- Physical examination
- Clear nasal drainage; reddened eyes and lacrimation

Clinical Decision-Making Questions

Using a separate sheet of paper, answer the following questions.

1. What immunoglobulins and chemical mediators are involved in M.W.'s allergic reaction?
2. Describe the procedure the nurse uses to perform the skin testing. What results indicate a positive response?
3. What precautions should be taken by the nurse during skin testing?
4. How do antihistamines act to relieve allergic symptoms? What information should the nurse include in teaching M.W. about using his antihistamines?
5. Skin testing indicates M.W. has an allergy to household dust. What information should the nurse include in teaching M.W. to control his exposure to this allergen?
6. M.W. is to begin immunotherapy. What precautions does the nurse use during the administration of the allergen extract?
7. *Priority Decision:* Based on the assessment data provided, what are the priority nursing diagnoses? Are there any collaborative problems?

CHAPTER 15

Infection and Human Immunodeficiency Virus Infection

1. The increase in emerging and untreatable infections is attributed to (select all that apply)
   a. the evolution of new infectious agents.
   b. use of antibiotics to treat viral infections.
   c. human population encroachment into wilderness areas.
   d. transmission of infectious agents from humans to animals.
   e. an increased number of immunosuppressed and chronically ill people.

2. The three antibiotic-resistant bacteria that are of most current concern are _____,
   _____, and _____.

3. *Priority Decision:* The priority teaching that the nurse should provide to a patient to prevent the development of antibiotic-resistant bacterial infections is to
   a. wash the hands after toileting and before eating.
   b. avoid crowds and contact with others with infections.
   c. take prescribed antibiotics at the frequency and for the duration directed.
   d. request antibiotic therapy when a cold or the flu does not resolve in 2 to 3 days.

4. The two recommended measures to prevent the transmission of hospital-acquired infections (HAIs) are
   _____ and _____.

5. Underline the situations in the following statements in which the risk for HIV transmission is highest.
   a. Transmission to women or to men during sexual intercourse
   b. Hollow-bore needle used for vascular access or used for IM injection
   c. Vaginal or anal intercourse
   d. Transfusion of whole blood or clotting factors
   e. First 2 to 6 months of infection or 1 year after infection
   f. Perinatal transmission from HIV-infected mothers taking antiretroviral therapy or HIV-infected mothers using no therapy
   g. A splash exposure of HIV-infected blood on skin with an open lesion or a needle-stick exposure to HIV-infected blood

6. Place the following events of HIV infection of a cell in sequence from 1 to 7.
   _____ a. Viral RNA is converted to single-strand viral DNA with assistance of reverse transcriptase
   _____ b. Viral DNA is spliced into cell genome using the enzyme integrase
   _____ c. gp 120 proteins on viral envelope combine with CD4 receptors of body cells
   _____ d. Cell replicates infected daughter cells and makes more HIV
   _____ e. Viral RNA and reverse transcriptase enzyme enter host cell
   _____ f. Long strands of viral RNA are cut in the presence of protease
   _____ g. Single-strand viral DNA replicates into double-stranded DNA

7. In the previous question, indicate what four events of HIV infection of a cell can be controlled with current drugs.
   a.

   b.

   c.

   d.

8. A primary reason that the normal immune response fails to contain HIV infection is that
   a. CD4+ T cells drawn to the viruses become infected and are destroyed.
   b. the virus inactivates B lymphocytes, preventing the production of HIV antibodies.
   c. natural killer cells are destroyed by the virus before the immune system can be activated.
   d. monocytes ingest infected cells, differentiate into macrophages, and shed viruses in body tissues.

9. Match the following characteristics with the corresponding stage of progression of HIV infection.
   _____ a. CD4+ T cells 200-500/μL
   _____ b. Flulike symptoms
   _____ c. Median length is about 11 years
   _____ d. HIV seroconversion
   _____ e. Median length is 2 years
   _____ f. CD4+ T-cell count usually normal
   _____ g. Temporary fall of CD4+ cells
   _____ h. Persistent fevers and night sweats
   _____ i. Cytomegalovirus retinitis
   _____ j. Oral hairy leukoplakia

   1. Acute HIV infection
   2. Early chronic infection
   3. Intermediate chronic infection
   4. AIDS or late chronic infection

10. Match the following characteristics with opportunistic diseases associated with AIDS.
    _____ a. Hyperpigmented lesions of skin, lungs, and gastrointestinal (GI) tract
    _____ b. Shingles with maculopapular, pruritic rash treated with acyclovir
    _____ c. Common yeast infection involving mouth, esophagus, GI tract
    _____ d. Oral and mucocutaneous vesicular and ulcerative lesions
    _____ e. May cause fungal meningitis
    _____ f. Diagnosed by lymph node biopsy
    _____ g. Pneumonia with dry, nonproductive cough
    _____ h. Viral retinitis, stomatitis, esophagitis, gastritis, colitis

    1. *Pneumocystis jiroveci* infection
    2. Herpes simplex 1 infection
    3. Kaposi sarcoma
    4. Cytomegalovirus infection
    5. *Cryptococcus* infection
    6. Varicella-zoster virus infection
    7. Non-Hodgkin's lymphoma
    8. *Candida albicans*

11. Opportunistic diseases develop in AIDS because these disorders are
    a. side effects of drug treatment of AIDS.
    b. sexually transmitted to individuals during exposure to HIV.
    c. characteristic in individuals with stimulated B and T lymphocytes.
    d. infections or tumors that rarely occur with a competent immune system.

12. A patient comes to the clinic and requests testing for HIV infection. Before administering testing, it is most important that the nurse
    a. ask the patient to identify all sexual partners.
    b. determine when the patient thinks exposure to HIV occurred.
    c. explain that all test results must be repeated at least twice to be valid.
    d. discuss prevention practices to prevent transmission of the HIV to others.

13. The "rapid" HIV antibody testing is performed on a patient at high risk for HIV infection. The nurse explains that
    a. the test measures the activity of the HIV and reports viral loads as real numbers.
    b. this test is highly reliable, and in 20 minutes the patient will know if HIV infection is present.
    c. if the results are positive, another blood test and a return appointment for results will be necessary.
    d. this test detects drug-resistant viral mutations that are present in viral genes to evaluate resistance to antiretroviral drugs.

14. Treatment with two nucleoside reverse transcriptase inhibitors (NRTIs) and a protease inhibitor (PI) is prescribed for a patient with HIV infection who has a CD4+ T cell count of <400/μL. The patient asks why so many drugs are necessary for treatment. The nurse explains that the primary rationale for combination therapy is that
    a. cross-resistance between specific antiretroviral drugs is reduced when drugs are given in combination.
    b. combinations of antiretroviral drugs decrease the potential for development of antiretroviral-resistant HIV variants.
    c. side effects of the drugs are reduced when smaller doses of three different drugs are used rather than large doses of one drug.
    d. when CD4+ T cell counts are <500/μL, a combination of drugs that have different actions is more effective in slowing HIV growth.

15. One of the most significant factors in determining when to start antiretroviral therapy in a patient with HIV infection is
    a. whether the patient has high levels of HIV antibodies.
    b. the confirmation that the patient has contracted HIV infection.
    c. the patient's readiness to commit to a complex, life-long, uncomfortable drug regimen.
    d. whether the patient has a support system to help manage the costs and side effects of the drugs.

16. After teaching a patient with HIV infection about using antiretroviral drugs, the nurse recognizes that further teaching is needed when the patient says,
    a. "I should never skip doses of my medication, even if I develop side effects."
    b. "If my viral load becomes undetectable, I will no longer be able to transmit HIV to others."
    c. "I should not use any over-the-counter drugs without checking with my health care provider."
    d. "If I develop a constant headache that is not relieved with aspirin or acetaminophen, I should report it within 24 hours."

17. Prophylactic measures that are routinely used as early as possible in HIV infection to prevent opportunistic and debilitating secondary problems include administration of
    a. isoniazid (INH) to prevent tuberculosis.
    b. trimethoprim-sulfamethoxazole (TMP-SMX) for toxoplasmosis.
    c. vaccines for pneumococcal pneumonia, influenza, and hepatitis A and B.
    d. varicella-zoster immune globulin (VZIG) to prevent chickenpox or shingles.

18. A patient identified as HIV-antibody–positive 1 year ago manifests early HIV infection but does not want to start antiretroviral therapy at this time. An appropriate nursing intervention for the patient at this stage of illness is to
    a. assist with end-of-life issues.
    b. provide care during acute exacerbations.
    c. provide physical care for chronic diseases.
    d. educate the patient regarding immune enhancement.

19. Identify three methods to eliminate or reduce the risk for HIV transmission related to sexual intercourse and drug use.

    Sexual Intercourse   **Drug Use**
    a.   a.

    b.   b.

    c.   c.

20. A patient with advanced AIDS has diarrhea and wasting syndrome. An appropriate nursing diagnosis for the patient is
    a. diarrhea related to opportunistic infection.
    b. risk for fluid volume deficit related to diarrhea.
    c. risk for infection related to immunosuppression.
    d. risk for impaired skin integrity related to altered nutritional status and frequent stools.

21. A patient with advanced AIDS has a nursing diagnosis of impaired memory related to neurologic changes. In planning care for the patient, the nurse sets the highest priority on
    a. maintaining a safe patient environment.
    b. providing a quiet, nonstressful environment to avoid overstimulation.
    c. using memory cues such as calendars and clocks to promote orientation.
    d. providing written instructions of directions to promote understanding and orientation.

CASE STUDY
HIV Infection
Patient Profile

A.K., a 28-year-old single man, had HIV antibody screening performed 2 weeks ago when he was seen at a health clinic for flulike symptoms. At that time, he revealed that he had a history of multiple sexual partners. He has returned to the clinic for the results of his screening.

Subjective Data

- Vague symptoms of fatigue and headache
- Reports occasional night sweats

Objective Data

- Positive Western blot test
- Temperature: 100° F (37.8° C)
- Enlarged cervical and femoral lymph nodes

Clinical Decision-Making Questions

Using a separate sheet of paper, answer the following questions.

1. *Priority Decision:* What are the priority posttest counseling activities that should be performed by the nurse during A.K.'s visit?
2. A.K.'s CD4$^+$ T cell count is 650/μL. What stage of HIV infection is he most likely experiencing?
3. What additional diagnostic tests might be performed at this visit?
4. What prophylactic treatments should be used at this time to prevent the development of opportunistic diseases?
5. The health care provider encourages A.K. to consider starting combination antiretroviral therapy. What can the nurse tell A.K. about the expected effect of this therapy?
6. If A.K. does not respond to treatment with an increased CD4$^+$ T cell count and a decreased viral load, what tests could be used to identify resistance to the antiretroviral agents?
7. *Priority Decision:* Based on the assessment data presented, what are the priority nursing diagnoses? Are there any collaborative problems?

16

Cancer

1. The nurse is presenting a community education program related to cancer prevention. Based on current cancer death rates, the nurse stresses that the most important preventive action for both women and men is
   a. smoking cessation.
   b. routine colonoscopies.
   c. protection from ultraviolet light.
   d. regular examination of reproductive organs.

2. The defect in cellular proliferation that occurs in the development of cancer involves
   a. a rate of cell proliferation that is more rapid than that of normal body cells.
   b. shortened phases of cell life cycles with occasional skipping of G_1 or S phases.
   c. rearrangement of stem cell RNA that causes abnormal cellular protein synthesis.
   d. indiscriminate and continuous proliferation of cells with loss of contact inhibition.

3. The presence of carcinoembryonic antigens (CEAs) and α-fetoprotein (AFP) on cell membranes is an indication that cells have
   a. shifted to more immature metabolic pathways and functions.
   b. spread from areas of original development to different body tissues.
   c. become more differentiated as a result of repression of embryonic functions.
   d. produced abnormal toxins or chemicals that indicate abnormal cellular function.

4. The major difference between benign tumors and malignant tumors is that malignant tumors
   a. grow at a faster rate.
   b. are often encapsulated.
   c. invade and metastasize.
   d. cause death whereas benign tumors do not.

5. Match the following precursors or malignancies with the carcinogenic factors associated with their initiation.
   _____ a. Skin cancer
   _____ b. Acute myelogenous leukemia
   _____ c. Familial adenomatous polyposis
   _____ d. Cervical cancer
   _____ e. Burkitt's lymphoma
   _____ f. Thyroid cancer

   1. Alkylating agents
   2. Mutation of tumor suppressor genes
   3. Epstein-Barr virus
   4. Ultraviolet light
   5. Ionizing radiation
   6. Human papillomavirus

6. Identify whether the following statements are true (*T*) or false (*F*). If a statement is false, correct the bold word(s) to make the statement true.
   _____ a. **Initiation** is the stage of cancer development in which there is an irreversible alteration in the cell's DNA.
   _____ b. Tobacco smoke is a complete carcinogen that is capable of both **initiation** and **promotion**.
   _____ c. The promotion stage of cancer is characterized by the **irreversible** proliferation of altered, initiated cells.
   _____ d. Obesity is an example of a **promoting factor**.
   _____ e. The latent period of cancer is the same as **promotion**.
   _____ f. Withdrawal of promoting factors will **reduce** the risk of cancer development.
   _____ g. BRCA-1 and BRCA-2 are genes that **suppress** the development of breast cancer.
   _____ h. During cancer progression, metastatic cells become more **homogenous**, making treatment more difficult.

7. List three capabilities of tumor cells that facilitate spread of the tumor from the original site.
   a.

   b.

   c.

8. Match the following terms related to cancer pathophysiology with their descriptions.
   _____ a. Mutations of protooncogenes that normally limit cell regulation
   _____ b. Substance that promotes blood vessel development within tumors
   _____ c. Tumor cell–surface antigens that stimulate an immune response
   _____ d. Capable of causing cellular alterations associated with cancer
   _____ e. Antigens on tumor cells that reflect a return to embryonic
            cell differentiation
   _____ f. Programmed cellular death
   _____ g. Lesion with histologic features of cancer except invasion
   _____ h. Evasion of the immune system by cancer cells

   1. Tumor-associated antigens
   2. Immunologic escape
   3. Apoptosis
   4. Oncofetal antigens
   5. Oncogenes
   6. Carcinoma in situ
   7. Oncogenic
   8. Tumor angiogenesis factor

9. Compare a meningioma and a meningeal sarcoma according to the anatomic site classification system for tumors.

	Meningioma	**Meningeal sarcoma**
Tissue of origin		
Anatomic site		
Behavior		

10. A patient's tumor has been classified as grade II, $T_1N_1M_0$ carcinoma of the breast. What does this tell the nurse about the tissue of origin and the extent of the disease process?
    a. Carcinoma

    b. Grade II

    c. $T_1N_1M_0$

11. The nurse is counseling a group of individuals over the age of 50 with average risk for cancer about screening tests for cancer. What are six specific tests that should be performed by health professionals for the people in this group and at what frequency?
    a.   d.

    b.   e.

    c.   f.

12. A small lesion is discovered in a patient's lung when an x-ray is performed for cervical spine pain. The definitive method of determining if the lesion is malignant is by
    a. lung scan.
    b. tissue biopsy.
    c. CT or PET scan.
    d. presence of oncofetal antigens in the blood.

13. A patient is admitted to the surgical unit where she is scheduled that day for a bilateral simple mastectomy. The nurse recognizes that this procedure is performed to (select all that apply)
    a. prevent breast cancer.
    b. diagnose breast cancer.
    c. cure or control breast cancer.
    d. provide palliative care for untreated breast cancer.

14. Match the surgical procedures with their primary purposes in cancer treatment (answers may be used more than once).
    _____ a. Colostomy to bypass bowel obstruction
    _____ b. Bowel resection
    _____ c. Mammoplasty
    _____ d. Debulking procedure to enhance radiation therapy
    _____ e. Insertion of suprapubic catheter
    _____ f. Cordotomy for pain control
    _____ g. Insertion of feeding tube into stomach

    1. Cure, control, or both
    2. Supportive care
    3. Palliation
    4. Rehabilitation

15. Chemotherapy for the treatment of cancer would be most effective in
    a. a small tumor of the bone.
    b. a young tumor of the brain.
    c. a large tumor in a highly vascular area.
    d. malignant changes in hemopoietic cells.

16. Match the following descriptions of chemotherapeutic drugs with their classifications.
    _____ a. Cell cycle phase–specific drugs that mimic essential cellular metabolites
    _____ b. Cell cycle phase–nonspecific drugs that break DNA strands
    _____ c. Cell cycle phase–specific drugs that cause mitotic arrest in metaphase
    _____ d. Bind with DNA to block RNA production
    _____ e. Cell cycle phase–nonspecific drugs that break DNA helix; cross blood-brain barrier

    1. Alkylating agents
    2. Antimetabolites
    3. Antitumor antibiotics
    4. Mitotic inhibitors
    5. Nitrosoureas

17. The nurse uses many precautions during IV administration of vesicant chemotherapeutic agents primarily to prevent
    a. septicemia.
    b. extravasation.
    c. catheter occlusion.
    d. anaphylactic shock.

18. Match the following malignancies with commonly used routes of regional chemotherapeutic administration.
    _____ a. Bladder
    _____ b. Osteogenic sarcoma
    _____ c. Metastasis to the brain
    _____ d. Metastasis from a primary colorectal cancer
    _____ e. Leukemia

    1. Intraperitoneal
    2. Intraarterial
    3. Intravenous
    4. Intravesical
    5. Intrathecal

19. When teaching the patient with cancer about chemotherapy, the nurse should
    a. avoid telling the patient about possible side effects of the drugs to prevent anticipatory anxiety.
    b. explain that antiemetics, antidiarrheals, and analgesics will be provided as needed to control side effects.
    c. assure the patient that the side effects from chemotherapy are merely uncomfortable, not life threatening.
    d. inform the patient that chemotherapy-related alopecia is usually permanent but can be managed with lifelong use of wigs.

20. Normal tissues that may manifest early, acute responses to radiation therapy include
    a. spleen and liver.
    b. kidney and nervous tissue.
    c. bone marrow and gastrointestinal mucosa.
    d. hollow organs such as the stomach and bladder.

21. The rationale for treatment of cancer with radiation includes the knowledge that
    a. radiation damages cellular DNA only in abnormal cells.
    b. malignant cells respond to the effects of radiation because they more frequently go through mitosis.
    c. damage to cells will occur only during M and G_2 phases of the cell cycle, necessitating a series of treatment.
    d. normal cells are able to repair radiation-induced damage to DNA and do not have permanent radiation damage.

22. When a patient is undergoing brachytherapy, it is important for the nurse to recognize that
    a. the patient will undergo simulation to identify and mark the field of treatment.
    b. the patient is a source of radiation and personnel must wear film badges during care.
    c. the goal of this treatment is only palliative and the patient should be aware of the expected outcome.
    d. computerized dosimetry is used to determine the maximum dose of radiation to the tumor within an acceptable dose to normal tissue.

23. To prevent the debilitating cycle of fatigue-depression-fatigue in patients receiving radiation therapy, the nurse encourages the patient to
    a. implement a walking program.
    b. ignore the fatigue as much as possible.
    c. do the most stressful activities when fatigue is tolerable.
    d. schedule rest periods throughout the day whether fatigue is present or not.

24. The late effects of chemotherapy and high-dose radiation may include
    a. third-space syndrome.
    b. chronic nausea and vomiting.
    c. persistent myelosuppression.
    d. secondary resistant malignancies.

25. The primary use of biologic therapy in cancer treatment is to
    a. prevent the fatigue associated with chemotherapy and high-dose radiation.
    b. enhance or supplement the effects of the host's immune responses to tumor cells.
    c. depress the immune system and circulating lymphocytes, as well as increasing a sense of well-being.
    d. protect normal rapidly reproducing cells of the gastrointestinal system from damage during chemotherapy.

26. A side effect common to biologic therapies is
    a. flulike syndrome.
    b. bone marrow suppression.
    c. central nervous system deficits.
    d. nausea, vomiting, anorexia, and diarrhea.

27. While caring for a patient who is at the nadir of chemotherapy, the nurse establishes the highest priority for the nursing diagnosis of
    a. diarrhea.
    b. grieving.
    c. risk for infection.
    d. imbalanced nutrition: less than body requirements.

28. An allogenic hematopoietic stem cell transplant is considered as treatment for a patient with acute myelogenous leukemia. The nurse explains that during this procedure
    a. there is no risk for graft-versus-host disease because the donated marrow is treated to remove cancer cells.
    b. bone marrow is obtained from a donor who has an HLA match with the patient.
    c. the patient's bone marrow will be removed, treated, stored, and then reinfused after intensive chemotherapy.
    d. there is no need for posttransplant protective isolation because the stem cells are infused directly into the blood.

29. During initial chemotherapy a patient with leukemia develops hyperkalemia and hyperuricemia. The nurse recognizes these symptoms as an oncologic emergency and anticipates that the priority treatment will be
    a. establishing ECG monitoring.
    b. increasing urine output with hydration therapy.
    c. administering a bisphosphonate such as pamidronate (Aredia).
    d. restricting fluids and administering hypertonic sodium chloride solution.

30. Identify five factors that will assist a patient in coping positively with having cancer.

    a.

    b.

    c.

    d.

    e.

CASE STUDY
Cancer

Patient Profile

R.M. is a 65-year-old patient who was recently diagnosed with metastatic colon cancer. He began treatment with chemotherapy through a peripherally inserted central venous catheter 5 days ago.

Subjective Data

- States he has almost continuous nausea, which becomes severe and causes vomiting following his dose of chemotherapy
- States he has no appetite
- Expresses no hope that the chemotherapy will have a positive effect

Objective Data

- Temperature: 99.4° F (37.4° C)
- WBC: 3200/μL (3.2 × 10⁹/L)
- Neutrophils: 500/μL (0.5 × 10⁹/L)
- Skin warm with decreased turgor

Clinical Decision-Making Questions

Using a separate sheet of paper, answer the following questions.

1. What factors may be responsible for R.M.'s decreased WBC and neutrophil count?
2. What assessment data indicate that R.M. may be experiencing an infection?
3. What additional assessment data should be collected from R.M. to determine the presence of an infection?
4. What factors may contribute to R.M.'s negative attitude toward the chemotherapy?
5. *Priority Decision:* What are the priority nursing measures that should be used to help control his anorexia, nausea, and vomiting?
6. *Priority Decision:* What are the priority teaching measures that should be included in the teaching plan for R.M. and his family to prevent infection?
7. *Priority Decision:* Based on the assessment data presented, what are the priority nursing diagnoses? Are there any collaborative problems?

CHAPTER

17

Fluid, Electrolyte, and Acid-Base Imbalances

1. Identify whether the following statements are true (*T*) or false (*F*). If a statement is false, correct the bold word(s) to make the statement true.
   - _____ a. A patient with consistent dietary intake who loses 1 kg of weight in 1 day has lost **500 mL** of fluid.
   - _____ b. A man who weighs 90 kg has a total body water content of approximately **60 L**.
   - _____ c. Major tissue damage that causes release of intracellular electrolytes into extracellular fluid will cause **hypernatremia**.
   - _____ d. The primary difference in the electrolyte composition of intravascular fluid and interstitial fluid is the higher content of **protein** in plasma.
   - _____ e. The different concentrations of sodium and potassium between interstitial fluid and intracellular fluid are maintained by the **sodium-potassium pump**.
   - _____ f. A cell surrounded by a hypoosmolar fluid will **shrink and die** as water moves **out of** the cell.
   - _____ g. Third spacing refers to the abnormal movement of fluid into **interstitial spaces**.
   - _____ h. The primary hypothalamic mechanism of water intake is **thirst**.

2. Match the following descriptions with the mechanisms of fluid and electrolyte movement.
   - _____ a. Pressure exerted by proteins
   - _____ b. ATP required
   - _____ c. Flow of water from low-solute concentration to high-solute concentration
   - _____ d. Force exerted by a fluid
   - _____ e. Passive movement of molecules from a high concentration to lower concentration
   - _____ f. Uses a carrier molecule
   - _____ g. Force determined by osmolality of a fluid

   1. Facilitated diffusion
   2. Diffusion
   3. Osmotic pressure
   4. Oncotic pressure
   5. Active transport
   6. Osmosis
   7. Hydrostatic pressure

3. A patient has a serum Na^+ of 147 mEq/L (147 mmol/L) and a blood glucose level of 126 mg/dL (7.0 mmol/L). Osmolality = (2 × Na concentration) + (glucose concentration/18). The patient's effective serum osmolality is _____ mOsm/kg. Is the patient's serum osmolality increased, decreased, or normal?

4. As fluid circulates through the capillaries, there is movement of fluid between the capillaries and the interstitium. In the following descriptions, match the direction of fluid movement and the location of the movement in the capillary.
   - _____ _____ a. Plasma hydrostatic pressure is less than plasma oncotic pressure
   - _____ _____ b. Interstitial hydrostatic pressure is lower than plasma hydrostatic pressure
   - _____ _____ c. Plasma hydrostatic pressure is less than interstitial hydrostatic pressure
   - _____ _____ d. Plasma hydrostatic pressure is higher than plasma oncotic pressure

   Direction of Movement
   1. Movement into capillary
   2. Movement into interstitium
   Location of Movement
   3. Occurs at arterial end
   4. Occurs at venous end

5. Fill in the blanks preceding a to g below with 1, 2, 3, or 4 to indicate whether fluid shifts (may use answer more than once)
   1. from blood vessels to interstitium.
   2. from extracellular compartment to the cell.
   3. from cell to extracellular compartment.
   4. from interstitium to vessels.

   In each of the blanks following a to g, identify which mechanism of fluid movement is involved.
   _____ a. Low serum albumin   a. _____
   _____ b. Hyponatremia   b. _____
   _____ c. Administration of 10% glucose   c. _____
   _____ d. Dehydration   d. _____
   _____ e. Burns   e. _____
   _____ f. Fluid overload   f. _____
   _____ g. Application of elastic bandages   g. _____

6. A woman has ham with gravy and green beans cooked with salt pork for dinner.
   a. What could happen to the woman's serum osmolality as a result of this meal?

   b. What fluid regulation mechanisms are stimulated by the intake of these foods?

7. Aldosterone is secreted by the adrenal cortex in response to
   a. excessive water intake.
   b. loss of serum potassium.
   c. loss of sodium and water.
   d. increased serum osmolality.

8. While caring for an 84-year-old patient, the nurse monitors the patient's fluid and electrolyte balance, recognizing that normal changes of aging are likely to cause
   a. hyperkalemia.
   b. hyponatremia.
   c. decreased insensible fluid loss.
   d. increased plasma oncotic pressures.

9. While obtaining an assessment and health history from a patient, which of the following statements by the patient will alert the nurse to a possible fluid volume excess?
   a. "I have been urinating a lot, and my urine is dark, almost brown."
   b. "I get light-headed and dizzy when I stand up too fast after sitting or lying down."
   c. "My heart feels like it is about to run away with me some of the time because it goes so fast."
   d. "I have been taking some salt tablets while working outdoors in the summer, but they sure make me thirsty."

10. A patient at risk for hypernatremia is one who
    a. has a deficiency of aldosterone.
    b. has prolonged vomiting and diarrhea.
    c. receives excessive 5% dextrose solution intravenously.
    d. has impaired consciousness and decreased thirst sensitivity.

11. Symptoms of sodium imbalances are primarily manifested through altered
    a. kidney function.
    b. cardiovascular function.
    c. neuromuscular function.
    d. central nervous system function.

12. Match the electrolyte imbalances with their associated causes (answers may be used more than once).
   _____ a. Alcohol withdrawal
   _____ b. Metabolic alkalosis
   _____ c. Parathyroidectomy
   _____ d. Diabetes insipidus
   _____ e. Fleet enemas
   _____ f. Primary polydipsia
   _____ g. Milk of Magnesia use in renal failure
   _____ h. Early burn stage
   _____ i. Chronic alcoholism
   _____ j. Vitamin D deficiency
   _____ k. Osmotic diuresis
   _____ l. Prolonged immobilization

   1. Hypernatremia
   2. Hyponatremia
   3. Hyperkalemia
   4. Hypokalemia
   5. Hypercalcemia
   6. Hypocalcemia
   7. Hyperphosphatemia
   8. Hypophosphatemia
   9. Hypermagnesemia
   10. Hypomagnesemia

13. Several conditions will cause multiple imbalances of electrolytes. Identify three electrolyte imbalances that are caused by the following.
   a. Hyperaldosteronism
      1.
      2.
      3.

   b. Chronic kidney disease
      1.
      2.
      3.

   c. Loop and thiazide diuretics
      1.
      2.
      3.

14. A patient is taking diuretic drugs that cause sodium loss from the kidney. The fluid or electrolyte imbalance most likely to occur in this patient is
   a. hyperkalemia.
   b. hyponatremia.
   c. hypocalcemia.
   d. isotonic fluid loss.

15. A common collaborative problem that is indicated for both hyperkalemia and hypokalemia is a
   a. potential complication: seizures.
   b. potential complication: paralysis.
   c. potential complication: dysrhythmias.
   d. potential complication: acute kidney injury.

16. Hyperkalemia is frequently associated with
   a. hypoglycemia.
   b. metabolic acidosis.
   c. respiratory alkalosis.
   d. decreased urine potassium levels.

17. In a patient with a positive Chvostek's sign, the nurse would anticipate the IV administration of
   a. calcitonin.
   b. vitamin D.
   c. loop diuretics.
   d. calcium gluconate.

18. A patient with chronic kidney disease has hyperphosphatemia. A commonly associated electrolyte imbalance is
    a. hypokalemia.
    b. hyponatremia.
    c. hypocalcemia.
    d. hypomagnesemia.

19. The normal pH range of the blood is _____ to _____. This reflects a ratio of base to acid

    of _____ to _____.

20. pH is a negative logarithm that is a measure of _____ in a solution.

21. Match the components of the buffer system with their characteristics (answers may be used more than once).
    _____ a. Neutralizes a strong base to a weak base and water
    _____ b. Free acid radicals dissociate into H^+ and CO_2, buffering
        excess base
    _____ c. Shifts chloride in and out of red blood cells in exchange
        for sodium bicarbonate, buffering both acids and bases
    _____ d. Resultant sodium biphosphate is eliminated by kidneys
    _____ e. Neutralizes HCl acid to yield carbonic acid and salt
    _____ f. Free basic radicals dissociate into ammonia and OH^- that
        combines with H^+ to form water
    _____ g. Resultant CO_2 is eliminated by the lungs
    _____ h. Neutralizes a strong acid to yield sodium biphosphate, a weak
        acid, and salt
    _____ i. Shifts H^+ in and out of cell in exchange for other cations such as
        potassium and sodium
    _____ j. H_2CO_3 formed by neutralization dissociates into H_2O and CO_2

    1. Carbonic acid–bicarbonate
    2. Phosphate buffer
    3. Hemoglobin buffer
    4. Protein buffer
    5. Cellular buffer

22. A patient who has a large amount of carbon dioxide in the blood has a
    a. large amount of carbonic acid and low hydrogen ion concentration.
    b. small amount of carbonic acid and low hydrogen ion concentration.
    c. large amount of carbonic acid and high hydrogen ion concentration.
    d. small amount of carbonic acid and high hydrogen ion concentration.

23. List the three ways that kidneys eliminate acids to maintain acid-base balance.
    a.

    b.

    c.

24. Match the acid-base imbalances with their mechanisms.
    _____ a. Increased base bicarbonate
    _____ b. Decreased carbonic acid (CO_2)
    _____ c. Increased carbonic acid (CO_2)
    _____ d. Decreased base bicarbonate

    1. Respiratory acidosis
    2. Respiratory alkalosis
    3. Metabolic acidosis
    4. Metabolic alkalosis

25. Identify the compensatory mechanism that occurs in each of the following.
    a. Respiratory acidosis
    b. Metabolic acidosis
    c. Metabolic alkalosis

26. Match the acid-base imbalances with their common causes (answers may be used more than once).

    _____ a. Prolonged vomiting
    _____ b. Renal failure
    _____ c. Response to anxiety, fear, and pain
    _____ d. Respiratory failure
    _____ e. Baking soda use as antacid
    _____ f. Severe shock
    _____ g. Diabetic ketosis
    _____ h. Mechanical overventilation
    _____ i. Sedative or opioid overdose

    1. Respiratory acidosis
    2. Respiratory alkalosis
    3. Metabolic acidosis
    4. Metabolic alkalosis

27. A patient with a pH of 7.29 has metabolic acidosis. A value that is useful in determining whether the cause of the acidosis is due to an acid gain or to a bicarbonate loss is the
    a. $PaCO_2$.
    b. anion gap.
    c. serum Na^+ level.
    d. bicarbonate level.

28. Identify the acid-base imbalances represented by the following laboratory values.

    a. pH: 7.50
       $PaCO_2$: 30 mm Hg
       HCO_3^-: 24 mEq/L
       Interpretation:

       _____

       _____

    b. pH: 7.2
       $PaCO_2$: 25 mm Hg
       HCO_3^-: 15 mEq/L
       Interpretation:

       _____

       _____

    c. pH: 7.26
       $PaCO_2$: 56 mm Hg
       HCO_3^-: 24 mEq/L
       Interpretation:

       _____

       _____

    d. pH: 7.62
       $PaCO_2$: 48 mm Hg
       HCO_3^-: 45 mEq/L
       Interpretation:

       _____

       _____

    e. pH: 7.44
       $PaCO_2$: 54 mm Hg
       HCO_3^-: 36 mEq/L
       Interpretation:

       _____

       _____

    f. pH: 7.35
       $PaCO_2$: 60 mm Hg
       HCO_3^-: 40 mEq/L
       Interpretation:

       _____

       _____

29. To provide free water and intracellular fluid hydration for a patient with acute gastroenteritis who is NPO, the nurse would expect administration of
    a. lactated Ringer's solution.
    b. dextrose 5% in water.
    c. dextrose 10% in water.
    d. dextrose 5% in normal saline (0.9%).

30. An example of an IV solution that would be appropriate to treat an extracellular fluid volume deficit is
    a. D_5W.
    b. 3% saline.
    c. D_5W in 1/2 normal saline (0.45%).
    d. lactated Ringer's solution.

31. On assessment of a central venous access device (CVAD) site, the nurse observes that the transparent dressing is loose along two sides. The nurse should
    a. wait and change the dressing when it is due.
    b. tape the two loose sides down and document.
    c. apply a gauze dressing over the transparent dressing and tape securely.
    d. remove the dressing and apply a new transparent dressing using sterile technique.

32. Indicate whether the following statements are true (*T*) or false (*F*). If a statement is false, correct the bold word(s) to make the statement true.
    _____ a. The recommended method for cleansing CVAD insertion sites with chlorhexidine is to cleanse with a **circular motion** and generate friction.
    _____ b. Accurate placement of a centrally inserted catheter must be verified by **chest x-ray** before use.
    _____ c. CVAD catheters should be flushed with normal saline using at least a **10-mL syringe** and the push-pause technique.
    _____ d. The two major disadvantages of CVADs are increased risk of systemic infection and **thrombosis**.

33. A patient is scheduled to have placement of a tunnelled catheter for administration of chemotherapy for breast cancer. When preparing the patient for the catheter insertion, the nurse explains that this method of administration
    a. decreases the risk for extravasation at the infusion site.
    b. reduces the incidence of systemic side effects of the drug.
    c. does not become occluded as peripherally inserted catheters can.
    d. allows continuous infusion of the drug directly to the area of the tumor.

34. The nurse is reviewing a patient's morning lab results. Which of these results is of highest concern?
    a. Serum K^+ of 2.8 mEq/L
    b. Serum Na^+ of 150 mEq/L
    c. Serum Mg^{++} of 1.1 mEq/L
    d. Serum Ca^{++} (total) of 8.6 mg/dL

CASE STUDY
Fluid and Electrolyte Imbalance
Patient Profile

F.E., a 74-year-old woman who lives alone, is admitted to the hospital because of weakness and confusion. She has a history of chronic heart failure and chronic diuretic use.

Objective Data

- Neurologic: Confusion, slow to respond to questioning, generalized weakness
- Cardiovascular: BP 90/62, HR 112 and irregular, peripheral pulses weak; ECG indicates sinus tachycardia
- Pulmonary: Respirations 12/min and shallow
- Additional findings: Decreased skin turgor; dry mucous membranes

Significant Laboratory Results

- Serum electrolytes
  - Na^+ 141 mEq/L (141 mmol/L)
  - K^+ 2.5 mEq/L (2.5 mmol/L)
  - Cl^- 85 mEq/L (85 mmol/L)
  - HCO_3^- 43 mEq/L (43 mmol/L)
- BUN 42 mg/dL (15 mmol/L)
- Hct 49%
- Arterial blood gases
  - pH   7.52
  - $PaCO_2$ 55 mm Hg
  - PaO_2 88 mm Hg
  - HCO_3^- 42 mEq/L (42 mmol/L)

Clinical Decision-Making Questions

Using a separate sheet of paper, answer the following questions.

1. Evaluate F.E.'s fluid volume and electrolyte status. Which physical assessment findings support your analysis? Which laboratory results support your analysis? What is the most likely etiology of these imbalances?
2. Explain the reasons for F.E.'s ECG changes.
3. Analyze the arterial blood gas results. What is the etiology of the primary imbalance? Is the body compensating for this imbalance?
4. Why has F.E.'s advanced age placed her at risk for her fluid imbalance?
5. Discuss the role of aldosterone in the regulation of fluid and electrolyte balance. How will changes in aldosterone affect F.E.'s fluid and electrolyte imbalances?
6. *Priority Decision:* Develop a plan of care for F.E. while she is in the hospital. What are the priority daily assessments that should be included in this plan of care?
7. *Priority Decision:* Based on the assessment data presented, what are the priority nursing diagnoses? Are there any collaborative problems?

Nursing Management: Preoperative Care

1. Indicate a common purpose of surgery in the following procedures:
   a. Gastroscopy
   b. Rhinoplasty
   c. Tracheotomy
   d. Herniorrhaphy
   e. Hysterectomy

2. A patient is scheduled for a hemorrhoidectomy at an ambulatory day-surgery center. An advantage of performing surgery at an ambulatory center is a decreased need for
   a. laboratory tests and perioperative medications.
   b. preoperative and postoperative teaching by the nurse.
   c. psychologic support to alleviate fears of pain and discomfort.
   d. preoperative nursing assessment related to possible risks and complications.

3. A patient who is being admitted for a hysterectomy to the surgical unit paces the floor, repeatedly saying, "I just want this over." To promote a positive surgical outcome for the patient, the nurse should
   a. ask the patient what her specific concerns are about the surgery.
   b. redirect the patient's attention to the necessary preoperative preparations.
   c. reassure the patient that the surgery will be over soon and she will be fine.
   d. tell the patient she has no reason to be so anxious because she is having a common, safe surgery.

4. List five herbal or supplementary products that the nurse should recognize as possibly increasing the risk for bleeding in a surgical patient.
   a.

   b.

   c.

   d.

   e.

5. When the nurse asks a preoperative patient about allergies, the patient reports a history of seasonal environmental allergies and allergies to a variety of fruits. The nurse should
   a. note this information in the patient's record as hay fever and food allergies.
   b. place an allergy alert wristband on the patient identifying the specific allergies.
   c. ask the patient to describe the nature and severity of any allergic responses experienced to these agents.
   d. notify the anesthetic care provider (ACP) because the patient may have an increased risk for allergies to anesthetics.

6. During preoperative assessment of a patient, the nurse obtains subjective data related to the patient's functional health patterns. Identify one finding and a related surgical risk factor or need for nursing intervention for the following patterns.

	Finding	Risk/Nursing Need
a. Health perception–health management		
b. Nutrition-metabolic		
c. Elimination		
d. Activity-exercise		
e. Sleep-rest		
f. Cognitive-perceptive		
g. Self-perception–self-concept		
h. Coping–stress tolerance		

7. During a preoperative systems review, the patient reveals a history of renal disease. This finding suggests the need for preoperative diagnostic tests of
   a. ECG and chest x-ray.
   b. Serum glucose and CBC.
   c. ABGs and coagulation tests.
   d. BUN, serum creatinine, and electrolytes.

8. During a preoperative physical examination, the nurse is alerted to the possibility of compromised respiratory function during or after surgery in the patient with
   a. obesity.
   b. dehydration.
   c. an enlarged liver.
   d. decreased peripheral pulse volume.

9. Procedural information that should be given to a patient in preparation for ambulatory surgery includes (select all that apply)
   a. how pain will be controlled.
   b. any fluid and food restrictions.
   c. characteristics of monitoring equipment.
   d. what odors and sensations may be experienced.
   e. the technique and practice of coughing and deep breathing, if appropriate.

10. The nurse asks a preoperative patient to sign a surgical consent form as specified by the surgeon and signs the form after the patient. By this action, the nurse is
    a. witnessing the patient's signature.
    b. obtaining informed consent from the patient for the surgery.
    c. verifying that the consent for surgery is truly voluntary and informed.
    d. ensuring that the patient is mentally competent to sign the consent form.

11. When the nurse prepares to administer a preoperative medication to a patient, the patient tells the nurse that she really does not understand what the surgeon plans to do.
    a. What action should be taken by the nurse?
    b. What criterion of informed consent has not been met in this situation?

12. A patient scheduled for hip-replacement surgery in the early afternoon receives and ingests a breakfast tray with clear liquids the morning of surgery. The nurse notifies the ACP with the expectation that the patient
    a. will be able to undergo surgery as scheduled.
    b. will have to have surgery rescheduled for the following day.
    c. should be rescheduled for surgery 8 hours after the fluid intake.
    d. should have a nasogastric tube inserted to remove the fluids from the stomach.

13. Preoperative checklists are used on the day of surgery to ensure that
    a. the patient is correctly identified.
    b. all preoperative orders and procedures have been carried out and records are complete.
    c. patients' families have been informed as to where they can accompany and wait for patients.
    d. preoperative medications are the last procedure carried out before the patient is transported to the operating room.

14. The nurse recognizes that extra time may be necessary when preparing an elderly adult for surgery because of
    a. ineffective coping.
    b. limited adaptation to stress.
    c. diminished vision and hearing.
    d. the need to include caregivers in preoperative activities.

15. The nurse is reviewing the lab results for a preoperative patient. Which of these results should be brought to the attention of the surgeon?
    a. Hemoglobin of 15 g/dL
    b. Serum K⁺ of 3.8 mEq/L
    c. Blood glucose of 100 mg/dL
    d. White blood cell count (WBC) of 18,500/μL

16. The nurse is preparing a patient for transport to the operating room. The patient is scheduled for a right knee arthroscopy. What actions should the nurse take at this time? (select all that apply)
    a. Ensure that the patient has voided.
    b. Verify that the informed consent is signed.
    c. Complete the preoperative nursing documentation.
    d. Verify that the right knee is marked with indelible marker.
    e. Ensure that the H&P, diagnostic reports, and vital signs are on the chart.

CASE STUDY
Preoperative Patient
Patient Profile

C.J., a 49-year-old construction worker, is scheduled for a bronchoscopy for biopsy of a right lung lesion. He initially sought medical care for hemoptysis and increasing fatigue. When the nurse asked him to sign the operative permit, he stated that he was not certain if he should go ahead with the procedure because he fears a diagnosis of cancer.

Subjective Data
- Has never been hospitalized
- Has had no medical problems except mild obesity
- Has a cigarette smoking history of 40 pack-years
- Is married with two children, ages 6 and 8; both children have cystic fibrosis
- Is fearful that his wife will not be able to manage without him

Objective Data
- Diagnostic studies: Chest x-ray revealed mass in upper lobe of right lung
- Hematocrit: 31%

Clinical Decision-Making Questions
Using a separate sheet of paper, answer the following questions.

1. What factors in C.J.'s background or personal situation might influence his emotional response and physical reactions to this surgery?
2. What should C.J. know if his consent for surgery is to be truly informed?
3. *Priority Decision:* C.J. will be an outpatient for this procedure. What is the priority preoperative teaching that should be done to prepare him for surgery?
4. What risk factors for surgical and anesthetic complications might you anticipate for C.J.? What are the potential interventions that might minimize the risks?
5. *Priority Decision:* Based on the assessment data provided, what are the priority nursing diagnoses? Are there any collaborative problems?

Nursing Management:
Intraoperative Care

1. The physical environment of a surgery suite is designed primarily to promote
   a. electrical safety.
   b. medical and surgical asepsis.
   c. comfort and privacy of the patient.
   d. communication among the surgical team.

2. When transporting an inpatient to the surgical department, the nurse from another area of the hospital has access to
   a. the clean core.
   b. the holding area.
   c. corridors of the surgical suite.
   d. an unprepared operating room.

3. Match the surgical team members with their appropriate roles (answers may be used more than once).
   _____ a. Provides gowns and gloves for self and other members of the surgical team
   _____ b. Admits patient to the operating room
   _____ c. Responsible for maintenance of physiologic homeostasis during surgery (MD)
   _____ d. Checks mechanical and electrical equipment
   _____ e. Passes instruments to surgeon and assistants
   _____ f. Supervises postanesthesia recovery of patient in PACU (nurse)
   _____ g. Coordinates all activities in room with team members
   _____ h. Works with surgeon, assisting with hemostasis and suturing
   _____ i. Chooses surgical procedure and management of patient
   _____ j. Prepares instrument table
   _____ k. Administers anesthesia and adjuvant drugs (nurse)

   1. Circulating nurse
   2. Scrub nurse
   3. Surgeon
   4. Anesthesiologist
   5. Nurse anesthetist
   6. Registered nurse first assistant

4. Identify five examples of data collected during the perioperative nurse's physical assessment of the patient that indicate special consideration of the patient's needs during surgery.
   a.

   b.

   c.

   d.

   e.

5. The primary goal of the circulating nurse during preparation of the operating room, transferring and positioning the patient, and assisting the anesthesia team is
   a. avoiding any type of injury to the patient.
   b. maintaining a clean environment for the patient.
   c. providing for patient comfort and sense of well-being.
   d. preventing breaks in aseptic technique by the sterile members of the team.

6. Goals for patient safety in the operating room (OR) include the Universal Protocol, in which
   a. all surgical centers of any type must submit reports on patient safety infractions to the accreditation agencies.
   b. the members of the surgical team stop whatever they are doing to check that all sterile items have been properly prepared.
   c. a surgical timeout is performed just before the procedure is started to verify patient identity, surgical procedure, and surgical site.
   d. all members of the surgical team pause right before surgery to meditate for 1 minute to decrease stress and possible errors.

7. A break in sterile technique during surgery would occur when the scrub nurse touches
   a. the mask with gloved hands.
   b. gloved hands to the gown at chest level.
   c. the drape at the incision site with gloved hands.
   d. the lower arms to the instruments on the instrument tray.

8. During surgery, a patient has a nursing diagnosis of risk for perioperative positioning injury. A common risk factor for this nursing diagnosis is
   a. skin lesions.
   b. break in sterile technique.
   c. musculoskeletal deformities.
   d. electrical or mechanical equipment failure.

9. At the end of the surgical procedure, the perioperative nurse evaluates the patient's response to the nursing care delivered during the perioperative period. Which of the following criteria reflects an outcome related to the patient's physical status?
   a. The patient's right to privacy is maintained.
   b. The patient's care is consistent with the perioperative plan of care.
   c. The patient receives consistent and comparable care regardless of the setting.
   d. The patient's respiratory function is consistent with or improved from baseline levels established preoperatively.

10. The two short-acting barbiturates most commonly used for induction of general anesthesia are
    _____ and _____.

11. Because of the rapid elimination of volatile liquids used for general anesthesia, the nurse should anticipate that early in the anesthesia recovery period, the patient will need
    a. warm blankets.
    b. analgesic medication.
    c. observation for respiratory depression.
    d. airway protection in anticipation of vomiting.

12. The primary advantage of the use of midazolam (Versed) as an adjunct to general anesthesia is its
    a. amnestic effect.
    b. analgesic effect.
    c. antiemetic effect.
    d. prolonged action.

13. Identify the rationale for the use of each of the following drugs during surgery and one nursing implication indicated in the care of the patient immediately postoperatively related to the drug.

	Use	Nursing Implication
a. desflurane (Suprane)		
b. ketamine (Ketalar)		
c. fentanyl (Sublimaze)		
d. succinylcholine (Anectine)		

14. Monitored anesthesia care (MAC) is being considered for a patient undergoing a cervical dilation and endometrial biopsy in the health care provider's office. The patient asks the nurse, "What is this MAC?" The nurse's response is based on the knowledge that MAC
    a. can be administered only by anesthesiologists or nurse anesthetists.
    b. enables the patient to respond to commands and accept painful procedures.
    c. should never be used outside of the OR because of the risk of serious complications.
    d. is so safe that it can be administered by nurses with direction from health care providers.

15. Match the methods of local anesthetic administration with their descriptions.
    _____ a. Injection of anesthetic agent directly into tissues
    _____ b. Injection of anesthetic agent into space around the vertebrae
    _____ c. Injection of a specific nerve with an anesthetic agent
    _____ d. Injection of agent into subarachnoid space
    _____ e. Injection of agent into veins of extremity after limb is exsanguinated

    1. Nerve block
    2. IV nerve block
    3. Spinal block
    4. Epidural block
    5. Local infiltration

16. During epidural and spinal anesthesia, the nurse should monitor the patient for
    a. spinal headache.
    b. hypotension and bradycardia.
    c. loss of consciousness and seizures.
    d. downward extension of nerve block.

17. A preoperative patient reveals that an uncle died during surgery because of a fever and cardiac arrest. The perioperative nurse alerts the surgical team, knowing that if the patient is at risk for malignant hyperthermia,
    a. the surgery will have to be cancelled.
    b. specific precautions can be taken to safely anesthetize the patient.
    c. dantrolene (Dantrium) must be given to prevent hyperthermia during surgery.
    d. the patient should be placed on a cooling blanket during the surgical procedure.

CASE STUDY

Intraoperative Patient

Patient Profile

T.M., a 76-year-old retired policeman, is admitted to the OR for an inguinal hernia repair. T.M. has a history of severe COPD and heart failure. Therefore the anesthesia care provider has decided to administer spinal anesthesia. The circulating nurse has verified the baseline data (VS, height, weight, age; allergies; level of consciousness; NPO status; and comfort level). A signed informed consent is on the chart. T.M. has no allergies.

Clinical Decision-Making Questions

Using a separate sheet of paper, answer the following questions.

1. *Priority Decision:* What are the priority nursing actions that should be taken when T.M. arrives in the OR?
2. What specific precautions should be taken when positioning T.M. for his surgery?
3. What complications of spinal anesthesia should T.M. be monitored for during surgery?
4. T.M. is 76 years old. What gerontologic considerations should be taken?
5. *Priority Decision:* Based on the data presented, what are the priority nursing diagnoses?

CHAPTER

20

Nursing Management: Postoperative Care

1. Progression of patients through various phases of care in a postanesthesia care unit (PACU) depends primarily on
   a. the condition of the patient.
   b. the type of anesthesia used.
   c. the preference of the surgeon.
   d. the type of surgical procedure.

2. *Priority Decision:* Upon admission of a patient to the PACU, the nurse's priority assessment is the patient's
   a. vital signs.
   b. surgical site.
   c. respiratory adequacy.
   d. level of consciousness.

3. The initial information given to the PACU nurses about the surgical patient is provided by
   a. a copy of the written operative report.
   b. a verbal report from the circulating nurse.
   c. a verbal report from the anesthesia care provider.
   d. an explanation of the surgical procedure from the surgeon.

4. To prevent agitation during the patient's recovery from anesthesia, the nurse should begin orientation explanations when the patient
   a. is awake.
   b. first arrives in the PACU.
   c. becomes agitated or frightened.
   d. can be aroused and recognizes where he or she is.

5. Routine assessment of the patient's cardiovascular function on admission to the PACU includes
   a. ECG monitoring.
   b. monitoring arterial blood gases.
   c. determining fluid and electrolyte status.
   d. direct arterial blood pressure monitoring.

6. Match the postoperative respiratory complications with their associated causes and mechanisms (answers may be used more than once).

   _____ a. Pain
   _____ b. Tongue falling back
   _____ c. Medullary depression
   _____ d. Retained secretions
   _____ e. Inhalation of gastric contents
   _____ f. Atelectasis
   _____ g. Laryngospasm
   _____ h. Obesity

   1. Airway obstruction
   2. Hypoxemia
   3. Hypoventilation

7. To prevent airway obstruction in the postoperative patient who is unconscious or semiconscious, the nurse
   a. encourages deep breathing.
   b. elevates the head of the bed.
   c. administers oxygen per mask.
   d. positions the patient in a side-lying position.

8. To promote effective coughing, deep breathing, and ambulation in the postoperative patient, it is most important for the nurse to
   a. teach the patient controlled breathing.
   b. explain the rationale for these activities.
   c. provide adequate and regular pain medication.
   d. use an incentive spirometer to motivate the patient.

9. While assessing a patient in the PACU, the nurse finds that the patient's blood pressure is below the preoperative baseline. The nurse determines that the patient has residual vasodilating effects of anesthesia upon finding
   a. an oxygen saturation of 88%.
   b. a urinary output >30 mL/hr.
   c. a normal pulse with warm, dry, pink skin.
   d. a narrowing pulse pressure with normal pulse.

10. A patient in the PACU has emergence delirium manifested by agitation and thrashing. The nurse should assess the patient first for
    a. hypoxemia.
    b. neurologic injury.
    c. a distended bladder.
    d. cardiac dysrhythmias.

11. The nurse applies warm blankets to a patient who is shivering and has a body temperature of 96.0°F (35.6°C). The nurse would also anticipate the administration of
    a. oxygen.
    b. vasodilating drugs.
    c. antidysrhythmic drugs.
    d. analgesics or sedatives.

12. List five criteria used to determine when a patient is ready for discharge from phase I PACU care to the clinical unit.
    a.

    b.

    c.

    d.

    e.

13. Identify six nursing diagnoses or collaborative problems common in postoperative patients for which ambulation of the patient is an appropriate intervention for the problem.
    a.

    b.

    c.

    d.

    e.

    f.

14. In the absence of postoperative vomiting, GI suctioning, and wound drainage, the physiologic responses to the stress of surgery are most likely to cause
    a. diuresis.
    b. hyperkalemia.
    c. fluid overload.
    d. impaired blood coagulation.

15. Describe two independent nursing interventions in addition to ambulation that could be implemented to prevent or treat the following postoperative complications.
    a. Syncope
       1.

       2.

    b. Urinary retention
       1.

       2.

    c. Abdominal distention
       1.

       2.

    d. Wound infection
       1.

       2.

16. Match the following tubes and drains with their expected drainage (answers may be used more than once).
    _____ a. Indwelling catheter   1. Wound drainage
    _____ b. Gastrostomy tube   2. Urine
    _____ c. Hemovac   3. Bile
    _____ d. T-tube   4. Gastric contents
    _____ e. Nasogastric tube

17. The nurse notes drainage on the surgical dressing when the patient is transferred from the PACU to the clinical unit. The nurse should
    a. change the dressing and assess the wound.
    b. notify the surgeon of the drainage type and amount.
    c. note and record the type, amount, and color of the drainage.
    d. observe the dressing every 15 minutes for an increase in drainage.

18. Thirty-six hours postoperatively, a patient has a temperature of 100°F (37.8°C). The nurse recognizes that this finding is most likely a result of
    a. dehydration.
    b. wound infection.
    c. lung congestion and atelectasis.
    d. the normal surgical stress response.

19. The health care provider has ordered IV morphine q2-4hr PRN for a patient following major abdominal surgery. The nurse would plan to administer the morphine
    a. before all planned painful activities.
    b. every 2 to 4 hours during the first 48 hours.
    c. every 4 hours as the patient requests the medication.
    d. after assessing the nature and intensity of the patient's pain.

20. Instructions given to the postoperative patient before discharge should include
    a. the need for follow-up care with home care nurses.
    b. directions for maintaining the routine postoperative diet.
    c. written information about his self-care during recuperation.
    d. the necessity to restrict all activity until surgical healing is complete.

CASE STUDY
Postoperative Patient
Patient Profile

S.B., a 28-year-old school teacher, is admitted to the PACU following a cystoscopy for recurrent bladder infections and hematuria. The procedure was scheduled as outpatient surgery and was performed under IV sedation.

Postoperative Orders

- Vital signs per routine
- D/C IV before discharge
- Patient to void before discharge
- Cipro 500 mg PO q6 hr for 10 days
- Tylenol #3 1-2 tabs q3-4 hr PRN for pain
- Patient to call office to schedule follow-up appointment

Clinical Decision-Making Questions

Using a separate sheet of paper, answer the following questions.

1. *Priority Decision:* What priority nursing actions will be required to progress S.B. toward discharge?
2. What precautions will be required in ambulating S.B. after surgery?
3. What problems might interfere with discharging S.B. to home in a timely manner?
4. How will the nurse determine that S.B. is ready to be discharged to home?
5. What are the unique needs of discharging a patient home as opposed to a clinical unit?
6. *Priority Decision:* Based on the data presented, what are the priority nursing diagnoses? Are there any collaborative problems?

1. Use the following terms to fill in the labels in the illustration below.

Terms

Anterior chamber   Optic nerve
Choroid   Posterior chamber
Ciliary body   Pupil
Cornea   Retina
Iris   Sclera
Lens   Vitreous cavity
Optic disc

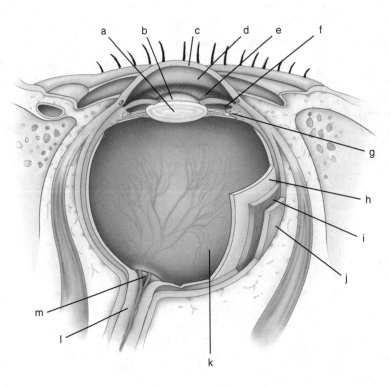

a. _____ h. _____

b. _____ i. _____

c. _____ j. _____

d. _____ k. _____

e. _____ l. _____

f. _____ m. _____

g. _____

2. Word Search. Find the words that are described by the clues given below. The words may be located horizontally, vertically, or diagonally, and may be reversed.

```
Q R I M K J E R S R C M O P
E A Q U E O U S H U M O R R
A V I T R E O U S H U M O R
D I O R O H C D L I I P O M
W T H U M T O U M E R O U S
E C E R T R E D L I P U P O
A N T C O R N E A T C N U P
Q U I R S E N T E L L I O N
S J S C U S S E L U N O Z T
E N I T B O P T I C D I S C
N O R A M I L T A R E L C S
O C I L I A R Y B O D Y E T
C A N A L O F S C H L E M M
S P C S C R E L O T M L E T
```

Clues

a. Fibers holding the lens in place
b. Fills the anterior cavity of the eye
c. Fills the posterior cavity of the eye
d. Clear outer layer of anterior eyeball
e. Secretes aqueous humor
f. Photoreceptor cells stimulated in dim environments
g. Focuses light rays on retina
h. Needed for color vision
i. Protective white outer layer of the eyeball
j. Junction of the cornea and sclera (see Fig. 21-2)
k. Transparent mucous membrane lining the eyelids
l. Drains tears from the surface of the eye into the lacrimal canals
m. Point where the optic nerve exits the eyeball
n. Nourishes ciliary body, iris, and part of retina
o. Drainage path for the aqueous humor
p. Colored portion of the eye
q. Opening in the center of the iris

3. Identify the cranial nerves that are responsible for the following eye functions.

a. Eyelid movement _____

b. Pupil constriction _____

c. Pupil dilation _____

d. Visual acuity _____

4. Identify the causes of the following assessment findings of the eye that are associated with aging.
   a. Ectropion
   b. Pinguecula
   c. Arcus senilis
   d. "Floaters"
   e. Changes in color perception
   f. Decreased pupil size
   g. Yellowish sclera
   h. Dry, irritated eyes

5. When obtaining a health history from a patient with cataracts, it is most important for the nurse to ask about the patient's use of
   a. corticosteroids.
   b. oral hypoglycemic agents.
   c. antihistamine/decongestants.
   d. β-adrenergic blocking agents.

6. Identify a specific finding identified by the nurse during assessment of each of the patient's functional health patterns that indicates either a risk factor for visual problems or the response of the patient to an eye problem.
   a. Health perception–health management
   b. Nutritional-metabolic
   c. Elimination
   d. Activity-exercise
   e. Sleep-rest
   f. Cognitive-perceptual
   g. Self-perception–self-concept
   h. Role-relationship
   i. Sexuality-reproductive
   j. Coping–stress tolerance
   k. Value-belief

7. Describe what is meant by the finding that the patient has a visual acuity of OD: 20/40; OS: 20/50.

8. The nurse documents PERRLA following assessment of a patient's eyes. One finding that supports these data is
   a. a slightly oval shape of the pupils.
   b. the presence of nystagmus on far lateral gaze.
   c. dilation of the pupil when a light is shined in the opposite eye.
   d. constriction of the pupils when an object is brought closer to the eyes.

9. Identify the assessment techniques used to obtain the following data.
   a. Peripheral vision field
   b. Extraocular muscle functions
   c. Near visual acuity
   d. Visual acuity
   e. Intraocular pressure

10. The nurse would expect to find a yellow cast to the sclera in
    a. infants.
    b. dark-skinned persons.
    c. persons with brown irises.
    d. patients with eye infections.

11. To determine the presence of corneal abrasions or defects in a patient with an eye injury, the nurse would provide
    a. a tonometer.
    b. fluorescein dye.
    c. a pocket pen light.
    d. an ophthalmoscope.

12. Match the following assessment abnormalities of the eye with their descriptions.
    _____ a. Anisocoria   1. Upper lid droop
    _____ b. Diplopia   2. Light intolerance
    _____ c. Exophthalmos   3. Unequal pupil size
    _____ d. Ptosis   4. Deviation of eye position
    _____ e. Blepharitis   5. Protrusion of eyeball
    _____ f. Strabismus   6. Double vision
    _____ g. Photophobia   7. Redness and crusting along lid margins

13. When examining the patient's eye with an ophthalmoscope, which of the following findings would be of most concern to the nurse?
    a. Depression at the center of the optic disc
    b. Blurring of the nasal margin of the optic disc
    c. A break in the retina at the site of the macula
    d. The presence of small pieces of liquefied vitreous in the vitreous chamber

14. To prepare a patient for a fluorescein angiography, the nurse explains that the test involves
    a. the measurement of the curvature of the cornea.
    b. IV injection of a dye to evaluate blood flow through epithelial and retinal blood vessels.
    c. application of eyedrops containing a dye that will localize arterial abnormalities in the retina.
    d. anesthetizing the eye so that probes can be inserted into the anterior chamber to measure intraocular pressure.

15. Match the structures of the ear with their functions.
    _____ a. Semicircular canals   1. Sets bones of the middle ear in motion
    _____ b. Tympanic membrane   2. Allows for equalization of pressure in the middle ear
    _____ c. Organ of Corti   3. Receives sound waves and transmits to the tympanic membrane
    _____ d. Cochlea   4. Converts mechanical sound waves into electrochemical impulse
    _____ e. Vestibular portion of CN VIII 5. Organ of balance and equilibrium
    _____ f. Acoustic portion of CN VIII   6. Transmits sound stimuli to the brain
    _____ g. External ear   7. Receptor organ of sound
    _____ h. Ossicular chain   8. Amplifies sound waves and transmits vibrations to the inner ear
    _____ i. Eustachian tube   9. Transmits stimuli from the semicircular canals to the brain

16. Identify one change in the external, middle, and inner ear that can impair hearing in the older adult.
    a. External ear
    b. Middle ear
    c. Inner ear

17. The nurse suspects a patient has presbycusis when she complains of
    a. ringing in the ears.
    b. a sensation of fullness in the ears.
    c. difficulty understanding the meaning of words.
    d. a decrease in the ability to hear high-pitched sounds.

18. Describe the significance of the following questions asked of the patient while obtaining subjective data during assessment of the auditory system.
    a. Do you have a history of childhood ear infections or ruptured eardrums?
    b. Do you use any over-the-counter or prescription medications on a regular basis?
    c. Have you ever been treated for a head injury?
    d. Is there a history of hearing loss in your parents?
    e. Have you been exposed to excessive noise levels in your work or recreational activities?
    f. Has the amount of social activities you are involved in changed?

19. Identify whether the following statements are true (*T*) or false (*F*). If a statement is false, correct the bold word(s) to make the statement true.
    _____ a. Examination of the external ear involves the techniques of **inspection and palpation**.
    _____ b. To straighten the ear canal in an adult before insertion of the otoscope, the nurse grasps the auricle and pulls **downward and backward**.
    _____ c. Major landmarks of the tympanic membrane include the **umbo, the handle of malleus, and the cone of light**.
    _____ d. A normal finding upon physical assessment of the ear is the ability to hear a low whisper at **30 cm**.
    _____ e. A patient has a negative Rinne test of the left ear. The nurse would expect that with Weber testing the patient would hear the tuning fork sound best in the **right** ear.
    _____ f. The presence of a retracted eardrum on otoscopic examination is indicative of **negative pressure in the middle ear**.
    _____ g. In **chronic otitis media,** the nurse would expect to find a lack of landmarks and a bulging eardrum on otoscopic examination.

20. Indicate whether conductive hearing loss (CHL) or sensorineural hearing loss (SHL) is associated with the following.
    _____ a. Positive Rinne test
    _____ b. Negative Rinne test
    _____ c. Weber lateralization to impaired ear
    _____ d. Weber lateralization to good ear
    _____ e. External or middle ear pathology
    _____ f. Inner ear or nerve pathway pathology

21. Results of an audiometry indicate that a patient has a 10-dB hearing loss at 8000 Hz. The most appropriate action by the nurse is to
    a. encourage the patient to start learning to lip read.
    b. speak at a normal speed and volume with the patient.
    c. avoid words in conversation that have many high-pitched consonants.
    d. discuss the advantages and disadvantages of various hearing aids with the patient.

22. Disease of the vestibular system of the ear is indicated with caloric testing when
    a. hearing is improved with irrigation of the external ear canal.
    b. no nystagmus is elicited with application of water in the external ear.
    c. the patient experiences intolerable pain with irrigation of the external ear.
    d. irrigation of the external ear with water produces nystagmus opposite the side of instillation.

Nursing Management:
Visual and Auditory Problems

1. Match the refractive conditions with their characteristics (answers may be used more than once).

_____ a. Corrected with cylinder lens
_____ b. Absence of crystalline lens
_____ c. Corrected with convex lens
_____ d. Image focused behind retina
_____ e. Abnormally long eyeball
_____ f. Excessive light refraction
_____ g. Corrected with concave lens
_____ h. Unequal corneal curvature
_____ i. Loss of accommodation associated with age
_____ j. Insufficient light refraction
_____ k. Abnormally short eyeball
_____ l. Image focused in front of retina

1. Myopia
2. Hyperopia
3. Presbyopia
4. Astigmatism
5. Aphakia

2. To determine if an unconscious patient has contact lenses in place, the nurse
   a. uses a pen light to shine a light obliquely over the eyeball.
   b. applies drops of fluorescein dye to the eye to stain the lenses yellow.
   c. touches the cornea lightly with a dry cotton ball to see if the patient reacts.
   d. tenses the lateral canthus to cause a lens to be ejected if it is present in the eye.

3. The choices for correction for a refractive error include (select all that apply)
   a. LASIK.
   b. Corneal molding.
   c. Laser thermal keratoplasty (LTK).
   d. Photorefractive keratectomy (PRK).
   e. Surgical implantation of intraocular lens.

4. A patient tells the nurse on admission to the health care facility that he recently has been classified as legally blind. The nurse recognizes that the patient
   a. has lost usable vision but has some light perception.
   b. will need time for grieving and adjusting to living with total blindness.
   c. will be dependent on others to ensure a safe environment for functioning.
   d. may be able to perform many tasks and activities with vision enhancement techniques.

5. Identify five nursing measures that should be implemented to increase a visually impaired patient's safety and comfort.
   a.

   b.

   c.

   d.

   e.

6. A patient is admitted to the emergency department with a wood splinter imbedded in the right eye. An appropriate intervention by the nurse is to
   a. irrigate the eye with a large amount of sterile saline.
   b. carefully remove the splinter with a pair of sterile forceps.
   c. cover the eye with a dry sterile patch and a protective shield.
   d. apply light pressure on the closed eye to prevent bleeding or loss of aqueous humor.

7. Word Search. Find the words that are defined by the clues given below. The words may be located horizontally, vertically, or diagonally and may be reversed.

```
I Q V S T P S E H J K J L B W Z O A E D
R P W T J F C D F Y E K C X O Y P C P N
C A J K Q F C F L J R F N U R L U U I S
E O M L J H O A P Y A U F X R U V T D I
V S R O J B V D U R T N T A B L B E E H
H B K N H N Y B O X I P Z J V E P B M B
P O N S E C I H H C T C B U L V T A I H
L T R T O A A G N X I S I H B A E C C Q
O I V D Z A L R R Z S J N S Y G Q T K C
N Q N N E C M U T I I I I K E O H E E R
G B A D H O A F L S H B G K E Z B R R M
U S F E I L L L N C O D D H Z G I I A L
J O W R N P P U I L E V G F D Q H A T H
W Z W X D W K Y M J Q R E P O S F L O Y
B L P J K P Y V M C G R C F H S R C C K
F L V W O U D G S R T P M K R X K O O A
X J E A N U W J E T F X J E J J I N N L
F C P P L D Q F E I H S O Z J U R J J V
I R E D H G O U R S G K Y V F Z B U U H
R D F E D A R B N B O U I U Z X A N N V
U N Y T G C R Q F K E D U V R P R C C N
X O E K J O W I R V O Z I X D S R T T K
L I X F X I X T T H N I Z V A T I I I O
P Z Q H T C Y H L I G G K C K M V V V U
W A V U H N V J Z N S V L R T K B I I W
Z L S I T I V I T C N U J N O C H T T X
G A P K X H L G O G B I Z K X E J I I L
F H I B F R R E T S Z E G W U G U S S I
M C B U Z P W E J J Q Q H S T N G Z O I
M S O D Z V P Y Z T J F O G H J O Z I A
```

Clues

a. Chronic inflammation of the sebaceous glands

b. Sty

c. Blindness-causing chlamydial conjunctivitis

d. Pinkeye

e. Infectious keratitis

f. Viral infection spread by direct and sexual contact

g. Inflammation of the cornea

h. Inflammation of lid margins bilaterally

i. Inflammation of the conjunctiva

8. The nurse teaches all patients with conjunctival infections to use

a. artificial tears to moisten and soothe the eyes.

b. dark glasses to prevent discomfort of photophobia.

c. warm moist compresses to the eyes to promote drainage and healing.

d. frequent and thorough hand washing to avoid spreading the infection.

9. A patient with early cataracts tells the nurse that he is afraid cataract surgery may cause permanent visual damage. The nurse informs the patient that

a. progression of the cataracts can be prevented by avoidance of UV light and good dietary management.

b. cataract surgery is very safe and with the implantation of an intraocular lens, the need for glasses will be eliminated.

c. the cataracts will only worsen with time and should be removed as early as possible to prevent blindness.

d. vision-enhancement techniques may improve vision until surgery becomes an acceptable option to maintain desired activities.

10. A 60-year-old patient is being prepared for outpatient cataract surgery. When obtaining admission data from the patient, the nurse would expect to find that the patient has a history of
    a. a painless, sudden, severe loss of vision.
    b. blurred vision, colored halos around lights, and eye pain.
    c. a gradual loss of vision with abnormal color perception and glare.
    d. light flashes, floaters, and a "cobweb" in the field of vision with loss of central or peripheral vision.

11. A patient with bilateral cataracts is scheduled for an extracapsular cataract extraction with an intraocular lens implantation of one eye. Preoperatively, the nurse should
    a. assess the visual acuity in the unoperated eye to plan the need for postoperative assistance.
    b. inform the patient that the operative eye will need to be patched for 3 to 4 days postoperatively.
    c. assure the patient that vision in the operative eye will be improved to near-normal on the first postoperative day.
    d. teach the patient routine coughing and deep-breathing techniques to use postoperatively to prevent respiratory complications.

12. Complete the following sentences.
    a. Retinal tears leading to retinal detachment are most often caused by _____.
    b. The leakage of vitreous humor into the subretinal space, separating the sensory retina from the pigment epithelium, is termed a _____ retinal detachment.
    c. Treatments for retinal detachment that are used to create an inflammation and scarring between the retina and the choroid include _____ and _____.
    d. The surgical procedure that involves physical indentation of the globe to bring the pigmented epithelium, the choroid, and sclera in contact with a detached retina is known as _____.

13. Following a pneumatic retinopexy, the nurse plans postoperative care of the patient based on the knowledge that
    a. specific positioning and activity restrictions are likely to be required for several days.
    b. the patient is frequently hospitalized for 7 to 10 days on bed rest until healing is complete.
    c. patients experience little or no pain, and development of pain indicates hemorrhage or infection.
    d. reattachment of the retina commonly fails and patients can be expected to grieve for loss of vision.

14. In caring for the patient with age-related macular degeneration (AMD), it is important for the nurse to
    a. teach the patient how to use topical eyedrops for treatment of AMD.
    b. emphasize the use of vision enhancement techniques to improve what vision is present.
    c. encourage the patient to undergo laser treatment to slow the deposit of extracellular debris.
    d. explain that nothing can be done to save the patient's vision because there is no treatment for AMD.

15. A patient with wet AMD is treated with photodynamic therapy. After the procedure the nurse instructs the patient to
    a. maintain the head in an upright position for 24 hours.
    b. avoid blowing the nose or causing jerking movements of the head.
    c. completely cover all the skin to avoid a thermal burn from sunlight.
    d. expect to experience blind spots where the laser has caused retinal damage.

16. Visual impairment occurring with glaucoma results from
    a. ischemic pressure on the retina and optic nerve.
    b. clouding of aqueous humor in the anterior chamber.
    c. deposition of drusen and degeneration of the macula.
    d. loss of accommodation from paralysis of the ciliary body.

17. An important health promotion nursing intervention that is relevant to glaucoma is
    a. teaching individuals at risk for glaucoma about early signs and symptoms of the disease.
    b. preparing patients with glaucoma for lifestyle changes necessary to adapt to eventual blindness.

    c. promoting regular measurements of intraocular pressure for early detection and treatment of glaucoma.

    d. informing patients that glaucoma is curable if eye medications are administered before visual impairment has occurred.

18. Indicate whether the following characteristics of glaucoma are associated with primary open-angle glaucoma (POAG) or primary angle-closure glaucoma (PACG).

    _____ a. Resistance to aqueous outflow through trabecular meshwork

    _____ b. Treated with iridotomy/iridectomy

    _____ c. Administration of hypertonic oral and IV fluids

    _____ d. Caused by lens blocking pupillary opening

    _____ e. May be caused by increased production of aqueous humor

    _____ f. Causes sudden, severe eye pain associated with nausea and vomiting

    _____ g. Treated with β-adrenergic blocking agents

    _____ h. Gradual loss of peripheral vision

    _____ i. Treated with trabeculoplasty/trabeculectomy

    _____ j. Causes loss of central vision with corneal edema

19. The health care provider has prescribed optic drops of betaxolol (Betoptic), dipivefrin (Propine), and carbachol (Isopto Carbachol) in addition to oral acetazolamide (Diamox) for treatment of a patient with chronic open-angle glaucoma. What is the rationale for the use of each of these drugs in the treatment of glaucoma?

    a. Betaxolol

    b. Dipivefrin

    c. Carbachol

    d. Acetazolamide

20. One of the nurse's roles in preservation of hearing includes

    a. advising patients to keep the ears clean of wax with cotton-tipped applicators.

    b. monitoring patients at risk for drug-induced ototoxicity for tinnitus and vertigo.

    c. promoting the use of ear protection in work and recreational activity with noise levels above 120 dB.

    d. advocating MMR (measles, mumps, rubella) immunization in susceptible women as soon as pregnancy is confirmed.

21. Number the following high-noise environments from the highest risk for ear injury to the lowest.

    _____ a. Noisy restaurant for 12 hours

    _____ b. Sitting in front of amplifiers at a rock concert

    _____ c. Working in a quiet home office for 8 hours

    _____ d. Guiding jet planes to and from airport gates

    _____ e. Heavy factory noise for 8 hours

    _____ f. Using a chain saw continuously for 2 hours

22. A 74-year-old man has moderate presbycusis and heart disease. He takes one aspirin a day as an antiplatelet agent and uses quinidine, furosemide (Lasix), and enalapril (Vasotec) for his heart condition. What risk factors are present for ototoxicity in this situation?

23. Nursing management of the patient with external otitis includes

    a. irrigating the ear canal with body temperature saline several hours after instilling lubricating eardrops.

    b. inserting an ear wick into the external canal before each application of eardrops to disperse the medication.

    c. teaching the patient to prevent further infections by instilling antibiotic drops into the ear canal before swimming.

    d. administering eardrops without touching the dropper to the auricle and positioning the ear upward for 2 minutes afterward.

24. Identify whether the following statements are true (*T*) or false (*F*). If a statement is false, correct the bold word(s) to make the statement true.
    _____ a. Acute otitis media is most commonly treated with **a myringotomy** to resolve the increased pressure and inflammation in the middle ear.
    _____ b. In chronic otitis media, formation of **an acoustic neuroma** may destroy the structures of the middle ear or invade the dura of the brain.
    _____ c. A **tympanoplasty** may be used to insert an ossicular prosthesis and a tympanic membrane graft in patients with chronic otitis media.
    _____ d. The patient who has had a myringotomy with placement of a tympanostomy tube should be instructed to **avoid getting water in the ear**.
    _____ e. **Acute** otitis media is an infection of the middle ear that frequently leads to mastoiditis and meningitis.
    _____ f. Impairment of the **eustachian tube** is most commonly associated with chronic otitis media with effusion.
    _____ g. Following middle ear surgery, the patient should be positioned **flat in bed**.

25. While caring for a patient with otosclerosis, the nurse would expect that the patient has
    a. a strong family history of the disease.
    b. symptoms of sensorineural hearing loss.
    c. a positive Rinne test and lateralization to the good or better ear on Weber testing.
    d. an immediate and consistent improvement in hearing at the time of surgical treatment.

26. The nurse identifies a nursing diagnosis of risk for injury for a patient following a stapedectomy based on the knowledge that
    a. nystagmus may result from perilymph disturbances caused by surgery.
    b. stimulation of the labyrinth during surgery may cause vertigo and loss of balance.
    c. blowing the nose or coughing may precipitate dislodgement of the tympanic graft.
    d. postoperative tinnitus may decrease the patient's awareness of environmental hazards.

27. List the triad of symptoms that occur with inner ear problems.
    a.

    b.

    c.

28. An appropriate nursing intervention for the patient during an acute attack of Ménière's disease includes providing
    a. frequent positioning.
    b. a quiet, darkened room.
    c. a television for diversion.
    d. padded side rails on the bed.

29. The nurse counsels the patient with an acoustic neuroma based on the knowledge that
    a. widespread metastasis usually occurs before symptoms of the tumor are noticed.
    b. facial nerve function will be sacrificed during surgical treatment to preserve hearing.
    c. early diagnosis and treatment of the tumor can preserve hearing and vestibular function.
    d. treatment is usually delayed until hearing loss is significant because a neuroma is a benign tumor.

30. Indicate whether the following characteristics of hearing loss are associated with conductive loss (*C*), sensorineural loss (*S*), or both (*B*).
    _____ a. Hears best in noisy environment
    _____ b. May be caused by impacted cerumen
    _____ c. Hearing aid is helpful
    _____ d. Speaks softly
    _____ e. Caused by noise trauma
    _____ f. Associated with otosclerosis
    _____ g. Presbycusis
    _____ h. Associated with Ménière's disease
    _____ i. Result of ototoxic drugs
    _____ j. Related to otitis media

31. When teaching a patient to use a hearing aid, the nurse encourages the patient to initially use the aid
    a. outdoors where sounds are distinct.
    b. at social functions where simultaneous conversations take place.
    c. in a quiet, controlled environment to experiment with tone and volume.
    d. in public areas such as malls or stores where others will not notice its use.

CASE STUDY
Chronic Open-Angle Glaucoma
Patient Profile

A.G., a 58-year-old African American woman, was seen in her ophthalmologist's office for a routine eye examination. Her last examination was 5 years ago.

Subjective Data

- Has no current ocular complaints
- Has not kept annually scheduled examinations because her eyes have not bothered her
- Takes metoprolol tartrate (Lopressor) for hypertension
- Has a family history of glaucoma
- Uses over-the-counter diphenhydramine (Benadryl) for her seasonal allergies

Objective Data

- Blood pressure: 130/78
- Heart rate: 72

Ophthalmic Examination

- Visual acuity: OD 20/20, OS 20/20
- Intraocular pressure: OD 25, OS 28; by Tono-pen tonometry
- Direct and indirect ophthalmoscopy: small, scattered retinal hemorrhages, optic discs appear normal with no cupping
- Visual field perimetry: early glaucomatous changes, OU

Collaborative Care

The health care provider prescribed betaxolol (Betoptic) gtt 1 OU. The nurse instructed A.G. on the reasons for the drug and how to do punctal occlusion.

Clinical Decision-Making Questions

Using a separate sheet of paper, answer the following questions.

1. Why should A.G. have been seeing an ophthalmologist on a yearly basis even though she had no ocular complaints?
2. Explain why the nurse instructed A.G. to use punctal occlusion when she uses the drops.
3. Why is it permissible for A.G. to use her antihistamine? What would the nurse have told her if gonioscopy had revealed narrow angles?
4. Will this patient be able to discontinue her eyedrops once her intraocular pressures are within the normal range? Explain your answer.
5. If topical therapy does not control A.G.'s intraocular pressures, what should she be told about alternative therapies?
6. Describe the probable appearance of A.G.'s optic discs in the future if her glaucoma is left untreated. What would her visual complaints be?
7. *Priority Decision:* Based on the assessment data presented, what are the priority nursing diagnoses? Are there any collaborative problems?

Nursing Assessment:
Integumentary System

1. Use the following terms to fill in the labels in the illustration below.

Terms

adipose tissue	connective tissue	hair shaft	stratum germinativum
apocrine sweat gland	hair follicle	stratum corneum	epidermis
arrector pili muscle	sebaceous gland	eccrine sweat gland	nerves
blood vessels	dermis	melanocyte	subcutaneous tissue

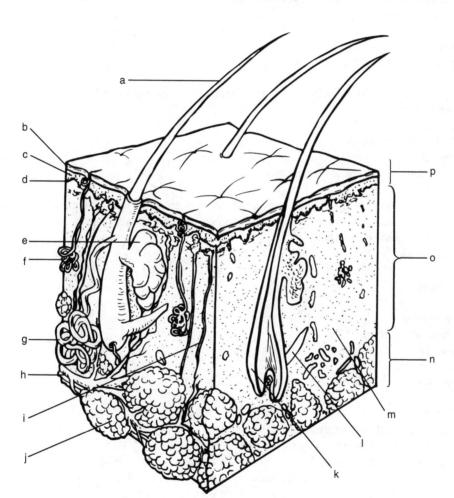

a. _____   g. _____   m. _____

b. _____   h. _____   n. _____

c. _____   i. _____   o. _____

d. _____   j. _____   p. _____

e. _____   k. _____

f. _____   l. _____

2. Match the following skin structures and substances with their descriptions (answers may be used more than once).

_____ a. Pigment-producing cells
_____ b. Attaches skin to muscle and bone
_____ c. Site of vitamin D synthesis
_____ d. Specialized protective protein
_____ e. Composed of collagen fibrils
_____ f. Produce collagen and elastin in dermis
_____ g. Form the basic cells of epidermis
_____ h. Form the stratum corneum
_____ i. Dermal layer responsible for skin ridging
_____ j. Location of skin glands and vessels
_____ k. Location of skin-producing cells

1. Epidermis
2. Dermis
3. Subcutaneous tissue
4. Keratinocytes
5. Melanocytes
6. Keratin
7. Papillary layer
8. Fibroblasts

3. Identify the causes of the following assessment findings of the skin associated with aging.
   a. Wrinkling and skin laxity
   b. Dryness
   c. Easy bruising
   d. Thick, ridged, brittle nails

4. When obtaining important health information from a patient during assessment of the skin, it is important for the nurse to ask about
   a. a history of freckles as a child.
   b. patterns of weight gain and loss.
   c. communicable childhood illnesses.
   d. skin problems related to the use of medications.

5. Identify one specific finding identified by the nurse during assessment of each of the patient's functional health patterns that would indicate a risk factor for skin problems or a patient response to a skin problem.
   a. Health perception–health management
   b. Nutritional-metabolic
   c. Elimination
   d. Activity-exercise
   e. Sleep-rest
   f. Cognitive-perceptual
   g. Self-perception–self-concept
   h. Role-relationship
   i. Sexuality-reproductive
   j. Coping–stress tolerance
   k. Value-belief

6. When performing a physical assessment of the skin, the nurse
   a. palpates the temperature of the skin with the fingertips.
   b. assesses the degree of turgor by pinching the skin on the forearm.
   c. inspects specific lesions before performing a general examination of the skin.
   d. asks the patient to undress completely so all areas of the skin can be inspected.

7. The nurse observes that redness remains after palpation of a discolored lesion on the patient's leg. This finding is characteristic of
   a. varicosities.
   b. intradermal bleeding.
   c. dilated blood vessels.
   d. erythematous lesions.

8. A woman calls the health clinic and describes a rash over the abdomen and chest. She tells the nurse it has raised, fluid-filled, small blisters that are distinct.
   a. Identify the type of primary skin lesion described by this patient.
   b. What is the distribution terminology for these lesions?
   c. What additional information does the nurse need to record the critical components of these lesions?

9. The primary difference between an excoriation and an ulcer is that
   a. ulcers do not penetrate below the epidermal junction.
   b. excoriations involve only thinning of the epidermis and dermis.
   c. excoriations will form crusts or scabs, whereas ulcers remain open.
   d. an excoriation heals without scarring because the dermis is not involved.

10. When assessing for changes in skin color in an African American patient, the best place for the nurse to use is the
    a. sclera.
    b. oral mucosa.
    c. soles of the feet.
    d. palms of the hands.

11. A patient has a plaque lesion on the dorsal forearm. The type of biopsy most likely to be used for diagnosis of the lesion is
    a. a punch biopsy.
    b. a shave biopsy.
    c. an incisional biopsy.
    d. an excisional biopsy.

12. The most common diagnostic test used to determine a causative agent of skin infections is
    a. a culture.
    b. the Tzanck test.
    c. immunofluorescent studies.
    d. potassium hydroxide slides.

13. Word Search. Find the words that are defined by the clues given below. The words may be located horizontally, vertically, or diagonally and may be reversed.

```
I C V R D D B H P B D N M C R P F T Z A
I N S E I F M X H W Q O G X W E S S I I
F C T O S A U I V S T I S T G T P Z P C
Z T L E C I R T A X U T L P S E O Q R E
Z E O U R S C C J K S A A U O C Q G Z P
K G L G U T U L F A E C S S X H M M Q O
O E S T I Q R B E A L I G T J I A V A L
X K I G K L T I N E A F Z U I A F I E A
W S Z L G Y I O G S C I M L E E S H A U
M O J U V V W T J O S N V E V A C M H L
A M O T A M E H I L E E Y M T E O G B C
F I S S U R E I F V R H E C I I X Q I E
E K C C M X V O K F P C E U G I Y E G R
A C O M E D O E B H E I D N Q G T S V N
I K O M C Z G D E C G L A H G A O X E F
W W U G J V W H Q N E L U P A P L V G A
U H E X C O R I A T I O N O J D U P H R
M X E D Z F X L W Y C C W L I S N H D S
I D A A A W E S I J C E N E N N T A Y S
D Z R A L T B D B R T G F U Z A V N L B
```

Clues

a. Firm plaque caused by fluid in dermis
b. A defined collection of free fluid up to 0.5 cm in diameter
c. Tiny purple spots resulting from tiny hemorrhage
d. A circumscribed, flat discoloration
e. Linear loss of epidermis and dermis
f. Circumscribed collection of leukocytes and free fluid
g. Elevated solid lesion up to 0.5 cm in diameter
h. Excess dead epidermal cells
i. Benign tumor of blood or lymph vessels
j. Circumscribed, elevated solid lesion formed by confluence of papules
k. Irregular, crater-like loss of the epidermis and dermis
l. Excavation of epidermis; dermis exposed
m. Small, superficial, dilated blood vessels
n. Loss of melanin
o. Excessive scar tissue
p. Abnormal hairiness in women
q. Thickening of skin
r. Mole
s. Swelling caused by bleeding
t. Overlying skin surfaces
u. Associated with acne vulgaris
v. Loss of hair

Nursing Management: Integumentary Problems

1. Identify whether the following statements are true (*T*) or false (*F*). If a statement is false, correct the bold word(s) to make the statement true.

_____ a. Exposure to **UVA rays** is believed to be the most important factor in the development of skin cancer.

_____ b. **Photosensitivity** results when certain chemicals in body cells and tissues absorb light from the sun and release energy that harms the tissues and cells.

_____ c. When teaching a patient about the use of sunscreens that protect against exposure to both UVA and UVB rays, the nurse advises the patient to look for the inclusion of **benzophenones**.

_____ d. The photosensitivity caused by various drugs can be blocked by the use of **topical hydrocortisone**.

_____ e. The nutrient that is critical in maintaining and repairing the structure of epithelial cells is **vitamin C**.

_____ f. One of the detrimental effects of obesity on the skin is **increased sweating**.

2. Match the following skin conditions with their most typical characteristics (answers may be used more than once).

_____ a. Skin cancer with highest mortality rate
_____ b. Slow-growing tumor with rare metastasis
_____ c. Neoplastic growth of melanocytes
_____ d. Precursor of squamous cell carcinoma
_____ e. Lesions keratitic and firm
_____ f. Condition treated with topical 5-FU
_____ g. Most common skin cancer
_____ h. Frequently occurs on previously damaged skin
_____ i. Irregular color and asymmetrical shape
_____ j. Precursor of malignant melanoma
_____ k. Noduloulcerative type has "pearly" borders

1. Actinic keratosis
2. Dysplastic nevus syndrome
3. Basal cell carcinoma
4. Squamous cell carcinoma
5. Malignant melanoma

3. Describe what is indicated by the ABCDEs of malignant melanoma.

A:

B:

C:

D:

E:

4. A 46-year-old African American patient is scheduled to have a basal cell carcinoma on his cheek excised in the health care provider's office. When reviewing the patient's history, it is important for the nurse to ask the patient about a history of

a. unprotected sun exposure.
b. radiation treatment for acne.
c. prior treatments for the lesion.
d. exposure to harsh irritants such as ammonia.

5. The nurse plans care for a patient with a newly diagnosed malignant melanoma based on the knowledge that initial treatment may involve (select all that apply)

a. Mohs' surgery.
b. surgical excision.
c. localized radiation.
d. topical nitrogen mustard.

6. The patient is a 78-year-old woman who has had chronic respiratory disease for 30 years. She weighs 212 lb (96.4 kg) and is 5 ft 1 in (152.5 cm) tall. She has recently completed corticosteroid and antibiotic treatment for an exacerbation of her respiratory disease. Identify four specific predisposing factors for bacterial skin infection in this patient.

   a.

   b.

   c.

   d.

7. Crossword Puzzle: Skin Conditions

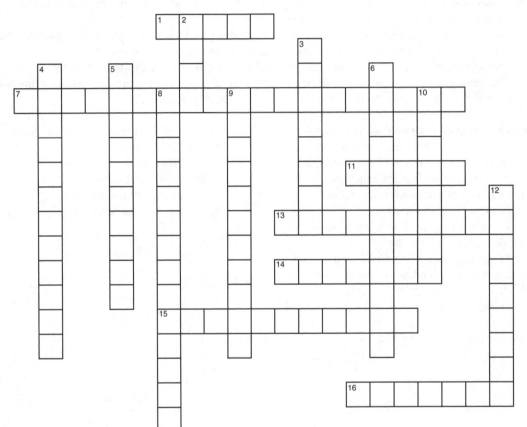

Across
1. Papillomavirus infection
7. Warty, irregular papules or plaques
11. Dermatophyte fungal infection
13. Deep inflammation of subcutaneous tissue
14. Increase in normal melanocytes
15. Head, body, or pubic lice
16. Allergic reaction to mite eggs

Down
2. Sebaceous gland inflammation
3. Deep follicular staphylococcal infection
4. Varicella infection of dermatome
5. Streptococcal infection of dermis
6. Small pustule at hair follicle
8. Viral oral vesicles
9. White, patchy yeast infection
10. Associated with poor hygiene
12. Excessive turnover of epithelial cells

8. Three conditions of the skin that more commonly occur in immunosuppressed patients are _____,

   _____, and _____.

9. The nurse should advise the patient with urticaria to
   a. apply topical benzene hexachloride.
   b. avoid contact with the causative agent.
   c. gradually expose the area to increasing amounts of sunlight.
   d. use over-the-counter antihistamines routinely to prevent the condition.

10. A nurse caring for a disheveled patient with poor hygiene observes that the patient has small red lesions flush with the skin on the head and body. The patient complains of severe itching at the sites. The nurse should further assess the patient for
    a. nits on the shafts of his head hair.
    b. a history of sexually transmitted diseases.
    c. the presence of ticks attached to the scalp.
    d. the presence of burrows in the interdigital webs.

11. A patient with a contact dermatitis is treated with calamine lotion. The nurse knows that the base for this topical preparation includes
    a. a suspension of oil and water to lubricate and prevent drying.
    b. an emulsion of oil and water used for lubrication and protection.
    c. insoluble powders suspended in water that leave a residual powder on the skin.
    d. a mixture of a powder and ointment that causes drying when moisture is absorbed.

12. A patient with psoriasis is being treated with psoralen plus UVA light (PUVA) phototherapy. During the course of therapy, the nurse teaches the patient to wear protective eyewear that blocks all UV rays
    a. continuously for 6 hours after taking the medication.
    b. until the pupils are able to constrict on exposure to light.
    c. for 12 hours following treatment to prevent retinal damage.
    d. for 24 hours following treatment when indoors near a bright window.

13. Identify one instruction the nurse should provide to a patient receiving the following medications for dermatologic problems.
    a. Topical antibiotics
    b. Topical corticosteroids
    c. Systemic antihistamines
    d. Topical fluorouracil

14. Match the surgical interventions with conditions that they are used to treat (interventions may be used for more than one condition).
    _____ a. Electrodessication/coagulation
    _____ b. Excision
    _____ c. Mohs' surgery
    _____ d. Curettage
    _____ e. Cryosurgery

    1. Cutaneous malignancies
    2. Common and genital warts
    3. Small basal and squamous cell carcinomas
    4. Telangiectasia
    5. Lesions involving the dermis
    6. Seborrheic keratoses

15. The most appropriate dressings to use to promote comfort for a patient with an inflamed, pruritic dermatitis are
    a. cool tap water dressings.
    b. cool acetic acid dressings.
    c. warm sterile saline dressings.
    d. warm potassium permanganate dressings.

16. An appropriate intervention to promote debridement and removal of scales and crusts of skin lesions is
    a. warm oatmeal baths.
    b. warm saline dressings.
    c. cool sodium bicarbonate baths.
    d. cool magnesium sulfate dressings.

17. Identify the rationale for using the following interventions to control pruritus.
    a. Cool environment
    b. Topical menthol, camphor, or phenol
    c. Soaks and baths

18. A female patient with chronic skin lesions of   face and arms tells the nurse that she cannot stand to look at herself in the mirror anymore because of her appearance. Ba   ' on this information, the nurse identifies the nursing diagnosis of
    a. anxiety related to personal appearance.
    b. disturbed body image related to perception nsightly lesions.
    c. social isolation related to decreased activities a result of poor self-image.
    d. ineffective self-health management related to l   of knowledge of cover-up techniques.

19. To prevent lichenification related to chronic skin pro   ns, the nurse encourages the patient to
    a. use measures to control itching.
    b. wear sterile gloves when touching the lesions.
    c. use careful hand washing and safe disposal of soiled   sings.
    d. use topical antibiotics with wet-to-dry dressings over t   sions.

20. The most common reason elective cosmetic surgery is reque   ' by patients is to
    a. improve self-image.
    b. remove deep acne scars.
    c. lighten the skin in pigmentation problems.
    d. prevent skin changes associated with aging.

21. Identify one cosmetic procedure indicated for each of the following   lems.
    a. Redundant soft tissue conditions
    b. Obesity with subcutaneous fat accumulation
    c. Reduce fine wrinkles or remove facial lesions

22. A skin graft that is used to transfer skin and subcutaneous tissue to large are   of deep tissue destruction is a
    a. skin flap.
    b. free graft.
    c. soft tissue extension.
    d. free graft with microscopic vascular anastomoses.

CASE STUDY

Cellulitis

Patient Profile

W.B., a 72-year-old, cut his lower arm on a kitchen knife. At the time of the injury, he did not seek medical attention. On the fourth day following the injury, he began to be concerned about the condition of the wound and the way he was feeling.

Subjective Data

- States he has a fever and has had a general feeling of malaise
- Has pain in the area of the cut and the entire lower arm

Objective Data

- 4-cm area around cut is hot, erythematous, and edematous with redness extending both up and down his arm
- Temperature: 100.8° F (38.2° C)

Clinical Decision-Making Questions

Using a separate sheet of paper, answer the following questions.

1. What care of the wound should W.B. have taken to prevent the occurrence of cellulitis?
2. What are the usual etiologies of this type of infection?
3. What would you tell W.B. about the usual treatment of cellulitis?
4. What could result if treatment is not initiated and maintained?
5. *Priority Decision:* Based on the assessment data presented, what are the priority nursing diagnoses? Are there any collaborative problems?

1. Match the following characteristics of burns with the types of burns (answers may be used more than once).

    _____ a. Risk for cardiac dysrhythmias or arrest   1. Thermal

    _____ b. Hot cooking oil   2. Chemical

    _____ c. Tissue adherence with protein hydrolysis   3. Smoke and inhalation

    _____ d. Causes coagulation necrosis   4. Electrical

    _____ e. Can be caused by explosive flare

    _____ f. May cause carbon monoxide poisoning

    _____ g. Indicated by facial burns and hoarseness

2. Identify whether the following statements are true (*T*) or false (*F*). If a statement is false, correct the bold word(s) to make the statement true.

    _____ a. Inhalation injury below the glottis may occur with **exposure to toxic fumes**.

    _____ b. **Acid substances** that cause chemical burns continue to cause tissue damage even after being neutralized.

    _____ c. Lavage with large amounts of water is important to stop the burning process in **scald** injuries.

    _____ d. The visible skin injury seen with **an electrical burn** often does not represent the full extent of tissue damage.

    _____ e. Metabolic acidosis occurs immediately following an **acid chemical burn**.

3. When assessing a patient's full-thickness burn injury during the emergent phase, the nurse would expect to find
    a. leathery, dry, hard skin.
    b. red, fluid-filled vesicles.
    c. massive edema at the injury site.
    d. serous exudate on a shiny, dark-brown wound.

4. A patient has the following mixed deep partial-thickness and full-thickness burn injuries: face, anterior neck, right anterior trunk, and anterior surfaces of the right arm and lower leg.
    a. According to the Lund-Browder chart, what is the extent of the patient's burns?

    _____% total body surface area (TBSA)
    b. According to the rule of nines chart, what is the extent of the patient's burns?

    _____% TBSA
    c. Is it possible to determine the actual extent and depth of burn injury during the emergent phase of the burn? Why or why not?

5. *Priority Decision:* The initial intervention in the emergency management of a burn of any type is to
    a. establish and maintain an airway.
    b. assess for other associated injuries.
    c. establish an IV line with a large-gauge needle.
    d. remove the patient from the burn source and stop the burning process.

6. Describe the criteria for each of the phases of burn injury and the approximate time frame of each phase.
    a. Emergent
    b. Acute
    c. Rehabilitation

7. During the early emergent phase of burn injury, the patient's laboratory results would most likely include
    a. ↑ Hct, ↓ serum Na, ↑ serum K.
    b. ↓ Hct, ↓ serum albumin, ↓ serum Na, ↑ serum K.
    c. ↓ Hct, ↑ serum Na, ↑ serum K.
    d. ↑ Hct, ↓ serum Na, ↓ serum K.

8. The initial cause of hypovolemia during the emergent phase of burn injury is
   a. increased capillary permeability.
   b. loss of sodium to the interstitium.
   c. decreased vascular oncotic pressure.
   d. fluid loss from denuded skin surfaces.

9. The response of the immune system to a burn injury includes
   a. bone marrow stimulation.
   b. impaired function of WBCs.
   c. an increase in immunoglobulin levels.
   d. becoming overwhelmed by microorganisms entering denuded tissue.

10. One clinical manifestation the nurse would expect to find during the emergent phase in a patient with a full-thickness burn over the lower half of the body is
    a. fever.
    b. shivering.
    c. severe pain.
    d. unconsciousness.

11. A patient has a 20% TBSA deep partial-thickness and full-thickness burn to the right anterior chest and entire right arm. It is most important that the nurse assess the patient for
    a. presence of pain.
    b. swelling of the arm.
    c. formation of eschar.
    d. presence of pulses in the arms.

12. Nasotracheal or endotracheal intubation is instituted in burn patients who have
    a. electrical burns causing cardiac dysrhythmias.
    b. thermal burn injuries to the face, neck, or airway.
    c. respiratory distress resulting from eschar formation around the chest.
    d. symptoms of hypoxia as a result of carbon monoxide poisoning.

13. A patient is admitted to the emergency department at 10:15 PM following a flame burn at 9:30 PM. The patient has 40% TBSA deep partial-thickness and full-thickness burns and weighs 132 lb.
    a. According to the Parkland formula, the type of fluid prescribed for the patient would be _____, and the total amount to be administered during the first 24 hours would be _____ mL.
    b. The schedule for the fluid administration would be _____ mL between _____ and _____ (time), _____ mL between _____ and _____, and _____ mL between _____ and _____.
    c. Colloidal solutions are given the second 24 hours. Based on the patient's body weight, what amount of these solutions will be given during this time? _____
    d. The adequacy of the patient's fluid replacement is determined by _____ and _____.

14. A patient's deep partial-thickness burns are treated with the open method. When caring for the patient, the nurse
    a. ensures that sterile water is used in the debridement tank.
    b. wears a cap, mask, gown, and gloves during patient contact.
    c. uses sterile gloves to remove the dressings and wash the wounds.
    d. applies topical antimicrobial ointment with clean gloves to prevent wound trauma.

15. A patient with deep partial-thickness burns over 45% of his trunk and legs is going for debridement in the cart shower 48 hours postburn. The drug of choice to control the patient's pain during this activity is
    a. IV morphine.
    b. midazolam (Versed).
    c. IM meperidine (Demerol).
    d. long-acting oral morphine.

16. The nurse assesses absent bowel sounds and abdominal distention in a patient 12 hours postburn. The nurse notifies the health care provider and prepares to
    a. withhold all oral intake except water.
    b. insert a nasogastric tube for decompression.
    c. administer a histamine-2 blocking agent such as cimetidine (Tagamet).
    d. administer nutritional supplements through a feeding tube placed in the duodenum.

17. The nurse positions the patient with ear, face, and neck burns
    a. prone.
    b. on the side.
    c. without pillows.
    d. with extra padding around the head.

18. Identify three factors that increase nutritional needs during the emergent and acute phases of burn injury.
    a.

    b.

    c.

19. At the end of the emergent phase and the initial acute phase of burn injury, a patient has a serum sodium level of 152 mEq/L (152 mmol/L) and a serum potassium level of 2.8 mEq/L (2.8 mmol/L). The nurse recognizes that these imbalances could occur as a result of
    a. free oral water intake.
    b. prolonged hydrotherapy.
    c. mobilization of fluid and electrolytes at the acute phase.
    d. excessive fluid replacement with dextrose in water without potassium supplementation.

20. A burn patient has a nursing diagnosis of impaired physical mobility related to a limited range of motion (ROM) resulting from pain. An appropriate nursing intervention for this patient is to
    a. have the patient perform ROM exercises when pain is not present.
    b. teach the patient the importance of exercise to prevent contractures.
    c. provide analgesic medications before physical activity and exercise.
    d. arrange for the physical therapist to encourage exercise during hydrotherapy.

21. The nurse suspects the possibility of sepsis in the burn patient based on changes in
    a. vital signs.
    b. urinary output.
    c. gastrointestinal function.
    d. burn wound appearance.

22. Identify one major complication of burns that is believed to be stress-related that may occur in each of the following systems during the acute burn phase.
    a. Neurologic
    b. Gastrointestinal
    c. Endocrine

23. Complete the following sentences.
    a. A permanent skin graft that may be available for the patient with large body surface area burns who has limited skin for donor harvesting is _____.
    b. Early excision and grafting of burn wounds involve excising _____ down to clean viable tissue and applying _____.
    c. Blebs can be removed from skin grafts by _____.

24. To help a burn patient who has developed an increasing dread of painful dressing changes, it would be most appropriate to ask the health care provider to prescribe
    a. midazolam (Versed) to be used with morphine before dressing changes.
    b. morphine in a dosage range so that more may be given before dressing changes.
    c. buprenorphine (Buprenex) to be administered with morphine before dressing changes.
    d. patient-controlled analgesia so that the patient may have control over analgesic administration.

25. During the rehabilitation phase of a burn injury, the contour of scarring can be controlled with
    a. pressure garments.
    b. avoidance of sunlight.
    c. splinting joints in extension.
    d. application of emollient lotions.

26. *Priority Decision:* The nurse has received the change of shift report on his group of patients. Indicate the priority order for the nurse to see these patients.
    _____ a. a 40-year-old female returning from the PACU following surgical debridement of her back and legs.
    _____ b. a 76-year-old male with partial-thickness burns of his arms and abdomen who is complaining of severe pain.
    _____ c. a 62-year-old female just admitted following partial-thickness burns to her anterior chest, face, and neck.
    _____ d. an 18-year-old male with full-thickness burns of his lower extremities who is refusing to go for his scheduled dressing change.

CASE STUDY
Burn Patient in Rehabilitation Phase
Patient Profile

D.K. is a 30-year-old woman who has been in the burn center for 3 weeks. She sustained partial- and full-thickness burns to both hands and forearms while cooking. She has undergone three surgeries for escharotomy and split-thickness skin grafting. D.K. is married and has three young children at home. Her health care providers feel she is nearly ready for discharge, but she has been tearful and noncompliant with therapy. D.K. and her husband refuse to look at her hand grafts, which continue to require light dressings. She has not seen her children since admission.

Clinical Decision-Making Questions

Using a separate sheet of paper, answer the following questions.

1. When should discharge planning be initiated with D.K.? Who should be involved in the planning and implementation of the educational process before discharge?
2. Describe the nutritional needs D.K. will have after discharge and interventions to meet those needs.
3. D.K. has been wearing hand and elbow splints at night while in the burn center. What instructions will D.K. need regarding her splinting and exercise routine at home?
4. D.K. complains of tightness in her hands, which restricts her motion. She uses this excuse to avoid exercise and independent performance of her activities of daily living. What activities and education would be beneficial to address this issue?
5. *Priority Decision:* D.K. and her husband have been extremely upset and anxious regarding D.K.'s discharge. They are not actively participating in the discharge planning process. What priority interventions should the staff implement to assist the couple?
6. What are some of the feelings D.K. and her family may experience following her return home? What can the nurse do to prepare the family?
7. *Priority Decision:* What are the priority needs that must be addressed with D.K. and her husband regarding dressing changes and graft care before discharge from the burn center? Discuss how this should be managed.
8. *Priority Decision:* Based on the assessment data presented, what are the priority nursing diagnoses? Are there any collaborative problems?

Nursing Assessment: Respiratory System

1. Identify the structures in the following illustration.

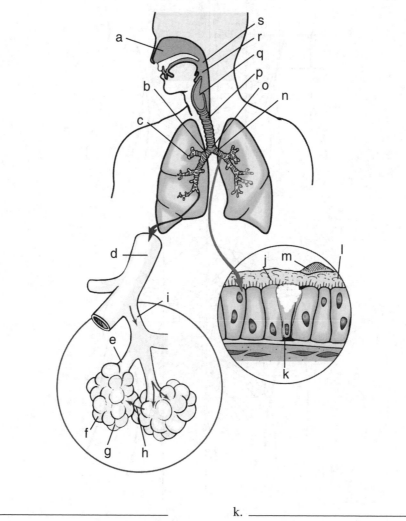

a. _____	k. _____
b. _____	l. _____
c. _____	m. _____
d. _____	n. _____
e. _____	o. _____
f. _____	p. _____
g. _____	q. _____
h. _____	r. _____
i. _____	s. _____
j. _____	

2. Identify the structures and the landmarks of the chest wall in the following illustrations.

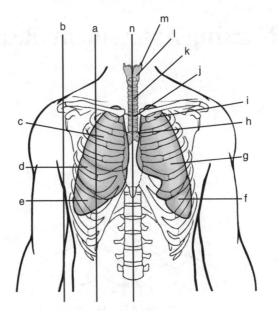

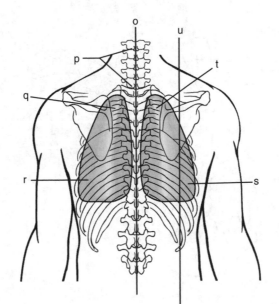

a. _____

b. _____

c. _____

d. _____

e. _____

f. _____

g. _____

h. _____

i. _____

j. _____

k. _____

l. _____

m. _____

n. _____

o. _____

p. _____

q. _____

r. _____

s. _____

t. _____

u. _____

3. Word Search. Find the words that are defined by the clues given below. The words may be located horizontally, vertically, or diagonally and may be reversed.

```
E  D  T  N  A  T  C  A  F  R  U  S  T  A
S  E  M  P  Y  E  M  A  N  I  C  U  R  T
E  A  R  O  C  A  R  I  N  A  L  U  A  H
T  D  I  P  W  M  I  R  S  D  E  M  C  O
A  S  V  I  S  C  E  R  A  L  O  C  H  N
N  P  I  M  T  A  A  Y  P  S  I  M  E  G
I  A  S  O  I  L  A  L  M  L  G  B  A  O
B  C  T  H  O  R  A  C  I  C  C  A  G  E
R  E  F  E  S  T  L  A  R  Y  N  X  I  T
U  L  V  T  E  P  I  G  L  O  T  T  I  S
T  L  S  I  U  O  L  F  U  E  L  G  N  A
A  E  R  O  C  O  M  P  L  I  A  N  C  E
W  A  E  V  R  E  N  C  I  N  E  R  H  P
P  F  B  W  E  T  I  S  R  A  M  D  E  S
```

Clues

a. Shapes and supports the chest wall
b. Covers the larynx during swallowing
c. Separates the larynx and the bronchi
d. Point of bifurcation of the trachea into bronchi
e. 150 ml of air in this area is not available for gas exchange
f. Keeps the alveoli from collapsing
g. Terminal structures of the respiratory tract
h. Elasticity of the lungs and thorax
i. Location of the vocal cords
j. Warm and moisturize inhaled air
k. Manubriosternal junction at level of carina
l. Membrane lining the chest cavity
m. Innervates the diaphragm
n. Small hairs that move mucus up the respiratory tract
o. The _____ pleura lines the lungs
p. Collection of pus in thoracic cavity

4. Identify whether the following statements are true (*T*) or false (*F*). If a statement is false, correct the bold word(s) to make the statement true.

   _____ a. **Partial pressure of oxygen** (PaO_2) is the amount of oxygen bound to hemoglobin in comparison with the amount of oxygen the hemoglobin can carry, expressed **in mm Hg**.

   _____ b. **Arterial oxygen saturation** (SaO_2) is the amount of oxygen dissolved in plasma and is expressed **as a percentage**.

   _____ c. If hemoglobin is **desaturated of oxygen**, more oxygen is released from the hemoglobin to provide oxygen to the tissues.

   _____ d. The oxygen-hemoglobin dissociation curve indicates that a patient is adequately oxygenated when PaO_2 is above 60 mm Hg because at this point hemoglobin O_2 saturation **remains above 90%**.

   _____ e. A patient has an oxyhemoglobin saturation of 90%. On the normal oxygen-hemoglobin dissociation curve with this saturation, he would have a PaO_2 of about **90 mm Hg**.

5. When providing oxygen therapy to a patient with a shift to the right in the oxygen-hemoglobin dissociation curve caused by an acidosis,
   a. low concentrations of oxygen are administered because more oxygen is delivered to the tissues.
   b. high concentrations of oxygen are necessary because blood picks up less oxygen from the lungs.
   c. low concentrations of oxygen are administered because blood picks up more oxygen from the lungs.
   d. high concentrations of oxygen may be administered to compensate for decreased unloading of oxygen in tissues.

6. A patient with an SaO_2 of 85% has a PaO_2 of 50 mm Hg. This indicates a
   a. shift to the left in the oxygen-hemoglobin dissociation curve that could be caused by acidosis.
   b. shift to the right in the oxygen-hemoglobin dissociation curve that could be caused by alkalosis.
   c. shift to the left in the oxygen-hemoglobin dissociation curve that could be caused by hypothermia.
   d. shift to the right in the oxygen-hemoglobin dissociation curve that could be caused by hyperthermia.

7. A 75-year-old patient breathing room air has the following arterial blood gas (ABG) results: pH 7.40, PaO_2 72 mm Hg, SaO_2 92%, $PaCO_2$ 40 mm Hg. An appropriate action by the nurse is to
   a. document the results in the patient's record.
   b. repeat the ABGs within an hour to validate the findings.
   c. encourage deep breathing and coughing to open the alveoli.
   d. initiate pulse oximetry for continuous monitoring of the patient's oxygen status.

8. A patient's ABGs include a PaO_2 of 88 mm Hg and a $PaCO_2$ of 38 mm Hg, and mixed venous blood gases include a PvO_2 of 40 mm Hg and $PvCO_2$ of 46 mm Hg. These findings indicate that the patient has
   a. impaired cardiac output.
   b. unstable hemodynamics.
   c. inadequate delivery of oxygen to the tissues.
   d. normal capillary oxygen–carbon dioxide exchange.

9. *Priority Decision:* A pulse oximetry monitor indicates that the patient has a drop in SpO_2 from 95% to 85% over several hours. The first action the nurse should take is to
   a. order stat ABGs to confirm the SpO_2 with a SaO_2.
   b. notify the health care provider of the change in baseline PaO_2.
   c. check the position of the probe on the finger or earlobe.
   d. start oxygen administration by nasal cannula at 2 L/min.

10. Pulse oximetry may not be a reliable indicator of oxygen saturation in the patient
    a. with a fever.
    b. who is anesthetized.
    c. in hypovolemic shock.
    d. receiving oxygen therapy.

11. A patient has an SpO$_2$ of 70%. What are four other assessments the nurse should consider in making a judgment about the adequacy of the patient's oxygenation?
    a.
    b.
    c.
    d.

12. Criteria for the use of continuous oxygen therapy include
    a. SpO$_2$ of 95%; PaO$_2$ of 70 mm Hg.
    b. SpO$_2$ of 90%; PaO$_2$ of 60 mm Hg.
    c. SpO$_2$ of 88%; PaO$_2$ of 55 mm Hg.
    d. SpO$_2$ of 75%; PaO$_2$ <40 mm Hg.

13. An excess of carbon dioxide in the blood causes an increased respiratory rate and volume because
    a. CO$_2$ displaces oxygen on hemoglobin, leading to a decreased PaO$_2$.
    b. CO$_2$ causes an increase in the amount of hydrogen ions available in the body.
    c. CO$_2$ combines with water to form carbonic acid, lowering the pH of cerebrospinal fluid.
    d. CO$_2$ directly stimulates chemoreceptors in the medulla to increase respiratory rate and volume.

14. The respiratory defense mechanism that is most impaired by smoking is
    a. filtration of air.
    b. the cough reflex.
    c. mucociliary clearance.
    d. reflex bronchoconstriction.

15. Identify two specific causes of each of the following age-related changes in the respiratory system.
    a. Decreased PaO$_2$
    b. Barrel-chest appearance
    c. Decreased secretion clearance
    d. Decreased resistance to infection

16. Identify one specific finding identified by the nurse during assessment of each of the patient's functional health patterns that indicates a risk factor for respiratory problems or a patient response to an actual respiratory problem.
    a. Health perception–health management
    b. Nutritional-metabolic
    c. Elimination
    d. Activity-exercise
    e. Sleep-rest
    f. Cognitive-perceptual
    g. Self-perception–self-concept
    h. Role-relationship
    i. Sexuality-reproductive
    j. Coping–stress tolerance
    k. Value-belief

17. Match the following abnormal assessment findings with the assessment technique used to detect them (answers may be used more than once).
    _____ a. Dullness
    _____ b. Limited chest expansion
    _____ c. Hyperresonance
    _____ d. Increased tactile fremitus
    _____ e. Finger clubbing
    _____ f. Tracheal deviation
    _____ g. Pleural friction rub
    _____ h. Wheeze
    _____ i. Use of accessory muscles
    _____ j. Barrel chest
    _____ k. Stridor

    1. Inspection
    2. Palpation
    3. Percussion
    4. Auscultation

18. To assess the patient's chest expansion, the nurse places
    a. the thumbs at the midline of the lower chest.
    b. the palms of the hands against the chest wall.
    c. the index fingers on either side of the trachea.
    d. one hand on the lower anterior chest and one hand on the upper abdomen.

19. The nurse records the presence of an increased anteroposterior (AP) diameter of the chest when
    a. there is a prominent protrusion of the sternum.
    b. the width of the chest is equal to the depth of the chest.
    c. there is equal but diminished movement of the two sides of the chest.
    d. the patient cannot fully expand the lungs because of kyphosis of the spine.

20. The presence of bronchovesicular breath sounds in the peripheral lung fields is described as
    a. rhonchi.
    b. crackles.
    c. adventitious sounds.
    d. abnormal lung sounds.

21. Match the descriptions or possible etiologies with the appropriate abnormal assessment findings.
    _____ a. Finger clubbing   1. Lung consolidation with fluid or exudate
    _____ b. Stridor   2. Air trapping
    _____ c. Wheezes   3. Atelectasis
    _____ d. Pleural friction rub   4. Interstitial filling with fluid
    _____ e. Increased tactile fremitus 5. Bronchoconstriction
    _____ f. Hyperresonance   6. Partial obstruction of trachea or larynx
    _____ g. Fine crackles   7. Chronic hypoxemia
    _____ h. Absent breath sounds   8. Pleurisy

22. A nurse has been exposed to tuberculosis (TB) during care of a patient with TB and has TB skin testing performed. The nurse is considered uninfected if
    a. there is no redness or induration at the injection site.
    b. there is an induration of only 5 mm at the injection site.
    c. testing causes a 10-mm reddened flat area at the injection site.
    d. a negative skin test is followed by another negative skin test in 3 weeks.

23. A primary nursing responsibility after obtaining a blood specimen for ABGs is
    a. adding heparin to the blood specimen.
    b. applying pressure to the puncture site for 2 full minutes.
    c. taking the specimen immediately to the laboratory in an iced container.
    d. avoiding any changes in oxygen intervention for 20 minutes following the procedure.

24. When preparing a patient for a pulmonary angiogram scan, the nurse
    a. assesses the patient for iodine allergy.
    b. implements NPO orders for 6 to 12 hours before the test.
    c. ensures that informed consent has been obtained from the patient.
    d. informs the patient that radiation isolation for 24 hours after the test is necessary.

25. To prepare the patient for a thoracentesis, the nurse positions the patient
    a. side-lying with the affected side up.
    b. flat in the bed with the arms extended out to the side.
    c. sitting upright with the elbows on an over-the-bed table.
    d. in semi-Fowler's position with the arms above the head.

26. The nurse observes the patient for symptoms of a pneumothorax following a
    a. thoracentesis.
    b. ventilation-perfusion scan.
    c. pulmonary function test.
    d. positron emission tomography scan.

27. The health care provider orders a pulmonary angiogram for a patient admitted with dyspnea and hemoptysis. The nurse recognizes that this test is most commonly used to diagnose
    a. TB.
    b. cancer of the lung.
    c. airway obstruction.
    d. pulmonary embolism.

28. Match the following pulmonary capacities and function tests with their descriptions.
    _____ a. Vt   1. Amount of air exhaled in first second of forced vital capacity
    _____ b. RV   2. Maximum amount of air lungs can contain
    _____ c. TLC   3. Volume of air inhaled and exhaled with each breath
    _____ d. VC   4. Maximum amount of air that can be exhaled after maximum inhalation
    _____ e. FVC   5. Amount of air that can be quickly and forcefully exhaled after maximum inspiration
    _____ f. PEFR   6. Maximum rate of airflow during forced expiration
    _____ g. FEV_1 7. Amount of air remaining in lungs after forced expiration
    _____ h. FRC   8. Volume of air in lungs after normal exhalation

1. Identify whether the following statements are true (*T*) or false (*F*). If a statement is false, correct the bold word(s) to make the statement true.

   _____ a. A major deviation in the nasal septum that causes obstruction of nasal airflow is usually corrected by a **rhinoplasty**.

   _____ b. In the patient who has suffered a major frontal blow with a nasal fracture, the nurse should monitor for **leakage of cerebrospinal fluid**.

   _____ c. Preoperative teaching for the patient planning an elective rhinoplasty for cosmetic effects includes informing the patient to avoid **aspirin-containing products** for 2 weeks before and immediately following the surgery.

   _____ d. An individual who has nasal reactions to pollen that last 3 to 4 weeks, several times a year, is said to have **intermittent** allergic rhinitis.

   _____ e. Nasal polyps are a complication of long-term **allergic rhinitis**.

2. A patient develops epistaxis upon removal of a nasogastric tube. The nurse should
   a. pinch the soft part of the nose.
   b. position the patient on the side.
   c. have the patient hyperextend the neck.
   d. apply an ice pack to the back of the neck.

3. *Priority Decision:* The nurse receives an evening report on a patient who underwent posterior nasal packing for epistaxis earlier in the day. The first assessment of the patient the nurse should make is the
   a. patient's temperature.
   b. the level of the patient's pain.
   c. the drainage on the nasal dressing.
   d. the oxygen saturation by pulse oximetry.

4. The nurse teaches the patient with allergic rhinitis that the most effective way to decrease allergic symptoms is to
   a. undergo weekly immunotherapy.
   b. identify and avoid triggers of the allergic reaction.
   c. use cromolyn nasal spray prophylactically year-round.
   d. use over-the-counter antihistamines and decongestants during an acute attack.

5. During assessment of the patient with a viral upper respiratory infection, the nurse recognizes that antibiotics may be indicated based on the finding of
   a. cough and sore throat.
   b. copious nasal discharge.
   c. dyspnea and purulent sputum.
   d. 100° F (38° C) temperature.

6. A 36-year-old patient asks the nurse whether an influenza vaccine is necessary every year. The best response by the nurse is,
   a. "You should get the live, attenuated flu vaccine that is inhaled nasally every year."
   b. "Only health care workers in contact with high-risk patients should be immunized each year."
   c. "Annual vaccination is not necessary because previous immunity will protect you for several years."
   d. "New antiviral drugs, such as zanamivir (Relenza), eliminate the need for vaccine except in the older adult."

7. The nurse identifies a nursing diagnosis of ineffective health maintenance related to lack of knowledge of therapeutic regimen for a patient with acute sinusitis who
   a. continues to take antibiotics for a week after symptoms are relieved.
   b. uses aspirin or aspirin-containing products to relieve headache and facial pain.
   c. uses over-the-counter antihistamines to relieve symptoms of congestion and drainage.
   d. reports a lack of improvement in symptoms after 3 days of taking broad-spectrum antibiotics.

8. A patient with an acute pharyngitis is seen at the clinic with fever and severe throat pain that affects swallowing. On inspection, the throat is reddened and edematous with patchy yellow exudates. The nurse anticipates that collaborative management will include
   a. treatment with antibiotics.
   b. treatment with antifungal agents.
   c. a throat culture or rapid strep antigen test.
   d. treatment with medication only if the pharyngitis does not resolve in 3 to 4 days.

9. While the nurse is feeding a patient, the patient appears to choke on the food. List four symptoms that indicate to the nurse that the patient has a partial airway obstruction.
   a.

   b.

   c.

   d.

10. An advantage of a tracheostomy over an endotracheal tube for long-term management of an upper airway obstruction is that a tracheostomy
    a. is safer to perform in an emergency.
    b. allows for more comfort and mobility.
    c. has a lower risk of tracheal pressure necrosis.
    d. is less likely to lead to lower respiratory tract infection.

11. Match the following descriptions with the types of tracheostomy tubes (answers may be used more than once).
    _____ a. Patient can speak with attached air source with cuff inflated
    _____ b. Patient can swallow without aspiration but requires suctioning of secretions
    _____ c. Cuff pressure monitoring not required
    _____ d. Two tubings, one opening just above the cuff
    _____ e. Most likely to cause airway obstruction if exact steps are not followed to produce speech
    _____ f. Pilot tubing not capped
    _____ g. Airflow around tube and through window allows speaking when the cuff is deflated and the plug is inserted
    _____ h. Patient does not require mechanical ventilation and can protect airway
    _____ i. Cuff fills passively with air

    1. Cuffless tracheostomy tube
    2. Speaking tracheostomy tube
    3. Fenestrated tracheostomy tube
    4. Tracheostomy tube with foam-filled cuff

12. During care of a patient with a cuffed tracheostomy, the nurse notes that the tracheostomy tube has an inner cannula. To care for the tracheostomy appropriately, the nurse
    a. deflates the cuff and removes and suctions the inner cannula.
    b. removes the inner cannula and cleans the mucus from the tube.
    c. removes the inner cannula if the patient shows signs of airway obstruction.
    d. keeps the inner cannula in place at all times to prevent dislodging the tracheostomy tube.

13. List three precautions related to prevention of dislodgement of a tracheostomy tube the first several days after its placement.
   a.

   b.

   c.

14. ***Delegation Decision:*** In planning the care for a patient with a tracheostomy who has been stable and is to be discharged later in the day, the RN may delegate which of the following interventions to the LPN? (select all that apply)
   a. Assess the need for suctioning.
   b. Suction the tracheostomy.
   c. Assess the patient's swallowing ability.
   d. Teach the patient about home tracheostomy care.
   e. Provide tracheostomy care.

15. Nursing care of the patient with a cuffed tracheostomy tube in place includes
   a. changing the tube every 3 days.
   b. recording cuff pressure every 8 hours.
   c. performing mouth care every 12 hours.
   d. assessing arterial blood gases every 8 hours.

16. ***Priority Decision:*** A patient's tracheostomy tube becomes dislodged with vigorous coughing. The first action by the nurse is to
   a. attempt to replace the tube.
   b. notify the health care provider.
   c. place the patient in high Fowler's position.
   d. ventilate the patient with a manual resuscitation bag until the health care provider arrives.

17. To determine when the patient with a tracheostomy tube can effectively swallow, the nurse deflates the cuff and
   a. checks for a gag reflex at the back of the tongue with a tongue blade.
   b. asks the patient to drink 30 ml of milk and suctions the tube for colored secretions.
   c. has the patient swallow a small amount of water and observes for symptoms of respiratory distress.
   d. has the patient drink a small amount of blue-colored water, observing for coughing and colored secretions.

18. When obtaining a health history from a patient with possible cancer of the mouth, the nurse would expect the patient to report
   a. long-term denture use.
   b. heavy tobacco and alcohol use.
   c. persistent swelling of the neck and face.
   d. chronic herpes simplex infections of the mouth and lips.

19. The patient has been diagnosed with an early vocal cord malignancy. The nurse explains that usual treatment includes
   a. radiation therapy that preserves the quality of the voice.
   b. a hemilaryngectomy that prevents the need for a tracheostomy.
   c. a radical neck dissection that removes possible sites of metastasis.
   d. a total laryngectomy to prevent development of second primary cancers.

20. During preoperative teaching for the patient scheduled for a total laryngectomy, the nurse includes information related to
   a. the postoperative use of nonverbal communication techniques.
   b. techniques that will be used to alleviate a dry mouth and prevent stomatitis.
   c. the need for frequent, vigorous coughing in the first 24 hours postoperatively.
   d. self-help groups and community resources for patients with cancer of the larynx.

21. When assessing the patient upon return to the surgical unit following a total laryngectomy and radical neck dissection, the nurse would expect to find
    a. a closed-wound drainage system.
    b. a nasal endotracheal tube in place.
    c. a tracheostomy tube and mechanical ventilation.
    d. placement of a nasogastric tube with orders for tube feedings.

22. Following a supraglottic laryngectomy, the patient is taught how to use the supraglottic swallow to minimize the risk of aspiration. In teaching the patient about this technique, the nurse instructs the patient to
    a. perform Valsalva maneuver immediately after swallowing.
    b. breathe between each Valsalva maneuver and cough sequence.
    c. cough after swallowing to remove food from the top of the vocal cords.
    d. practice swallowing thin, watery fluids before attempting to swallow solid foods.

23. Discharge teaching by the nurse for the patient with a total laryngectomy includes
    a. how to use esophageal speech to communicate.
    b. how to use a mirror to suction the tracheostomy.
    c. the necessity of never covering the laryngectomy stoma.
    d. the need to use baths instead of showers for personal hygiene.

24. The most normal functioning method of speech restoration in the patient with a total laryngectomy is
    a. a voice prosthesis.
    b. esophageal speech.
    c. an electrolarynx held to the neck.
    d. an electrolarynx placed in the mouth.

CASE STUDY
Rhinoplasty
Patient Profile

F.N. is a 28-year-old married accountant who sustained bilateral fractures of the nose, three rib fractures, and a comminuted fracture of the tibia in an automobile crash 5 days ago. An open reduction and internal fixation of the tibia were performed the day of the trauma, and he is now scheduled for a rhinoplasty to reestablish an adequate airway and improve cosmetic appearance.

Subjective Data

- Reports facial pain at a level of 6 on a 0-10 point scale
- Expresses concern about his facial appearance
- Complains of dry mouth

Objective Data

- Oral respirations at 24 minutes; pulse 68 beats/min
- Bilateral ecchymosis of eyes (raccoon eyes)
- Periorbital edema and edema of face reduced by about half since second hospital day
- Has been NPO since midnight in preparation for surgery

Clinical Decision-Making Questions

Using a separate sheet of paper, answer the following questions.

1. When F.N. was admitted, examination of his nose revealed clear drainage. What is the significance of the drainage? What testing is indicated?
2. What is the reason for delaying repair of his nose for several days after the trauma?
3. What measures should be taken to maintain his airway before and after surgery?
4. *Priority Decision:* When F.N. arrives in the postanesthesia care unit (PACU) following surgery, what priority assessments should the nurse make in the immediate postoperative period?
5. *Priority Decision:* F.N.'s nasal packing is removed in 24 hours, and he is to be discharged. What priority predischarge teaching should the nurse perform?
6. *Priority Decision:* Based on the assessment data presented, what are the priority nursing diagnoses? Are there any collaborative problems?

CHAPTER 28

Nursing Management: Lower Respiratory Problems

1. List the three methods by which microorganisms that cause pneumonia reach the lungs.

    a.

    b.

    c.

2. The classification of pneumonia as community-acquired pneumonia (CAP) or hospital-acquired pneumonia (HAP) is clinically useful because
    a. atypical pneumonia syndrome is more likely to occur in HAP.
    b. diagnostic testing does not have to be used to identify causative agents.
    c. causative agents can be predicted, and empiric treatment is often effective.
    d. IV antibiotic therapy is necessary for HAP, but oral therapy is adequate for CAP.

3. Match the following microorganisms to the type of pneumonia with which they are most commonly associated (answers may be used more than once).

    _____ a. *Pneumocystis jiroveci*   1. Community-acquired pneumonia
    _____ b. *Escherichia coli*   2. Hospital-acquired pneumonia
    _____ c. *Pseudomonas aeruginosa*   3. Opportunistic pneumonia
    _____ d. *Legionella pneumophila*
    _____ e. *Staphylococcus aureus*
    _____ f. *Streptococcus pneumoniae*
    _____ g. *Enterobacter* sp.
    _____ h. *Klebsiella* sp.
    _____ i. *Haemophilus influenzae*
    _____ j. Cytomegalovirus
    _____ k. *Mycoplasma pneumoniae*

4. Identify the pathophysiologic stages of pneumococcal pneumonia.
    a. Massive dilation of capillaries with alveolar filling with organisms, neutrophils, and fibrin

    _____

    b. Exudate becomes lysed and processed by macrophages, and normal lung tissue is restored

    _____

    c. Outpouring of fluid into alveoli that supports microorganism growth and spread

    _____

    d. Blood flow decreases and leukocytes and fibrin consolidate in affected lung tissue

    _____

5. When obtaining a health history from a patient at the clinic with suspected CAP, the nurse expects the patient to report
    a. a dry, hacking cough.
    b. a recent loss of consciousness.
    c. an abrupt onset of fever and chills.
    d. a gradual onset of headache and sore throat.

124 Chapter 28 Nursing Management: Lower Respiratory Problems

6. Initial antibiotic treatment for pneumonia is usually based on
   a. the severity of symptoms.
   b. the presence of characteristic leukocytes.
   c. Gram stains and cultures of sputum specimens.
   d. history and physical examination and characteristic chest radiographic findings.

7. *Priority Decision:* After the health care provider sees a patient hospitalized with a stroke who developed a fever and adventitious lung sounds, the following orders are written. Which will the nurse implement first?
   a. Anterior/posterior and lateral chest x-rays
   b. Start IV levofloxacin (Levaquin) 500 mg q24 hr
   c. Sputum specimen for Gram stain and culture and sensitivity
   d. Complete blood count (CBC) with white blood cell (WBC) count and differential

8. Identify four clinical situations in which hospitalized patients are at risk for aspiration pneumonia and one nursing intervention for each situation that is indicated to prevent pneumonia.

Situation	Intervention
a.	
b.	
c.	
d.	

9. Following assessment of a patient with pneumonia, the nurse identifies a nursing diagnosis of impaired gas exchange based on the findings of
   a. SpO$_2$ of 86%.
   b. crackles in both lower lobes.
   c. temperature of 101.4° F (38.6° C).
   d. production of greenish purulent sputum.

10. A patient is admitted to the hospital with fever, chills, a productive cough with rusty sputum, and pleuritic chest pain. Pneumococcal pneumonia is suspected. An appropriate nursing diagnosis for the patient based on the patient's manifestations is
    a. hyperthermia related to acute infectious process.
    b. chronic pain related to ineffective pain management.
    c. risk for injury related to disorientation and confusion.
    d. ineffective airway clearance related to retained secretions.

11. A patient with pneumonia has a nursing diagnosis of ineffective airway clearance related to pain, fatigue, and thick secretions. An appropriate nursing intervention for the patient is to
    a. encourage a fluid intake of at least 3 L/day.
    b. administer oxygen as prescribed to maintain SpO$_2$ of 95%.
    c. place the patient in semi-Fowler's position to maximize lung expansion.
    d. teach the patient to take three or four shallow breaths before coughing to minimize pain.

12. During an annual health assessment of a 65-year-old clinic patient, the patient tells the nurse he had the pneumonia vaccine when he was age 58. The nurse advises the patient that the best way for him to prevent pneumonia now is to
    a. seek medical care and antibiotic therapy for all upper respiratory infections.
    b. obtain the pneumococcal vaccine this year with an annual influenza vaccine.
    c. obtain the pneumococcal vaccine if he is exposed to individuals with pneumonia.
    d. obtain only the influenza vaccine every year because he has immunity to the pneumococcus.

13. The resurgence in tuberculosis (TB) resulting from the emergence of multidrug-resistant strains of *Mycobacterium tuberculosis* was primarily the result of
    a. a lack of effective means to diagnose TB.
    b. poor compliance with drug therapy in patients with TB.
    c. the increased population of immunosuppressed individuals with AIDS.
    d. indiscriminate use of antitubercular drugs in treatment of other infections.

14. ***Priority Decision:*** A patient diagnosed with class 3 TB 1 week ago is admitted to the hospital with symptoms of chest pain. Initially, the nurse gives the highest priority to
    a. administering the patient's antitubercular drugs.
    b. admitting the patient to an airborne-infection isolation room.
    c. preparing the patient's room with suction equipment and extra linens.
    d. placing the patient in an intensive care unit where he can be closely monitored.

15. When obtaining a health history from a patient suspected of having early TB, the nurse asks the patient about experiencing
    a. chest pain, hemoptysis, and weight loss.
    b. fatigue, low-grade fever, and night sweats.
    c. cough with purulent mucus and fever with chills.
    d. pleuritic pain, nonproductive cough, and temperature elevation at night.

16. List the components of the four-drug therapy that is recommended for the initial 2-month treatment of clinically active TB.

    _____

    _____

    _____

    _____

17. A patient with active TB continues to have positive sputum cultures after 6 months of treatment because she says she cannot remember to take the medication all the time. The best action by the nurse is to
    a. schedule the patient to come to the clinic every day to take the medication.
    b. have a patient who has recovered from TB tell the patient about his successful treatment.
    c. schedule more teaching sessions so the patient will understand the risks of noncompliance.
    d. arrange for directly observed therapy by a responsible family member or a public health nurse.

18. A patient receiving chemotherapy for breast cancer develops a cryptococcus infection of the lungs and is treated with IV amphotericin B. The nurse monitors the patient carefully during the drug's administration with the knowledge that this drug increases the patient's risk for (select all that apply)
    a. renal impairment.
    b. immunosuppression.
    c. nausea and vomiting.
    d. hypersensitivity reactions.
    e. malignant hyperthermia reaction.

19. To reduce the risk for most occupational lung diseases, the most important measure promoted by the occupational nurse is
    a. maintaining smoke-free work environments for all employees.
    b. using masks and effective ventilation systems to reduce exposure to irritants.
    c. inspection and monitoring of workplaces by national occupational safety agencies.
    d. requiring periodic chest x-rays and pulmonary function tests for exposed employees.

20. During a health-promotion program, the nurse plans to target women in a discussion of lung cancer prevention because (select all that apply)
    a. women develop lung cancer at a younger age than men.
    b. more women die of lung cancer than die from breast cancer.
    c. women have a worse prognosis from lung cancer than do men.
    d. women who smoke are at greater risk to develop lung cancer than men who smoke.
    e. women are more likely to develop small cell carcinoma than men

21. A patient with a 40-pack-year history of smoking has recently stopped because of the fear of developing lung cancer. The patient asks the nurse what he can do to learn about whether he develops lung cancer. The best response by the nurse is,
    a. "You should get a chest x-ray every 6 months to screen for any new growths."
    b. "It would be very rare for you to develop lung cancer now that you have stopped smoking."
    c. "You should monitor for any persistent cough, wheezing, or difficulty breathing, which could indicate tumor growth."
    d. "Screening measures for lung cancer are controversial, but we can discuss the advantages and disadvantages of various measures."

22. A patient with a lung mass found on chest x-ray is undergoing further testing. The nurse explains that a diagnosis of lung cancer can be confirmed by
    a. CT scans.
    b. lung tomograms.
    c. pulmonary angiography.
    d. biopsy positive for malignant cells.

23. Match the following treatments for lung cancer with their descriptions.
    _____ a. Considered primary treatment for small cell lung cancer (SCLC)
    _____ b. Dye activated by laser light that destroys cancer cells
    _____ c. Freezes bronchial tumors with use of bronchoscope
    _____ d. Palliative treatment for airway collapse or compression therapy
    _____ e. Best procedure for cure of lung cancer
    _____ f. Medications that block growth of cancer cells
    _____ g. Palliative treatment by bronchoscope to remove obstructing bronchial tumors
    _____ h. Improves survival when combined with chemotherapy and surgery
    _____ i. Used to prevent metastasis to the brain

    1. Surgical therapy
    2. Radiation therapy
    3. Chemotherapy
    4. Prophylactic cranial radiation
    5. Bronchoscopic laser
    6. Photodynamic therapy
    7. Airway stenting
    8. Cryotherapy
    9. Biologic and targeted therapy

24. A patient with advanced lung cancer refuses pain medication, saying, "I deserve everything this cancer can give me." The nurse's best response to the patient is
    a. "Would talking to a counselor help you?"
    b. "Can you tell me what the pain means to you?"
    c. "Are you using the pain as a punishment for your smoking?"
    d. "Pain control will help you to deal more effectively with your feelings."

25. Complete the following statements.
    a. Collapse of the lung from accumulation of air in the intrapleural space caused by a sucking chest wound is a(n) _____.

    b. Collapse of the lung from accumulation of blood in the intrapleural space is a(n) _____.

    c. Collapse of the lung from accumulation of air in the intrapleural space caused by an injury to the lungs from closed rib fractures is known as a(n) _____.

    d. When air in the intrapleural space progressively increases intrathoracic pressure because it cannot escape during expiration, a(n) _____ occurs.

    e. Accumulation of lymphatic fluid in the pleural space from a leak in the thoracic duct is known as _____.

    f. The usual treatment for large pneumothorax or hemothorax of any cause is a(n) _____ connected to _____.

26. To determine whether a tension pneumothorax is developing in a patient with chest trauma, the nurse assesses the patient for
    a. dull percussion sounds on the injured side.
    b. severe respiratory distress and tracheal deviation.
    c. muffled and distant heart sounds with decreasing blood pressure.
    d. decreased movement and diminished breath sounds on the affected side.

27. Following a motor vehicle accident, the nurse assesses the driver for which distinctive sign of flail chest?
    a. Severe hypotension
    b. Chest pain over ribs
    c. Absence of breath sounds
    d. Paradoxical chest movement

28. On the figure below, locate and label the water-seal chamber, the suction control chamber, and the collection chamber.

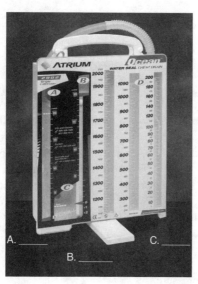

29. Describe the function of each chamber:
    a. Water-seal
    b. Suction control
    c. Collection

30. The nurse should check for leaks in the chest tube and pleural drainage system when
    a. there is constant bubbling of water in the suction control chamber.
    b. there is continuous bubbling in the water-seal chamber.
    c. the water levels in the water-seal and suction control chambers are decreased.
    d. fluid in the tubing in the water-seal chamber fluctuates with the patient's breathing.

31. When caring for the patient with a chest tube, the nurse should intervene when the nursing assistant is
    a. looping the drainage tubing on the bed.
    b. securing the drainage container in an upright position.
    c. stripping or milking the chest tube to promote drainage.
    d. reminding the patient to cough and deep-breathe every 2 hours.

32. Match the following chest surgeries with their descriptions.

   _____ a. Thoracotomy   1. Removal of a small lesion
   _____ b. Lobectomy   2. Removal of a lung
   _____ c. Wedge resection   3. Incision into the thorax
   _____ d. Segmental resection   4. Stripping of a fibrous membrane
   _____ e. Lung volume–reduction surgery   5. Removal of one lung lobe
   _____ f. Decortication   6. Removal of lung segment
   _____ g. Pneumonectomy   7. Removal of lung tissue by multiple wedge excisions

33. Following a thoracotomy, the patient has a nursing diagnosis of ineffective airway clearance related to inability to cough as a result of pain and positioning. The best nursing intervention for this patient is to
   a. have the patient drink 16 oz of water before attempting to deep-breathe.
   b. auscultate the lungs before and after deep-breathing and coughing regimens.
   c. place the patient in the Trendelenburg position for 30 minutes before the coughing exercises.
   d. medicate the patient with analgesics 20 to 30 minutes before assisting to cough and deep-breathe.

34. Match the following restrictive lung conditions with the mechanisms that cause decreased vital capacity (VC) and decreased total lung capacity (TLC).

   _____ a. Pleural effusion   1. Central depression of respiratory rate and depth
   _____ b. Empyema   2. Lung expansion restricted by fluid in pleural space
   _____ c. Pleurisy   3. Paralysis of respiratory muscles
   _____ d. Atelectasis   4. Excess fat restricts chest wall and diaphragmatic excursion
   _____ e. Idiopathic pulmonary fibrosis   5. Inflammation of the pleura restricting lung movement
   _____ f. Kyphoscoliosis   6. Lung expansion restricted by pus in intrapleural space
   _____ g. Opioid and sedative overdose   7. Presence of collapsed, airless alveoli
   _____ h. Muscular dystrophy   8. Spinal angulation restricting ventilation
   _____ i. Pickwickian syndrome   9. Excessive connective tissue in lungs

35. ***Priority Decision:*** Two days after undergoing pelvic surgery, a patient develops marked dyspnea and anxiety. The first action the nurse should take is to
   a. raise the head of the bed.
   b. notify the health care provider.
   c. take the patient's pulse and blood pressure.
   d. determine the patient's SpO_2 with an oximeter.

36. A pulmonary embolus is suspected in a patient with a deep-vein thrombosis who develops hemoptysis, tachycardia, and pleuritic chest pain, and diagnostic testing is scheduled. The nurse plans to teach the patient about
   a. chest radiographs.
   b. spiral (helical) CT scan.
   c. pulmonary angiography.
   d. ventilation-perfusion lung scan.

37. Match the following conditions with their related mechanisms of pulmonary hypertension.

   _____ a. Chronic obstructive pulmonary disease (COPD)   1. Stiffening of pulmonary vasculature
   _____ b. Pulmonary fibrosis   2. Obstruction of pulmonary blood flow
   _____ c. Pulmonary embolism   3. Pulmonary capillary/alveolar damage

38. While caring for a patient with primary pulmonary hypertension, the nurse observes that the patient has exertional dyspnea and chest pain, in addition to fatigue. The nurse knows that these symptoms are related to
   a. decreased left ventricular output.
   b. right ventricular hypertrophy and dilation.
   c. increased systemic arterial blood pressure.
   d. development of alveolar interstitial edema.

39. The primary treatment for cor pulmonale is directed toward
    a. controlling dysrhythmias.
    b. dilating the pulmonary arteries.
    c. strengthening the cardiac muscle.
    d. treating the underlying pulmonary condition.

40. Six days after a heart-lung transplant, the patient develops a low-grade fever and a decreased SpO_2 with exercise. The nurse recognizes that this may indicate
    a. a normal response to extensive surgery.
    b. a frequently fatal cytomegalovirus infection.
    c. acute rejection that can be treated with corticosteroids.
    d. obliterative bronchiolitis that plugs terminal bronchioles.

CASE STUDY
Pulmonary Hypertension

Patient Profile

T.S. is a 46-year-old patient who was diagnosed with primary pulmonary hypertension at the age of 42. At that time she presented to her primary care health care provider with a history of increasing fatigue and recent onset of swelling in her feet and ankles. A chest x-ray revealed severe cardiomegaly with pulmonary congestion. She underwent a right-sided cardiac catheterization, which showed very high pulmonary artery pressures. Since then, she has been treated with several drugs, but her pulmonary hypertension has never been controlled and her peripheral edema has progressively worsened.

Subjective Data

- Short of breath at rest and exercise intolerant to the extent that she had to quit her job
- Recently divorced from her husband
- Has two children: a girl, 10 years old, and a boy, 4 years old

Objective Data

- 3+ pitting edema from her feet to her knees
- Respirations: 28 at rest
- Heart rate: 92 and bounding

Clinical Decision-Making Questions

Using a separate sheet of paper, answer the following questions.

1. What drugs might T.S. have been given to treat her pulmonary hypertension?
2. Is T.S. a candidate for heart-lung or lung transplantation? Why or why not?
3. What transplantation procedure would be considered for T.S.? What is the rationale?
4. *Priority Decision:* What priority preoperative counseling would be necessary for T.S. to prepare for a transplantation procedure?
5. *Priority Decision:* Based on the assessment data presented, what are the priority nursing diagnoses? Are there any collaborative problems?

CHAPTER
29

Nursing Management:
Obstructive Pulmonary Diseases

1. While assisting a patient with asthma to identify specific triggers of the asthma, the nurse explains that
   a. food and drug allergies do not manifest in respiratory symptoms.
   b. exercise-induced asthma is seen only in individuals with sensitivity to cold air.
   c. asthma attacks are psychogenic in origin and can be controlled with relaxation techniques.
   d. viral upper respiratory infections are a common precipitating factor in acute asthma attacks.

2. A patient is admitted to the emergency department with an acute asthma attack. Which of the following assessments of the patient is of greatest concern to the nurse?
   a. The presence of a pulsus paradoxus
   b. Markedly diminished breath sounds with no wheezing
   c. Use of accessory muscles of respiration and a feeling of suffocation
   d. A respiratory rate of 34 breaths/min and increased pulse and blood pressure

3. A patient with asthma has the following arterial blood gas (ABG) results early in an acute asthma attack: pH 7.48, $PaCO_2$ 30 mm Hg, PaO_2 78 mm Hg. The most appropriate action by the nurse is to
   a. prepare the patient for mechanical ventilation.
   b. have the patient breathe in a paper bag to raise the $PaCO_2$.
   c. document the findings and monitor the ABGs for a trend toward acidosis.
   d. reduce the patient's oxygen flow rate to keep the PaO_2 at the current level.

4. Indicate the role or relationship of the following agents to asthma.
   a. Salicylates
   b. β-adrenergic blocking agents
   c. Beer and wine

5. Marked bronchoconstriction with air trapping and hyperinflation of the lungs in the patient with asthma is indicated by
   a. SaO_2 of 85%.
   b. PEFR of <150 L/min.
   c. FEV_1 of 85% of predicted.
   d. chest x-ray showing a flattened diaphragm.

6. Match the following drugs, first with their use in promoting quick relief of asthma symptoms or long-term control of symptoms and then with their primary mode of action (answers may be used more than once).

Use	Action		
_____	_____	a. albuterol nebulizer	1. Long-term control
_____	_____	b. oral prednisone	2. Quick-relief agent
_____	_____	c. triamcinolone inhaler	*Primary Mechanism of Action*
_____	_____	d. ipratropium inhaler	3. β₂-adrenergic agonist
_____	_____	e. oral theophylline	4. Mast-cell stabilizer
_____	_____	f. cromolyn inhaler	5. Leukotriene inhibitor
_____	_____	g. budesonide inhaler	6. Steroid antiinflammatory
_____	_____	h. montelukast	7. Methylxanthine bronchodilator
_____	_____	i. omalizumab	8. Anticholinergic
_____	_____	j. zileuton	9. Anti-IgE
_____	_____	k. beclomethasone inhaler	
_____	_____	l. nedocromil inhaler	
_____	_____	m. salmeterol inhaler	

7. Of the following instructions for patients about the use of asthma medications, check all those that are correct.

_____ a. When using pirbuterol (Maxair) and fluticasone (Flovent) inhalers, it does not make any difference which you use first.

_____ b. Cromolyn (Intal) inhalers should be used before exercise or when anticipating exposure to allergens known to cause asthma.

_____ c. The mouth should be rinsed thoroughly after using the ipratropium (Atrovent) inhaler to prevent oral candidiasis.

_____ d. The salmeterol (Serevent) inhaler should not be used more than every 12 hours.

_____ e. The best way to use a metered-dose inhaler is to hold it about 1 to 2 inches in front of your mouth before depressing the inhaler.

_____ f. You should wait 5 minutes before taking a second puff of any inhaled medication.

_____ g. If you use a spacer with your inhaler, depress the inhaler before starting to inhale.

_____ h. You should take zafirlukast (Accolate) tablets on an empty stomach.

_____ i. To use your dry powder inhaler (DPI), empty your lungs of air, close your lips around the mouthpiece, and inhale quickly and deeply.

8. To decrease the patient's sense of panic during an acute asthma attack, the best action of the nurse is to
   a. leave the patient alone to rest in a quiet, calm environment.
   b. stay with the patient and encourage slow, pursed-lip breathing.
   c. reassure the patient that the attack can be controlled with treatment.
   d. let the patient know his or her status is being closely monitored with frequent measurement of vital signs and SpO_2.

9. When a patient with asthma is admitted to the emergency department in severe respiratory distress, the nurse anticipates that initial drug treatment will most likely include administration of
   a. IV aminophylline.
   b. IV hydrocortisone.
   c. inhaled ipratropium.
   d. aerosolized albuterol.

10. When teaching the patient with asthma about the use of the peak flow meter, the nurse instructs the patient to
    a. carry the flow meter with the patient at all times in case an asthma attack occurs.
    b. follow written asthma action plan (e.g., increasing quick relief drugs) if the peak expiratory flow rate is in the yellow zone.
    c. use the flow meter to check the status of the patient's asthma every time the patient takes quick-relief medication.
    d. use the flow meter by emptying the lungs, closing the mouth around the mouthpiece, and inhaling through the meter as quickly as possible.

11. The nurse recognizes that additional teaching is needed when the patient with asthma says,
    a. "I should exercise every day if my symptoms are controlled."
    b. "I may use over-the-counter bronchodilator drugs occasionally if I develop chest tightness."
    c. "I should inform my spouse about my medications and how to get help if I have a severe asthma attack."
    d. "A diary to record my medication use, symptoms, peak expiratory flow rate (PEFR) levels, and activity level will help in adjusting my therapy."

12. Indicate whether the statement is true (*T*) or false (*F*). If it is false, correct the bold word(s) to make the statement true.

_____ a. The mortality rate from asthma is **greater** in men than in women.

_____ b. The incidence of COPD is **increasing** in women.

_____ c. Women with COPD respond better to **oxygen therapy** than do men.

_____ d. Cystic fibrosis has the **highest** incidence in whites.

_____ e. Female **whites** have the highest mortality rates from asthma.

13. Tobacco smoke causes defects in multiple areas of the respiratory system. For each of the areas listed below, identify one acute effect and one long-term effect of smoking.

	Acute Effect	**Long-Term Effect**
a. Alveolar macrophages		
b. Tongue		
c. Cilia		
d. Vocal cords		
e. Mucous glands		
f. Nasopharyngeal		
g. Bronchioles		

14. Indicate whether the following clinical manifestations are most characteristic of asthma (A), COPD (C), or both (B).
    _____ a. Barrel chest
    _____ b. Persistent cough
    _____ c. Flattened diaphragm
    _____ d. Polycythemia
    _____ e. Decreased breath sounds
    _____ f. Cor pulmonale
    _____ g. Weight loss
    _____ h. Wheezing
    _____ i. Increased fractional exhaled nitric oxide (FENO)
    _____ j. Increased total lung capacity
    _____ k. Frequent sputum production

15. The pulmonary vasoconstriction leading to the development of cor pulmonale in the patient with COPD results from
    a. increased viscosity of the blood.
    b. alveolar hypoxia and hypercapnia.
    c. long-term low-flow oxygen therapy.
    d. administration of high concentrations of oxygen.

16. In addition to smoking cessation, treatment for COPD that is indicated to slow the progression of the disease includes
    a. use of bronchodilator drugs.
    b. use of inhaled corticosteroids.
    c. lung-volume–reduction surgery.
    d. prevention of respiratory tract infections.

17. Match the following characteristics with their methods of oxygen administration.
    _____ a. Provides highest oxygen concentrations
    _____ b. May cause aspiration of condensed fluid
    _____ c. Safest system to use in patient with COPD
    _____ d. Most comfortable and causes the least restriction on activities
    _____ e. Reservoir bag conserves oxygen
    _____ f. Used to give oxygen quickly for short time

    1. Nasal cannula
    2. Simple face mask
    3. Partial rebreathing mask
    4. Nonrebreathing mask
    5. Venturi mask
    6. Tracheostomy collar

18. A patient is being discharged with plans for home oxygen therapy provided by a liquid oxygen reservoir with a refillable portable unit. In preparing the patient to use the equipment, the nurse teaches the patient that
    a. the portable tank filled from the reservoir will last about 6 to 8 hours at 2 L/min.
    b. the unit concentrates oxygen from the air, providing a continuous oxygen supply.
    c. the unit should be kept out of the bedroom and extension tubing used at night because of the noise.
    d. weekly delivery of one large cylinder of oxygen will be necessary for a 7- to 10-day supply of oxygen.

19. A breathing technique the nurse should teach the patient with COPD to promote exhalation is
    a. huff coughing.
    b. thoracic breathing.
    c. pursed-lip breathing.
    d. diaphragmatic breathing.

20. In planning for postural drainage for the patient with COPD, the nurse
    a. schedules the procedure 1 hour before and after meals.
    b. has the patient cough before positioning to clear the lungs.
    c. assesses the patient's tolerance for dependent (head-down) positions.
    d. ensures that percussion and vibration are performed before positioning the patient.

21. A dietary modification that helps meet the nutritional needs of patients with COPD is
    a. eating a high-carbohydrate, low-fat diet.
    b. avoiding foods that require a lot of chewing.
    c. preparing most foods of the diet to be eaten hot.
    d. drinking fluids with meals to promote digestion.

22. ***Delegation Decision:*** The nurse is caring for a patient with COPD. Which of these interventions could be delegated to nursing assistive personnel (NAP)?
    a. Assist the patient to get up out of bed
    b. Auscultate breath sounds every 4 hours
    c. Plan patient activities to minimize exertion
    d. Teach the patient pursed-lip breathing technique

23. Which of the following oxygen delivery systems delivers a precise oxygen concentration and is often used for COPD patients?
    a. Nasal cannula
    b. Simple face mask
    c. Venturi face mask
    d. Nonrebreather face mask

24. During an acute exacerbation of COPD, the patient is severely short of breath and the nurse identifies a nursing diagnosis of ineffective breathing pattern related to obstruction of airflow and anxiety. The best action by the nurse is to
    a. prepare and administer bronchodilator medications.
    b. perform chest physiotherapy to promote removal of secretions.
    c. administer oxygen at 5 L/min until the shortness of breath is relieved.
    d. position the patient upright with the elbows resting on the over-the-bed table.

25. The husband of a patient with COPD tells the nurse that they have not had any sexual activity since the patient was diagnosed with COPD because she becomes too short of breath. The best response by the nurse is,
    a. "You need to discuss your feelings and needs with your wife so she knows what you expect of her."
    b. "There are other ways to maintain intimacy besides sexual intercourse that will not make her short of breath."
    c. "You should explore other ways to meet your sexual needs since your wife is no longer capable of sexual activity."
    d. "Would you like for me to talk to you and your wife about some modifications that can be made to maintain sexual activity?"

26. In teaching the patient with COPD about the need for physical exercise, the nurse informs the patient that
    a. all patients with COPD should be able to increase walking gradually up to 20 min/day.
    b. a bronchodilator inhaler should be used to relieve exercise-induced dyspnea immediately after exercise.
    c. shortness of breath is expected during exercise but should return to baseline within 5 minutes after the exercise.
    d. monitoring the heart rate before and after exercise is the best way to determine how much exercise can be tolerated.

27. The pathophysiologic mechanism of cystic fibrosis leading to obstructive lung disease is
    a. fibrosis of mucous glands and destruction of bronchial walls.
    b. destruction of lung parenchyma from inflammation and scarring.
    c. production of abnormally thick, copious secretions from mucous glands.
    d. increased serum levels of pancreatic enzymes that are deposited in the bronchial mucosa.

28. The primary treatment for cystic fibrosis is
    a. heart-lung transplantation.
    b. administration of prophylactic antibiotics.
    c. administration of nebulized bronchodilators.
    d. vigorous and consistent chest physiotherapy.

29. Meeting the developmental tasks of young adulthood becomes a major problem for young adults with cystic fibrosis primarily because
    a. they have an expected shortened life span.
    b. any children they have will develop cystic fibrosis.
    c. they must also adapt to a newly diagnosed chronic disease.
    d. their illness keeps them from becoming financially independent.

30. The nursing assessment of a patient with bronchiectasis is most likely to reveal a history of
    a. chest trauma.
    b. childhood asthma.
    c. smoking or oral tobacco use.
    d. recurrent lower respiratory tract infections.

31. In planning care for the patient with bronchiectasis, the nurse includes measures that will
    a. relieve or reduce pain.
    b. prevent paroxysmal coughing.
    c. prevent spread of the disease to others.
    d. promote drainage and removal of mucus.

CASE STUDY
Asthma
Patient Profile

E.S. is a 35-year-old mother of two school-age boys who arrives via ambulance in the emergency department (ED) with severe wheezing, dyspnea, and anxiety. She was in the ED 6 hours earlier with an asthma attack.

Subjective Data
- Treated during previous ED visit with nebulized albuterol and responded quickly
- Allergic to cigarette smoke
- Began to experience increasing tightness in her chest and shortness of breath when she returned home following her previous ED visit.
- Used the albuterol several times after she returned home with no relief
- Diagnosed with asthma 2 years ago
- Does not have a health care provider and is not on any medications

Objective Data
Physical Examination
- Sitting upright and using accessory muscles to breathe
- Talks in one- to three-word sentences
- Respiratory rate is 34 shallow breaths/min
- Audible wheezing
- Auscultation of lung fields reveals no air movement in lower lobes
- Heart rate is 126 beats/min
- Noted to be extremely anxious and restless

Diagnostic Studies
- ABGs: pH 7.46, $PaCO_2$ 36 mm Hg, PaO_2 76 mm Hg, O_2 saturation 88%
- Chest x-ray: bilateral lung hyperinflation with lower lobe atelectasis
- CBC and electrolytes: within normal limits

An IV is started in her left forearm with normal saline infusing at 100 ml/hr.

Clinical Decision-Making Questions
Using a separate sheet of paper, answer the following questions.

1. *Priority Decision:* What is the priority collaborative intervention for E.S.?
2. What data obtained from the brief history, physical examination, and diagnostic studies indicate that E.S. is experiencing a severe or life-threatening asthma attack?
3. Identify two classifications of medications the nurse should expect will be administered to this patient? What effect is expected of these medications?
4. In addition to medication administration and close monitoring of the patient, what other key role can the nurse take in helping the patient through this episode?
5. What value would PEFR measures have during the care of E.S.?
6. *Priority Decision:* Based on the assessment data presented, what are the priority nursing diagnoses? What are the collaborative problems?

Nursing Assessment: Hematologic System

1. Match the following characteristics with the appropriate blood cells (answers may be used more than once).

   _____ a. May become tissue macrophages
   _____ b. 30% of volume stored in spleen
   _____ c. Primarily responsible for immune response
   _____ d. 4%-8% of white blood cell (WBC) count
   _____ e. Production stimulated by hypoxia
   _____ f. 0%-2% of WBCs
   _____ g. Immature cell is a band
   _____ h. Increased in individuals with allergies
   _____ i. Responds first at injury site
   _____ j. 20%-40% of WBCs
   _____ k. Releases granules that increase allergic and inflammatory responses
   _____ l. Arises from megakaryocyte
   _____ m. 50%-70% of WBCs
   _____ n. Increases indicate an increased rate of erythropoiesis
   _____ o. Make up 2%-4% of WBCs
   _____ p. Also known as "segs"

   1. Erythrocyte
   2. Reticulocyte
   3. Neutrophil
   4. Basophil
   5. Eosinophil
   6. Lymphocyte
   7. Monocyte
   8. Platelet

2. Complete the following statements.
   a. Granulocytic leukocytes include _____, _____, and _____.
   b. Red blood cell production is stimulated by the release of the growth factor, _____, from the kidney.
   c. Nutrients essential for red blood cell production include _____, _____, and _____.
   d. Obstruction of the lymph flow results in accumulation of lymph fluid known as _____.
   e. Organs of the hematologic system that have filtering functions include the _____, _____, and _____.
   f. Iron is stored in the body in the form of _____ and _____.

3. Match the following processes with the appropriate components that contribute to normal hemostasis (answers may be used more than once).

   _____ a. Thrombin converts fibrinogen to fibrin
   _____ b. Platelets interact with collagen
   _____ c. Release of adenosine diphosphate
   _____ d. Thrombin catalyzes conversion of plasminogen to plasmin
   _____ e. Release of PF3 and serotonin
   _____ f. Fibrin split products formed with action of plasmin
   _____ g. Action of protein C and protein S
   _____ h. Vasoconstriction and spasm
   _____ i. Prothrombin converted to thrombin
   _____ j. Damaged vascular surface
   _____ k. Serum calcium activity as factor IV
   _____ l. Platelet agglutination

   1. Vascular response
   2. Platelet plug formation
   3. Plasma clotting factors
   4. Lysis of clot

4. A patient's laboratory test results indicate increased fibrin split products (FSP). An appropriate nursing action is to monitor the patient for
   a. fever.
   b. bleeding.
   c. faintness.
   d. thrombotic episodes.

5. When reviewing the results of an 83-year-old patient's blood tests, which of the following findings would be of most concern to the nurse?
   a. Platelets of 150,000/μL
   b. Serum iron of 50 mcg/dL
   c. Partial thromboplastin time (PTT) of 60 seconds
   d. Erythrocyte sedimentation rate (ESR) of 35 mm in 1 hour

6. A patient with a bone marrow disorder has an overproduction of myeloblasts. The nurse would expect the results of a complete blood cell count (CBC) to include increased (select all that apply)
   a. basophils.
   b. monocytes.
   c. neutrophils.
   d. eosinophils.
   e. lymphocytes.

7. During the nursing assessment of a patient with anemia, the nurse asks the patient about a history of
   a. stomach surgery.
   b. recurring infections.
   c. corticosteroid therapy.
   d. oral contraceptive use.

8. Identify one specific finding identified by the nurse during assessment of each of the patient's functional health patterns that indicates a risk factor for hematologic problems or a patient response to an actual hematologic problem.
   a. Health perception–health management
   b. Nutritional-metabolic
   c. Elimination
   d. Activity-exercise
   e. Sleep-rest
   f. Cognitive-perceptual
   g. Self-perception–self-concept
   h. Role-relationship
   i. Sexuality-reproductive
   j. Coping–stress tolerance
   k. Value-belief

9. Using light pressure with the index and middle fingers, the nurse cannot palpate any of the patient's superficial lymph nodes. The nurse
   a. records this finding as normal.
   b. should reassess the lymph nodes using deeper pressure.
   c. asks the patient about any history of any radiation therapy.
   d. notifies the health care provider that x-rays of the nodes will be necessary.

10. During physical assessment of a patient with thrombocytopenia, the nurse would expect to find
    a. sternal tenderness.
    b. petechiae and purpura.
    c. jaundiced sclera and skin.
    d. tender, enlarged lymph nodes.

11. A patient with a hematologic disorder has a smooth, shiny red tongue. The nurse would expect the patient's laboratory results to include
    a. neutrophils: 45%.
    b. Hb: 9.6 g/dL (96 g/L).
    c. white blood cell (WBC) count: 13,500/μL.
    d. red blood cell (RBC) count: 6.4×10^6/μL.

12. A patient is being treated with chemotherapeutic agents. The nurse revises the patient's care plan based on the CBC results of
    a. WBC: 4000/μL.
    b. RBC: 3.8×10^6/μL.
    c. platelets: 50,000/μL.
    d. hematocrit (Hct): 38%.

13. Identify the type of condition indicated by each of the following laboratory study results.
    a. Serum iron: 40 mcg/dL (7 μmol/L)
    b. ESR: 30 mm/hr
    c. Increased band neutrophils
    d. Activated partial thromboplastin time: 60 sec
    e. Indirect bilirubin: 2.0 mg/dL (34 μmol/L)
    f. Bence-Jones protein in urine

14. If a patient with blood type O Rh⁺ is given AB Rh⁻ blood, the nurse would expect
    a. the patient's Rh factor to react with the RBCs of the donor blood.
    b. no adverse reaction because the patient has no antibodies against the donor blood.
    c. the anti-A and anti-B antibodies in the patient's blood to hemolyze the donor blood.
    d. the anti-A and anti-B antibodies in the donor blood to hemolyze the patient's blood.

15. A patient is undergoing a contrast CT of the spleen. Before this test, it is important for the nurse to ask the patient about
    a. iodine sensitivity.
    b. prior blood transfusions.
    c. phobia of confined spaces.
    d. internal metal implants or appliances.

16. When teaching a patient about a bone marrow examination, the nurse explains that
    a. the procedure will be done under general anesthesia because it is so painful.
    b. the patient will not have any pain after the area at the puncture site is anesthetized.
    c. the patient will experience a brief, very sharp pain during aspiration of the bone marrow.
    d. there will be no pain during the procedure, but an ache will be present several days afterward.

17. A lymph node biopsy is most often performed to diagnose
    a. leukemias.
    b. hemorrhagic tendencies.
    c. the cause of lymphedema.
    d. neoplastic cells in the lymph nodes.

18. Word Search. Find the words that are defined by the clues given below. The words may be located horizontally, vertically, or diagonally, and may be reversed.

```
A S R S Q K R U I Y I H B B E T H B E A
S I I E E M O C C K E E I L R H N S C P
P I N S T C J N N X N M L O Y R K I C I
I E S E E I O P D W F O F E T O Q S H O
J E T Y P I C I I R T L L Y H M I O Y N
Z D R E L O O U Y O U Y S F R B W T M U
G H B L C O T P L Z H S R W O O Z Y O H
S Y N A Z H N Y O O T I C Q P C P C S N
D M A F X Y I I C T C S S C O Y A O I O
D X L A P Z W A R O A Y U G I T N G S J
D J Y K Q W L B E B B M T R E O C A F L
A I N E P O K U E L I M E E S S Y H D L
D D G W Q Q A B U B F F O H I I T P O S
O S P L E N O M E G A L Y R S S O I L N
U P Y F L Y F W G B B B H S H F P K D U
L Y M P H A D E N O P A T H Y T E G T E
W S K E D K E Q O R B K K B J F N X G E
W C F Q N H O C A H D Z Y E Y F I H H L
S B I Q J N Y A Y D I E M N H F A Y S H
A I N E P O R T U E N X Y P B N X X D N
```

Clues

a. Bruising
b. RBC production
c. Dissolution of fibrin clot
d. Blood cell production
e. RBC destruction
f. WBC <4000/μL
g. Absolute neutrophil count <1000/μL
h. Marked decrease of RBCs, WBCs, and platelets
i. Small purplish pinpoint lesions
j. Immature RBC
k. Platelet count <100,000/μL
l. Excessive platelets
m. Ingestion and digestion of unwanted substances
n. Enlarged lymph nodes
o. Palpable spleen

1. Match each of the anemic states with both etiologic and morphologic classification systems (answers may be used more than once).

   _____ _____ a. Acute trauma
   _____ _____ b. Malaria
   _____ _____ c. Anemia of gastritis
   _____ _____ d. Anemia of renal failure
   _____ _____ e. Aplastic anemia
   _____ _____ f. Glucose-6-phosphate (G6PD)
   _____ _____ g. Iron deficiency anemia
   _____ _____ h. Thalassemia
   _____ _____ i. Pernicious anemia
   _____ _____ j. Sickle cell anemia
   _____ _____ k. Anemia of leukemia
   _____ _____ l. Anemia associated with prosthetic heart valve

   Etiologic
   1. Decreased RBC production
   2. Blood loss
   3. Increased RBC destruction

   Morphologic
   4. Normocytic, normochromic
   5. Macrocytic, normochromic
   6. Microcytic, hypochromic

2. A patient with a hemoglobin (Hb) level of 7.8 g/dL (78 g/L) has cardiac palpitations, a heart rate of 102, and an increased reticulocyte count. At this severity of anemia, the nurse would also expect the patient to manifest
   a. pallor.
   b. dyspnea.
   c. a smooth tongue.
   d. sensitivity to cold.

3. *Priority Decision:* A 76-year-old woman has an Hb of 7.3 g/dL (73 g/L) and is experiencing ataxia and confusion on admission to the hospital. A priority nursing intervention for this patient is to
   a. provide a darkened, quiet room.
   b. have the family stay with the patient.
   c. keep top bedside rails up and call bell in close reach.
   d. question the patient about possible causes of anemia.

4. During the physical assessment of the patient with severe anemia, which of the following findings is of the most concern to the nurse?
   a. Anorexia
   b. Bone pain
   c. Hepatomegaly
   d. Dyspnea at rest

5. A nursing diagnosis that is appropriate for patients with moderate to severe anemia of any etiology is
   a. impaired skin integrity related to edema and pruritus.
   b. disturbed body image related to changes in appearance and body function.
   c. imbalanced nutrition: less than body requirements related to lack of knowledge of adequate nutrition.
   d. activity intolerance related to decreased hemoglobin and imbalance between oxygen supply and demand.

6. Match the following descriptions with their associated types of anemia (answers may be used more than once).

   _____ a. Autosomal recessive genetic basis
   _____ b. Hypoxia-induced change in RBCs
   _____ c. Responds to treatment with erythropoietin
   _____ d. Most common type of anemia
   _____ e. Megaloblastic cells without neurologic involvement
   _____ f. Autoimmune-related disease
   _____ g. May occur with removal of the duodenum
   _____ h. May occur with removal of the stomach
   _____ i. Altered globin synthesis of hemoglobin
   _____ j. Lack of intrinsic factor
   _____ k. Associated with vascular occlusion and tissue infarction
   _____ l. Decrease in all blood cells
   _____ m. May be caused by adrenal hypofunction
   _____ n. Associated with chronic blood loss
   _____ o. Treatment causing chronic iron toxicity
   _____ p. Oral contraceptives a contributing factor

   1. Iron deficiency
   2. Thalassemia
   3. Cobalamin deficiency
   4. Folic acid deficiency
   5. Anemia of chronic disease
   6. Aplastic anemia
   7. Sickle cell

7. Explain the following laboratory findings in anemia.
   a. Reticulocyte counts are increased in chronic blood loss but decreased in cobalamin (vitamin B_{12}) deficiency.
   b. Bilirubin levels are increased in sickle cell anemia but are normal in acute blood loss.
   c. Mean cell volume (MCV) is increased in folic acid deficiency but decreased in iron deficiency anemia.

8. When teaching the patient about a new prescription for oral iron supplements, the nurse instructs the patient to
   a. take the iron preparations with meals.
   b. increase fluid and dietary fiber intake.
   c. report the presence of black stools to the health care provider.
   d. use enteric-coated preparations taken with orange juice.

9. In teaching the patient with pernicious anemia about the disease, the nurse explains that it results from a lack of
   a. folic acid.
   b. intrinsic factor.
   c. extrinsic factor.
   d. cobalamin intake.

10. During the assessment of a patient with cobalamin deficiency, the nurse would expect to find that the patient has
    a. icteric sclera.
    b. hepatomegaly.
    c. paresthesia of the hands and feet.
    d. intermittent heartburn with acid reflux.

11. The nurse determines that teaching about pernicious anemia has been effective when the patient says,
    a. "This condition can kill me unless I take injections of the vitamin the rest of my life."
    b. "My symptoms can be completely reversed if I take cobalamin (vitamin B_{12}) supplements."
    c. "If my anemia does not respond to cobalamin therapy, my only other alternative is a bone marrow transplant."
    d. "The least expensive and most convenient treatment of pernicious anemia is to use a diet with foods high in cobalamin."

12. The strict vegetarian is at highest risk for the development of
    a. thalassemias.
    b. iron deficiency anemia.
    c. folic acid deficiency anemia.
    d. cobalamin deficiency anemia.

13. A patient with aplastic anemia has a nursing diagnosis of impaired oral mucous membrane. The etiology of this diagnosis can be related to the effects of a deficiency of (select all that apply)
   a. platelets.
   b. RBCs.
   c. WBCs.
   d. coagulation factor VIII.

14. Nursing interventions for the patient with aplastic anemia are directed toward the prevention of the complications of
   a. fatigue and dyspnea.
   b. hemorrhage and infection.
   c. thromboemboli and gangrene.
   d. cardiac dysrhythmias and heart failure.

15. Identify whether the following statements are true (*T*) or false (*F*). If a statement is false, correct the bold word(s) to make the statement true.
   _____ a. The most reliable way to evaluate the effect and degree of blood loss in a patient with hemorrhage is with **laboratory data**.
   _____ b. A patient who has acute blood loss but normal vital signs at rest and increased heart rate and postural hypotension with exercise has lost approximately **30%** of the total blood volume.
   _____ c. The anemia that follows acute blood loss is most frequently treated with **increased dietary iron intake**.
   _____ d. In addition to the general symptoms of anemia, the patient with a hemolytic anemia also manifests **jaundice**.
   _____ e. A major concern in hemolytic anemia is maintenance of **liver** function.

16. The anemia of sickle cell disease is caused by
   a. intravascular hemolysis of sickled RBCs.
   b. accelerated breakdown of abnormal RBCs.
   c. autoimmune antibody destruction of RBCs.
   d. isoimmune antibody-antigen reactions with RBCs.

17. A patient with sickle cell anemia asks the nurse why the sickling crisis does not stop when oxygen therapy is started. The nurse explains that
   a. sickling occurs in response to decreased blood viscosity, which is not affected by oxygen therapy.
   b. when RBCs sickle, they occlude small vessels, which causes more local hypoxia and more sickling.
   c. the primary problem during a sickle cell crisis is destruction of the abnormal cells, resulting in fewer RBCs to carry oxygen.
   d. oxygen therapy does not alter the shape of the abnormal erythrocytes but only allows for increased oxygen concentration in hemoglobin.

18. A nursing intervention that is indicated for the patient during a sickle cell crisis is
   a. frequent ambulation.
   b. application of antiembolism hose.
   c. restriction of sodium and oral fluids.
   d. administration of large doses of continuous opioid analgesics.

19. During discharge teaching with a patient with newly diagnosed sickle cell disease, the nurse teaches the patient to
   a. limit fluid intake.
   b. avoid hot, humid weather.
   c. eliminate exercise from the lifestyle.
   d. seek early medical intervention for upper respiratory infections.

20. Identify whether the following statements are true (*T*) or false (*F*). If a statement is false, correct the bold word(s) to make the statement true.

_____ a. Genetic counseling and family planning is indicated for a couple when one of them has **thalassemia**.

_____ b. Immune thrombocytopenic purpura is characterized by increased platelet destruction by the **spleen**.

_____ c. The most common acquired thrombocytopenia is **thrombotic thrombocytopenic purpura (TTP)**.

_____ d. TTP is characterized by **decreased** platelets, **decreased** RBCs, and **decreased** agglutination function of platelets.

_____ e. A classic clinical manifestation of thrombocytopenia that the nurse would expect to find on physical examination of the patient is **ecchymosis**.

_____ f. Patients with platelet deficiencies usually bleed from **superficial sites**, whereas those with diminished clotting factors experience **deep or internal** bleeding.

_____ g. Treatment of **hemachromatosis** involves weekly phlebotomy for 2 to 3 years.

_____ h. The nurse suspects heparin-induced thrombocytopenia and thrombosis syndrome when a patient receiving heparin requires **decreased** heparin to maintain therapeutic activated thromboplastin times.

21. In providing care for a patient hospitalized with an acute exacerbation of polycythemia vera, the nurse gives priority to which of the following activities?
    a. Maintaining protective isolation
    b. Promoting leg exercises and ambulation
    c. Protecting the patient from injury or falls
    d. Promoting hydration with a large fluid intake

22. A patient has a platelet count of 50,000/µL and is diagnosed with immune thrombocytopenic purpura. The nurse anticipates that initial treatment will include
    a. splenectomy.
    b. corticosteroids.
    c. administration of platelets.
    d. immunosuppressive therapy.

23. *Priority Decision:* A patient is admitted to the hospital for evaluation and treatment of thrombocytopenia. Which of the following actions is most important for the nurse to implement?
    a. Taking the temperature every 4 hours to assess for fever
    b. Maintaining the patient on strict bed rest to prevent injury
    c. Monitoring the patient for headaches, vertigo, or confusion
    d. Removing the oral crusting and scabs with a soft brush four times a day

24. The nurse caring for a patient with heparin-induced thrombocytopenia (HIT) identifies risk for bleeding as the priority nursing diagnosis. Identify/list at least five nursing interventions that should be implemented.

25. In reviewing the laboratory results of a patient with hemophilia A (classic), the nurse would expect to find
    a. an absence of factor IX.
    b. a decreased platelet count.
    c. a prolonged bleeding time.
    d. a prolonged partial thromboplastin time (PTT).

26. A patient with hemophilia comes to the clinic for treatment. The nurse will prepare to administer
    a. whole blood.
    b. thromboplastin.
    c. factor concentrates.
    d. fresh frozen plasma.

27. A patient with hemophilia is hospitalized with acute knee pain and swelling. An appropriate nursing intervention for the patient includes
    a. wrapping the knee with an elastic bandage.
    b. placing the patient on bed rest and applying ice to the joint.
    c. administering nonsteroidal antiinflammatory drugs (NSAIDs) as needed for pain.
    d. gently performing range-of-motion (ROM) exercises to the knee to prevent adhesions.

28. Number in sequence the events that occur in disseminated intravascular coagulation (DIC).
    _____ a. Activation of fibrinolytic system
    _____ b. Uncompensated hemorrhage
    _____ c. Widespread fibrin and platelet deposition in capillaries and arterioles
    _____ d. Release of fibrin-split products
    _____ e. Fibrinogen converted to fibrin
    _____ f. Inhibition of normal blood clotting
    _____ g. Production of intravascular thrombin
    _____ h. Depletion of platelets and coagulation factors

29. A patient has a WBC count of 2300/μL and a neutrophil percentage of 40%.
    a. Does the patient have leukopenia?
    b. What is the patient's neutrophil count?
    c. Does the patient have a neutropenia?
    d. What is the patient's risk for developing a bacterial infection?

30. The most important method for identifying the presence of infection in a neutropenic patient is
    a. frequent temperature monitoring.
    b. routine blood and sputum cultures.
    c. assessing for redness and swelling.
    d. monitoring white blood cell (WBC) count.

31. The major method of preventing infection in the patient with neutropenia is use of
    a. HEPA filtration rooms.
    b. prophylactic antibiotics.
    c. a diet that eliminates fresh fruits and vegetables.
    d. strict hand washing by all persons in contact with the patient.

32. Myelodysplastic syndrome (MDS) differs from acute leukemias in that MDS
    a. has a slower disease progression.
    b. does not result in bone marrow failure.
    c. is a clonal disorder of hematopoietic cells.
    d. affects only the production and function of platelets and WBCs.

33. Match the following characteristics with their related types of leukemia (answers may be used more than once).
    _____ a. Neoplasm of activated B lymphocytes   1. acute myelogenous leukemia (AML)
    _____ b. Mature-appearing but functionally inactive lymphocytes   2. acute lymphocytic leukemia (ALL)
    _____ c. 85% of acute leukemia in adults   3. chronic myelogenous leukemia (CML)
    _____ d. Most common in children   4. chronic lymphocytic leukemia (CLL)
    _____ e. Only cure is bone marrow transplant
    _____ f. Proliferation of immature lymphocytes in bone marrow
    _____ g. Increased incidence in atomic bomb survivors
    _____ h. Proliferation of precursors of granulocytes
    _____ i. Associated with Philadelphia chromosome
    _____ j. Central nervous system (CNS) manifestations common
    _____ k. Most common leukemia of adults

34. Lymphadenopathy, splenomegaly, and hepatomegaly are common clinical manifestations of leukemia that are due to
    a. the development of infection at these sites.
    b. increased compensatory production of blood cells by these organs.
    c. infiltration of the organs by increased numbers of WBCs in the blood.
    d. normal hypertrophy of the organs in an attempt to destroy abnormal cells.

35. A patient with acute myelogenous leukemia is considering a hematopoietic stem cell transplant and asks the nurse what is involved. The best response by the nurse is,
    a. "Your bone marrow is destroyed by radiation, and new bone marrow cells from a matched donor are injected into your bones."
    b. "A specimen of your bone marrow may be aspirated and treated to destroy any leukemic cells and then reinfused when your disease becomes worse."
    c. "During chemotherapy and total body radiation to destroy all your blood cells, you are given transfusions of red blood cells and platelets to prevent complications."
    d. "Leukemic cells and bone marrow stem cells are eliminated with chemotherapy and total body radiation, and new bone marrow cells from a donor are infused."

36. ***Priority Decision:*** What are the priority nursing diagnoses for the patient with newly diagnosed chronic lymphocytic leukemia?
    a. pain and hopelessness
    b. anxiety and risk for infection
    c. self-care deficit and ineffective health maintenance
    d. decisional conflict: treatment options and risk for injury

37. Indicate whether the following characteristics are associated with Hodgkin's lymphoma (HL), non-Hodgkin's lymphoma (NHL), or both (B).
    _____ a. Multiple histopathologic classifications
    _____ b. Presence of Reed-Sternberg cells
    _____ c. Treated with radiation and chemotherapy
    _____ d. Affects all ages
    _____ e. Originates in lymph nodes in most patients
    _____ f. Often widely disseminated at time of diagnosis
    _____ g. Alcohol-induced pain at the site of disease
    _____ h. Primary initial clinical manifestation is painless lymph node enlargement
    _____ i. Greater than 90% cure rate in stage I disease
    _____ j. Associated with Epstein-Barr virus

38. Identify whether the following statements are true (*T*) or false (*F*). If a statement is false, correct the bold word(s) to make the statement true.
    _____ a. Staging of lymphomas is important to **predict prognosis**.
    _____ b. Nursing management of the patient undergoing treatment for Hodgkin's disease includes measures to prevent **infection**.
    _____ c. Multiple myeloma is characterized by proliferation of malignant activated **T cells** that destroy the **kidneys**.
    _____ d. Two important nursing interventions in the care of patients with multiple myeloma are increasing fluids to manage **hypercalcemia** and careful handling of the patient to prevent **pathologic** fractures.

39. Following a splenectomy for the treatment of immune thrombocytopenic purpura (ITP), the nurse would expect the patient's laboratory test results to reveal
    a. decreased RBCs.
    b. decreased WBCs.
    c. increased platelets.
    d. increased immunoglobulins.

40. While receiving a unit of packed RBCs, the patient develops chills and a temperature of 102.2° F (39° C). The priority action for the nurse to take is
    a. notify the health care provider and the blood bank.
    b. stop the transfusion and removes the IV catheter.
    c. add a leukocyte reduction filter to the blood administration set.
    d. recognize this as a mild allergic transfusion reaction and slow the transfusion.

41. A patient with thrombocytopenia with active bleeding is to receive two units of platelets. To administer the platelets, the nurse
    a. checks for ABO compatibility.
    b. agitates the bag periodically during the transfusion.
    c. takes vital signs every 15 minutes during the procedure.
    d. refrigerates the second unit until the first unit has transfused.

42. Match the following characteristics with their related transfusion reactions (answers may be used more than once).

    _____ a. May restart transfusion with antihistamine therapy in mild cases
    _____ b. May be avoided by leukocyte reduction filters
    _____ c. Acute renal failure may occur
    _____ d. Destruction of donor RBCs
    _____ e. Hypothermia common
    _____ f. Leukocyte or plasma protein incompatibility
    _____ g. ABO incompatibility
    _____ h. Hypocalcemia and hyperkalemia
    _____ i. Epinephrine used for severe reaction
    _____ j. May occur in cardiac and renal insufficiency

    1. Acute hemolytic reaction
    2. Febrile reaction
    3. Allergic reaction
    4. Circulatory overload
    5. Massive blood transfusion reaction

43. *Delegation Decision:* While administering an infusion of packed RBCs, the RN may delegate which of the following actions to nursing assistive personnel (NAP) (select all that apply)?
    a. Verify that the IV is patent.
    b. Obtain the blood products from the blood bank.
    c. Monitor the blood transfusion rate and adjust as needed.
    d. Obtain vital signs before and after the first 15 minutes.
    e. Assist with checking patient identification and blood product identification data with the RN.

44. The nurse is preparing to administer a blood transfusion. Number the actions in order of priority (1 is first priority; 10 is last priority action).
    _____ a. Verify the order for the transfusion.
    _____ b. Ensure the patient has a patent IV.
    _____ c. Prime the transfusion tubing/filter with normal saline.
    _____ d. Verify the consent for the transfusion is signed.
    _____ e. Obtain the blood product from the blood bank.
    _____ f. Ask another licensed person (nurse or MD) to assist in verifying the product identification and the patient identification.
    _____ g. Document outcomes in the patient record. Document vital signs, names of personnel, and starting/ending times.
    _____ h. Adjust the infusion rate and continue to monitor the patient every 30 minutes for up to an hour after the product is infused.
    _____ i. Infuse the first 50 mL over 15 minutes, staying with the patient.
    _____ j. Obtain the patient's vital signs before starting the transfusion.

CASE STUDY

Disseminated Intravascular Coagulation

Patient Profile

M.G., a 35-year-old mother of two, is admitted in active labor to the labor and delivery department for delivery of her third child. She delivers a 9-lb boy following an unusually difficult, prolonged labor.

Objective Data

- During her recovery period she continues to have heavy uterine bleeding and a boggy fundus
- Her skin is pale and diaphoretic
- BP 70/40; HR 150 beats/min
- Although the placenta appeared intact on examination, she is suspected of having retained placental fragments, causing disseminated intravascular coagulation (DIC)

Clinical Decision-Making Questions

Using a separate sheet of paper, answer the following questions.

1. What is the pathologic mechanism that triggers DIC in this case?
2. What additional clinical findings would indicate the presence of DIC?
3. Describe the common laboratory findings that are indicative of DIC.
4. What therapeutic modalities are most appropriate for this patient and why?
5. *Priority Decision:* Based on the assessment data presented, what are the priority nursing diagnoses? Are there any collaborative problems?

Nursing Assessment: Cardiovascular System

1. Using the list of terms below, identify the structures in the following illustration.

   Terms

   chordae tendineae   tricuspid valve
   mitral valve   interventricular septum
   papillary muscle

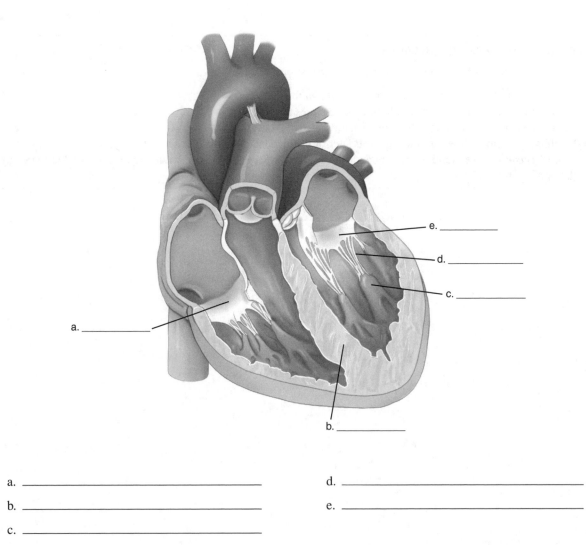

a. _____   d. _____

b. _____   e. _____

c. _____

2. Identify the structures in the following illustrations by placing the correct term from the list below in the corresponding answer blank at the bottom of the page (some terms will be used more than once).

Terms

left anterior descending artery	middle cardiac vein
aorta	posterior descending artery
aortic semilunar valve	posterior vein
circumflex artery	pulmonary trunk
coronary sinus	right atrium
great cardiac vein	right coronary artery
left atrium	right marginal artery
left coronary artery	right ventricle
left marginal artery	small cardiac vein
left ventricle	superior vena cava

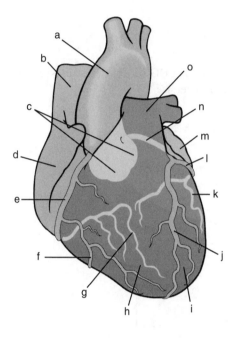 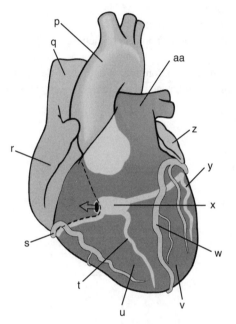

a. _____ o. _____

b. _____ p. _____

c. _____ q. _____

d. _____ r. _____

e. _____ s. _____

f. _____ t. _____

g. _____ u. _____

h. _____ v. _____

i. _____ w. _____

j. _____ x. _____

k. _____ y. _____

l. _____ z. _____

m. _____ aa. _____

n. _____

3. Complete the following statements.
   a. The three main coronary arteries are the _____,

   _____, and _____.

   b. In most people, the _____ artery supplies the AV node.

   c. Blood flow into the coronary arteries occurs primarily during the _____
   phase of the cardiac cycle.

4. Number in sequence the path of the action potential along the conduction system of the heart.
   _____ a. AV node
   _____ b. Purkinje fibers
   _____ c. Internodal pathways
   _____ d. Bundle of His
   _____ e. Ventricular cells
   _____ f. SA node
   _____ g. Right and left atrial cells
   _____ h. Right and left bundle branches

5. On the following illustration, locate and letter the following normal ECG pattern deflections and indicate where to
   locate/measure the intervals. (Use Table 36-2 to assist with this exercise.)
   P
   PR interval
   Q
   QRS interval
   QT interval
   R
   S
   T

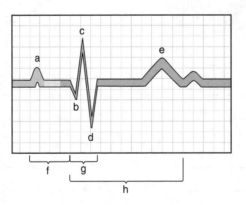

a. _____	e. _____
b. _____	f. _____
c. _____	g. _____
d. _____	h. _____

6. Match the cardiac activity and time frames characteristic of the waveforms of the electrocardiogram (answers may be used more than once).

   _____ a. Measured from beginning of P wave to beginning of QRS complex
   _____ b. Repolarization of the ventricles
   _____ c. 0.12-0.20 sec
   _____ d. 0.16 sec
   _____ e. Time of depolarization and repolarization of ventricles
   _____ f. <0.12 sec
   _____ g. Depolarization from the atrioventricular (AV) node throughout ventricles
   _____ h. 0.06-0.12 sec

   1. P wave
   2. PR interval
   3. QRS interval
   4. T wave
   5. QT interval

7. Indicate what factor of stroke volume (i.e., preload, afterload, or contractility) is primarily affected by the following situations and whether cardiac output (CO) is increased or decreased by the factor.

	Stroke Volume Factor	**Cardiac Output**
a. Valsalva maneuver		
b. Venous dilation		
c. Hypertension		
d. Administration of epinephrine		
e. Obstruction of pulmonary artery		
f. Hemorrhage		

8. Match the effects of the autonomic nervous system stimulation with the receptors responsible for the effects (answers may be used more than once).

   _____ a. Increased force of cardiac contraction
   _____ b. Decreased rate of impulse conduction
   _____ c. Vasoconstriction
   _____ d. Increased heart rate (HR)
   _____ e. Increased rate of impulse conduction
   _____ f. Decreased HR

   1. α-adrenergic stimulation
   2. β-adrenergic stimulation
   3. Parasympathetic stimulation

9. Identify the age-related physiologic changes that occur in the older adult that result in the following:
   a. Widened pulse pressure
   b. Decreased cardiac reserve
   c. Increased cardiac dysrhythmias
   d. Decreased response to sympathetic stimulation
   e. Aortic systolic murmur

10. Information related to the patient's health and medication history that the nurse identifies as significant during assessment of the cardiovascular system is a history of
    a. metastatic cancer.
    b. calcium supplementation.
    c. frequent viral pharyngitis.
    d. use of recreational/abused drugs.

11. Identify one specific finding identified by the nurse during assessment of each of the patient's functional health patterns that indicates a risk factor for cardiovascular disease or a patient response to an actual cardiovascular problem.
    a. Health perception–health management
    b. Nutritional-metabolic
    c. Elimination
    d. Activity-exercise
    e. Sleep-rest
    f. Cognitive-perceptual
    g. Self-perception–self-concept
    h. Role-relationship
    i. Sexuality-reproductive
    j. Coping–stress tolerance
    k. Value-belief

12. When palpating the patient's popliteal pulse, the nurse feels a vibration at the site. This finding is recorded as a
    a. thready, weak pulse.
    b. bruit at the artery site.
    c. bounding pulse volume.
    d. thrill of the popliteal artery.

13. Locate the following points/locations that are inspected and palpated on the chest wall.

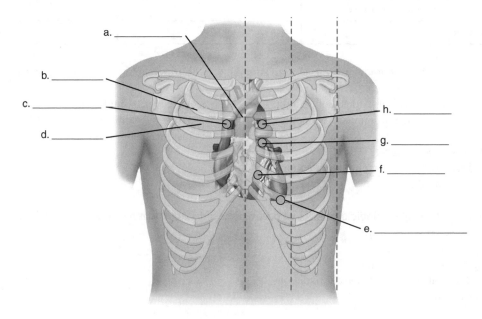

Angle of Louis	Pulmonic area
Aortic area	Tricuspid area
Erb's point	Second ICS
Mitral area (apex) and PMI	Second rib

14. Indicate whether the following are characteristic of the first heart sound (S_1) or the second heart sound (S_2).
    _____ a. Indicates the onset of diastole
    _____ b. Associated with closure of tricuspid and mitral valves
    _____ c. Loudest at pulmonic and aortic areas
    _____ d. Soft lub sound
    _____ e. Heard when carotid pulse felt
    _____ f. Indicates beginning of systole
    _____ g. Associated with closure of semilunar valves
    _____ h. Sharp dup sound
    _____ i. Is loudest at tricuspid and mitral areas

15. Match the following abnormal assessment findings with their descriptions or significance.

_____ a. Splinter hemorrhage
_____ b. Pulsus alternans
_____ c. Central cyanosis
_____ d. S_3
_____ e. Cardiac murmurs
_____ f. Finger clubbing
_____ g. Jugular vein distention
_____ h. Delayed capillary filling time
_____ i. S_4
_____ j. Peripheral cyanosis

1. Associated with increased right atrial pressure
2. Flattening of angle of nail base and finger
3. Decreased peripheral perfusion
4. Strength of pulse varies with each beat
5. Blue tinge around the nose and ears
6. Extra heart sound heard in late diastole
7. Small red/black streaks under fingernails
8. Common with heart valve disorders
9. Blue tinge around the lips and conjunctiva
10. Extra heart sound heard in early diastole

16. A patient is scheduled for exercise nuclear imaging stress testing. The nurse explains to the patient that this test involves
    a. placement of electrodes inside the right-sided heart chambers through a vein to record the electrical activity of the heart directly.
    b. exercising on a treadmill or stationary bicycle with continuous electrocardiographic (ECG) monitoring to detect ischemic changes during exercise.
    c. intravenous (IV) administration of a radioisotope of technetium-99 sestamibi at the maximum heart rate during exercise to identify areas of cardiac damage.
    d. placement of a small transducer in four positions on the chest to record the direction and flow of blood through the heart by the reflection of sound waves.

17. *Priority Decision:* The nurse caring for a patient immediately following a transesophageal echocardiogram (TEE) should consider which of these actions the highest priority?
    a. Monitor the ECG.
    b. Monitor pulse oximetry.
    c. Assess vital signs (BP, HR, RR, temperature).
    d. Maintain NPO status until gag reflex has returned.

18. Evaluation of ECG responses to normal activity over a period of a day or two is performed with
    a. serial ECGs.
    b. Holter monitoring.
    c. electrophysiology studies.
    d. positron emission tomography (PET).

19. When caring for a patient after a cardiac catheterization with coronary angiography, which of the following findings would be of most concern to the nurse?
    a. Swelling at the catheter insertion site
    b. Development of raised wheals on the patient's trunk
    c. Absence of pulses distal to the catheter insertion site
    d. Patient assessment of pain at the insertion site as 4 on a 1-to-10 scale

20. A female patient has a total cholesterol level of 232 mg/dL (6.0 mmol/L) and a high-density lipoprotein (HDL) of 65 mg/dL (1.68 mmol/L). A male patient has a total cholesterol level of 200 and an HDL of 32. Based on these findings, the patient with the highest cardiac risk is
    a. the man, because his HDL is lower.
    b. the woman, because her HDL is higher.
    c. the woman, because her cholesterol is higher.
    d. the man, because his cholesterol-to-HDL ratio is higher.

21. Which of the following factors have value as predictors of increased risk for coronary artery disease or evidence of myocardial injury (select all that apply)?
    a. Increased BNP
    b. Increased C-reactive protein
    c. Increased troponin T (cTnT)
    d. Increased creatine kinase (CK)-MM
    e. Increased lipoprotein-associated phospholipase A_2

CHAPTER 33

Nursing Management: Hypertension

1. In the regulation of normal blood pressure (BP), indicate whether the following mechanisms elevate BP by increasing cardiac output (CO), increasing systemic vascular resistance (SVR), or increasing both, and identify how these mechanisms cause the increases indicated.

	Increasing Cardiac Output	Increasing Systemic Vascular Resistance	Mechanisms Causing Increases
a. β_1-Adrenergic stimulation			
b. α_1-Adrenergic stimulation			
c. α_2-Adrenergic stimulation			
d. Endothelin release			
e. Angiotensin II			
f. Aldosterone release			
g. Antidiuretic hormone (ADH) release			

2. A patient is given an α_1-adrenergic agonist and experiences a reflex bradycardia. What normal mechanism of BP control is stimulated in this situation?

3. A patient uses a mixed β-adrenergic blocking agent for treatment of migraine headaches. What effect might this drug have on BP and why?

4. Identify four risk factors for primary hypertension that are not related to lifestyle behaviors.

   a.

   b.

   c.

   d.

5. Secondary hypertension is differentiated from primary hypertension in that secondary hypertension
   a. has a more gradual onset than primary hypertension.
   b. does not cause the target-organ damage that occurs with primary hypertension.
   c. has a specific cause, such as renal disease, that often can be corrected by medicine or surgery.
   d. is caused by age-related changes in BP regulatory mechanisms in individuals over 65 years of age.

6. The patient with primary hypertension is likely to report
   a. no symptoms.
   b. cardiac palpitations.
   c. dyspnea on exertion.
   d. dizziness and vertigo.

7. Most organ damage that occurs from hypertension is related to
   a. increased fluid pressure exerted against organ tissue.
   b. atherosclerotic changes in vessels that supply the organs.
   c. erosion and thinning of blood vessels from constant pressure.
   d. increased hydrostatic pressure causing leakage of plasma into organ interstitial spaces.

8. The organ that is damaged most directly as a result of high SVR is the
   a. brain.
   b. heart.
   c. retina.
   d. kidney.

9. Identify the significance of the following laboratory test results found in patients with hypertension.
   a. Blood urea nitrogen (BUN): 48 mg/dL (17.1 mmol/L); creatinine: 4.3 mg/dL (380 µmol/L)
   b. Serum K^+: 3.1 mEq/L (3.1 mmol/L)
   c. Fasting blood glucose: 183 mg/dL (10.2 mmol/L)
   d. Serum uric acid: 9.2 mg/dL (547 µmol/L)
   e. Low-density lipoproteins (LDL): 154 mg/dL (4.0 mmol/L)

10. A 42-year-old man has been diagnosed with primary hypertension with an average BP of 162/92 on three consecutive clinic visits. What are four priority lifestyle modifications that should be explored in the initial treatment of the patient?

    a.

    b.

    c.

    d.

11. Match the following primary effects in reducing BP with the classifications of drugs used to treat hypertension.

    _____ a. Decrease extracellular fluid volume by decreasing Na^+ and water reabsorption in the loop of Henle and distal tubule

    _____ b. Decrease CO by decreasing rate and strength of heart and decreasing renin secretion by the kidneys

    _____ c. Act directly on smooth muscle of arterioles to cause vasodilation

    _____ d. Cause vasodilation of arterioles by blocking movement of calcium into cells

    _____ e. Decrease Na^+ and water reabsorption by blocking the effect of aldosterone

    _____ f. Block peripheral α-adrenergic receptors to cause arteriole and venous dilation

    _____ g. Cause vasodilation by inhibiting sympathetic outflow from the central nervous system (CNS)

    _____ h. Interfere with enzyme conversion necessary for production of angiotensin II

    1. Central adrenergic antagonists
    2. Spironolactone
    3. ACE inhibitors
    4. Thiazide diuretics
    5. β-Adrenergic blockers
    6. Calcium-channel blockers
    7. α-Adrenergic blockers
    8. Direct vasodilators

12. Teaching to include dietary sources of potassium is indicated for the hypertensive patient taking
    a. enalapril (Vasotec).
    b. labetalol (Normodyne).
    c. spironolactone (Aldactone).
    d. hydrochlorothiazide (HydroDiuril).

13. A patient with stage 2 hypertension who is taking hydrochlorothiazide (HydroDiuril) and lisinopril (Prinivil) has prazosin (Minipress) added to the medication regimen. It is most important for the nurse to teach the patient to
    a. weigh every morning to monitor for fluid retention.
    b. change position slowly and avoid prolonged standing.
    c. use sugarless gum or candy to help relieve dry mouth.
    d. take the pulse daily to note any slowing of the heart rate.

14. A 38-year-old man is treated for hypertension with amiloride/hydrochlorothiazide (Maxide) and metaprolol (Lopressor). Four months after his last clinic visit, his BP returns to pretreatment levels and he admits he has not been taking his medication regularly. The best response by the nurse is,
    a. "Try always to take your medication when you carry out another daily routine so you do not forget to take it."
    b. "If you would exercise more and stop smoking, you probably would not need to be taking medications for hypertension."
    c. "The drugs you are taking cause sexual dysfunction in many patients. Are you experiencing any problems in this area?"
    d. "You need to remember that hypertension can be only controlled with medication, not cured, and you must always take your medication."

15. When teaching a patient for whom clonidine (Catapres) has been prescribed, the nurse stresses that
    a. the drug should never be stopped abruptly.
    b. the drug should be taken early in the day to prevent nocturia.
    c. the first dose should be taken when the patient is in bed for the night.
    d. aspirin will decrease the drug's effectiveness, and acetaminophen should be substituted for aspirin use.

16. The correct technique for BP measurements includes
    a. always taking the BP in both arms.
    b. positioning the patient supine for all readings.
    c. placing the cuff loosely around the upper arm.
    d. taking readings at least two times at least 1 minute apart.

17. A patient would be diagnosed with a hypertensive emergency when experiencing
    a. symptoms of a stroke with an elevated BP.
    b. a systolic BP >200 mm Hg and a diastolic BP >120 mm Hg.
    c. a sudden rise in BP accompanied by neurologic impairment.
    d. a severe elevation of BP that occurs over several days or weeks.

18. Drugs that are most commonly used to treat hypertensive crises include
    a. enalaprilat (Vasotec) and minoxidil (Loniten).
    b. labetalol (Normodyne) and diazoxide (Hyperstat).
    c. hydralazine (Apresoline) and captopril (Catapres).
    d. nitroglycerin (Tridil) and sodium nitroprusside (Nipride).

19. During treatment of a patient with a BP of 210/148 mm Hg, the nurse titrates the medications to
    a. lower the BP to the patient's normal within the second to third hour.
    b. decrease the mean arterial pressure (MAP) no more than 42 mm Hg in the first hour.
    c. decrease the systolic BP (SBP) to 158 mm Hg and the diastolic BP (DBP) to 111 within the first 2 hours.
    d. reduce the SBP to 160 mm Hg and the DBP to between 100 and 110 mm Hg as quickly as possible.

20. A nursing responsibility in the management of the patient with a hypertensive urgency often includes
    a. monitoring hourly urine output for drug effectiveness.
    b. providing for continuous ECG monitoring to detect side effects of the drugs.
    c. titrating intravenous drug dosages based on BP measurements every 2 to 3 minutes.
    d. instructing the patient to follow up with a health care professional 24 hours after outpatient treatment.

CASE STUDY
Isolated Systolic Hypertension

Patient Profile

K.J. is a 73-year-old white woman with no history of hypertension. She came to the doctor's office for a flu shot.

Subjective Data

- Says she has gained 20 lb over the past year since her husband died
- Has never smoked and uses no alcohol
- Only medication is one multivitamin per day
- Eats a lot of canned food
- Does not exercise

Objective Data

- Height: 64 in (162.6 cm); weight: 170 lb (77.1 kg)
- BP: 170/82 mm Hg
- Physical examination shows no abnormalities
- Serum potassium: 3.3 mEq/L (3.3 mmol/L)
- The health care provider diagnosed isolated systolic hypertension (ISH) and prescribed lifestyle modifications.

Clinical Decision-Making Questions

Using a separate sheet of paper, answer the following questions.

1. What contributing factors to the development of ISH are present?
2. What additional risk factors are present?
3. What specific dietary changes would the nurse recommend for K.J.?
4. *Priority Decision:* What other priority teaching measures should be instituted by the nurse?
5. If drug therapy became necessary to treat K.J.'s hypertension, what diuretic would be indicated on her laboratory results?
6. *Priority Decision:* Based on the assessment data presented, what are the priority nursing diagnoses? Are there any collaborative problems?

CHAPTER
34

Nursing Management: Coronary Artery Disease and Acute Coronary Syndrome

1. Identify the three stages of lesions that occur in the development of coronary artery disease (CAD) and the ages at which the stages are often present.

             Stage   **Age**

   a.

   b.

   c.

2. Identify whether the following statements are true (*T*) or false (*F*). If a statement is false, correct the bold word(s) to make the statement true.
   _____ a. The leading theory of atherogenesis proposes that **inflammation and endothelial injury** are the basic underlying causes of atherosclerosis.
   _____ b. Endothelial alteration may be caused by chemical irritants such as hyperlipidemia or by **tobacco use**.
   _____ c. Partial or total occlusion of the coronary artery occurs during the stage of raised **fibrous plaque**.
   _____ d. Collateral circulation in the coronary circulation is more likely to be present in the **young patient with CAD**.

3. While obtaining patient histories, the nurse identifies that the patient with the highest risk for CAD is
   a. a white man, age 54, who is a smoker and has a stressful lifestyle.
   b. an African American man, age 65, with obesity and a blood pressure (BP) of 130/86.
   c. a white woman, age 72, with a BP of 172/100 and who is physically inactive.
   d. an Asian woman, age 45, with a cholesterol level of 240 mg/dL and a BP of 130/75.

4. While teaching women about the risks and incidence of CAD, the nurse stresses that
   a. women have an increased incidence of sudden death compared with men.
   b. smoking is not as significant a risk factor for CAD in women as it is in men.
   c. estrogen replacement therapy in postmenopausal women decreases the risk for CAD.
   d. CAD is the leading cause of death in women, with a higher mortality rate following myocardial infarction (MI) than in men.

5. Match the following characteristics with their associated lipoproteins (answers may be used more than once).
   _____ a. Contains most of the triglycerides
   _____ b. Contains the most cholesterol
   _____ c. The higher the level, the lower the risk for CAD
   _____ d. Carries lipids away from arteries to liver
   _____ e. Increases are associated with obesity
   _____ f. Increases with exercise
   _____ g. High levels correlate most closely with CAD
   _____ h. Has an affinity for arterial walls

   1. High-density lipoproteins (HDL)
   2. Low-density lipoproteins (LDL)
   3. Very-low-density lipoproteins (VLDL)

6. Identify at what level the following serum lipoproteins become risk factors for CAD in individuals without risk factors for CAD.
   a. Total cholesterol
   b. Triglycerides
   c. LDL
   d. HDL

7. The nurse is encouraging a sedentary patient with major risks for CAD to perform physical exercise on a regular basis. In addition to decreasing the risk factor of physical inactivity, the nurse tells the patient that exercise will also directly contribute to reducing the risk factors of
   a. hyperlipidemia and obesity.
   b. diabetes mellitus and hypertension.
   c. elevated serum lipids and stressful lifestyle.
   d. hypertension and elevated serum homocysteine.

8. During a routine health examination, a 48-year-old patient is found to have a total cholesterol level of 224 mg/dL (5.8 mmol/L) and an LDL level of 140 mg/dL (3.6 mmol/L). The nurse teaches the patient that the diet of Therapeutic Lifestyle Changes recommends that the patient (select all that apply)
   a. use fat-free milk.
   b. abstain from alcohol use.
   c. eliminate red meat from the diet.
   d. eliminate intake of simple sugars.
   e. avoid egg yolks and foods prepared with whole eggs.

9. While providing information to patients to decrease the risk of CAD, the nurse uses the Therapeutic Lifestyle Changes diet for
   a. all patients to reduce CAD risk.
   b. patients who have experienced an MI.
   c. individuals with two or more risk factors for CAD.
   d. individuals with a cholesterol level >200 mg/dL (5.2 mmol/L).

10. A 62-year-old woman has hypertension and smokes a pack of cigarettes per day. She has no symptoms of CAD, but a recent LDL level is 154 mg/dL (3.98 mmol/L). Based on these findings, the nurse would expect that treatment for the patient would include
    a. diet therapy only.
    b. drug therapy only.
    c. diet and drug therapy.
    d. exercise instruction only.

11. Complete the following sentences.
    a. When myocardial ischemia is temporary and reversible, the condition is called

    _____ .

    b. The three conditions that are included as manifestations of acute coronary syndrome are _____,

    _____ , and _____ .

    c. When myocardial cells die as a result of ischemia, the area of cellular necrosis is known as an _____ .

12. Use the following terms to complete the statements.
    increased oxygen demand
    decreased oxygen supply

    a. Myocardial ischemia occurs as a result of two factors: _____ and _____ .

    b. Any factor that increases cardiac workload causes _____ .

    c. Narrowing of coronary arteries by atherosclerosis is the primary reason for _____ .

    d. Prinzmetal's angina results in _____ .

    e. Low blood volume or a decreased hemoglobin leads to _____ .

    f. Left ventricular hypertrophy caused by chronic hypertension leads to _____ .

    g. Sympathetic nervous system stimulation by drugs, emotions, or exertion constricts blood vessels and increases

    HR, resulting in _____ .

    h. In the patient with atherosclerotic coronary arteries, anything that causes _____ may precipitate angina.

13. Angina occurs with myocardial ischemia as a result of
    a. death of myocardial tissue.
    b. dysrhythmias caused by cellular irritability.
    c. lactic acid accumulation during anaerobic metabolism.
    d. elevated pressure in the ventricles and pulmonary vessels.

14. Match the following types of angina with their characteristics (answers may be used more than once).
    _____ a. Occurs only when the person is recumbent
    _____ b. Usually precipitated by exertion
    _____ c. Unpredictable and unrelieved by rest
    _____ d. Prevalent in persons with diabetes
    _____ e. Characterized by progressive severity
    _____ f. Occurs with same pattern of onset, duration, and intensity
    _____ g. Asymptomatic myocardial ischemia
    _____ h. Usually occurs in response to coronary artery spasm
    _____ i. Occurs only at night
    _____ j. May occur in the absence of CAD

    1. Silent ischemia
    2. Prinzmetal's angina
    3. Chronic stable angina
    4. Nocturnal angina
    5. Unstable angina
    6. Angina decubitus
    7. Microvascular angina

15. Tachycardia that is a response of the sympathetic nervous system to the pain of ischemia is detrimental because not only does it increase oxygen demand, but it
    a. increases CO.
    b. causes reflex hypotension.
    c. may lead to ventricular dysrhythmias.
    d. impairs perfusion of the coronary arteries.

16. The following are effects of drugs used to prevent and treat angina. Identify the classes of the drugs used to promote these effects.
    a. Decrease preload _____.

    b. Dilate coronary arteries _____.

    c. Prevent thrombosis of plaques _____.

    d. Decrease HR _____.

    e. Decrease afterload _____.

    f. Decrease myocardial contractility _____.

17. When teaching the patient with angina about taking sublingual nitroglycerin tablets, the nurse instructs the patient
    a. to lie or sit and place one tablet under the tongue when chest pain occurs.
    b. to take the tablet with a large amount of water so it will dissolve right away.
    c. that if one tablet does not relieve the pain in 15 minutes, the patient should go to the hospital.
    d. that if the tablet causes dizziness and a headache, the medication should be stopped and the doctor notified.

18. When teaching an older adult with CAD how to manage the treatment program for angina, the nurse instructs the patient
    a. to sit for 3 to 5 minutes before standing when getting out of bed.
    b. to exercise only twice a week to avoid unnecessary strain on the heart.
    c. that lifestyle changes are not as necessary as they would be in a younger person.
    d. that aspirin therapy is contraindicated in older adults because of the risk for bleeding.

19. When a patient reports chest pain, unstable angina must be identified and treated because
    a. the pain may be severe and disabling.
    b. ECG changes and dysrhythmias may occur during an attack.
    c. atherosclerotic plaque deterioration may cause complete thrombus of the vessel lumen.
    d. the spasm of a major coronary artery may cause total occlusion of the vessel with progression to MI.

20. The nurse suspects stable angina rather than MI pain in the patient who reports chest pain that
    a. is relieved by nitroglycerin.
    b. is a sensation of tightness or squeezing.
    c. does not radiate to the neck, back, or arms.
    d. is precipitated by physical or emotional exertion.

21. A patient admitted to the hospital for evaluation of chest pain has no abnormal serum cardiac markers 4 hours after the onset of pain. A noninvasive diagnostic test that can differentiate angina from other types of chest pain is a(n)
    a. ECG.
    b. exercise stress test.
    c. coronary angiogram.
    d. transesophageal echocardiogram.

22. A 52-year-old man is admitted to the emergency department with severe chest pain. The nurse suspects an MI on finding that the patient
    a. has pale, cool, clammy skin.
    b. reports nausea and vomited once at home.
    c. is anxious and has a feeling of impending doom.
    d. has had no relief of the pain with rest or position change.

23. The point in the healing process of the myocardium following an infarct where early scar tissue results in an unstable heart wall is
    a. 2 to 3 days after MI.
    b. 4 to 10 days after MI.
    c. 10 to 14 days after MI.
    d. 6 weeks after MI.

24. To detect and treat the most common complication of MI, the nurse
    a. measures hourly urine output.
    b. auscultates the chest for crackles.
    c. uses continuous cardiac monitoring.
    d. takes vital signs q2hr for the first 8 hours.

25. Match the following complications of MI with the clinical manifestations that commonly indicate its occurrence.
    _____ a. Heart failure
    _____ b. Cardiogenic shock
    _____ c. Papillary muscle dysfunction
    _____ d. Ventricular aneurysm
    _____ e. Pericarditis

    1. Intractable dysrhythmias and heart failure
    2. Systolic murmur at the cardiac apex radiating toward the axilla
    3. Persistent or intermittent pericardial friction rub
    4. Crackles in lungs and S_3 or S_4 heart sound
    5. Decreased CO with falling BP

26. In the patient with chest pain, unstable angina can be differentiated from an MI by
    a. ECG changes present at onset of the pain.
    b. a chest x-ray indicating left ventricular hypertrophy.
    c. CK-MB enzyme elevations that peak 18 hours after the infarct.
    d. the appearance of troponin in the blood 48 hours after the infarct.

27. A second 12-lead ECG performed on a patient 4 hours after the onset of chest pain reveals ST-segment elevation. The nurse recognizes that this finding indicates a
    a. transient ischemia typical of unstable angina.
    b. lack of permanent damage to myocardial cells.
    c. myocardial infarction associated with prolonged and complete coronary thrombosis.
    d. myocardial infarction associated with transient or incomplete coronary artery occlusion.

28. Match the following descriptions with the procedures used to treat CAD (answers may be used more than once).
    _____ a. Surgical construction of new vessels to carry blood beyond obstructed coronary artery
    _____ b. Requires anticoagulation following the procedure
    _____ c. Most common alternative to a coronary artery bypass graft (CABG)
    _____ d. Structure applied to hold vessels open
    _____ e. Laser-created channels between left ventricular cavity and coronary circulation
    _____ f. Compression of atherosclerotic plaque with a balloon

    1. Percutaneous coronary intervention (PCI)
    2. Stent placement
    3. Transmyocardial laser revascularization (TMR)
    4. CABG

29. *Delegation Decision:* In planning care for a patient who has just returned to the unit following a percutaneous coronary intervention (PCI), the nurse may delegate which of the following actions to nursing assistive personnel (NAP)?
    a. Monitor the IV fluids and measure urine output.
    b. Explain to the patient the need for frequent vital signs (VS) and pulse checks.
    c. Check VS and report increases or decreases in HR and/or BP.
    d. Assess the circulation to the extremity used by checking pulses, skin temperature, and color.

30. The nurse explains to the patient who is to undergo a coronary artery bypass graft that the procedure most often involves
    a. using a synthetic graft as a tube for blood flow from the aorta to a coronary artery distal to an obstruction.
    b. resecting a stenosed coronary artery and inserting a synthetic arterial tube graft to replace the diseased artery.
    c. loosening the internal mammary artery from the chest wall and attaching it to a coronary artery distal to a stenosis.
    d. anastomosing reversed segments of a saphenous artery from the aorta to the coronary artery distal to an obstruction.

31. Collaborative care of the patient with non–ST-segment–elevation myocardial infarction (NSTEMI) differs from that of a patient with ST-segment–elevation myocardial infarction (STEMI) in that NSTEMI is more frequently treated initially with
    a. PCI.
    b. CABG.
    c. acute intensive drug therapy.
    d. reperfusion therapy with fibrinolytics.

32. During treatment with tissue plasminogen activator (tPA) for a patient with a STEMI, the nurse is most concerned on finding
    a. BP of 102/60 with an HR of 78.
    b. oozing of blood from the IV site.
    c. a decrease in the responsiveness of the patient.
    d. the presence of intermittent accelerated idioventricular dysrhythmias.

33. The nurse recognizes that fibrinolytic therapy for the treatment of an MI has not been successful when the patient
    a. continues to have chest pain.
    b. develops major GI or genitourinary (GU) bleeding during treatment.
    c. has a marked increase in CK enzyme levels within 3 hours of therapy.
    d. develops premature ventricular contractions and ventricular tachycardia during treatment.

34. Match the following characteristics with the drugs used to treat myocardial infarction.
    _____ a. Controls ventricular dysrhythmias
    _____ b. Relieves pain by decreasing O_2 demand and increasing O_2 supply
    _____ c. Helps prevent ventricular remodeling
    _____ d. Relieves anxiety and cardiac workload
    _____ e. Associated with decreased reinfarction and increased survival
    _____ f. Minimizes bradycardia from vagal stimulation

    1. β-Adrenergic blockers
    2. IV morphine
    3. Stool softeners
    4. IV amiodarone (Cordarone)
    5. IV nitroglycerin
    6. ACE inhibitors

35. A patient with an MI has a nursing diagnosis of anxiety related to possible lifestyle changes and perceived threat of death. The nurse determines that outcome criteria have been met when the patient states,
    a. "I'm going to take this recovery one step at a time."
    b. "I feel much better and am ready to get on with my life."
    c. "How soon do you think I will be able to go back to work?"
    d. "I know you are doing everything possible to save my life."

36. ***Priority Decision:*** A patient hospitalized for evaluation of unstable angina experiences severe chest pain and calls the nurse. Prioritize the interventions below from 1 (highest priority) to 6 (lowest priority). These are the appropriate medical orders and/or protocols available to the nurse.
    _____ a. Notify the physician.
    _____ b. Perform a focused assessment of the chest.
    _____ c. Assess pain (PQRST) and medicate as ordered.
    _____ d. Administer oxygen per nasal cannula.
    _____ e. Obtain a 12-lead ECG.
    _____ f. Check patient's VS.

37. Indicate what emotional responses (denial, anger, etc.) to acute MI are indicated by the following statements by patients.
    a. "I don't think I can take care of myself at home yet."
    b. "What's going to happen if I have another heart attack?"
    c. "I'll never be able to enjoy life again."
    d. "I hope my wife is happy now after harping at me about my eating habits all these years."
    e. "Yes, I'm having a little chest pain. It's no big deal."

38. The nurse and patient set a patient outcome that at the time of discharge after an MI the patient will be able to tolerate moderate-energy activities similar to
    a. golfing.
    b. walking at 5 mph.
    c. cycling at 13 mph.
    d. mowing the lawn by hand.

39. A 58-year-old patient is in a cardiac rehabilitation program. The nurse teaches the patient to stop exercising if
    a. pain or dyspnea develop.
    b. the HR exceeds 150 beats/min.
    c. the HR is 30 beats over the resting HR.
    d. the respiratory rate increases to 30 beats/min.

40. In counseling the patient about sexual activity following an MI, the nurse
    a. should wait for the patient to ask about resuming sexual activity.
    b. may discuss sexual activity while teaching about other physical activity.
    c. should have the patient ask the health care provider when sexual activity can be resumed.
    d. should inform the patient that impotence is a common long-term complication following MI.

41. The nurse advises the male patient who has had an MI that during sexual activity
    a. the patient should use the superior position.
    b. foreplay may cause too great an increase in heart rate.
    c. prophylactic nitroglycerin may be used if angina occurs.
    d. performance can be enhanced with the use of sildenafil (Viagra).

42. A patient is hospitalized after a successful resuscitation of an episode of sudden cardiac death. During the care of the patient, which of the following assessments by the nurse is most important?
    a. Continuous ECG monitoring
    b. Frequent assessment heart sounds
    c. Auscultation of the carotid arteries
    d. Monitoring of airway status and respiratory patterns

CASE STUDY
Coronary Artery Disease

Patient Profile

H.C., a 47-year-old Navaho woman, comes to the emergency department with a burning sensation in her epigastric area extending into her sternum.

Subjective Data

- Has had chest pain with activity that is relieved with rest for the past 3 months
- Has had type 2 diabetes mellitus since she was 35
- Has a smoking history of one pack a day for 27 years
- Is more than 30% over her ideal body weight
- Has no regular exercise program
- Expresses frustration with physical problems
- Is reluctant to get medical therapy because it will interfere with her life
- Has no health insurance

Objective Data

Physical Examination
- Anxious, clutching fists
- Appears overweight and withdrawn

Diagnostic Studies

- 12 lead ECG
- Cholesterol 248 mg/dL (6.41 mmol/L)
- LDL 160 mg/dL (4.14 mmol/L)
- Glucose 210 mg/dL (11.7 mmol/L)

Collaborative Care

- metoprolol (Toprol) XL 100 mg
- nifedipine (Procardia) 10 mg tid
- nitroglycerin 0.4 mg sublingual PRN for chest pain
- Exercise treadmill testing

Clinical Decision-Making Questions

Using a separate sheet of paper, answer the following questions

1. What are H.C.'s risk factors for CAD?
2. *Priority Decision:* What are the priority nursing measures that should be instituted to help H.C. decrease her risk factors?
3. What symptoms would lead you to suspect the pain may be angina?
4. What kind of ECG changes would indicate myocardial ischemia?
5. What information should the nurse provide for H.C. before the treadmill testing?
6. *Priority Decision:* Based on the assessment data presented, what are the priority nursing diagnoses? Are there any collaborative problems?

Nursing Management: Heart Failure

1. Identify whether the following statements are true (*T*) or false (*F*). If a statement is false, correct the bold word(s) to make the statement true.

_____ a. **Systolic failure** is characterized by abnormal resistance to ventricular filling.

_____ b. A primary risk factor for heart failure is **coronary artery disease**.

_____ c. A common cause of diastolic failure is **left ventricular hypertrophy**.

_____ d. The mechanisms by which **hypervolemia** acts as a precipitating cause of heart failure include decreasing cardiac output (CO) and increasing the workload and oxygen requirements of the myocardium.

_____ e. Systolic heart failure results in a **normal** left ventricular ejection fraction.

2. Describe the primary ways in which each of the following compensatory mechanisms of heart failure increases CO, and identify at least one effect of the mechanism that is detrimental to cardiac function.

a. Cardiac dilation

↑ CO:

Detrimental effect:

b. Cardiac hypertrophy

↑ CO:

Detrimental effect:

c. Sympathetic nervous system stimulation

↑ CO:

Detrimental effect:

d. Neurohormonal response

(1) Renin-angiotensin-aldosterone system

↑ CO:

Detrimental effect:

(2) ADH

↑ CO:

Detrimental effect:

3. Identify the trigger for the release of the following counterregulatory mechanisms and describe the mechanism of action by which these substances attempt to maintain balance in heart failure.

	Substances	Trigger	Mechanism of Action
ANP			
BNP			
NO			

4. The acronym FACES is used to help educate patients to identify symptoms of heart failure. What does FACES signify?

F _____

A _____

C _____

E _____

S _____

5. The pathophysiologic mechanism that results in the pulmonary edema of left-sided heart failure is
   a. increased right ventricular preload.
   b. increased pulmonary hydrostatic pressure.
   c. impaired alveolar oxygen and carbon dioxide exchange.
   d. increased lymphatic flow of pulmonary extravascular fluid.

6. A physical assessment finding that the nurse would expect to be present in the patient with acute left-sided heart failure is
   a. bubbling crackles and tachycardia.
   b. hepatosplenomegaly and tachypnea.
   c. peripheral edema and cool, diaphoretic skin.
   d. frothy blood-tinged sputum and distended jugular veins.

7. The nurse assesses the patient with chronic biventricular heart failure for paroxysmal nocturnal dyspnea by questioning the patient regarding
   a. the presence of difficulty breathing at night.
   b. frequent awakening to void during the night.
   c. the presence of a dry, hacking cough when resting.
   d. the use of two or more pillows to help breathing during sleep.

8. *Priority Decision:* The nurse reviews the following vital signs recorded by a nursing assistive personnel (NAP) on a patient with acute decompensated heart failure.

BP	98/60
HR	102
RR	24
Temp	98.2° F
SpO_2	84% on 2 L/nasal cannula

   a. Which of these findings is of highest priority?
   b. What should the nurse do next?

9. A patient with chronic heart failure has atrial fibrillation and an LV ejection fraction (LVEF) of 18%. To decrease the risk of complications from these conditions, the nurse anticipates the administration of
   a. diuretics.
   b. anticoagulants.
   c. β-adrenergic blockers.
   d. potassium supplements.

10. The diagnostic test that is most useful in differentiating dyspnea related to pulmonary effects of heart failure from dyspnea related to pulmonary disease is
    a. exercise stress testing.
    b. a cardiac catheterization.
    c. b-type natriuretic peptide (BNP) levels.
    d. determination of blood urea nitrogen (BUN).

11. Crossword Puzzle: Cardiac medications used in the treatment of acute and chronic heart failure with their therapeutic effects.

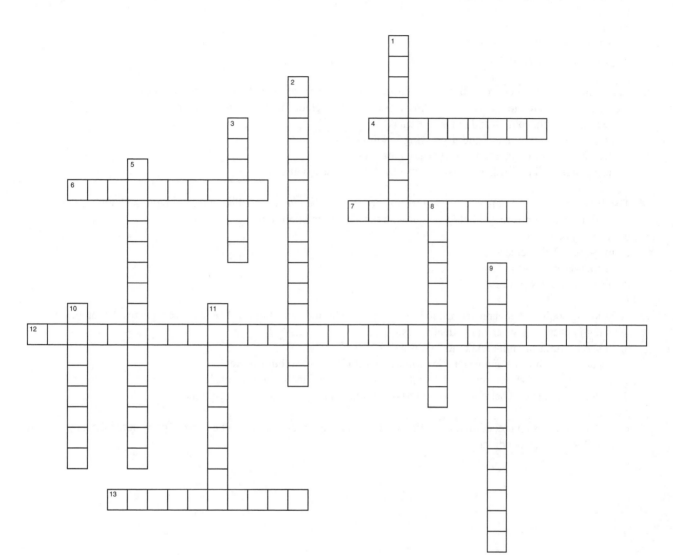

Across

4. Prevents vasoconstriction and blocks aldosterone; used for patient that cannot tolerate angiotensin-converting enzyme inhibitors

6. Directly blocks sympathetic nervous system's negative effects on the failing heart

7. Improves cardiac contractions, decreases afterload, and increases CO

12. Combination antihypertensive and antianginal agent; used only with African Americans

13. Primary effect is to decrease intravascular fluid volume, thus decreasing preload and improving left ventricular function

Down

1. Decreases afterload by reducing levels of angiotensin II and aldosterone

2. Primarily reduces preload and increases myocardial oxygen supply

3. Increases cardiac contractility and output and slows heart rate

5. Potent vasodilator that decreases both preload and afterload, increasing cardiac contractility and output

8. Dilates arterial and venous blood vessels in addition to relieving anxiety

9. Blocks action of aldosterone, decreasing intravascular volume by sodium excretion, but retains potassium

10. Increases cardiac contractility but may increase ventricular irritability

11. Recombinant form of a natriuretic peptide that decreases preload and afterload

12. A patient with chronic heart failure is treated with hydrochlorothiazide, digoxin, and lisinopril (Prinivil). To prevent the risk of digitalis toxicity with these drugs, it is most important that the nurse monitor the patient's
    a. HR.
    b. BP.
    c. potassium levels.
    d. gastrointestinal function.

13. The health care provider prescribes spironolactone (Aldactone) for the patient with chronic heart failure. Diet modifications related to the use of this drug that the nurse includes in patient teaching include
    a. decreasing both sodium and potassium intake.
    b. increasing calcium intake and decreasing sodium intake.
    c. decreasing sodium intake and increasing potassium intake.
    d. decreasing sodium intake and using salt substitutes for seasoning.

14. The nurse monitors the patient receiving treatment for acute decompensated heart failure with the knowledge that marked hypotension is most likely to occur with the IV administration of
    a. furosemide (Lasix).
    b. milrinone (Primacor).
    c. nitroglycerin (Tridil).
    d. nitroprusside (Nipride).

15. A 2400-mg sodium diet is prescribed for a patient with chronic heart failure. The nurse recognizes that additional teaching is necessary when the patient states,
    a. "I should limit my milk intake to 2 cups a day."
    b. "I can eat fresh fruits and vegetables without worrying about sodium content."
    c. "I can eat most foods as long as I do not add salt when cooking or at the table."
    d. "I need to read the labels on prepared foods and medicines for their sodium content."

16. List four cardiovascular conditions that may lead to heart failure and what can be done to prevent the development of heart failure in each condition.
    a.

    b.

    c.

    d.

17. The nurse determines that treatment of heart failure has been successful when the patient experiences
    a. weight loss and diuresis.
    b. warm skin and less fatigue.
    c. clear lung sounds and decreased heart rate (HR).
    d. absence of chest pain and improved level of consciousness (LOC).

18. A patient with heart failure has tachypnea, severe dyspnea, and an SpO_2 of 84%. The nurse identifies a nursing diagnosis of impaired gas exchange related to increased preload and mechanical failure. An appropriate nursing intervention for this diagnosis is to
    a. assist the patient to cough and deep-breathe q2hr.
    b. assess intake and output q8hr and weigh the patient daily.
    c. encourage alternate rest and activity periods to reduce cardiac workload.
    d. place the patient in high Fowler's position with the feet dangling over the bedside.

19. The nurse determines that additional discharge teaching is needed when the patient with chronic heart failure says,
    a. "I will take my pulse every day and call the clinic if it is irregular or less than 50."
    b. "I should hold my digitalis and call the doctor if I experience nausea and vomiting."
    c. "I plan to organize my household tasks so I don't have to constantly go up and down the stairs."
    d. "I should weigh myself every morning and go on a diet if I gain more than 2 or 3 pounds in 2 days."

20. The evaluation team for cardiac transplantation determines that the patient who would most benefit from a new heart is
    a. a 24-year-old man with Down syndrome who has received excellent care from parents in their 60s.
    b. a 46-year-old single woman with a limited support system who has alcohol-induced cardiomyopathy.
    c. a 60-year-old man with inoperable coronary artery disease who has not been compliant with lifestyle changes and rehabilitation programs.
    d. a 52-year-old woman with end-stage coronary artery disease who has limited financial resources but is emotionally stable and has strong social support.

21. The nurse plans long-term goals for the patient who has had a heart transplant with the knowledge that a common cause of death in heart transplant patients during the first year is
    a. infection.
    b. heart failure.
    c. embolization.
    d. malignant conditions.

CASE STUDY
Acute Decompensated Heart Failure

Patient Profile

L.J. is a 63-year-old man who has a history of hypertension, chronic heart failure, and sleep apnea. He has been smoking two packs of cigarettes a day for 40 years and has refused to quit. Three days ago he had an onset of flu with fever, pharyngitis, and malaise. He has not taken his antihypertensive medications or his medications to control his heart failure for 4 days. Today he has been admitted to the hospital intensive care area with acute decompensated heart failure.

Subjective Data

• Is very anxious and asks, "Am I going to die?"
• Denies pain but says he feels like he cannot get enough air
• Says his heart feels like it is "running away"
• Reports that he is so exhausted he can't eat or drink by himself

Objective Data

• Height: 5 ft 10 in (175 cm); weight: 210 lb (95.5 kg)
• Vital signs: T 99.6° F (37.6° C), HR 118 and irregular, RR 34, BP 90/58
• Cardiovascular: Distant S_1, S_2; S_3, S_4 present; PMI at sixth ICS and faint; all peripheral pulses are 1+; bilateral jugular vein distention; initial cardiac monitoring indicates atrial fibrillation with a ventricular rate of 132
• Respiratory: Pulmonary crackles; decreased breath sounds right lower lobe; coughing frothy blood-tinged sputum; SpO_2 82% on room air
• Gastrointestinal: BS present; hepatomegaly 4 cm below costal margin
• Laboratory work and diagnostic testing are scheduled.

Clinical Decision-Making Questions

Using a separate sheet of paper, answer the following questions

1. What signs and symptoms of right-sided and left-sided heart failure is L.J. experiencing?
2. What diagnostic procedures and findings would help to establish a diagnosis of acute decompensated heart failure with pulmonary edema?
3. What monitoring will be used to evaluate L.J.'s condition?
4. *Priority Decision:* What priority nursing interventions are appropriate for L.J. at the time of his admission?
5. During L.J.'s hospitalization, basic standards of evidence-based care for patients with HF are set forth in four core measures. Which two of these measures should be implemented by the nurse?
6. The physician mentions the possibility of inserting a pacemaker called cardiac resynchronization therapy (CRT). L.J. asks the nurse what CRT is. What response would be appropriate from the nurse?
7. *Priority Decision:* Based on the assessment data presented, what are the priority nursing diagnoses for L.J.? Are there any collaborative problems?

1. Identify whether the following statements are true (*T*) or false (*F*). If a statement is false, correct the bold word(s) to make the statement true.
    _____ a. During **repolarization** of cardiac cells, sodium migrates rapidly into the cell, making the cell positive compared with the outside of the cell.
    _____ b. Depolarization of the cells in the ventricles produces the **T wave** on the ECG.
    _____ c. A patient with a regular heart rate (HR) has four QRS complexes between every 3-second marker on the ECG paper. The patient's HR is **40 beats/min.**
    _____ d. The ECG pattern of a patient with a regular HR reveals 20 small squares between each R-R interval. The patient's heart rate is **75 beats/min.**
    _____ e. Lead placement for MCL$_1$ monitoring is the positive electrode at the **fourth intercostal space at the right sternal border** and the negative electrode at the **left midclavicular line just below the clavicle.**
    _____ f. If the SA node fails to discharge an impulse or discharges very slowly, a secondary pacemaker in the AV node is able to discharge at a rate of **30 to 40** times per minute.
    _____ g. **Reentrant excitation** causing premature beats may occur when areas of the heart do not repolarize at the same rate because of depressed conduction.
    _____ h. An abnormal cardiac impulse that arises in the atria, ventricles, or AV junction that creates a premature beat is known as **an artifact.**

2. Match the following terms with their definitions.
    _____ a. Conductivity   1. Ability to discharge an electrical impulse spontaneously
    _____ b. Excitability   2. Abnormal electrical impulses
    _____ c. Automaticity   3. Period in which heart tissue cannot be stimulated
    _____ d. Ectopic foci   4. Ability to respond mechanically to an impulse
    _____ e. Refractoriness   5. Property of myocardial tissue that enables it to be depolarized by an impulse
    _____ f. Contractility   6. Ability to transmit an impulse along a membrane

3. The patient's PR interval comprises six small boxes on the ECG graph. The nurse determines that this indicates
    a. a normal finding.
    b. a problem with ventricular depolarization.
    c. a disturbance in the repolarization of the atria.
    d. a problem with conduction from the SA node to the ventricular cells.

4. The nurse plans close monitoring for the patient during electrophysiologic testing because this test
    a. requires the use of dyes that irritate the myocardium.
    b. causes myocardial ischemia, resulting in dysrhythmias.
    c. involves the use of anticoagulants to prevent thrombus and embolism.
    d. induces dysrhythmias that may require cardioversion/defibrillation to correct.

5. Word Search. Find the words that are defined by the clues given on the next page. The words may be located horizontally, vertically, or diagonally and may be reversed.

```
Q K C I A O F Y R O P J V U K T N K I P N J L M D R D W S H
A B S H F L B U O G J V Q R J V P E T D Y A V B T J L M C Z
R B N L Z N D P N G I C X O E S R U V K F B W P R U B Y N A
S G O C X G E E N G W X V B P P E Q K F R W K Q N N T R Z C
F I I K C S V I G M E L J R W A M P M U M E S K A C L O A S
E C T R L M F E Q A Q I Q D D I A J B J Z T S I S T U K G E
U D C W Y Y O F N K L J U Z M D T E A N W Q I Y X I X Q K Q
K A A G G I H R P T Y U G C Z R U H A Z V M Q R K O T V G H
U C R P C B Q J X O R P K F P A R O K A G C V Y B N I Z E P
V L T X X N U T D A H I U R P C E E J K F B U F U A W M L U
X X N C N X R O V Y R L C V N Y V U E U C S N M E L A J Z D
M B O R E F E K Z C C B R U A H E K E S L D O C R E T L S J
T R C Y N H F W G T N D M N L C N U R B I B G O P S R D L C
S Q L O Z T X D O J J O A Y Q A T V W Z E H N C X C I G L I
P I A F B E I D A P L B I T J T R V D B V H K H J A A L T Z
C V I D S Q L Z K C P Z D T J R I F Q W X M T K Z P L M I I
G A R O Q T F M S K X M R U A A C I I A T H B K D E F V P S
Y I T O G K C S C X T O A O J L U T E B X G E G J R L J T F
T D A J J P B M F P H X C V W U L W Y O R P N M D H U R C F
S R E R W V J S E W I R Y Y L C A I P P C I Z L G Y T I Y W
K A R W I Y U A K R R C H V U I R X R I E U L K Y T T C F H
G C U M E D P Y U W D D C J K R C I C B V I K L L H E K Z B
Q Y T U D O F C P O D I A O W T O T A Y I O I S A M R F D C
C H A Y K A G X S T E J T S T N N M Z X N F N A A T P D M U
D C M V C G E U K Z G Z R H K E T H W J T A L S V J I I Z F
G A E L O B B Z D B R O A P J V R F M S Q Z Y A V B H O N V
Y T R X V R J A U D E J L L O A A A G C V S P O I D L W N K
U S P A R R A G L F E D U Z G R C A D B T C O R J R Y O D W
F U H N M G X X D I A Q C V Z P T Y U O Y K N J H I T L C B
I N F U W E Z Y P V V O I S E U I Z L D J G R K Q K R A F K
V I D U I N J K M D B H R N W S O E E B V L H F A B Y A Q I
A S G T B B Z F S H L C T A J L N G I Y V Q J K R E O U G Y
D L C Y U V H T H X O S N Q J A P R O U C J G U E C L M T U
J W H I M L V Y G U C K E U D M V C U X C L K J A X N Q P E
T E N E T J O G C T K J V I Q S C F F L S U A O E O U L A P
D E V Q C K S I N U S B R A D Y C A R D I A B M G G W A Y J
Z I B C Z C Q Z R E C Q V P M X S D P D C J C J M X G S H L
F I R S T D E G R E E A V B L O C K L D H U I R H I J E L E
A E P Y T I V I T C A L A C I R T C E L E S S E L E S L U P
F N Y S E C O N D D E G R E E A V B L O C K T Y P E I E W V
G Q S D F O V C N G V D T X M P V Z L C J L A T M V D D L Z
```

Clues

a. Absence of ventricular activity
b. Wide, distorted QRS
c. Usual spontaneous onset and termination
d. Associated with bundle branch blocks
e. Chaotic ventricular rhythm
f. Normal rhythm pattern with rate <60
g. Heart rate of 40-60 beats/min
h. May precipitate supraventricular tachycardia
i. Atria and ventricles dissociated
j. A run of PVCs
k. Prolonged PR interval
l. Chaotic P wave
m. Sinus rate >100
n. Electrical activity with no mechanical response
o. Recurring, sawtooth flutter waves
p. Gradually lengthening PR interval

6. Complete the following statements.

   a. A patient with an acute myocardial infarction (MI) develops the following ECG pattern: atrial rate of 82 and regular; ventricular rate of 46 and regular; P wave and QRS complex are normal, but there is no relationship between the P wave and the QRS complex. The nurse identifies the dysrhythmia as _____,

      and the treatment indicated is _____ .

   b. A common dysrhythmia the nurse would expect to find in a patient with hypoxemia and hypovolemia is

      _____.

   c. Vagal stimulation induced by carotid massage may be used to treat the dysrhythmia of

      _____.

   d. A dysrhythmia characterized by progressive lengthening of the PR interval until an atrial impulse is not conducted and a QRS complex is dropped is known as _____.

   e. PVCs that occur on the T wave of a preceding contraction are always treated because they may precipitate

      _____ or _____.

7. A patient with an acute MI has a sinus tachycardia of 126 beats/min. The nurse recognizes that if this dysrhythmia is not treated, the patient is likely to experience
   a. hypertension.
   b. escape rhythms.
   c. ventricular tachycardia.
   d. an increase in infarct size.

8. A patient with no history of heart disease has a rhythm strip that shows an occasional distorted P wave followed by normal AV and ventricular conduction. The nurse questions the patient about
   a. the use of caffeine.
   b. the use of sedatives.
   c. any aerobic training.
   d. holding of breath during exertion.

9. A patient's rhythm strip indicates a normal HR and rhythm with normal P wave and QRS complex, but the PR interval is 0.26 sec. The most appropriate action by the nurse is to
   a. continue to assess the patient.
   b. administer atropine per protocol.
   c. prepare the patient for synchronized cardioversion.
   d. prepare the patient for placement of a temporary pacemaker.

10. In the patient with a dysrhythmia, the nurse identifies a nursing diagnosis of decreased CO related to dysrhythmias when the patient experiences
    a. hypertension and bradycardia.
    b. chest pain and decreased mentation.
    c. abdominal distention and hepatomegaly.
    d. bounding pulses and a ventricular heave.

11. *Priority Decision:* A patient with an acute MI is having multifocal PVCs and ventricular couplets. He is alert and has a BP of 118/78 with an irregular pulse of 86 beats/min. The priority nursing action at this time is to
    a. continue to assess the patient.
    b. ask the patient to perform Valsalva maneuver.
    c. prepare to administer antidysrhythmic drugs per protocol.
    d. be prepared to administer cardiopulmonary resuscitation (CPR).

12. PVCs are indicated by a rhythm pattern finding of
    a. a QRS complex of >0.12 sec followed by a P wave.
    b. continuous wide QRS complexes with a ventricular rate of 160 beats/min.
    c. sawtooth P waves with no measurable PR interval and an irregular rhythm.
    d. P waves hidden in QRS complexes with a regular rhythm of 120 beats/min.

13. Cardiac defibrillation
    a. enhances repolarization and relaxation of ventricular myocardial cells.
    b. provides an electrical impulse that stimulates normal myocardial contractions.
    c. depolarizes the cells of the myocardium to allow the SA node to resume pacemaker function.
    d. delivers an electrical impulse to the heart at the time of ventricular contraction to convert the heart to a sinus rhythm.

14. Initial treatment of asystole and pulseless electrical activity is
    a. CPR.
    b. defibrillation.
    c. administration of atropine.
    d. administration of epinephrine.

15. The nurse's responsibilities in preparing to administer defibrillation include
    a. applying gel pads to the patient's chest.
    b. setting the defibrillator to deliver 50 joules.
    c. setting the defibrillator to a synchronized mode.
    d. sedating the patient with midazolam (Versed) before defibrillation.

16. While providing discharge instructions to the patient who has had an implantable cardioverter-defibrillator (ICD) inserted, the nurse teaches the patient that if he or she is alone when the ICD fires, he or she should (select all that apply)
    a. lie down.
    b. call the health care provider.
    c. push the reset button on the pulse generator.
    d. immediately take his or her antidysrhythmic medication.

17. A patient with a sinus node dysfunction has a permanent pacemaker inserted. Before discharge, the nurse teaches the patient to
    a. avoid cooking with microwave ovens.
    b. avoid high-voltage electrical generators.
    c. use mild analgesics to control the chest spasms caused by the pacing current.
    d. start lifting the arm above the shoulder right away to prevent a "frozen shoulder."

18. *Priority Decision:* A patient on the cardiac telemetry unit goes into ventricular fibrillation and is unresponsive. Following initiation of the emergency call system (Code Blue), the next priority for the nurse is to
    a. get the crash cart.
    b. administer amiodarone IV.
    c. defibrillate with 360 joules.
    d. begin cardiopulmonary resuscitation (CPR).

19. The use of catheter ablation therapy to "burn" areas of the cardiac conduction system is indicated for treatment of
    a. sinus arrest.
    b. heart blocks.
    c. tachydysrhythmias.
    d. premature ventricular tachycardia.

20. A patient with chest pain that is unrelieved by nitroglycerin is admitted to the coronary care unit for observation and diagnosis. While the patient has continuous ECG monitoring, the nurse would be most concerned with the presence of
    a. occasional PVCs.
    b. an inverted T wave.
    c. ST segment elevation.
    d. a PR interval of 0.18 sec.

21. A 54-year-old patient who has no structural heart disease has an episode of syncope. Upright tilt-table testing is performed to rule out neurocardiogenic syncope. The nurse explains to the patient that if neurocardiogenic syncope is the problem, the patient will experience
    a. no change in HR or BP.
    b. palpitations and dizziness.
    c. tachydysrhythmias and chest pain.
    d. marked bradycardia and hypotension.

22. Identify the following cardiac rhythms using the systematic approach to assessing cardiac rhythms found in Table 36-5 in the textbook. All rhythm strips are 6 seconds.
    a.

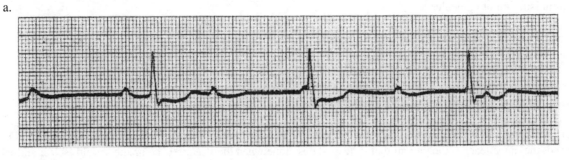

b.

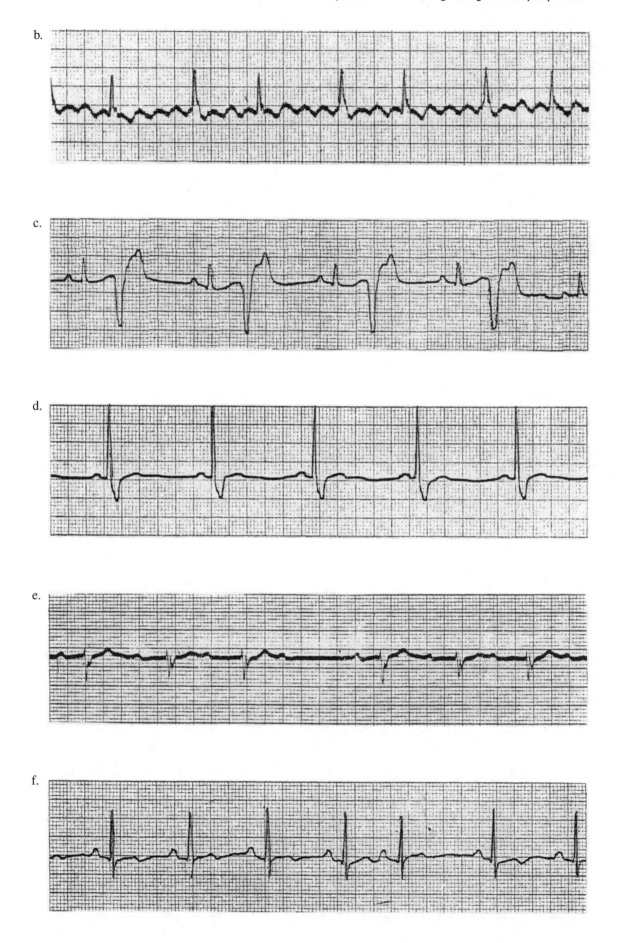

c.

d.

e.

f.

g.

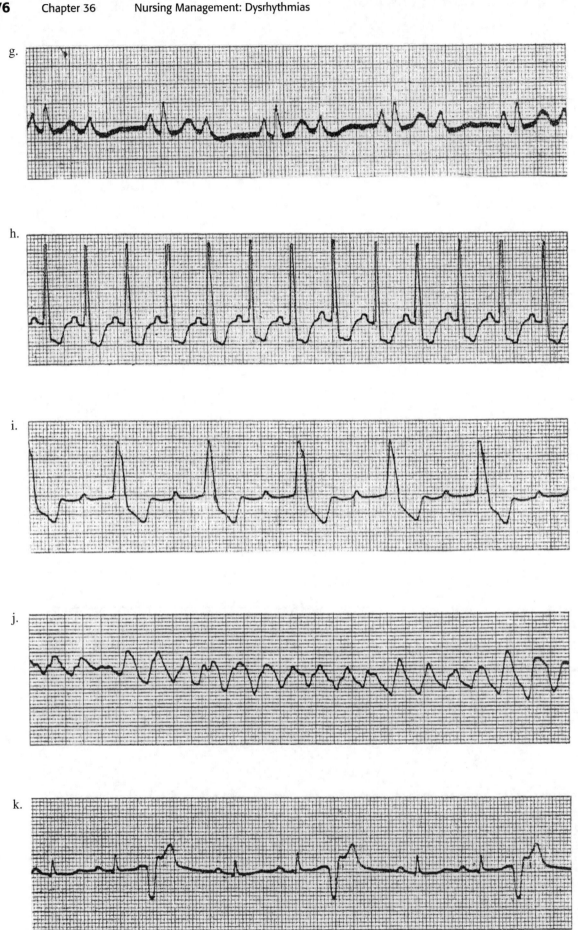

h.

i.

j.

k.

l.

m.

n.

o.

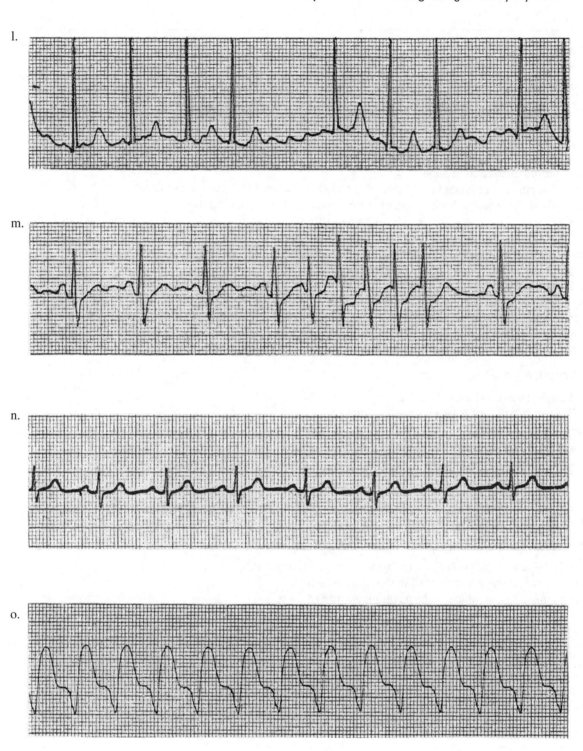

CASE STUDY
Dysrhythmia
Patient Profile

R.S. is a 75-year-old woman admitted to the telemetry unit with a diagnosis of new onset atrial fibrillation.

Subjective Data

- Has a history of hypothyroidism and hypertension
- Has no history of atrial fibrillation
- Is taking levothyroxin (Synthroid) 0.125 mg PO daily and enalapril (Vasotec) 5 mg PO bid
- Complains of palpitations, dizziness, shortness of breath, and mild chest pressure

Objective Data

Physical Examination
- Alert, anxious, older woman
- BP: 100/70, HR 150/min, RR 32/min
- Lungs: Bibasilar crackles
- Heart: S_1 and S_2, irregular

Diagnostic Study
- 12-lead ECG: Atrial fibrillation with an uncontrolled ventricular response

Collaborative Care

- Discontinue enalapril (Vasotec)
- IV diltiazem (Cardizem) bolus and then IV drip
- digoxin 0.25 mg PO daily
- enoxaparin (Lovenox) subcutaneous BID
- warfarin (Coumadin) 5 mg PO daily

Clinical Decision-Making Questions

Using a separate sheet of paper, answer the following questions.

1. What is the immediate goal of antidysrhythmic drug therapy for R.S.?
2. What nondrug therapy may be used to treat the dysrhythmia?
3. Explain the rationale for use of the medications ordered for R.S.
4. Explain the pathophysiology of her symptoms on admission to the telemetry unit.
5. Describe the characteristics of her ECG waveform.
6. *Priority Decision:* Based on the assessment data presented, what are the priority nursing diagnoses? Are there any collaborative problems?

37 Nursing Management: Inflammatory and Structural Heart Disorders

1. A 20-year-old patient has acute infective endocarditis. While obtaining a nursing history, the nurse should ask the patient about which of the following (select all that apply)?
   a. renal dialysis
   b. IV drug abuse
   c. recent dental work
   d. cardiac catheterization
   e. recent urinary tract infection

2. A patient has an admitting diagnosis of acute left-sided infective endocarditis. The nurse explains to the patient that this diagnosis is best confirmed with
   a. blood cultures.
   b. a complete blood count.
   c. a cardiac catheterization.
   d. a transesophageal echocardiogram.

3. Match the following manifestations of infective endocarditis with their descriptions.
   _____ a. Splinter hemorrhages   1. Hemorrhagic retinal lesions
   _____ b. Janeway's lesions   2. Painful red or purple lesions on fingers or toes
   _____ c. Osler's nodes   3. Black longitudinal streaks in nail beds
   _____ d. Roth's spots   4. Small hemorrhages in conjunctiva, lips, and buccal mucosa
   _____ e. Petechiae   5. Flat, red, painless spots on the palms and soles of feet

4. A patient with infective endocarditis of a prosthetic mitral valve develops a left hemiparesis and visual changes. The nurse expects that collaborative management of the patient will include
   a. an embolectomy.
   b. surgical valve replacement.
   c. administration of anticoagulants.
   d. higher than usual antibiotic dosages.

5. A patient with aortic valve endocarditis develops dyspnea, crackles in the lungs, and restlessness. The nurse suspects that the patient is experiencing
   a. vegetative embolization to the coronary arteries.
   b. pulmonary embolization from valve vegetations.
   c. nonspecific manifestations that accompany infectious diseases.
   d. valvular incompetence with possible infectious invasion of the myocardium.

6. *Priority Decision:* A patient hospitalized for 1 week with subacute infective endocarditis is afebrile and has no signs of heart damage. Discharge with outpatient antibiotic therapy is planned. During discharge planning with the patient, it is most important for the nurse to
   a. plan how his needs will be met while he continues on bed rest.
   b. teach the patient to avoid crowds and exposure to upper respiratory infections.
   c. encourage the use of diversional activities to relieve boredom and restlessness.
   d. assess the patient's home environment in terms of family assistance and hospital access.

7. When teaching a patient with endocarditis how to prevent recurrence of the infection, the nurse instructs the patient to
   a. start on antibiotic therapy when exposed to persons with infections.
   b. take one aspirin a day to prevent vegetative lesions from forming around the valves.
   c. always maintain continuous antibiotic therapy to prevent the development of any systemic infection.
   d. obtain prophylactic antibiotic therapy before certain invasive medical or dental procedures (e.g., dental cleaning).

8. A patient is admitted to the hospital with a suspected acute pericarditis. To establish the presence of a pericardial friction rub, the nurse listens to the patient's chest
   a. while timing the sound with the respiratory pattern.
   b. with the bell of the stethoscope at the apex of the heart.
   c. with the diaphragm of the stethoscope at the lower left sternal border of the chest.
   d. with the diaphragm of the stethoscope to auscultate a high-pitched continuous rumbling sound.

9. A patient with acute pericarditis has markedly distended jugular veins, decreased BP, tachycardia, tachypnea, and muffled heart sounds. The nurse recognizes that these symptoms occur when
   a. the pericardial space is obliterated with scar tissue and thickened pericardium.
   b. excess pericardial fluid compresses the heart and prevents adequate diastolic filling.
   c. the parietal and visceral pericardial membranes adhere to each other, preventing normal myocardial contraction.
   d. fibrin accumulation on the visceral pericardium infiltrates into the myocardium, creating generalized myocardial dysfunction.

10. Identify whether the following statements are true (*T*) or false (*F*). If a statement is false, correct the bold word(s) to make the statement true.
    _____ a. To measure a pulsus paradoxus, the nurse determines the difference between the systolic pressure **at inspiration** and the systolic pressure **at expiration**.
    _____ b. A pulsus paradoxus of >10 mm Hg occurs with **cardiac tamponade**.
    _____ c. A pericardiocentesis is indicated for the patient with pericarditis when there is **pericardial effusion of any amount**.
    _____ d. Acute pericarditis may be diagnosed with **ECG showing diffuse ST segment elevation**.
    _____ e. Treatment of chronic constrictive pericarditis may include a **pericardiectomy**.

11. A patient with acute pericarditis has a nursing diagnosis of pain related to pericardial inflammation. An appropriate nursing intervention for the patient is
    a. administering opioids as prescribed on an around-the-clock schedule.
    b. promoting progressive relaxation exercises with the use of deep, slow breathing.
    c. positioning the patient on the right side with the head of the bed elevated 15 degrees.
    d. positioning the patient in Fowler's position with a padded over-the-bed table for the patient to lean on.

12. When obtaining a nursing history for a patient with myocarditis, the nurse specifically questions the patient about
    a. a history of CAD with or without an MI.
    b. prior use of digoxin for treatment of cardiac problems.
    c. recent symptoms of a viral illness, such as fever and malaise.
    d. a recent streptococcal infection requiring treatment with penicillin.

13. The most important role of the nurse in preventing rheumatic fever is to
    a. teach patients with infective endocarditis to adhere to antibiotic prophylaxis.
    b. identify patients with valvular heart disease who are at risk for rheumatic fever.
    c. encourage the use of antibiotics for treatment of all infections involving a sore throat.
    d. promote the early diagnosis and immediate treatment of group A streptococcal pharyngitis.

14. The diagnosis of acute rheumatic fever is most strongly supported in the patient with
    a. carditis, polyarthritis, and erythema marginatum.
    b. polyarthritis, chorea, and increased antistreptolysin O titer.
    c. positive C-reactive protein, elevated WBC, subcutaneous nodules.
    d. organic heart murmurs, fever, and elevated erythrocyte sedimentation rate (ESR).

15. Identify the rationale for the use of the following drugs in the treatment of acute rheumatic fever:
    a. Antibiotics
    b. Aspirin
    c. Corticosteroids
    d. NSAIDs

16. A patient with rheumatic heart disease with carditis asks the nurse how long his activity will be restricted. The best answer by the nurse is that he
    a. can perform nonstrenuous activities as soon as antibiotics are started.
    b. will be confined to bed until symptoms of heart failure are controlled.
    c. will be able to have full activity as soon as acute symptoms have subsided.
    d. must be on bed rest until antiinflammatory therapy has been discontinued.

17. Identify whether the following statements are true *(T)* or false *(F)*. If a statement is false, correct the bold word(s) to make the statement true.
    _____ a. Valvular stenosis leads to **backward** flow of blood and **dilation** of the preceding chamber.
    _____ b. **Valvular regurgitation** causes a pressure gradient difference across an open valve.
    _____ c. The heart valve most commonly affected by stenosis or regurgitation is the **tricuspid** valve.
    _____ d. The most common form of valvular disease in the United States is **mitral stenosis**.

18. *Delegation Decision*: An RN is working with an LPN in caring for a group of patients on a cardiac telemetry unit. A patient with aortic stenosis has the nursing diagnosis of activity intolerance related to fatigue and exertional dyspnea. Which of these nursing activities could be delegated to the LPN?
    a. Explain the reason for planning frequent periods of rest.
    b. Evaluate the patient's understanding of his disease process.
    c. Monitor BP, HR, RR and SpO_2 before, during, and after ambulation.
    d. Teach the patient which activities to choose that will gradually increase endurance.

19. Match the following characteristics with the related type of valvular disease (answers may be used more than once).
    _____ a. Sudden onset of cardiovascular collapse
    _____ b. May be caused by pulmonary hypertension
    _____ c. Rapid development of pulmonary edema and cardiogenic shock
    _____ d. Dyspnea is a prominent symptom
    _____ e. Loud pansystolic or holosystolic murmur
    _____ f. Ballooning of valve into left atrium during ventricular systole
    _____ g. Characteristic systolic crescendo-decrescendo murmur
    _____ h. Water-hammer pulses
    _____ i. Angina and syncope result from decreased CO
    _____ j. Embolization may result from chronic atrial fibrillation
    _____ k. Major symptoms related to elevated systemic venous pressures
    _____ l. Rapid onset prevents left chamber dilation
    _____ m. Brisk carotid pulses present

    1. Mitral stenosis
    2. Acute mitral regurgitation hypertension
    3. Chronic mitral regurgitation
    4. Mitral valve prolapse
    5. Aortic stenosis
    6. Acute aortic regurgitation
    7. Chronic aortic regurgitation
    8. Tricuspid valve disease

20. Drugs that the nurse would expect to be prescribed for patients with a mechanical valve replacement include
    a. oral nitrates.
    b. anticoagulants.
    c. atrial antidysrhythmics.
    d. β-adrenergic blocking agents.

21. A patient with symptomatic mitral valve prolapse has atrial and ventricular dysrhythmias. In addition to monitoring for decreased cardiac output related to the dysrhythmias, an appropriate nursing diagnosis related to the dysrhythmias identified by the nurse is
    a. ineffective breathing pattern related to hypervolemia.
    b. risk for injury related to dizziness and lightheadedness.
    c. disturbed sleep pattern related to paroxysmal nocturnal dyspnea.
    d. ineffective self-health management related to lack of knowledge of prevention and treatment strategies.

22. A patient is scheduled for a percutaneous transluminal balloon valvuloplasty. The nurse understands that this procedure is indicated for
    a. any patient with aortic regurgitation.
    b. older patients with aortic regurgitation.
    c. older patients with stenosis of any valve.
    d. young adult patients with mild mitral valve stenosis.

23. A patient is scheduled for an open surgical valvuloplasty of the mitral valve. In preparing the patient for surgery, the nurse recognizes that
    a. cardiopulmonary bypass is not required with this procedure.
    b. valve repair is a palliative measure, whereas valve replacement is curative.
    c. the operative mortality rate is lower in valve repair than in valve replacement.
    d. patients with valve repair do not require postoperative anticoagulation as they do with valve replacement.

24. A mechanical prosthetic valve is most likely to be preferred over a biologic valve for valve replacement in a
    a. 41-year-old man with peptic ulcer disease.
    b. 22-year-old woman who desires to have children.
    c. 35-year-old man with a history of seasonal asthma.
    d. 62-year-old woman with early Alzheimer's disease.

25. When performing discharge teaching for the patient following a mechanical valve replacement, the nurse determines that further instruction is needed when the patient says,
    a. "I may begin an exercise program to gradually increase my cardiac tolerance."
    b. "I will always need to have my blood checked once a month for its clotting function."
    c. "I should wear a Medic Alert bracelet to identify my valve and anticoagulant therapy."
    d. "The biggest risk I have during invasive health procedures is bleeding because of my anticoagulants."

26. Indicate whether the following characteristics of cardiomyopathies are associated with dilated cardiomyopathy (D), hypertrophic cardiomyopathy (H), or restrictive cardiomyopathy (R).
    _____ a. The hyperdynamic systolic function creates a diastolic failure
    _____ b. Systemic embolization may occur because of stasis of blood in the ventricles
    _____ c. The most uncommon type of cardiomyopathy
    _____ d. Often requires a heart transplant
    _____ e. About one half of the cases have a genetic basis
    _____ f. Differs from chronic heart failure in that there is no ventricular hypertrophy
    _____ g. Echocardiogram reveals cardiomegaly with thin ventricular walls
    _____ h. Often results in syncope during increased activity resulting from an obstructed aortic valve outflow
    _____ i. Often follows an infective myocarditis or exposure to toxins or drugs
    _____ j. Surgery to remove myocardial tissue may be indicated for symptoms refractory to treatment
    _____ k. Characterized by ventricular stiffness
    _____ l. Characterized by massive thickening of intraventricular septum and ventricular wall

27. When performing discharge teaching for the patient with any type of cardiomyopathy, the nurse instructs the patient to (select all that apply)
    a. eat a low-sodium diet.
    b. suggest that caregivers learn CPR.
    c. engage in stress reduction activities.
    d. abstain from alcohol and caffeine intake.
    e. avoid strenuous activity and allow for periods of rest.

CASE STUDY
Infective Endocarditis
Patient Profile

N.B. is a 60-year-old man who is hospitalized with a suspected stroke.

Subjective Data

• Had a laparoscopic cholecystectomy a few weeks ago

Objective Data

• Neurologic signs typical of a stroke (paralysis on right side involving right arm and leg, slurred speech)
• Petechiae over the chest
• Crescendo-decrescendo murmur present
• Rectal temperature 103° F (39.4°C)

Clinical Decision-Making Questions

Using a separate sheet of paper, answer the following questions.

1. Why is N.B. at risk for infective endocarditis?
2. What asymptomatic underlying cardiac conditions might N.B. have had that contributed to his infectious endocarditis?
3. Explain the cause of N.B.'s assessment findings.
4. What is the relevance of the endoscopic surgery N.B. had a few weeks before this hospital admission?
5. What treatment would the nurse anticipate for N.B.?
6. Discuss how N.B.'s infective endocarditis could have been prevented.
7. *Priority Decision:* Based on the assessment data presented, what are the priority nursing diagnoses? Are there any collaborative problems?

Nursing Management: Vascular Disorders

1. When obtaining a health history from a 72-year-old man with peripheral arterial disease (PAD) of the lower extremities, the nurse asks about a history of related conditions such as
   a. venous thrombosis.
   b. venous stasis ulcers.
   c. pulmonary embolism.
   d. carotid artery disease.

2. Match the following descriptions with the related types of aneurysms.
   _____ a. Pouchlike bulge of an artery
   _____ b. Disruption of all layers of an artery with bleeding
   _____ c. Uniform, circumferential dilation of artery

   1. Fusiform aneurysm
   2. Saccular aneurysm
   3. Pseudoaneurysm

3. A surgical repair is planned for a patient who has a 5-cm abdominal aortic aneurysm (AAA). On physical assessment of the patient, the nurse would expect to find
   a. hoarseness and dysphagia.
   b. severe back pain with flank ecchymosis.
   c. the presence of a bruit in the periumbilical area.
   d. weakness in the lower extremities progressing to paraplegia.

4. A thoracic aortic aneurysm is found when a patient has a routine chest radiograph. The nurse anticipates that additional diagnostic testing to determine the size and structure of the aneurysm will include
   a. angiography.
   b. ultrasonography.
   c. echocardiography.
   d. a computed tomography (CT) scan.

5. A patient with a small AAA is not a good surgical candidate. The nurse teaches the patient that one of the best ways to prevent expansion of the lesion is to
   a. avoid strenuous physical exertion.
   b. control hypertension with prescribed therapy.
   c. comply with prescribed anticoagulant therapy.
   d. maintain a low-calcium diet to prevent calcification of the vessel.

6. During preoperative preparation of the patient scheduled for an AAA, the nurse establishes baseline data for the patient knowing that
   a. all physiologic processes will be altered postoperatively.
   b. the cause of the aneurysm is a systemic vascular disease.
   c. surgery will be cancelled if any physiologic function is not normal.
   d. BP and heart rate (HR) will be maintained well below baseline levels during the postoperative period.

7. Complete the following statements.

   a. A _____ aneurysm may be surgically treated by excising only the weakened area and suturing the artery closed.

   b. During conventional aortic aneurysm repair, a _____ is sutured to the aorta above and below the aneurysm, and the native aorta is replaced around the site.

   c. Repair of _____ aneurysms requires cross-clamping of the artery proximal and distal to the aneurysm.

   d. A synthetic bifurcation graft is used in aneurysm repair when an AAA extends into the

   _____ arteries.

   e. Repair of an aortic aneurysm by placing an aortic graft inside the aneurysm through the femoral artery is called

   the _____ procedure.

   f. Major complications of aortic aneurysm repair are associated with involvement or obstruction of the

   _____ arteries.

8. During the patient's acute postoperative period following repair of an aneurysm, the nurse should ensure that
   a. hypothermia is maintained to decrease oxygen need.
   b. the BP and all peripheral pulses are evaluated at least every hour.
   c. IV fluids are administered at a rate to maintain hourly urine output of 100 mL.
   d. the patient's BP is kept lower than baseline to prevent leaking at the suture line.

9. Following an ascending aortic aneurysm repair, which of the following findings should the nurse report immediately to the health care provider?
   a. A change in level of consciousness (LOC) and ability to speak
   b. Shallow respirations and poor coughing
   c. Decreased drainage from the chest tubes
   d. Lower-extremity pulses that are decreased from preoperative baseline

10. Identify at least one observation made by the nurse that would indicate the presence of the following complications of aortic aneurysm repair.
    a. Graft thrombosis
    b. Myocardial ischemia
    c. Bowel infarction
    d. Graft infection

11. **Priority Decision:** A patient who is postoperative following repair of an AAA has been receiving intravenous fluids at 125 mL/hr continuously for the last 12 hours. Urine output for the last 4 hours has been 60 mL, 42 mL, 28 mL, and 20 mL (the last hour). The priority action that the nurse should take is to
    a. monitor for a couple more hours.
    b. contact the physician and report the decrease in urine output.
    c. check that the infusion device is set at the correct rate and infusing correctly.
    d. send blood for electrolytes, blood urea nitrogen (BUN), and creatinine.

12. Following discharge teaching with a male patient with an AAA repair, the nurse determines that further instruction is needed when the patient says,
    a. "I should avoid heavy lifting."
    b. "I may have some permanent sexual dysfunction as a result of the surgery."
    c. "I should maintain a low-fat and low-cholesterol diet to help keep the new graft open."
    d. "I should take the pulses in my extremities and let the doctor know if they get too fast or too slow."

13. During the nursing assessment of the patient with a distal descending aortic dissection, the nurse would expect the patient to manifest
    a. a cardiac murmur characteristic of aortic valve insufficiency.
    b. altered LOC with dizziness and weak carotid pulses.
    c. severe hypertension and orthopnea and dyspnea of pulmonary edema.
    d. severe "ripping" back or abdominal pain with decreasing urine output.

14. A patient with a dissection of the arch of the aorta has a decreased LOC and weak carotid pulses. The nurse anticipates that initial treatment of the patient will include
    a. immediate surgery to replace the torn area with a graft.
    b. administration of anticoagulants to prevent embolization.
    c. administration of packed red blood cells (RBCs) to replace blood loss.
    d. administration of antihypertensives to maintain a mean arterial pressure of 70 to 80 mm Hg.

15. The nurse evaluates that treatment for the patient with an uncomplicated aortic dissection is successful when
    a. pain is relieved.
    b. BP is within normal range.
    c. surgical repair is completed.
    d. renal output is maintained at 30 mL/hr.

16. Indicate whether the following findings are characteristic of arterial disease (A) or venous disease (V).
    _____ a. Paresthesia
    _____ b. Heavy ulcer drainage
    _____ c. Edema around the ankles
    _____ d. Ulcers over bony prominences on toes and feet
    _____ e. Decreased peripheral pulses
    _____ f. Brown pigmentation of the legs
    _____ g. Thickened, brittle nails
    _____ h. Ulceration around the medial malleolus
    _____ i. Pallor on elevation of the legs
    _____ j. Dull ache in calf or thigh
    _____ k. Pruritus

17. Complete the following statements.
    a. The classic ischemic pain of PAD is known as _____.
    b. Two serious complications of PAD that frequently lead to lower limb amputation are
       _____ and _____.
    c. A patient with chronic arterial disease has a brachial SBP of 132 mm Hg and an ankle SBP of 102 mm Hg. The ankle-brachial index is _____ and indicates _____ (mild/moderate/severe) arterial disease.
    d. Surgery for PAD is indicated when the patient has limb pain during _____.

18. Following teaching about medications for PAD, the nurse determines that additional instruction is necessary when the patient says,
    a. "I should take one aspirin a day to prevent clotting in my legs."
    b. "The lisinopril (Zestril) I use for my blood pressure may help me walk further without pain."
    c. "I will need to have frequent blood tests to evaluate the effect of the oral anticoagulant I will be taking."
    d. "Pletal should help me be able to increase my walking distance and keep clots from forming in my legs."

19. A patient with PAD has a nursing diagnosis of ineffective peripheral tissue perfusion. Appropriate teaching for the patient includes instructions to (select all that apply)
    a. keep legs and feet warm.
    b. walk at least 30 min/day to the point of discomfort.
    c. apply cold compresses when the legs become swollen.
    d. use nicotine replacement therapy as a substitute for smoking.
    e. inspect lower extremities for pulses, temperature, and any swelling.

20. When teaching the patient with peripheral artery disease about modifying risk factors associated with the condition, the nurse emphasizes that
    a. amputation is the ultimate outcome if the patient does not alter lifestyle behaviors.
    b. modifications will reduce the risk of other atherosclerotic conditions such as stroke.
    c. risk-reducing behaviors initiated after angioplasty can stop the progression of the disease.
    d. maintenance of normal body weight is the most important factor in controlling arterial disease.

21. During care of the patient following femoral bypass graft surgery, the nurse immediately notifies the health care provider if the patient experiences
    a. fever and redness at the incision site.
    b. 2+ edema of the extremity and pain at the incision site.
    c. a loss of palpable pulses and numbness and tingling of the feet.
    d. decreasing ankle-brachial indices and serous drainage from the incision.

22. A patient has chronic atrial fibrillation and develops an acute arterial occlusion at the iliac artery bifurcation. What are the six Ps of acute arterial occlusion the nurse may find in the patient?
    a.

    b.

    c.

    d.

    e.

    f.

23. Indicate whether the following manifestations and treatments are characteristic of thromboangiitis obliterans (Buerger's disease) (B) or arteriospastic disease (Raynaud's phenomenon) (R).
    _____ a. Involves small cutaneous arteries of the fingers and toes
    _____ b. Inflammation of midsized arteries and veins
    _____ c. Treated with calcium-channel blockers, especially nifedipine (Procardia)
    _____ d. Strongly associated with smoking
    _____ e. Predominant in young females
    _____ f. Episodes involve white, blue, and red color changes of fingertips
    _____ g. Amputation of digits or legs below the knee may be necessary for ulceration and gangrene
    _____ h. Precipitated by exposure to cold, caffeine, and tobacco
    _____ i. Intermittent claudication of feet, arms, and hands may be present
    _____ j. Frequently associated with autoimmune disorders

24. Identify the factor(s) of Virchow's triad present in each of the following conditions associated with venous thromboembolism (VTE).
    a. IV therapy
    b. Prolonged immobilization
    c. Estrogen therapy
    d. Orthopedic surgery
    e. Smoking
    f. Pregnancy

25. Identify whether the following statements are true (*T*) or false (*F*). If a statement is false, correct the bold word(s) to make the statement true.
    _____ a. The most common cause of superficial thrombophlebitis in the legs is **IV therapy**.
    _____ b. A tender, red, inflamed induration along the course of a subcutaneous vein is characteristic of a **venous thromboembolism (VTE)**.
    _____ c. A patient with VTE is scheduled for surgical treatment. The nurse recognizes that surgery is most commonly performed for this condition to **insert a vena cava interruption device** to prevent pulmonary embolism.

26. To help prevent embolization of the thrombus in a patient with a VTE, the nurse teaches the patient to
    a. dangle the feet over the edge of the bed q2-3hr.
    b. ambulate for short periods three to four times a day.
    c. keep the affected leg elevated above the level of the heart.
    d. maintain bed rest until edema is relieved and anticoagulation is established.

27. Match the following anticoagulant drugs with their characteristics (answers may be used more than once).
    _____ a. Is only administered intravenously
    _____ b. No antidote for anticoagulant effect
    _____ c. Vitamin K is antidote
    _____ d. Is administered subcutaneously only
    _____ e. Routine coagulation tests not usually required
    _____ f. Protamine sulfate is antidote
    _____ g. May be administered intravenously or subcutaneously
    _____ h. Is only administered orally
    _____ i. International normalized ratio (INR)
    _____ j. Activated partial thromboplastin time (aPTT)

    1. Unfractionated heparin (Heparin)
    2. Low-molecular-weight heparin (Lovenox)
    3. Hirudin derivatives
    4. Warfarin (Coumadin)
    5. Thrombin inhibitor (argatroban [Acova])

28. The patient with VTE is receiving therapy with heparin and asks the nurse whether the drug will dissolve the clot in her leg. The best response by the nurse is
    a. "This drug will break up and dissolve the clot so that circulation in the vein can be restored."
    b. "The purpose of the heparin is to prevent growth of the clot or formation of new clots where the circulation is slowed."
    c. "Heparin won't dissolve the clot, but it will inhibit the inflammation around the clot and delay the development of new clots."
    d. "The heparin will dilate the vein, preventing turbulence of blood flow around the clot that may cause it to break off and travel to the lungs."

29. A patient with VTE is to be discharged on long-term warfarin (Coumadin) therapy and is taught about prevention and continuing treatment of VTE. The nurse determines that discharge teaching for the patient has been effective when the patient states,
    a. "I should expect that Coumadin will cause my stools to be somewhat black."
    b. "I should avoid all dark green and leafy vegetables while I am taking Coumadin."
    c. "Massaging my legs several times a day will help increase my venous circulation."
    d. "Swimming is a good activity to include in my exercise program to increase my circulation."

30. The nurse teaches the patient with any venous disorder that the best way to prevent venous stasis and increase venous return is to
    a. walk.
    b. sit with the legs elevated.
    c. frequently rotate the ankles.
    d. continuously wear graduated compression stockings.

31. Number in sequence the processes that occur as venous stasis precipitates varicose veins leading to venous stasis ulcers.
    _____ a. Venous blood flow reverses
    _____ b. Edema forms
    _____ c. Venous pressure increases
    _____ d. Additional venous distention occurs
    _____ e. Blood supply to local tissues decreases
    _____ f. Venous valves become incompetent
    _____ g. Ulceration occurs
    _____ h. Capillary pressure increases
    _____ i. Veins dilate

32. The most important measure in the treatment of venous stasis ulcers is
    a. elevation of the limb.
    b. extrinsic compression.
    c. application of moist dressings.
    d. application of topical antibiotics.

CASE STUDY
Abdominal Aortic Aneurysm
Patient Profile

C.S. is a 73-year-old man who was brought to the local emergency department complaining of severe back pain.

Subjective Data

- Has a known AAA, which has been followed with yearly abdominal ultrasounds
- Has smoked a pack of cigarettes per day for 52 years
- Has had occasional bouts of angina for the past 3 years

Objective Data

- Has a pulsating abdominal mass
- BP: 88/68 mm Hg
- Extremities are cool and clammy

Clinical Decision-Making Questions

Using a separate sheet of paper, answer the following questions.

1. What are C.S.'s risk factors for AAA?
2. Define the etiology of an AAA.
3. Which signs or symptoms make the nurse suspect that C.S. has a ruptured AAA rather than a nonruptured AAA?
4. *Priority Decision:* What is the first priority in this patient's care?
5. What is the nurse's role in assisting the family in this critical situation?
6. What steps, if any, could have been taken to prevent the rupture of the AAA?
7. *Priority Decision:* Based on the assessment data presented, what are the priority nursing diagnoses? Are there any collaborative problems?

Nursing Assessment: Gastrointestinal System

1. Identify the structures in the following illustration:

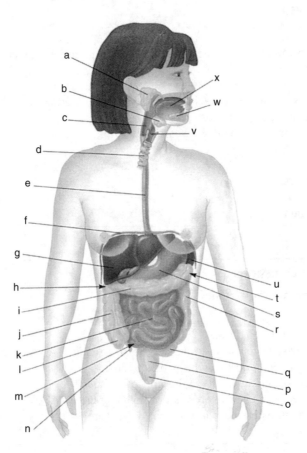

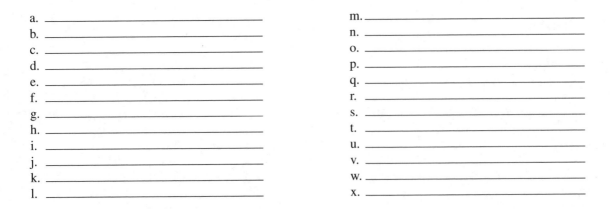

a. _____

b. _____

c. _____

d. _____

e. _____

f. _____

g. _____

h. _____

i. _____

j. _____

k. _____

l. _____

m. _____

n. _____

o. _____

p. _____

q. _____

r. _____

s. _____

t. _____

u. _____

v. _____

w. _____

x. _____

2. Identify the structures in the following illustration using the following terms:

Terms

ampulla of Vater	duodenum	pancreas (body)
common bile duct	gallbladder	pancreas (head)
common hepatic duct	left hepatic duct	pancreas (tail)
cystic duct	main pancreatic duct	right hepatic duct

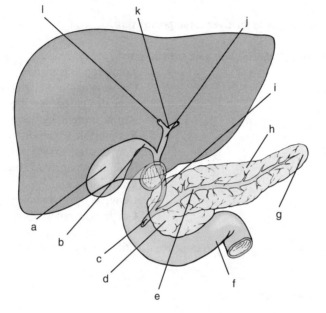

a. _____   g. _____
b. _____   h. _____
c. _____   i. _____
d. _____   j. _____
e. _____   k. _____
f. _____   l. _____

3. A patient receives atropine, an anticholinergic drug, in preparation for surgery. The nurse expects this drug to affect the gastrointestinal (GI) tract by
   a. increasing gastric emptying.
   b. relaxing pyloric and ileocecal sphincters.
   c. decreasing secretions and peristaltic action.
   d. stimulating the nervous system of the GI tract.

4. After eating, a patient with an inflamed gallbladder experiences pain caused by contraction of the gallbladder. The mechanism responsible for this action is
   a. production of bile by the liver.
   b. production of secretin by the duodenum.
   c. release of gastrin from the stomach antrum.
   d. production of cholecystokinin by the duodenum.

5. When caring for a patient who has had most of the stomach surgically removed, the nurse plans to teach the patient
   a. that extra iron will need to be taken to prevent anemia.
   b. to avoid foods with lactose to prevent bloating and diarrhea.
   c. that lifelong supplementation of cobalamin (vitamin B$_{12}$) will be needed.
   d. that, because of the absence of digestive enzymes, protein malnutrition is likely.

6. Identify whether the following statements are true (*T*) or false (*F*). If a statement is false, correct the bold word(s) to make the statement true.

  _____ a. The structure that prevents reflux of stomach contents into the esophagus is the **upper esophageal sphincter**.

  _____ b. The nurse encourages the patient with chronic constipation to attempt defecation after the first meal of the day because **gastrocolic and duodenocolic reflexes** increase colon peristalsis at that time.

  _____ c. A drug that blocks the release of secretions from the stomach's **chief cells** will decrease gastric acidity.

  _____ d. The secretion of hydrochloric acid and pepsinogen is stimulated by the **sight, smell, and taste** of food.

  _____ e. Obstruction of the biliary tract is indicated by increased **unconjugated (indirect)** bilirubin levels in the blood.

  _____ f. The major blood supply to the liver is the **portal vein.**

7. Match the following digestive substances with their descriptions:

  _____ a. Gastrin

  _____ b. Intrinsic factor

  _____ c. Secretin

  _____ d. Bile

  _____ e. Amylase

  _____ f. Enterokinase

  _____ g. Pepsinogen

  _____ h. Pepsin

  _____ i. Maltase

  _____ j. Lipase

  1. Converted to pepsin by acidity
  2. Converts maltose to glucose
  3. Increases gastric motility and secretion
  4. Begins protein digestion
  5. Responsible for absorption of cobalamin
  6. Converts fats to fatty acids (fat digestion)
  7. Stimulates pancreatic bicarbonate secretion
  8. Emulsifies fats
  9. Converts trypsinogen to trypsin
  10. Converts starch to disaccharides

8. The destruction of normal bowel bacteria by prolonged antibiotic therapy may cause
  a. coagulation problems.
  b. elevated serum ammonia levels.
  c. impaired absorption of amino acids.
  d. increased mucus and bicarbonate secretion.

9. An obstruction at the sphincter of Oddi will affect the digestion of all nutrients because
  a. bile is responsible for emulsification of all nutrients and vitamins.
  b. intestinal digestive enzymes are released through the ampulla of Vater.
  c. both bile and pancreatic enzymes enter the duodenum at the ampulla of Vater.
  d. gastric contents can only pass to the duodenum when the sphincter of Oddi is open.

10. A patient experiences increased red blood cell (RBC) destruction from a mechanical heart-valve prosthesis. Describe what happens to the bilirubin that is released from the breakdown of hemoglobin (Hb) from the RBCs.

11. A clinical manifestation of age-related changes in the GI system that the nurse may find in an older patient is
  a. gastric hyperacidity.
  b. intolerance to fatty foods.
  c. yellowish tinge to the skin.
  d. reflux of gastric contents into the esophagus.

12. Identify one specific finding identified by the nurse during assessment of each of the patient's functional health patterns that indicates a risk factor for GI problems or the response of the patient to a GI disorder.
  a. Health perception–health management
  b. Nutritional-metabolic
  c. Elimination
  d. Activity-exercise
  e. Sleep-rest
  f. Cognitive-perceptual
  g. Self-perception–self-concept
  h. Role-relationship
  i. Sexuality-reproductive
  j. Coping–stress tolerance
  k. Value-belief

13. A normal finding during physical assessment of the mouth is
    a. a red, slick appearance of the tongue.
    b. uvular deviation to the side on saying "Ahh."
    c. a thin, white coating of the dorsum of the tongue.
    d. scattered red, smooth areas on the dorsum of the tongue.

14. A normal finding on physical examination of the abdomen is
    a. auscultation of bruits.
    b. observation of visible pulsations.
    c. percussion of liver dullness in the left midclavicular line.
    d. palpation of the spleen 1 to 2 cm below the left costal margin.

15. A patient is admitted to the hospital with upper left quadrant (ULQ) pain. A possible source of the pain may be the
    a. liver.
    b. pancreas.
    c. appendix.
    d. gallbladder.

16. During auscultation of the abdomen
    a. the presence of borborygmi indicates hyperperistalsis.
    b. the bell of the stethoscope is used to auscultate high-pitched sounds.
    c. high-pitched, rushing, and tinkling bowel sounds are heard after eating.
    d. absence of bowel sounds for 3 minutes in each quadrant is reported as abnormal.

17. Following inspection of the abdomen, the nurse's next action would be to
    a. lightly percuss over all four quadrants.
    b. have the patient empty his/her bladder.
    c. perform light palpation to assess for tenderness.
    d. auscultate over all four quadrants and the epigastric area.

18. Complete the table below by indicating with check marks which of the following preparations are required for each of the diagnostic procedures listed.
    (1) NPO up to 8 or more hours
    (2) Bowel emptying with laxatives, enemas, or both
    (3) Informed consent
    (4) Allergy to iodine ascertained

	(1) NPO	(2) Bowel	(3) Consent	(4) Allergy
Upper GI series				
Barium enema				
Percutaneous transhepatic cholangiogram				
Gallbladder ultrasound				
Hepatobiliary scintigraphy				
Upper GI endoscopy				
Colonoscopy				
Endoscopic retrograde cholangiopancreatography (ERCP)				

19. A patient's serum liver enzyme tests reveal an elevated aspartate aminotransferase (AST). The nurse recognizes that the elevated AST
    a. eliminates infection as a cause of liver damage.
    b. is diagnostic for liver inflammation and damage.
    c. may reflect tissue damage in organs other than the liver.
    d. may cause nervous system symptoms related to hepatic encephalopathy.

20. Match the nursing responsibilities indicated for the diagnostic procedures (answers may be used more than once).
    _____ a. Ensure no smoking morning of test
    _____ b. Monitor for LUQ pain and nausea/vomiting
    _____ c. Observe for white stools
    _____ d. Monitor for rectal bleeding
    _____ e. Position to right side after test
    _____ f. Check for return of gag reflex
    _____ g. Monitor for internal bleeding
    _____ h. Check coagulation status before test
    _____ i. Check temperature every 15 to 30 minutes for signs of perforation
    _____ j. Ensure bowel preparation was done

    1. Barium swallow
    2. Colonoscopy
    3. Liver biopsy
    4. EGD
    5. ERCP

CHAPTER 40

Nursing Management: Nutritional Problems

1. A 30-year-old man's diet consists of 3000 calories with 120 g of protein, 160 g of fat, and 270 g of carbohydrate. He weighs 176 lb and is 5 ft 11 in tall.
   a. What percentage of total calories does each of the nutrients contribute to the man's diet?
      Protein
      Fat
      Carbohydrate
   b. Nutritional guidelines recommend how many grams of each of the nutrients for this man?
      Protein
      Fat
      Carbohydrate
   c. How many kilocalories would be recommended for him as an average adult?
   d. Using the food pyramid as a guide, what changes could the nurse suggest to bring the man's diet more in line with nutrition recommendations?

2. Identify whether the following statements are true (*T*) or false (*F*). If a statement is false, correct the bold word(s) to make the statement true.
   _____ a. A food high in iron that could be recommended to an iron-deficient vegan is **soybeans**.
   _____ b. The two nutrients most often lacking in the diet of a vegan are **vitamin B$_6$** and **folic acid**.
   _____ c. The major nutritional problem in the United States today is the high intake of **sugar** in the diet.
   _____ d. **Marasmus** is a type of malnutrition that results from a deficiency of protein intake.

3. The most common cause of secondary protein-calorie malnutrition in the United States is
   a. the unavailability of foods high in protein.
   b. a lack of knowledge about nutritional needs.
   c. a lack of money to purchase high-protein foods.
   d. an alteration in ingestion, digestion, absorption, or metabolism.

4. Describe the metabolism of nutrients used for energy during starvation within the given approximate time frames.
   a. First 18 hours
   b. 18 hours to 5 to 9 days
   c. 9 days to 6 weeks
   d. Over 6 weeks

5. Failure of the sodium-potassium pump during severe protein depletion may lead to
   a. ascites.
   b. anemia.
   c. hyperkalemia.
   d. hypoalbuminemia.

6. Identify whether the following statements are true (*T*) or false (*F*). If a statement is false, correct the bold word(s) to make the statement true.
   _____ a. A patient with an elevated temperature will need approximately **12%** more calories per Fahrenheit degree to meet the increased basal metabolic rate (BMR) caused by the fever.
   _____ b. Vitamin deficiencies in adults most commonly are clinically manifested by disorders of the **skin**.
   _____ c. Surgery on the GI tract may contribute to **vitamin deficiencies** because of impaired absorption.

7. During assessment of the patient with protein-calorie malnutrition, the nurse would expect to find (select all that apply)
   a. decreased bowel sounds.
   b. prominent bony structures.
   c. a flat or concave abdomen.
   d. cool, rough, dry, scaly skin.
   e. decreased reflexes and inattention.

8. The nurse determines that the patient with the highest risk for the nursing diagnosis of imbalanced nutrition: less than body requirements related to decreased ingestion is the patient with
   a. tuberculosis infection.
   b. malabsorption syndrome.
   c. draining decubitus ulcers.
   d. severe anorexia resulting from radiation therapy.

9. The nurse monitors the laboratory results of the patient with protein-calorie malnutrition during treatment. An indication of improvement in the patient's condition is
   a. decreased lymphocytes.
   b. increased serum potassium.
   c. increased serum transferrin.
   d. decreased serum prealbumin.

10. To evaluate the effect of nutritional interventions with a patient with protein-calorie malnutrition, the best indicator for the nurse to use is the patient's
    a. height and weight.
    b. body mass index (BMI).
    c. weight in relation to ideal body weight.
    d. mid-upper arm circumference and triceps skinfold.

11. The nurse evaluates that patient teaching about a high-calorie, high-protein diet has been effective when the patient selects for breakfast from the hospital menu
    a. two poached eggs, hash brown potatoes, and whole milk.
    b. two slices of toast with butter and jelly, orange juice, and skim milk.
    c. three pancakes with butter and syrup, two slices of bacon, and apple juice.
    d. cream of wheat with 2 tbsp of skim milk powder, one-half grapefruit, and a high-protein milkshake.

12. When teaching the older adult about nutritional needs during aging, the nurse emphasizes that
    a. the need for all nutrients decreases as one ages.
    b. fewer calories, but the same amount of protein, are required as one ages.
    c. fats, carbohydrates, and protein should be decreased, but vitamin and mineral intake should be increased.
    d. high-calorie oral supplements should be taken between meals to ensure that recommended nutrient needs are met.

13. When planning nutritional interventions for a healthy 83-year-old man, the nurse recognizes that the factor most likely to affect his nutritional status is
    a. living alone on a fixed income.
    b. changes in cardiovascular function.
    c. an increase in GI motility and absorption.
    d. snacking between meals, resulting in obesity.

14. When considering tube feedings for a patient with severe protein-calorie malnutrition, the nurse knows that an advantage of a gastrostomy tube over a nasogastric (NG) tube is that
    a. there is less irritation to the nasal and esophageal mucosa.
    b. the patient experiences the sight and smells associated with eating.
    c. aspiration resulting from reflux of formulas into the esophagus is less common.
    d. routine checking for placement is not required because gastrostomy tubes do not become displaced.

15. Identify one nursing intervention indicated for each of the following desired outcomes of tube feeding.
    a. Prevention of aspiration
    b. Prevention of diarrhea
    c. Maintenance of tube patency
    d. Maintenance of tube placement
    e. Administration of medication

16. Before administering a bolus of intermittent tube feeding to a patient with a percutaneous endoscopic gastrostomy (PEG), the nurse aspirates 220 mL of gastric contents. The nurse should
    a. return the aspirate to the stomach and recheck the volume of aspirate in an hour.
    b. return the aspirate to the stomach and continue with the tube feeding as planned.
    c. discard the aspirate to prevent overdistending the stomach when the new feeding is given.
    d. notify the health care provider that the feedings have been scheduled too frequently to allow for stomach emptying.

17. *Delegation Decision:* Indicate whether the following nursing actions must be performed by the RN or if they can be delegated to nursing assistive personnel (NAP).
    _____ a. Insert NG tube for stable patients.
    _____ b. Weigh the patient receiving enteral feedings.
    _____ c. Teach the patient about home gastric tube care.
    _____ d. Remove an NG tube.
    _____ e. Provide oral care to the patient with an NG tube.
    _____ f. Position patient receiving enteral feedings.
    _____ g. Monitor a patient with continuous feeding for complications.
    _____ h. Respond to infusion pump alarm by reporting it to an RN or LPN.

18. Indicate whether the following characteristics of parenteral nutrition (PN) apply more to central parenteral nutrition (CPN) or peripheral parenteral nutrition (PPN).
    _____ a. Limited to 20% glucose
    _____ b. Tonicity of 1600 mOsm/L
    _____ c. Nutrients can be infused using smaller volumes
    _____ d. Supplements oral feedings
    _____ e. Long-term nutritional support
    _____ f. Phlebitis more common
    _____ g. May use peripherally inserted catheter

19. An indication for parenteral nutrition that is not appropriate for enteral tube feedings is
    a. head and neck cancer.
    b. hypermetabolic states.
    c. malabsorption syndrome.
    d. protein-calorie malnutrition.

20. What nursing interventions are indicated during parenteral nutrition to prevent the following complications?
    a. Infection
    b. Hyperglycemia
    c. Air embolism

21. The nurse is caring for a patient receiving 1000 mL of PN solution over 24 hours. When it is time to change the solution, 150 mL remain in the bottle. The most appropriate action by the nurse is to
    a. hang the new solution and discard the unused solution.
    b. notify the health care provider for instructions regarding the infusion rate.
    c. open the IV line and infuse the remaining solution as quickly as possible.
    d. wait to change the solution until the remaining solution infuses at the prescribed rate.

22. Identify the following characteristics of eating disorders as associated with anorexia nervosa (A), bulimia (B), or both (AB).
    _____ a. Treated with psychotherapy
    _____ b. Ignores feelings of hunger
    _____ c. Binge eating with purging
    _____ d. Conceals abnormal eating habits
    _____ e. Concerned about body image
    _____ f. Self-induced starvation

23. An 18-year-old female patient with anorexia nervosa is admitted to the hospital for treatment. On admission she weighs 82 lb (37 kg) and is 5 ft 3 in (134.6 cm). Her laboratory test results include the following: K^+ 2.8 mEq/L (2.8 mmol/L), Hb 8.9 g/dL (89 g/L), and BUN 64 mg/dL (22.8 mmol/L). In planning care for the patient, the nurse gives the highest priority to the nursing diagnosis of
    a. risk for injury related to dizziness and weakness resulting from anemia.
    b. risk for decreased CO related to dysrhythmias resulting from hypokalemia.
    c. imbalanced nutrition: less than body requirements related to inadequate food intake.
    d. risk for impaired urinary elimination related to elevated BUN resulting from renal failure.

CASE STUDY
Malnutrition
Patient Profile

R.M., a 62-year-old Hispanic widow, recently underwent radiation and chemotherapy following surgery for breast cancer. On a follow-up visit to the clinic, the nurse notes that R.M. appears thinner and more tired than usual.

Subjective Data

- Says she has not had an appetite since the treatment for cancer was started
- Feels "weak" and "worn out"
- Thinks the treatment for cancer has not been effective
- Lives alone in an apartment in the inner city
- Is a nationalized citizen from Honduras
- Speaks English but does not read English very well

Objective Data

- Height: 62 in (155 cm); weight: 92 lb (41.8 kg)
- BP: 98/60, HR: 60, RR: 12
- Ulcerations of her buccal mucosal membranes and tongue

Laboratory test results:
- Serum albumin: 2.8 g/dL (28 g/L)
- Hb: 10 g/dL (100 g/L); Hct: 32%

Clinical Decision-Making Questions

Using a separate sheet of paper, answer the following questions.

1. What additional assessment data should the nurse obtain from R.M. related to her nutritional status?
2. What physical and psychosocial factors have contributed to R.M.'s malnutrition?
3. What additional symptoms would the nurse expect to see based on R.M.'s laboratory test results?
4. What complications of malnutrition are most likely to occur in R.M. because of her history and clinical manifestations?
5. *Priority Decision:* What are the priority teaching instructions that the nurse should give to R.M. regarding her diet that would be most therapeutic?
6. *Priority Decision:* Based on the assessment data presented, what are the priority nursing diagnoses? Are there any collaborative problems?

Nursing Management: Obesity

1. Identify whether the following statements are true (*T*) or false (*F*). If a statement is false, correct the bold word(s) to make the statement true.
   _____ a. The highest prevalence of obesity occurs in the **18-40** age range.
   _____ b. **Primary** obesity results from the consumption of more food than required for normal physiologic functions and growth.
   _____ c. Obesity is the **third** leading cause of preventable death after smoking and liver failure.
   _____ d. The physiology of obesity suggests there is a **genetic factor** to obesity.

2. Using the body mass index (BMI) chart (Figure 41-2) in the textbook or the BMI formula:

$$\text{BMI (kg/m}^2) = \frac{\text{weight (pounds)} \times 703}{\text{height (inches)}^2}$$

   a. Determine the BMI for a patient who is 5 ft 5 in (164 cm) and weighs 202 lb (91.8 kg). _____

      What is the patient's weight classification? _____
   b. Calculate the waist-to-hip ratio of a woman who has a waist measurement of 32 in and hip measurement of 36 in

      _____

   c. What does this value indicate? _____

3. Which of the following patients is most at risk for complications of obesity?
   a. A 30-year-old woman who is 5 ft (151 cm), weighs 140 lb (63.6 kg), and carries weight in her thighs.
   b. A 56-year-old woman with a BMI of 38, a waist measurement of 38 in (96 cm), and a hip measurement of 36 in (91 cm).
   c. A 42-year-old man with a waist measurement of 36 in (91 cm) and a hip measurement of 36 in (91 cm), who is 5 ft 6 in (166 cm) and weighs 150 lb (68.2 kg).
   d. A 68-year-old man with a waist measurement of 38 in (96 cm) and a hip measurement of 42 in (76 cm), who is 5 ft 11 in (179 cm) and weighs 200 lb (90.9 kg).

4. A woman is 5 ft 6 in (166 cm) and weighs 200 lb (90.9 kg) with a waist-to-hip ratio of 0.7. The nurse counsels the patient with the knowledge that the patient is at greatest risk for
   a. heart disease.
   b. osteoporosis.
   c. diabetes mellitus.
   d. endometrial cancer.

5. Before selecting a weight-reduction plan with an obese patient, it is most important for the nurse to first assess
   a. the patient's motivation to lose weight.
   b. the length of time that the patient has been obese.
   c. whether financial considerations will affect the patient's choices.
   d. the patient's anthropometric measures of height, weight, BMI, waist-to-hip ratio, and skinfold thickness.

6. Explain the rationale for the following interventions in the management of obesity.
   a. 800- to 1200-calorie diet
   b. 1-2 lb/wk weight loss
   c. Support group
   d. Determine portion sizes
   e. Limit/avoid alcohol
   f. Exercise program
   g. Behavioral modification

7. Describe how the nurse would explain to the obese patient about the following:
   a. The rapid weight loss of first few days of dieting
   b. Why to weigh weekly rather than daily
   c. How gender influences weight loss

8. A patient has been on a 1000-calorie diet with a daily exercise routine. In 2 months, the patient has lost 20 lb (9 kg) of a goal of 50 lb (23 kg) but is now discouraged that no weight has been lost for the last 2 weeks. The nurse informs the patient that
   a. plateaus where no weight is lost normally occur during a weight-loss program.
   b. a weight considered by the body to be most efficient for functioning has been reached.
   c. a return to former eating habits is the most common cause of not continuing to lose weight.
   d. the steady weight that has occurred may be due to water gain from eating foods high in sodium.

9. When teaching a patient about weight-reduction diets, the nurse informs the patient that an appropriate single serving of a food is
   a. a 6-inch bagel.
   b. 1 cup of chopped vegetables.
   c. a piece of cheese the size of three dice.
   d. a chicken breast the size of a deck of cards.

10. When medications are used in the treatment of obesity, it is important for the nurse to teach the patient that
    a. over-the-counter (OTC) diet aids are safer than other agents and can be useful in controlling appetite.
    b. drugs should be used only as adjuncts to a diet and exercise program as treatment for a chronic condition.
    c. all drugs used for weight control are capable of altering central nervous system (CNS) function and should be used with caution.
    d. the primary effect of the medications is psychologic, controlling the urge to eat in response to stress or feelings of rejection.

11. When a patient asks the nurse about taking Meridia for weight loss, it is important for the nurse to determine whether the patient has a history of
    a. depression.
    b. hypertension.
    c. valvular heart disease.
    d. irritable bowel disease.

12. The nurse has completed initial instruction with a patient regarding a weight-loss program. The nurse determines that the teaching has been effective when the patient says,
    a. "I will keep a diary of daily weight to illustrate my weight loss."
    b. "I plan to lose 4 lb a week until I have lost the 60 lb I want to lose."
    c. "I should not exercise more than what is required so I don't increase my appetite."
    d. "I plan to join a behavior-modification group to help establish long-term behavior changes."

13. Match the following characteristics with the appropriate surgical procedures used for treatment of morbid obesity (answers may be used more than once).
    _____ a. Stomach restrictions can be reversed
    _____ b. Partition stomach into a small pouch with restricted outlet
    _____ c. Provides the greatest long-term weight loss
    _____ d. Malabsorption of fat-soluble vitamins
    _____ e. Allows for modification of gastric stoma size
    _____ f. Stomach size with a gastric pouch anastomosed to the jejunum.
    _____ g. Distention of wall of pouch is a complication
    _____ h. Increases the risk of gallstones.

    1. Vertical banded gastroplasty
    2. Adjustable gastric banding
    3. Biliopancreatic diversion
    4. Roux-en-Y gastric bypass

14. During care of the morbidly obese patient, it is important that the nurse
    a. avoid reference to the patient's weight to avoid embarrassing the patient.
    b. emphasize to the patient how important it is to lose weight to maintain health.
    c. plan for necessary modifications in equipment and nursing techniques before initiating care.
    d. recognize that a full assessment of each body system might not be possible because of numerous layers of skinfolds.

15. A postoperative nursing intervention for the obese patient who has undergone bariatric surgery is
    a. irrigating and repositioning the nasogastric (NG) tube as needed.
    b. delaying ambulation until the patient has enough strength to support self.
    c. keeping the patient positioned on the side to facilitate respiratory function.
    d. providing adequate support to the incision during coughing, deep breathing, and turning.

16. The nurse admitting a patient for bariatric surgery obtains the following information from the patient. Which of these findings should be brought to the surgeon's attention before proceeding with further patient preparation?
    a. history of hypertension
    b. history of untreated depression
    c. history of sleep apnea treated with CPAP
    d. history of multiple attempts at weight loss

17. Dietary teaching for the patient following a Roux-en-Y gastric bypass includes information regarding the need to
    a. avoid sugary foods and limit fluids to prevent dumping syndrome.
    b. gradually increase the amount of food ingested to preoperative levels.
    c. maintain a long-term liquid diet to prevent damage to the surgical site.
    d. consume foods high in complex carbohydrate, protein, and fiber to add bulk to intestinal contents.

18. Which of the following teaching points are important when providing information to a patient with metabolic syndrome (select all that apply)?
    a. Monitor weight daily.
    b. Increase level of activity.
    c. Decrease saturated fat intake.
    d. Reduce weight and maintain lower weight.
    e. Check blood sugar each morning prior to eating.

19. The main underlying risk factor for metabolic syndrome is
    a. age.
    b. heart disease.
    c. insulin resistance.
    d. high cholesterol levels.

CASE STUDY
Morbid Obesity
Patient Profile

L.C., a 32-year-old single man, is seeking information at the outpatient center regarding possible bariatric surgery for his obesity. He reports that he has always been heavy, even as a small child, but he has gained about 100 lb in the last 2 to 3 years. Previous medical evaluations have not indicated any metabolic disease, but he says he has sleep apnea and high BP, which he tries to control with sodium restriction. He currently works at a catalog telephone center.

Subjective Data

- Says he is constantly dieting, but eventually hunger takes over and he eats to satisfy his appetite.
- Reports that he used fenfluramine (Pondimin) for about 2 months before it was taken off the market, but he only lost about 5 lb.
- Admits to being treated for depression when he felt that he had no quality of life.
- Lives alone in an apartment and has several good friends in the building, but rarely socializes with them outside of the complex because of his size.

Objective Data

- Height: 68 in (171 cm); weight: 296 lb (134.5 kg)
- BP: 172/96, HR 88, RR 24
- Waist measure: 56 in (141 cm)
- Laboratory test results
  - Fasting blood glucose: 146 mg/dL (8.1 mmol/L)
  - Total cholesterol: 250 mg/dL (6.5 mmol/L)
  - Triglycerides: 312 mg/dL (3.5 mmol/L)
  - HDL: 30 mg/dL (0.77 mmol/L)

Clinical Decision-Making Questions

Using a separate sheet of paper, answer the following questions.

1. What is L.C.'s estimated BMI?
2. What health risks associated with obesity does L.C. have?
3. Does L.C. qualify for bariatric surgery? Why or why not?
4. L.C. says he has read about Roux-en-Y gastric bypass surgery and the vertical banded surgery and asks which is best. What advantages and disadvantages of these procedures can the nurse explain to L.C.?
5. *Priority Decision:* After an extensive workup by the health care provider, L.C. is scheduled for Roux-en-Y bypass surgery. What priority preoperative teaching should the nurse provide for L.C. before he is admitted to the hospital?
6. *Priority Decision:* Based on the assessment data presented, what are the priority nursing diagnoses? Are there any collaborative problems?

1. Identify whether the following statements are true (*T*) or false (*F*). If a statement is false, correct the bold word(s) to make the statement true.

_____ a. Immediately before the act of vomiting, activation of the **sympathetic nervous system** causes increased salivation, increased gastric mobility, and relaxation of the lower esophageal sphincter (LES).

_____ b. Stimulation of the vomiting center by the chemoreceptor trigger zone (CTZ) is commonly caused by **stretch and distention of hollow organs**.

_____ c. The acid-base imbalance most commonly associated with persistent vomiting is **metabolic acidosis** caused by loss of **bicarbonate**.

2. Laboratory findings that the nurse would expect in the patient with persistent vomiting include
   a. ↓ pH, ↑ sodium, ↓ hematocrit.
   b. ↑ pH, ↓ chloride, ↓ hematocrit.
   c. ↑ pH, ↓ potassium, ↑ hematocrit.
   d. ↓ pH, ↓ potassium, ↑ hematocrit.

3. A patient who has been vomiting for several days from an unknown cause is admitted to the hospital. The nurse anticipates collaborative care to include
   a. insertion of a nasogastric (NG) tube to suction.
   b. oral administration of broth and tea.
   c. administration of parenteral antiemetics.
   d. IV replacement of fluid and electrolytes.

4. A patient treated for vomiting is to begin oral intake when the symptoms have subsided. To promote rehydration, the nurse plans to administer
   a. water.
   b. hot tea.
   c. Gatorade.
   d. warm broth.

5. Ondansetron (Zofran) is prescribed for a patient with cancer chemotherapy–induced vomiting. The nurse understands that this drug
   a. is a derivative of cannabis and has a potential for abuse.
   b. has a strong antihistamine effect that provides sedation and induces sleep.
   c. is used only when other therapies are ineffective because of side effects of anxiety and hallucinations.
   d. relieves vomiting centrally by action in the vomiting center and peripherally by promoting gastric emptying.

6. Older patients may have cardiac or renal insufficiency and may be more susceptible to antiemetic drug side effects. List at least three nursing interventions that should be implemented.

   a.

   b.

   c.

7. Match the following characteristics of inflammations and infections of the mouth with their types (answers may be used more than once).

_____ a. Viral infection related to upper respiratory system

_____ b. Staphylococcal infection that may occur with prolonged NPO status

_____ c. Painful bleeding gums with gingival necrosis and metallic-tasting saliva

_____ d. Associated with prolonged high-dose antibiotic or corticosteroid therapy

_____ e. Formation of abscesses with loosening of teeth

_____ f. Infectious ulcers of mouth and lips with a defined erythematous base occurs as a result of systemic disease.

_____ g. White membranous lesions of mucosa of mouth and throat

_____ h. Inflammation of mouth related to systemic disease and cancer chemotherapy

_____ i. Shallow, painful vesicular ulcerations of lips and mouth

_____ j. Results in decreased salivation and ear pain

_____ k. Bacterial infection predisposed by fatigue, stress, and poor oral hygiene

1. Gingivitis infections.
2. Vincent's infection
3. Oral candidiasis
4. Herpes simplex
5. Aphthous stomatitis
6. Parotitis
7. Stomatitis

8. A patient is scheduled for biopsy of a painful tongue ulcer. Based on knowledge of risk factors for oral cancer, the nurse specifically asks the patient about a history of
   a. excessive exposure to sunlight.
   b. recurrent herpes simplex infections.
   c. use of any type of tobacco products.
   d. difficulty swallowing and pain in the ear.

9. When caring for a patient following a glossectomy with dissection of the floor of the mouth and a radical neck dissection for cancer of the tongue, the nurse's primary concern is maintaining
   a. relief of pain.
   b. a patent airway.
   c. a positive body image.
   d. tube feedings to provide nutrition.

10. A patient with oral cancer has a history of heavy smoking, excessive alcohol intake, and personal neglect. During the patient's early postoperative course, the nurse anticipates that the patient may need
    a. oral nutritional supplements.
    b. drug therapy to prevent substance withdrawal symptoms.
    c. counseling about lifestyle changes to prevent recurrence of the tumor.
    d. less pain medication because of cross-tolerance with central nervous system (CNS) depressants.

11. Identify four foods or beverages that decrease LES pressure that the nurse should teach the patient with gastroesophageal reflux disease (GERD) to avoid.

    a.

    b.

    c.

    d.

12. The nurse teaches the patient with a hiatal hernia or GERD to control symptoms by
    a. drinking 10 to 12 oz of water with each meal.
    b. spacing six small meals a day between breakfast and bedtime.
    c. sleeping with the head of the bed elevated on 4- to 6-in blocks.
    d. performing daily exercises of toe-touching, sit-ups, and weight lifting.

13. A patient with esophageal cancer is scheduled for a partial esophagectomy. A nursing diagnosis that is likely to be of highest priority preoperatively is
    a. deficient fluid volume related to inadequate intake.
    b. impaired oral mucous membrane related to inadequate oral hygiene.
    c. imbalanced nutrition: less than body requirements related to dysphagia.
    d. ineffective self-health management related to lack of knowledge of disease process.

14. Following a patient's esophagogastrostomy for cancer of the esophagus, it is important for the nurse to
    a. report any bloody drainage from the NG tube.
    b. maintain the patient in semi-Fowler's or Fowler's position.
    c. monitor for abdominal distention that may disrupt the surgical site.
    d. expect to find decreased breath sounds bilaterally because of the surgical approach.

15. Match the following esophageal disorders with their descriptions.
    _____ a. Esophagitis   1. Absence of peristalsis of lower two thirds of esophagus
    _____ b. Esophageal diverticula   with nonrelaxing LES
    _____ c. Esophageal strictures   2. Inflammation of the esophagus from irritants or gastric reflux
    _____ d. Achalasia   3. Narrowing of the esophagus from scarring
    _____ e. Barrett's esophagus   4. Precancerous esophageal metaplasia associated with GERD
                                             5. Common site above the upper esophageal sphincter

16. Identify what type of bleeding is indicated by the following findings:
    a. Profuse bright-red hematemesis
    b. Coffee-ground emesis
    c. Melena
    d. Occult

17. A patient is admitted to the emergency department with profuse bright-red hematemesis. During the initial care of the patient, the nurse's first priority is to
    a. establish two IV sites with large-gauge catheters.
    b. perform a nursing assessment of the patient's status.
    c. obtain a thorough health history to assist in determining the cause of the bleeding.
    d. perform a gastric lavage with cool tap water in preparation for endoscopic examination.

18. A patient with upper GI bleeding is treated with several drugs. The nurse recognizes that an agent that is used to decrease bleeding and decrease gastric acid secretions is
    a. ranitidine (Zantac).
    b. omeprazole (Prilosec).
    c. vasopressin (Pitressin).
    d. octreotide (Sandostatin).

19. In teaching patients at risk for upper GI bleeding to prevent bleeding episodes, the nurse stresses that
    a. all stools and vomitus must be tested for the presence of blood.
    b. the use of over-the-counter (OTC) medications of any kind should be avoided.
    c. antacids should be taken with all prescribed medications to prevent gastric irritation.
    d. misoprostol (Cytotec) should be used to protect the gastric mucosa in individuals with peptic ulcers.

20. The nurse evaluates that management of the patient with upper GI bleeding is effective when assessment and laboratory findings reveal a
    a. decreasing blood urea nitrogen (BUN).
    b. hematocrit (Hct) of 35%.
    c. urinary output of 20 mL/hr.
    d. urine-specific gravity of 1.030.

21. Complete the following sentences.
    a. The self-limiting type of gastritis most likely to occur in a college student who has an isolated drinking binge is

       _____ gastritis.

    b. _____ gastritis is associated with an increased risk for stomach cancer.

    c. A definite diagnosis of gastritis is made with the use of _____.

    d. The microorganism that has a strong causative relationship with both diffuse antral and multifocal gastritis is

       _____.

    e. A complication of chronic gastritis that results from the destruction and atrophy of acid-secreting cells is the loss

       of _____, leading to pernicious anemia.

    f. _____ drugs and _____ drugs reduce irritation of the mucosa, relieve symptoms, and promote healing of erosive gastritis.

22. Nursing management of the patient with chronic gastritis includes teaching the patient to
    a. take antacids before meals to decrease stomach acidity.
    b. maintain a nonirritating diet with six small meals a day.
    c. eliminate alcohol and caffeine from the diet when symptoms occur.
    d. use nonsteroidal antiinflammatory drugs (NSAIDs) instead of aspirin for any minor pain relief.

23. Indicate whether the following characteristics are associated with gastric ulcers (G), duodenal ulcers (D), or both (B).
    _____ a. Increased gastric secretion
    _____ b. Superficial with smooth margins
    _____ c. High recurrence rate
    _____ d. Burning and cramping in midepigastric area
    _____ e. Increased incidence with smoking and drug and alcohol use
    _____ f. Higher incidence in women in fifth and sixth decade of life
    _____ g. Burning and gaseous pressure in high epigastrium
    _____ h. May cause hemorrhage, perforation, and obstruction
    _____ i. Pain 1 to 2 hours after meals
    _____ j. Increased incidence in persons from lower socioeconomic class
    _____ k. Associated with *Helicobacter pylori* infection
    _____ l. Relief of pain with food

24. Match the following factors associated with the development of peptic ulcers with their probable pathophysiologic mechanisms.
    _____ a. *H. pylori*   1. Decrease(s) the rate of mucous cell renewal
    _____ b. Aspirin and NSAIDs   2. Produce(s) the enzyme urease.
    _____ c. Corticosteroids   3. Inhibit(s) the synthesis of mucus and prostaglandins
    _____ d. Alcohol   4. Increase(s) secretion of hydrochloric acid

25. Regardless of the precipitating factor, the injury to mucosal cells in peptic ulcers is caused by
    a. acid back-diffusion into the mucosa.
    b. the release of histamine from GI cells.
    c. ammonia formation in the mucosal wall.
    d. breakdown of the gastric mucosal barrier.

26. The nurse expects a patient with an ulcer of the posterior portion of the duodenum to experience
    a. pain that occurs after not eating all day.
    b. back pain that occurs 2 to 4 hours following meals.
    c. midepigastric pain that is unrelieved with antacids.
    d. high epigastric burning that is relieved with food intake.

27. The nurse teaches a patient with newly diagnosed peptic ulcer disease to
    a. maintain a bland, soft, low-residue diet.
    b. use alcohol and caffeine in moderation and always with food.
    c. eat as normally as possible, eliminating foods that cause pain or discomfort.
    d. avoid milk and milk products because they stimulate gastric acid production.

28. Identify the rationale for treatment with NG intubation for each of the following situations associated with peptic ulcer disease.
    a. Acute exacerbation
    b. Peritonitis
    c. Gastric outlet obstruction

29. Match the following characteristics with the drugs used to treat or prevent peptic ulcer disease (answers may be used more than once).
    _____ a. Prevents conversion of pepsinogen to pepsin
    _____ b. Used in patients with verified *H. pylori*
    _____ c. Covers the ulcer, protecting it from erosion by acids
    _____ d. Decreases gastric acid secretion by blocking adenosine triphosphatase (ATPase) enzyme
    _____ e. High incidence of side effects and contraindications
    _____ f. High dose and frequency stimulate release of gastrin
    _____ g. Reduce HCl acid secretion by blocking action of histamine
    _____ h. Antisecretory effects in patients using antiprostaglandin drugs
    _____ i. Has the greatest noncompliance
    _____ j. Decrease HCl acid secretion and gastric motility

    1. Famotidine (Pepcid)
    2. Omeprazole (Prilosec)
    3. Aluminum/magnesium hydroxide
    4. Sucralfate (Carafate)
    5. Misoprostol (Cytotec) mixture
    6. Amoxicillin/clarithromycin/omeprazole
    7. Anticholinergics

30. The nurse determines that teaching for the patient with peptic ulcer disease has been effective when the patient states,
    a. "I should stop all my medications if I develop any side effects."
    b. "I should continue my treatment regimen as long as I have pain."
    c. "I have learned some relaxation strategies that decrease my stress."
    d. "I can buy whatever antacids are on sale because they all have the same effect."

31. A patient with a history of peptic ulcer disease is hospitalized with symptoms of a perforation. During the initial assessment, the nurse would expect the patient to report
    a. vomiting of bright-red blood.
    b. projectile vomiting of undigested food.
    c. sudden, severe upper abdominal pain and shoulder pain.
    d. hyperactive stomach sounds and upper abdominal swelling.

32. A patient with a gastric outlet obstruction has been treated with NG decompression. After the first 24 hours, the patient develops nausea and increased upper abdominal bowel sounds. An appropriate action by the nurse is to
    a. check the patency of the NG tube.
    b. place the patient in a recumbent position.
    c. assess the patient's vital signs and circulatory status.
    d. encourage the patient to deep-breathe and consciously relax.

33. When caring for a patient with an acute exacerbation of a peptic ulcer, the nurse finds the patient doubled up in bed with shallow, grunting respirations. The initial appropriate action by the nurse is to
    a. notify the health care provider.
    b. irrigate the patient's NG tube.
    c. place the patient in high-Fowler's position.
    d. assess the patient's abdomen and vital signs.

34. Match the descriptions with the following surgical procedures used to treat peptic ulcer disease.
    _____ a. Often performed with a vagotomy to increase gastric emptying
    _____ b. Severing of a parasympathetic nerve to decrease gastric secretion
    _____ c. Removal of distal two thirds of stomach with anastomosis to jejunum
    _____ d. Removal of distal two thirds of stomach with anastomosis to duodenum

    1. Billroth I
    2. Billroth II
    3. Pyloroplasty
    4. Vagotomy

35. Following a Billroth II procedure, a patient develops dumping syndrome. The nurse explains that the symptoms associated with this problem are caused by
    a. distention of the smaller stomach by too much food and fluid intake.
    b. hyperglycemia caused by uncontrolled gastric emptying into the small intestine.
    c. irritation of the stomach lining by reflux of bile salts because the pylorus has been removed.
    d. movement of fluid into the small bowel because concentrated food and fluids move rapidly into the intestine.

36. The nurse determines that further dietary teaching is needed when a patient with dumping syndrome says,
    a. "I should eat bread with every meal."
    b. "I should avoid drinking fluids with my meals."
    c. "I should eat smaller meals about six times a day."
    d. "I need to lie down for 30 to 60 minutes after my meals."

37. While caring for a patient following a subtotal gastrectomy with a gastroduodenostomy anastomosis, the nurse determines that the NG tube is obstructed. The nurse should
    a. replace the tube with a new one.
    b. irrigate the tube until return can be aspirated.
    c. reposition the tube and then attempt irrigation.
    d. notify the surgeon to reposition or replace the tube.

38. A patient with cancer of the stomach at the lesser curvature undergoes a total gastrectomy with an esophagojejunostomy. Postoperatively, the nurse teaches the patient to expect
    a. rapid healing of the surgical wound.
    b. lifelong administration of cobalamin.
    c. to be able to return to normal dietary habits.
    d. close follow-up for development of peptic ulcers in the jejunum.

39. A large number of children at a public school have developed profuse diarrhea and bloody stools. The school nurse suspects food poisoning from the school cafeteria and requests analysis and culture of
    a. chicken.
    b. ground beef.
    c. commercially canned fish.
    d. salads with mayonnaise dressing.

CASE STUDY
Gastric Cancer
Patient Profile

S.E. is a 75-year-old retired garment worker who was diagnosed with gastric cancer 2 weeks ago. The home health nurse assigned to her case reads the following on her medical record:

Subjective Data

- 6-month history of epigastric discomfort, anorexia, nausea, vomiting, and a 25-lb weight loss
- Stated she has had "stomach problems" for a long time and was diagnosed with gastritis 20 years ago
- Stated she was told that the tumor could not be removed because it was too advanced
- Stated, "I've always been a strong person, but now I'm just too tired to eat or do anything."

Objective Data

- Physical examination: Palpable mass in left upper quadrant of the abdomen
- Diagnostic tests: Barium swallow, gastroscopy, and biopsy/cytology all confirmed the presence of a well-advanced tumor in the fundus of the stomach
- Laboratory tests:
  - Decreased hemoglobin and hematocrit
  - Serum albumin 2.4 g/dL (24 g/L)
- Appears emaciated with areas of skin discoloration on her forearms

When the nurse visits S.E., she has just returned from a radiation treatment and is holding a plastic emesis basin and tissues in her lap.

Clinical Decision-Making Questions

Using a separate sheet of paper, answer the following questions.

1. What pathophysiologic changes occur in gastric cancer that lead to the symptoms experienced by S.E.?
2. What subjective and objective data indicate the presence of malnutrition in S.E.?
3. What other factors might be contributing to S.E.'s malnutrition besides those described?
4. What other complications may develop as a result of S.E.'s malnutrition?
5. *Priority Decision:* What priority interventions should the nurse include in the treatment plan for S.E. and her family?
6. S.E. asks the nurse if anyone with her stage of gastric cancer has ever recovered. What is the nurse's best response to S.E.?
7. *Priority Decision:* Based on the assessment data presented, what are the priority nursing diagnoses? Are there any collaborative problems?

1. The nurse identifies a need for additional teaching when a patient with acute infectious diarrhea states,
   a. "I can use A&D ointment or Vaseline jelly around the anal area to protect my skin."
   b. "Gatorade is a good liquid to drink because it replaces the fluid and salts I have lost."
   c. "I must wash my hands after every bowel movement to prevent spreading the diarrhea to my family."
   d. "I may use over-the-counter loperamide (Imodium) or Parepectolin (paregoric, pectin, kaolin) as needed to control the diarrhea."

2. In instituting a bowel training program for a patient with fecal incontinence, the nurse plans to
   a. teach the patient to use a perianal pouch.
   b. place the patient on a bedpan 30 minutes before breakfast.
   c. insert a rectal suppository at the same time every morning.
   d. assist the patient to the bathroom at the time of the patient's normal defecation.

3. Explain the significance of each of the following pieces of information obtained from the patient with chronic constipation during the nursing assessment.
   a. Suppressing the urge to defecate while at work
   b. A history of diverticulosis
   c. Belief in necessity of daily bowel movement
   d. History of hemorrhoids and hypertension
   e. High dietary fiber with low fluid intake

4. The nurse teaches the patient with chronic constipation that, of the following foods, dietary fiber is highest in
   a. bananas.
   b. popcorn.
   c. dried beans.
   d. shredded wheat.

5. The preferred immediate treatment for an acute episode of constipation is the administration of
   a. an enema.
   b. increased fluid.
   c. stool-softeners.
   d. bulk-forming medication.

6. *Priority Decision:* A patient is admitted to the emergency department with acute abdominal pain. The nursing intervention that should be implemented first is
   a. measurement of vital signs.
   b. administration of prescribed analgesics.
   c. assessment of the onset, location, intensity, duration, and character of the pain.
   d. physical assessment of the abdomen for distention, masses, abnormal pulsations, bowel sounds, and pigmentation changes.

7. For the following causes of acute abdomen, select those for which surgery would be indicated.
   _____ a. Foreign-body perforation
   _____ b. Pancreatitis
   _____ c. Ruptured abdominal aneurysm
   _____ d. Ruptured ectopic pregnancy
   _____ e. Pelvic inflammatory disease
   _____ f. Acute ischemic bowel

8. *Priority Decision:* A patient returns to the surgical unit with a nasogastric (NG) tube to low intermittent suction, IV fluids, and a Jackson-Pratt drain at the surgical site following an exploratory laparotomy and repair of a bowel perforation. Four hours after admission, the patient experiences nausea and vomiting. A priority nursing intervention for the patient is to
   a. assess the abdomen for distention and bowel sounds.
   b. inspect the surgical site and drainage in the Jackson-Pratt.
   c. administer prescribed hydroxine (Vistaril) to control the nausea and vomiting.
   d. check the amount and character of gastric drainage and the patency of the NG tube.

9. A postoperative patient has a nursing diagnosis of pain related to effects of medication and decreased GI motility as evidenced by abdominal pain and distention and inability to pass flatus. An appropriate nursing intervention for the patient is to
   a. ambulate the patient more frequently.
   b. assess the abdomen for bowel sounds.
   c. place the patient in high Fowler's position.
   d. withhold opioids because they decrease bowel motility.

10. A 22-year-old patient calls the outpatient clinic complaining of nausea and vomiting and right lower abdominal pain. The nurse advises the patient to
    a. use a heating pad to relax the muscles at the site of the pain.
    b. drink at least 2 quarts of juice to replace the fluid lost in vomiting.
    c. take a laxative to empty the bowel before examination at the clinic.
    d. have the symptoms evaluated by a health care provider right away.

11. When caring for a patient with irritable bowel syndrome (IBS), it is most important for the nurse to
    a. recognize that IBS is a psychogenic illness that cannot be definitively diagnosed.
    b. develop a trusting relationship with the patient to provide support and symptomatic care.
    c. teach the patient that a diet high in fiber will relieve the symptoms of both diarrhea and constipation.
    d. inform the patient that new medications for IBS are available and effective for treatment of IBS manifested by either diarrhea or constipation

12. *Priority Decision:* A patient with a gunshot wound to the abdomen complains of increasing abdominal pain several hours after surgery to repair the bowel. What action should the nurse take first?
    a. Take the patient's vital signs.
    b. Notify the health care provider.
    c. Position the patient with the knees flexed.
    d. Determine the patient's IV intake since the end of surgery.

13. Identify whether the following statements are true (*T*) or false (*F*). If a statement is false, correct the bold word(s) to make the statement true.
    _____ a. The nurse recognizes that surgery is indicated for the patient with abdominal trauma when positive findings are obtained with **peritoneal lavage**.
    _____ b. The major complication of appendicitis is **colitis**.
    _____ c. The site of pain localization in appendicitis is known as **Grey Turner's sign**.
    _____ d. Regardless of the cause of peritonitis, the nurse would anticipate that treatment of the patient would include **IV fluid replacement**.
    _____ e. The nurse advises the patient with gastroenteritis to start increasing fluid intake as soon as **vomiting subsides**.

14. Indicate whether the following characteristics of inflammatory bowel disease are most likely to be associated with ulcerative colitis (UC), Crohn's disease (CD), or both conditions (B).

_____ a. Presence of diarrhea

_____ b. Confined to large intestine

_____ c. Involves the entire thickness of the bowel wall

_____ d. Has periods of remission and exacerbation

_____ e. Can be cured with surgical colectomy

_____ f. Has segmented distribution

_____ g. Rectal bleeding

_____ h. Extraintestinal complications

_____ i. Risk of colon cancer

_____ j. Bowel perforation

_____ k. Formation of fistulas

_____ l. Unknown cause

_____ m. Abdominal pain

15. Indicate what laboratory findings are expected in ulcerative colitis as a result of the following:

a. Bloody diarrhea

b. Hypoalbuminemia

c. Diarrhea and vomiting

d. Toxic megacolon

16. Extraintestinal symptoms that are seen in both ulcerative colitis and Crohn's disease are

a. osteoporosis and conjunctivitis.

b. peptic ulcer disease and uveitis.

c. erythema nodosum and arthritis.

d. gluten intolerance and gallstones.

17. Match the following treatment modalities for inflammatory bowel disease (IBD) with the appropriate rationale (answers may be used more than once).

_____ a. Corticosteroids

_____ b. Parenteral nutrition

_____ c. Cobalamin injections

_____ d. Antidiarrheal agents

_____ e. Sulfasalazine (Azulfidine)

_____ f. IV fluids

_____ g. Sedatives

_____ h. 6-Mercaptopurine

_____ i. Nasogastric suction

_____ j. Iron injections

_____ k. NPO

1. Promote(s) bowel rest

2. Control(s) inflammation

3. Prevent(s) secondary infection

4. Correct(s) malnutrition

5. Alleviate(s) stress

6. Relieve(s) symptoms

18. A patient with ulcerative colitis undergoes the first phase of a total colectomy with ileoanal anastomosis and formation of an ileal reservoir. On postoperative assessment of the patient, the nurse would expect to find

a. an unopened loop ileostomy.

b. a rectal tube set to low continuous suction.

c. an ileostomy stoma with a catheter in place to provide pouch irrigations.

d. a permanent ileostomy stoma in the right lower quadrant of the abdomen.

19. A patient with ulcerative colitis has a total colectomy with formation of a terminal ileum stoma. An important nursing intervention for this patient postoperatively is to

a. measure the ileostomy output to determine the status of the patient's fluid balance.

b. change the ileostomy appliance every 3 to 4 hours to prevent leakage of drainage onto the skin.

c. emphasize that the ostomy is temporary and the ileum will be reconnected when the large bowel heals.

d. teach the patient about the high-fiber, low-carbohydrate diet required to maintain normal ileostomy drainage.

20. A patient with IBD has a nursing diagnosis of imbalanced nutrition: less than body requirements related to decreased nutritional intake and decreased intestinal absorption. Assessment data that support this nursing diagnosis are
    a. pallor and hair loss.
    b. frequent diarrhea stools.
    c. anorectal excoriation and pain.
    d. hypotension and urine output below 30 mL/hr.

21. Match the following intestinal obstructions with their descriptions.
    _____ a. Adhesions   1. Nervous paralysis of the bowel
    _____ b. Volvulus   2. Protrusion of bowel in weak or abnormal opening
    _____ c. Intussusception   3. Bands of scar tissue constrict the intestine
    _____ d. Hernia   4. Twisting of bowel on itself
    _____ e. Vascular obstruction   5. Bowel folding on itself
    _____ f. Adynamic ileus   6. Emboli of arterial supply to the bowel

22. Identify whether the following statements are true (*T*) or false (*F*). If a statement is false, correct the bold word(s) to make the statement true.
    _____ a. A rapid onset of projectile vomiting occurs with a **large bowel obstruction**.
    _____ b. Abdominal distention is the most apparent in an obstruction of the **large bowel**.
    _____ c. Fecal vomiting is most likely to occur in a **lower small** bowel obstruction.
    _____ d. **Metabolic alkalosis** is most likely to occur with prolonged vomiting.
    _____ e. Sudden, severe, constant abdominal pain is indicative of an **upper small** bowel obstruction.
    _____ f. Abdominal pain that is colicky and crampy, coming and going in waves, is characteristic of a **paralytic ileus**.

23. An important nursing intervention for the patient with a small bowel obstruction who has an NG tube is to
    a. offer ice chips to suck PRN.
    b. provide mouth care every 1 to 2 hours.
    c. irrigate the tube with normal saline every 8 hours.
    d. keep the patient supine with the head of the bed elevated 30 degrees.

24. During a routine screening colonoscopy on a 56-year-old patient, a rectosigmoidal polyp was identified and removed. The patient asks the nurse if his risk for colon cancer is increased because of the polyp. The best response by the nurse is,
    a. "It is very rare for polyps to become malignant, but you should continue to have routine colonoscopies."
    b. "Individuals with polyps have a 100% lifetime risk of developing colorectal cancer, and at an earlier age than those without polyps."
    c. "All polyps are abnormal and should be removed, but the risk for cancer depends on the type and if malignant changes are present."
    d. "All polyps are premalignant and a source of most colon cancer. You will need to have a colonoscopy every 6 months to check for new polyps."

25. When obtaining a nursing history from the patient with colorectal cancer, the nurse asks the patient specifically about
    a. dietary intake.
    b. history of smoking.
    c. history of alcohol intake.
    d. environmental exposure to carcinogens.

26. Describe how the structures of the colon are altered during an abdominal-perineal resection.

27. On examining a patient 8 hours after formation of a colostomy, the nurse would expect to find
    a. hypoactive, high-pitched bowel sounds.
    b. a brick-red, puffy stoma that oozes blood.
    c. a purplish stoma, shiny and moist with mucus.
    d. a small amount of liquid fecal drainage from the stoma.

28. ***Delegation Decision:*** The RN coordinating the care for a patient who is 2 days postoperative following an anterior-posterior resection with colostomy may delegate which of the following interventions to the LPN (select all that apply)?
    a. irrigate the colostomy
    b. teach ostomy and skin care
    c. assess and document stoma appearance
    d. monitor and record the volume, color, and odor of the drainage
    e. empty the ostomy bag and measure and record the amount of drainage.

29. A male patient who has undergone an abdominal-perineal resection has a nursing diagnosis of ineffective sexuality pattern. An appropriate nursing intervention for the patient is to
    a. have the patient's sexual partner reassure the patient that he is still desirable.
    b. reassure the patient that sexual function will return when healing is complete.
    c. remind the patient that affection can be expressed in other ways besides sexual intercourse.
    d. explain that physical and emotional factors can affect sexual function but not necessarily the patient's sexuality.

30. Describe the type of drainage expected from the stoma of each of the following:
    a. Ileostomy
    b. Descending colostomy
    c. Transverse loop colostomy

31. The nurse plans teaching for the patient with a colostomy, but the patient refuses to look at the nurse or the stoma, stating, "I just can't see myself with this thing." An appropriate nursing diagnosis for the patient is
    a. self-care deficit related to refusal to care for colostomy.
    b. disturbed body image related to presence of colostomy stoma.
    c. ineffective coping related to feelings of helplessness and lack of coping skills.
    d. ineffective self-health management related to lack of knowledge for care of colostomy.

32. In teaching a patient about colostomy irrigation, the nurse tells the patient to
    a. infuse 1500 to 2000 mL of warm tap water as irrigation fluid.
    b. allow 30 to 45 minutes for the solution and feces to be expelled.
    c. insert a firm plastic catheter 3 to 4 inches into the stoma opening.
    d. hang the irrigation bag on a hook about 36 inches above the stoma.

33. The nurse teaches the patient with diverticulosis to
    a. use anticholinergic drugs routinely to prevent bowel spasm.
    b. have an annual colonoscopy to detect malignant changes in the lesions.
    c. maintain a high-fiber diet and use bulk laxatives to increase fecal volume.
    d. exclude whole grain breads and cereals from the diet to prevent irritating the bowel.

34. During an acute attack of diverticulitis, the patient is
    a. monitored for signs of peritonitis.
    b. treated with daily medicated enemas.
    c. prepared for surgery to resect the involved colon.
    d. provided with a heating pad to apply to the left lower quadrant.

35. Match the types of hernias with their descriptions.
   _____ a. Reducible   1. Obstructed intestinal flow and blood supply
   _____ b. Incarcerated   2. Follows the spermatic cord or round ligament
   _____ c. Strangulated   3. Weakness at the site of previous incision
   _____ d. Femoral   4. Cannot be placed back into abdominal cavity
   _____ e. Inguinal   5. Protrusion into femoral canal
   _____ f. Ventral   6. Can be placed back into abdominal cavity

36. A nursing intervention that is indicated for a male patient following an inguinal herniorrhaphy is
   a. applying heat to the inguinal area.
   b. elevating the scrotum with a scrotal support.
   c. applying a truss to support the operative site.
   d. encouraging the patient to cough and deep-breathe.

37. The most common form of malabsorption syndrome is treated with
   a. administration of antibiotics.
   b. avoidance of milk and milk products.
   c. supplementation with pancreatic enzymes.
   d. avoidance of gluten found in wheat, barley, oats, and rye.

38. A patient is diagnosed with celiac disease following a workup for iron-deficiency anemia and decreased bone
   density. The nurse identifies that additional teaching about disease management is needed when the patient says,
   a. "I should ask my close relatives to be screened for celiac disease."
   b. "If I do not follow the gluten-free diet, I might develop a lymphoma."
   c. "I don't need to restrict gluten intake because I don't have diarrhea or bowel symptoms."
   d. "It is going to be difficult to follow a gluten-free diet because it is found in so many foods."

39. Short bowel syndrome is most likely to occur in the patient with
   a. ulcerative colitis.
   b. irritable bowel syndrome.
   c. an extensive resection of the ileum.
   d. a colectomy performed for cancer of the bowel.

40. Match the following anorectal conditions with their descriptions.
   _____ a. Pilonidal sinus   1. Engorged rectal vein around anal sphincter
   _____ b. Anorectal abscess   2. Ulcer in anal wall
   _____ c. Anal fissure   3. Tunnel leading from the anus or rectum
   _____ d. Hemorrhoid   4. Collection of perianal pus
   _____ e. Anorectal fistula   5. Sacrococcygeal hairy tract

41. Following anal surgery, the nurse advises the patient to
   a. use daily laxatives to facilitate bowel emptying.
   b. use ice packs to the perineum to prevent swelling.
   c. avoid having a bowel movement for several days until healing occurs.
   d. take warm sitz baths several times a day to promote comfort and cleaning.

CASE STUDY
Cancer of the Rectum
Patient Profile

C.D., a 63-year-old married insurance salesman, has undergone an abdominal-perineal resection for cancer of the rectum. He is 1 day postoperative on the general surgical unit.

Subjective Data

- Complains of pain in his abdominal and perineal incisions that is not well controlled even with his patient-controlled analgesia (PCA) machine
- Jokes about his stoma winking at him when the dressings are removed the first time and a temporary colostomy bag is applied
- Refers to his stoma as "Jake"
- Tells his wife that "Jake" will be watching her

Objective Data

- Bright red stoma on left lower quadrant of abdomen; colostomy bag has small amount of pink mucus drainage
- Midline abdominal incision; no signs of infection; sutures intact
- Perineal incision partially closed; two Penrose drains with bulky dressings with a large amount of serosanguineous drainage
- All vital signs normal
- PCA orders of 1 mg morphine sulfate every 10 minutes, with 17 attempts in the past hour

Clinical Decision-Making Questions

Using a separate sheet of papaer, answer the following questions.

1. What symptoms may have alerted C.D. to seek medical care for his cancer of the rectum?
2. What care is indicated for C.D.'s perineal wound?
3. What are the primary goals of care for C.D.'s colostomy?
4. What would be the nurse's evaluation of C.D.'s adjustment to his colostomy?
5. What factors may be influencing the pain that C.D. is experiencing?
6. *Priority Decision:* What are the priority teaching needs for C.D. before his discharge?
7. *Priority Decision:* Based on the assessment data presented, what are the priority nursing diagnoses? Are there any collaborative problems?

44   Nursing Management: Liver, Pancreas, and Biliary Tract Problems

1. Complete the following statements.
   a. The type of jaundice associated with gallstones is _____ jaundice, and the type of serum bilirubin that is elevated is most likely _____.
   b. Hemolytic jaundice is caused by _____, and the type of bilirubin elevated in the blood is _____.
   c. Jaundice resulting from failure of the liver to conjugate and excrete bilirubin is known as _____ jaundice and causes serum elevations of _____ bilirubin.

2. Match the following characteristics of viral hepatitis with their related types (answers may be used more than once).
   _____ a. IV drug use is method of greatest transmission
   _____ b. Uncommon in United States
   _____ c. Exists only with hepatitis B
   _____ d. Caused by a DNA virus
   _____ e. Most common cause of chronic hepatitis
   _____ f. Often causes asymptomatic anicteric hepatitis
   _____ g. Chronic carriers have increased risk for hepatocellular cancer
   _____ h. Has no chronic carrier state
   _____ i. No readily available diagnostic serology tests
   _____ j. Usual cause of hepatitis epidemics

   1. Hepatitis A (HAV)
   2. Hepatitis B (HBV)
   3. Hepatitis C (HCV)
   4. Hepatitis D (HDV)
   5. Hepatitis E (HEV)

3. Serologic findings in viral hepatitis include both the presence of viral antigens and antibodies produced in response to the viruses. Identify the three antigens associated with active HBV and the corresponding antibodies for those antigens. (One of the antigens stimulates two antibodies.)

Antigen	Antibodies
a. (surface)	
b. (e)	
c. (core)	

4. Complete the following sentences related to serologic findings in viral hepatitis.
   a. In addition to HBV antigens and antibodies, the best indicator of active, ongoing HBV replication is the presence of _____ in the blood.
   b. The HBV antibody that is a marker of response to the HBV vaccine is _____.
   c. The HBV antibody that does not appear after immunization is _____.
   d. The HBV antigen that persists in chronic carrier states is _____.
   e. HAV antigens are not tested in the blood; like HBV, they stimulate specific IgM and IgG antibodies. Acute HAV infection is indicated by _____ antibodies, whereas prior infection is indicated by _____ antibodies.
   f. Co-infection of HDV with HBV can be detected by testing for the _____ antibody.
   g. Several tests are used to determine the presence of HCV. The initial screening for acute or chronic HCV includes testing for the _____ antibody.
   h. A patient with anti-HCV antibodies can have active, chronic, or prior HCV infection. The test that best indicates active disease and can also detect HCV in an immunosuppressed patient is _____.
   i. A more sensitive antibody test for HCV includes the use of the _____.

5. The systemic effects of viral hepatitis are caused primarily by
   a. cholestasis.
   b. impaired portal circulation.
   c. toxins produced by the infected liver.
   d. activation of the complement system by antigen-antibody complexes.

6. During the incubation period of viral hepatitis, the nurse would expect the patient to report
   a. pruritus and malaise.
   b. dark urine and easy fatigability.
   c. anorexia and right upper quadrant discomfort.
   d. constipation or diarrhea with light-colored stools.

7. Fulminant viral hepatitis as a complication of viral hepatitis is highest in those individuals with
   a. hepatitis A.
   b. hepatitis C.
   c. hepatitis B accompanied with hepatitis C.
   d. hepatitis B accompanied with hepatitis D.

8. Identify the prophylactic immunologic agents that are used for the following.
   a. Preexposure protection to HBV
   b. Postexposure protection to HBV

9. The family members of a patient with hepatitis A ask if there is anything that will prevent them from developing the disease. The best response by the nurse is
   a. "No immunization is available for hepatitis A, nor are you likely to get the disease."
   b. "Only individuals who have had sexual contact with the patient should receive immunization."
   c. "All family members should receive the hepatitis A vaccine to prevent or modify the infection."
   d. "Those who have had household or close contact with the patient should receive immune globulin."

10. A patient newly diagnosed with acute hepatitis B asks about drug therapy to treat the disease. The most appropriate response by the nurse is informing the patient that
    a. there are no specific drug therapies that are effective for treating acute viral hepatitis.
    b. only chronic hepatitis C is treatable, primarily with antiviral agents and α-interferon.
    c. no drugs can be used for treatment of viral hepatitis because of the risk of additional liver damage.
    d. α-interferon combined with lamivudine (Epivir) will decrease viral load and liver damage if taken for 1 year.

11. The nurse identifies a need for further teaching when the patient with hepatitis B states,
    a. "I should avoid alcohol completely for as long as a year."
    b. "I must avoid all physical contact with my family until the jaundice is gone."
    c. "I should use a condom to prevent spread of the disease to my sexual partner."
    d. "I will need to rest several times a day, gradually increasing my activity as I tolerate it."

12. One of the most challenging nursing interventions to promote healing in the patient with viral hepatitis is
    a. providing adequate nutritional intake.
    b. promoting strict bed rest during the icteric phase.
    c. providing pain relief without using liver-metabolized drugs.
    d. providing quiet diversional activities during periods of fatigue.

13. When caring for a patient with autoimmune hepatitis, the nurse recognizes that, unlike viral hepatitis, the patient
    a. does not manifest hepatomegaly or jaundice.
    b. experiences less liver inflammation and damage.
    c. is treated with corticosteroids or other immunosuppressant agents.
    d. is usually an older adult who has used a wide variety of prescription and over-the-counter drugs.

14. Match the following clinical manifestations with the pathophysiologic changes that occur in cirrhosis (answers may be used more than once).

_____ a. Jaundice
_____ b. Testicular atrophy
_____ c. Anorexia and dyspepsia
_____ d. Spider angiomas
_____ e. Amenorrhea
_____ f. Peripheral neuropathy
_____ g. Anemia, leukopenia, thrombocytopenia
_____ h. Dull, heavy, right upper quadrant (RUQ) pain
_____ i. Male gynecomastia
_____ j. Petechiae and purpura

1. Decreased prothrombin production
2. Vascular congestion of spleen
3. Decreased estrogen metabolism
4. Stretching of liver capsule
5. Decreased bilirubin conjugation and excretion
6. Altered carbohydrate, protein, and fat metabolism
7. Decreased testosterone metabolism
8. Vitamin B deficiencies

15. Describe the pathophysiologic changes of cirrhosis that cause the following.
    a. Portal hypertension
    b. Esophageal varices

16. Complete the following statements related to formation of ascites using these terms.

Terms

antidiuretic hormone (ADH)   hypoalbuminemia
aldosterone   hypokalemia
decreased albumin production   peripheral edema

a. Fluid moves into the abdominal cavity, producing ascites because of decreased serum oncotic colloidal pressure. The decreased serum oncotic pressure is caused by _____.

b. Fluid sequestering in the peritoneal cavity results in (increased/decreased) _____ vascular volume, (increased/decreased) _____ blood return to the heart, and (increased/decreased) _____ cardiac output (CO).

c. The change in CO results in (increased/decreased) _____ kidney perfusion and secretion of _____ and _____, both of which increase fluid retention.

d. The retained fluid has low oncotic colloidal pressure, and it escapes into the interstitial spaces, causing _____.

e. Excessive fluid continues to be reabsorbed from the kidney because of the altered kidney perfusion and because _____ is not metabolized by the impaired liver.

f. The changes in laboratory test results that relate to this process are _____ and _____.

17. Laboratory test results that the nurse would expect to find in a patient with cirrhosis include
    a. serum albumin: 7.0 g/dL (70 g/L).
    b. bilirubin: total 3.2 mg/dL (54.7 μmol/L).
    c. serum cholesterol: 260 mg/dL (6.7 mmol/L).
    d. aspartate aminotransferase (AST): 6.0 U/L (0.1 μkat/L).

18. Identify the rationales for the following interventions in treating the cirrhotic patient with ascites.
    a. Bed rest
    b. Salt-poor albumin
    c. Diuretic therapy
    d. Low-sodium diet
    e. Paracentesis
    f. Peritoneovenous shunts

19. The nurse recognizes early signs of hepatic encephalopathy in the patient who
    a. manifests asterixis.
    b. becomes unconscious.
    c. has increasing oliguria.
    d. is irritable and lethargic.

20. Identify the rationales for the following interventions in treating the cirrhotic patient with hepatic encephalopathy.
    a. Lactulose (Cephulac)
    b. Neomycin
    c. Eliminating blood from the GI tract

21. A patient with advanced cirrhosis has a nursing diagnosis of imbalanced nutrition: less than body requirements related to anorexia and inadequate food intake. An appropriate midday snack for the patient would be
    a. peanut butter and salt-free crackers.
    b. a fresh tomato sandwich with salt-free butter.
    c. popcorn with salt-free butter and herbal seasoning.
    d. canned chicken noodle soup with low-protein bread.

22. During the treatment of the patient with bleeding esophageal varices, it is most important that the nurse
    a. prepare the patient for immediate portal shunting surgery.
    b. perform guaiac testing on all stools to detect occult blood.
    c. maintain the patient's airway and prevent aspiration of blood.
    d. monitor for the cardiac effects of IV vasopressin and nitroglycerin.

23. A patient with cirrhosis that is refractory to other treatments for esophageal varices undergoes a peritoneovenous shunt. As a result of this procedure, the nurse would expect the patient to experience
    a. an improved survival rate.
    b. decreased serum ammonia levels.
    c. improved metabolism of nutrients.
    d. improved hemodynamic function and renal perfusion.

24. In discussing long-term management with the patient with alcoholic cirrhosis, the nurse advises the patient that
    a. a daily exercise regimen is important to increase the blood flow through the liver.
    b. cirrhosis can be reversed if the patient follows a regimen of proper rest and nutrition.
    c. abstinence from alcohol is the most important factor in improvement of the patient's condition.
    d. the only over-the-counter analgesic that should be used for minor aches and pains is acetaminophen.

25. A patient is hospitalized with metastatic cancer of the liver. The nurse plans care for the patient based on the knowledge that
    a. chemotherapy is highly successful in the treatment of liver cancer.
    b. the patient will undergo surgery to remove the involved portions of the liver.
    c. supportive care that is appropriate for all patients with severe liver damage is indicated.
    d. metastatic cancer of the liver is more responsive to treatment than primary carcinoma of the liver.

26. A patient with cirrhosis asks the nurse about the possibility of a liver transplant. The best response by the nurse is,
    a. "Liver transplants are only indicated in children with irreversible liver disease."
    b. "If you are interested in a transplant, you really should talk to your doctor about it."
    c. "Rejection is such a problem in liver transplants that it is seldom attempted in patients with cirrhosis."
    d. "Cirrhosis is an indication for transplantation in some cases. Have you talked to your doctor about this?"

27. Match the complications of acute pancreatitis with the pathophysiologic mechanisms.
    _____ a. Pseudocyst
    _____ b. Pancreatic abscess
    _____ c. Pleural effusion
    _____ d. Tetany
    _____ e. Hypovolemia

    1. Combining of calcium with fatty acids during fat necrosis
    2. Cavity continuous with pancreas filled with necrotic products and secretions
    3. Pancreatic enzymes pass from peritoneal cavity through diaphragmatic lymph channels
    4. Exudation of blood and plasma into retroperitoneal space
    5. Extensive pancreatic necrosis with resultant fluid-filled cavity

28. When assessing a patient with acute pancreatitis, the nurse would expect to find
    a. hyperactive bowel sounds.
    b. hypertension and tachycardia.
    c. severe midepigastric or left upper quadrant (LUQ) pain.
    d. a temperature greater than 102° F (38.9° C).

29. Combined with clinical manifestations, the laboratory finding that is most commonly used to diagnose acute pancreatitis is
    a. increased serum calcium.
    b. increased serum amylase.
    c. increased urinary amylase.
    d. decreased serum glucose.

30. Management of the patient with acute pancreatitis includes
    a. surgery to remove the inflamed pancreas.
    b. pancreatic enzymes administered with meals.
    c. NG suction to prevent gastric contents from entering the duodenum.
    d. endoscopic pancreatic sphincterotomy using endoscopic retrograde cholangiopancreatography (ERCP).

31. A patient with acute pancreatitis has a nursing diagnosis of pain related to distention of pancreas and peritoneal irritation. In addition to effective use of analgesics, the nurse should
    a. provide diversional activities to distract the patient from the pain.
    b. provide small frequent meals to increase the patient's tolerance to food.
    c. position the patient on the side with the head of the bed elevated 45 degrees for pain relief.
    d. ambulate the patient every 3 to 4 hours to increase circulation and decrease abdominal congestion.

32. The nurse determines that further discharge instruction is needed when the patient with acute pancreatitis states,
    a. "I should observe for fat in my stools."
    b. "I must not use alcohol to prevent future attacks of pancreatitis."
    c. "I shouldn't eat salty foods or foods with high amounts of sodium."
    d. "I will need to continue to monitor my blood glucose levels until my pancreas is healed."

33. The patient with chronic pancreatitis is more likely than the patient with acute pancreatitis to
    a. need to abstain from alcohol.
    b. experience acute abdominal pain.
    c. have malabsorption and diabetes mellitus.
    d. require a high-carbohydrate, high-protein, low-fat diet.

34. The nurse is instructing a patient with chronic pancreatitis on measures to prevent further attacks. What information should be provided (select all that apply)?
    a. Avoid nicotine
    b. Eat bland foods
    c. Observe stools for steatorrhea
    d. Eat high-fat, low-protein, high-carbohydrate meals.
    e. Take prescribed pancreatic enzymes immediately following meals.

35. A risk factor associated with cancer of the pancreas is
    a. alcohol intake.
    b. cigarette smoking.
    c. exposure to asbestos.
    d. increased dietary intake of milk and milk products.

36. In a radical pancreaticoduodenectomy (Whipple's procedure) for treatment of cancer of the pancreas, what anatomic structures are completely resected?

    a.

    b.

    What anatomic structures are partially resected?

    c.

    d.

    What anastomoses are made?

    e.

    f.

    g.

37. Identify whether the following statements are true (*T*) or false (*F*). If a statement is false, correct the bold word(s) to make the statement true.

    _____ a. **Cholelithiasis** is the most common disorder of the biliary system.

    _____ b. Most gallstones are composed primarily of **calcium and bile salts**.

    _____ c. If a gallstone blocks the cystic duct, the patient will have symptoms of **biliary colic**.

    _____ d. Obstructive jaundice occurs when gallstones obstruct the **common bile duct**.

38. Of the following characteristics, identify those that are associated with cholelithiasis.

    _____ a. Family history of gallbladder disease

    _____ b. History of excessive alcohol intake

    _____ c. Multiparous female

    _____ d. Obesity

    _____ e. High-serum, high-density lipoproteins

    _____ f. African American men

    _____ g. Age over 40

    _____ h. Use of estrogen or oral contraceptives

39. The patient with an obstruction of the common bile duct has the following signs and symptoms. Identify the pathophysiologic changes that cause these clinical manifestations.

    a. Jaundice

    b. Clay-colored stools

    c. Dark urine

    d. Steatorrhea

    e. Pain with fatty food intake

40. The patient with suspected gallbladder disease is scheduled for an ultrasound of the gallbladder. The nurse explains to the patient that this test

    a. is noninvasive and is a very reliable method of detecting gallstones.

    b. is used only when other tests cannot be used because of allergy to contrast media.

    c. is an adjunct to liver function tests to determine whether the gallbladder is inflamed.

    d. will outline the gallbladder and the ductal system to enable visualization of stones.

41. Identify the rationale for the treatment of acute cholecystitis with the following interventions:

    a. NPO with NG suction

    b. Administration of antibiotics

    c. Administration of anticholinergics

42. Match the following descriptions with the treatments used for cholelithiasis.
    _____ a. External shock waves disintegrate stones
    _____ b. Stones removed through sphincter of Oddi
    _____ c. Gallbladder removed
    _____ d. Administered orally to dissolve stones and reduce cholesterol saturation

    1. Endoscopic retrograde cholangio-pancreatography (ERCP) with sphincterotomy
    2. Extracorporeal shock-wave lithotripsy (ESWL)
    3. Laparoscopic cholecystectomy
    4. Chenodeoxycholic acid (chenodiol)

43. Following a laparoscopic cholecystectomy, the nurse would expect the patient to
    a. return to work in 2 to 3 weeks.
    b. be hospitalized for 3 to 5 days postoperatively.
    c. have four small abdominal incisions covered with small dressings.
    d. have a T-tube placed in the common bile duct to provide bile drainage.

44. A patient with chronic cholecystitis asks the nurse whether she will need to continue a low-fat diet after she has a cholecystectomy. The best response by the nurse is,
    a. "A low-fat diet will prevent the development of further gallstones and should be continued."
    b. "Yes, because you will not have a gallbladder to store bile, you will not be able to digest fats adequately."
    c. "A low-fat diet is recommended for a few weeks after surgery until the intestine adjusts to receiving a continuous flow of bile."
    d. "Removal of the gallbladder will eliminate the source of your pain associated with fat intake, so you may eat whatever you like."

45. To care for a T-tube in a patient following a cholecystectomy, the nurse
    a. keeps the tube supported and free of kinks.
    b. attaches the tube to low continuous suction.
    c. clamps the tube when ambulating the patient.
    d. irrigates the tube with 10-mL sterile saline every 2 to 4 hours.

46. During discharge instructions for a patient following a laparoscopic cholecystectomy, the nursing advises the patient to
    a. keep the incision areas clean and dry for at least a week.
    b. report the need to take pain medication for shoulder pain.
    c. report any bile-colored or purulent drainage from the incisions.
    d. expect some postoperative nausea and vomiting for a few days.

CASE STUDY

Acute Pancreatitis

Patient Profile

V.A. is a 55-year-old man admitted to the hospital with acute pancreatitis.

Subjective Data

- Has severe abdominal pain in the LUQ, radiating to the back
- States he is nauseated and has been vomiting

Objective Data

- Vital signs: Temp 101° F (38.3° C); HR 114; RR 26; BP 92/58
- Jaundice noted in sclera
- Laboratory values
  - Serum amylase 400 U/L (6.67 μkat/L)
  - Urinary amylase 3800 U/day
  - WBC count 20,000/μL
  - Blood glucose 180 mg/dL (10 mmol/L)
  - Serum calcium 7 mg/dL (1.7 mmol/L)

Collaborative Care

- NPO status
- NG tube to low, intermittent suction
- IV therapy with lactated Ringer's solution
- Morphine PCA
- Ranitidine (Zantac) IVPB

Clinical Decision-Making Questions

Using a separate sheet of paper, answer the following questions.

1. Explain the pathophysiology of acute pancreatitis.
2. What are the most common causes of acute pancreatitis?
3. How do the results of V.A.'s laboratory values relate to the pathophysiology of acute pancreatitis?
4. What causes hypocalcemia in acute pancreatitis? How does the nurse assess for hypocalcemia?
5. Describe the characteristics of the pain that occurs in acute pancreatitis.
6. What complications can occur with acute pancreatitis?
7. Identify the purpose of each medication V.A. is taking.
8. Why is V.A. NPO? What is the purpose of the NG tube?
9. *Priority Decision:* Based on the assessment data presented, what are the priority nursing diagnoses? Are there any collaborative problems?

Nursing Assessment:
Urinary System

1. Using the following list of terms, identify the structures in the illustrations below (some of the terms will be used in both illustrations).

Terms

adrenal gland	major calyx	right renal artery
aorta	medulla	right renal vein
bladder	minor calyx	ureter
cortex	papilla	urethra
fibrous capsule	pyramid	vena cava
kidney	renal pelvis	

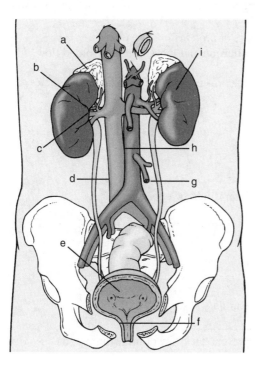

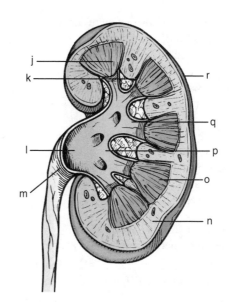

a. _____

b. _____

c. _____

d. _____

e. _____

f. _____

g. _____

h. _____

i. _____

j. _____

k. _____

l. _____

m. _____

n. _____

o. _____

p. _____

q. _____

r. _____

2. Match the following functions with the appropriate site in the nephron (answers may be used more than once).

_____ a. Active reabsorption of Cl⁻ and passive reabsorption of Na⁺

_____ b. Formed from capillary network of afferent arterioles

_____ c. Secretion of H⁺ into filtrate

_____ d. Reabsorption of water without ADH

_____ e. Blood filtered into Bowman's capsule

_____ f. Reabsorption of Na⁺ in exchange for K⁺

_____ g. Reabsorption of most of electrolytes

_____ h. Reabsorption of bicarbonate

_____ i. Reabsorption of Ca⁺⁺ under parathormone influence

_____ j. Reabsorption of glucose and amino acids

_____ k. Reabsorption of water under ADH influence

1. Glomerulus
2. Proximal convoluted tubule
3. Descending loop of Henle
4. Ascending loop of Henle
5. Distal convoluted tubule

3. Identify whether the following statements are true (*T*) or false (*F*). If a statement is false, correct the bold word(s) to make the statement true.

_____ a. Glomerular filtration rate is primarily dependent on adequate **blood flow** and adequate **hydrostatic pressure**.

_____ b. The primary function of the kidney is to **excrete nitrogenous waste products**.

_____ c. **Water** is the primary substance reabsorbed in the collecting duct.

_____ d. Atrial natriuretic factor (ANF) is secreted by the right atrium when atrial blood pressure is low, and it inhibits the action of **aldosterone**.

_____ e. Increased permeability in the **glomerulus** causes loss of proteins into the urine.

_____ f. Prostaglandin synthesis by the kidneys causes **vasodilation** and **increased** renal blood flow.

4. A patient with an obstruction of the renal artery causing renal ischemia exhibits hypertension. One factor that may contribute to the hypertension is
   a. increased renin release.
   b. increased antidiuretic hormone (ADH) secretion.
   c. decreased aldosterone secretion.
   d. increased synthesis and release of prostaglandins.

5. A clinical situation in which the increased release of erythropoietin would be expected is
   a. hypoxemia.
   b. hypotension.
   c. hyperkalemia.
   d. fluid overload.

6. Complete the following statements.
   a. The sites where urinary stones are most likely to obstruct the urinary system are at the

   _____ and the _____.
   b. The ureteral muscle fiber attachments into the bladder help prevent backflow of urine through the

   _____ junction.
   c. The volume of urine in the bladder that usually causes the urge to urinate is _____ mL.
   d. Total bladder capacity ranges from _____ mL to _____ mL.
   e. Absorption or leakage of urine wastes out of the urinary system is prevented by the cellular characteristics of the

   _____.

7. One factor that contributes to an increased incidence of urinary tract infections in women is
   a. the shorter length of the urethra.
   b. the larger capacity of the bladder.
   c. relaxation of pelvic floor muscles.
   d. the tight muscular support at the rhabdosphincter.

8. An age-related change in the kidney that leads to nocturia in an older adult is
   a. decreased renal mass.
   b. decreased detrusor muscle tone.
   c. decreased ability to conserve sodium.
   d. decreased ability to concentrate urine.

9. List one specific finding identified by the nurse during assessment of each of the patient's functional health patterns that indicates a risk factor for urinary problems or a patient response to a urinary disorder.
   a. Health perception–health management
   b. Nutritional-metabolic
   c. Elimination
   d. Activity-exercise
   e. Sleep-rest
   f. Cognitive-perceptual
   g. Self-perception–self-concept
   h. Role-relationship
   i. Sexuality-reproductive
   j. Coping–stress tolerance
   k. Value-belief

10. During physical assessment of the urinary system, the nurse
    a. auscultates the lower abdominal quadrants for fluid sounds.
    b. palpates an empty bladder at the level of the symphysis pubis.
    c. percusses the kidney with a firm blow at the posterior costovertebral angle.
    d. positions the patient prone to palpate the kidneys with a posterior approach.

11. Word Search: Find the words that are described by the clues on the next page. The words may be located horizontally, vertically, or diagonally or may be reversed.

```
A O C B V W K T A B N Y P E X L X D N E
I E L B S X G I G H F E C C O G U Z G K
R P V I B Z R U E H C Y C N E U Q E R F
U T N T G U Z M I N B U G E A Q F K L E
T Q K E Y U A A E C B P H N C T Y R Y P
C D I L U T R N V A T P M I X D I U Y O
O E O X U M I I N F D K N T R P R S I O
N P J R W T A U A G J P N N E D N C E V
V B I L N D R T G Z J N O O T Y N L O H
C A I O A I A F U V D C D C E S A C S V
J X C C A N Z L Q R X E E N N U W D Z D
V N M I C T U R I T I O N I T R V J Y T
I E N U R E S I S E F A U S I I O V I B
J R B C X K Z H T W S U F S O A Q Q C D
S Z S P R R G F I G D G K E N S X S F E
D G W G V P U Y V D R P W R W R H B V N
Y T B A A B Q E G M H Q N T V W F G O J
T T C X C O J O N S S K S S G F T G D G
O Z K D C D A F H N E H V A R G A L P A
G N L P M C B O D U K Q C P X N F Z T G
```

Clues

a. Blood in the urine
b. Scanty urine output
c. Can be caused by sneezing
d. Evacuation of urine
e. Urine containing gas
f. Incontinence during sleep
g. Painful urination
h. No urine formation
i. Frequent urination at night
j. Inability to void
k. Inability to voluntarily control urination
l. Increased incidence of urination
m. Large amount of urine output
n. Difficulty starting urine stream

12. A urinalysis of a urine specimen that is not processed within 1 hour may result in erroneous measurement of
    a. glucose.
    b. bacteria.
    c. specific gravity.
    d. white blood cells.

13. Urinalysis results that most likely indicate a urinary tract infection (UTI) include
    a. yellow, protein: 6 mg/dL; pH: 6.8; 10^2 bacteria.
    b. cloudy, yellow; WBC: >5/hpf; pH: 8.2; numerous casts.
    c. cloudy, brown; ammonia odor; specific gravity: 1.030; RBC: 3/hpf.
    d. clear; colorless; glucose: trace; ketones: trace; osmolality: 500 mOsm/kg (500 mmol/kg).

14. Which of the following urine specific gravity values would indicate to the nurse that the patient is receiving excessive IV fluid therapy?
    a. 1.002
    b. 1.010
    c. 1.025
    d. 1.030

15. After a patient has a renal arteriogram, it is important that the nurse
    a. observe for gross bleeding in the urine.
    b. place the patient in high Fowler's position.
    c. monitor the patient for signs of allergy to the contrast medium.
    d. assess peripheral pulses in the involved leg every 30 to 60 minutes.

16. A patient with an elevated blood urea nitrogen (BUN)
    a. has decreased urea in the urine.
    b. may have nonrenal tissue destruction.
    c. definitely has impaired renal function.
    d. will always have a rise in serum creatinine.

17. The test that is most specific for renal function is the
    a. renal scan.
    b. serum creatinine.
    c. BUN.
    d. creatinine clearance.

18. Identify the kidney function that is impaired in the following lab findings in a patient with kidney disease.
    a. Serum Ca^{2+}: 7.2 mg/dL (1.8 mmol/L)
    b. Hb: 9.6 g/dL (96 g/L)
    c. Serum creatinine: 3.2 mg/dL (283 μmol/L)

19. Following a renal biopsy, it is important that the nurse
    a. offer warm sitz baths to relieve discomfort.
    b. test urine for microscopic bleeding with a dipstick.
    c. expect the patient to experience burning on urination.
    d. monitor the patient for symptoms of a urinary infection.

20. Match the following nursing responsibilities with the appropriate diagnostic test (answers may be used more than once).

    _____ a. Use dipstick and read results with color chart
    _____ b. Ensure informed consent was obtained
    _____ c. Explain that bladder will be filled with water to measure tone and stability
    _____ d. Must start the test with full bladder
    _____ e. May notice salty taste during procedure
    _____ f. Insert catheter immediately after voiding
    _____ g. Clean meatus before voiding
    _____ h. First morning specimen is best
    _____ i. Explain that postprocedure pink urine is normal
    _____ j. Have the patient void, stop, void in container
    _____ k. Discard first specimen at start; include voided specimen 24 hours later
    _____ l. Use sterile container
    _____ m. Assess for iodine sensitivity

    1. Urinalysis
    2. Creatinine clearance
    3. Clean-catch urine specimen
    4. Residual urine
    5. Protein determination
    6. Cystoscopy
    7. Intravenous pyelogram (IVP)
    8. Cystometrogram
    9. Urinary flow study

1. Match the following characteristics with the appropriate classifications of urinary tract infection (UTI).

   _____ a. Occurs in otherwise normal urinary tract
   _____ b. Initially resistant to antibiotics
   _____ c. Exists in presence of obstruction or stones
   _____ d. Infection of kidney, kidney pelvis, or ureter
   _____ e. Infection of bladder and/or urethra
   _____ f. Continuing infection because of development resistance
   _____ g. Reinfection following successful treatment of prior UTI

   1. Upper UTI
   2. Lower UTI
   3. Complicated UTI
   4. Uncomplicated UTI
   5. Recurrent UTI
   6. Unresolved bacteriuria
   7. Bacterial persistence

2. While caring for a 77-year-old woman who has a urinary catheter, the nurse monitors the patient for the development of a UTI. The clinical manifestations the patient is most likely to experience include
   a. cloudy urine and fever.
   b. urethral burning and bloody urine.
   c. vague abdominal pain and disorientation.
   d. suprapubic pain and slight decline in body temperature.

3. A woman with no history of UTIs who is experiencing urgency, frequency, and dysuria comes to the clinic, where a dipstick and microscopic urinalysis indicate a bacteriuria. The nurse anticipates that the patient will
   a. need to have a blood specimen drawn for a complete blood count (CBC) and kidney function tests.
   b. not be treated with medication unless she develops fever, chills, and flank pain.
   c. be requested to obtain a clean-catch midstream urine specimen for culture and sensitivity.
   d. be treated empirically with trimethoprim-sulfamethoxazole (TMP-SMX, Bactrim) for 3 days.

4. A female patient with a UTI has a nursing diagnosis of risk for infection related to lack of knowledge regarding prevention of recurrence. The nurse includes in the teaching plan instructions to
   a. empty the bladder at least 4 times a day.
   b. drink at least 2 quarts of water every day.
   c. wait to urinate until the urge is very intense.
   d. clean the urinary meatus with an antiinfective agent after voiding.

5. Acute pyelonephritis resulting from an ascending infection from the lower urinary tract occurs most often when
   a. the kidney is scarred and fibrotic.
   b. the organism is resistant to antibiotics.
   c. there is a preexisting abnormality of the urinary tract.
   d. the patient does not take all of the antibiotics for treatment of a UTI.

6. The patient with acute pyelonephritis is more likely than the patient with a lower UTI to have a nursing diagnosis of
   a. hyperthermia related to infection.
   b. acute pain related to dysuria and bladder spasms.
   c. impaired urinary elimination related to infection.
   d. risk for infection related to lack of knowledge regarding prevention of recurrence.

7. Identify whether the following statements are true (*T*) or false (*F*). If a statement is false, correct the bold word(s) to make the statement true.
   _____ a. **Acute** pyelonephritis causes progressive destruction of nephrons, resulting in chronic renal insufficiency.
   _____ b. In a patient with acute pyelonephritis, an **IVP** may be performed **after** the infection is resolved to evaluate the urinary system for abnormalities.
   _____ c. Diagnosis of acute pyelonephritis always requires a **urine culture and sensitivity test**.
   _____ d. Following initial treatment of acute pyelonephritis, the patient must have a follow-up **CBC**.
   _____ e. The most common cause of urethritis in men is **sexually transmitted diseases (STDs)**.

8. A patient with suprapubic pain and symptoms of urinary frequency and urgency has two negative urine cultures. One assessment finding that would indicate interstitial cystitis is
   a. residual urine >200 mL.
   b. a large, atonic bladder on urodynamic testing.
   c. a voiding pattern that indicates psychogenic urinary retention.
   d. pain with bladder filling that is transiently relieved by urination.

9. When caring for the patient with interstitial cystitis, the nurse teaches the patient to
   a. avoid foods that make the urine more alkaline.
   b. use high-potency vitamin therapy to decrease the autoimmune effects of the disorder.
   c. always keep a voiding diary to document pain, voiding frequencies, and patterns of nocturia.
   d. use the dietary supplement calcium glycerophosphate (Prelief) to decrease bladder irritation.

10. Glomerulonephritis is characterized by glomerular damage caused by
    a. growth of microorganisms in the glomeruli.
    b. release of bacterial substances toxic to the glomeruli.
    c. hemolysis of RBCs circulating through the glomeruli.
    d. accumulation of immune complexes and complement in the glomeruli.

11. Restriction of dietary protein may be indicated in management of acute poststreptococcal glomerulonephritis (APSGN) when the patient has
    a. hematuria.
    b. proteinuria.
    c. hypertension.
    d. elevated blood urea nitrogen (BUN).

12. The nurse plans care for the patient with APSGN based on the knowledge that
    a. most patients with APSGN recover completely or rapidly improve with conservative management.
    b. chronic glomerulonephritis leading to renal failure is a common sequela to acute glomerulonephritis.
    c. pulmonary hemorrhage may occur as a result of antibodies also attacking the alveolar basement membrane.
    d. a large percentage of patients with APSGN develop rapidly progressive glomerulonephritis resulting in kidney failure.

13. The edema associated with nephrotic syndrome occurs as a result of
    a. hypercoagulability.
    b. hyperalbuminemia.
    c. decreased plasma oncotic pressure.
    d. decreased glomerular filtration rate.

14. An appropriate nursing diagnosis for the patient with nephrotic syndrome is
    a. risk for injury related to decreased clotting function.
    b. risk for impaired skin integrity related to immobility.
    c. risk for infection related to altered immune responses.
    d. imbalanced nutrition: more than body requirements related to high cholesterol intake.

15. Number in sequence the following ascending pathologic changes that occur in the urinary tract in the presence of a bladder outlet obstruction.
    _____ a. Hydronephrosis
    _____ b. Reflux of urine into ureter
    _____ c. Bladder detrusor muscle hypertrophy
    _____ d. Ureteral dilation
    _____ e. Renal atrophy
    _____ f. Trabeculation of muscle cells
    _____ g. Hydroureter
    _____ h. Diverticula formation
    _____ i. Chronic pyelonephritis

16. Crossword Puzzle: Kidneys/Ureter/Bladder/Urethra

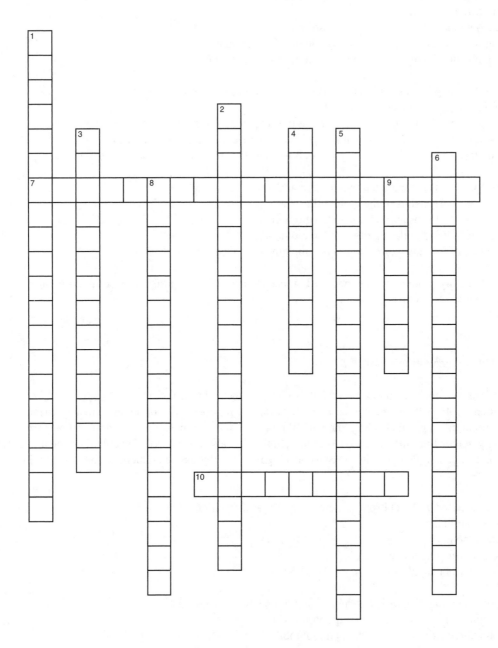

Across

7. Rupture of periurethral gland with tissue regrowth
10. UTI that has spread systemically

Down

1. Urine backup from lower to upper urinary tract
2. Autoimmune disease that may also involve the lungs
3. Inflammation of renal parenchyma and collecting system
4. Inflammation of the urethra
5. Chronic, painful inflammation of the bladder
6. Inflammation of the glomeruli
8. Kidney infiltrated with bacilli 5-8 years after primary infection
9. Inflammation of bladder wall

17. Patients at risk for renal lithiasis can prevent the stones in many cases by
   a. leading an active lifestyle.
   b. limiting protein and acid foods in the diet.
   c. drinking enough fluids to produce a urine output of 2 L/day.
   d. taking prophylactic antibiotics to control UTIs.

18. Match the following characteristics with their associated urinary tract calculi (answers may be used more than once).
   _____ a. More common in women
   _____ b. Genetic autosomal recessive defect
   _____ c. Often mixed with struvite and oxalate stones
   _____ d. Frequently obstruct the ureter
   _____ e. Always associated with UTI
   _____ f. Associated with gout
   _____ g. Defective GI and kidney absorption
   _____ h. Most common type of stone
   _____ i. Often staghorn formation in kidney pelvis
   _____ j. High incidence in Jewish men
   _____ k. Associated with alkaline urine

   1. Calcium oxalate
   2. Calcium phosphate
   3. Struvite
   4. Uric acid
   5. Cystine

19. On assessment of the patient with a renal calculus passing down the ureter, the nurse would expect the patient to report
   a. dull, costovertebral flank pain.
   b. a history of chronic UTIs.
   c. severe, colicky back pain radiating to the groin.
   d. a feeling of bladder fullness with urgency and frequency.

20. Prevention of calcium oxalate stones would include dietary restriction of
   a. milk and milk products.
   b. dried beans and dried fruits.
   c. liver, kidney, and sweetbreads.
   d. spinach, cabbage, and tomatoes.

21. Following lithotripsy for treatment of renal calculi, the patient has a nursing diagnosis of risk for infection related to the introduction of bacteria following manipulation of the urinary tract. An appropriate nursing intervention for the patient is to
   a. monitor for hematuria.
   b. encourage high fluid intake.
   c. apply moist heat to the flank area.
   d. strain all urine through gauze or a special strainer.

22. Identify whether the following statements are true (*T*) or false (*F*). If a statement is false, correct the bold word(s) to make the statement true.
   _____ a. Kidney injury should be suspected when a patient suffering a sports injury has **gross hematuria**.
   _____ b. Benign and accelerated nephrosclerosis cause necrosis of the renal parenchyma and are treated with **anticoagulants**.
   _____ c. The most common manifestations of renal artery stenosis include flank pain and **hematuria**.
   _____ d. Renal vein thrombosis is most commonly treated with **surgical revascularization**.
   _____ e. Patients with urethral strictures may be taught to dilate the urethra by **self-catheterization** every few days.

23. In providing care for the patient with adult-onset polycystic kidney disease, the nurse
   a. helps the patient cope with the rapid progression of the disease.
   b. suggests genetic counseling resources for the children of the patient.
   c. expects the patient to have polyuria and poor concentration ability of the kidneys.
   d. implements appropriate measures for the patient's deafness and blindness in addition to the renal problems.

24. Match the following metabolic and connective tissue diseases with the pathologic renal changes that occur in the diseases.

    _____ a. Diabetes mellitus
    _____ b. Gout
    _____ c. Amyloidosis
    _____ d. Systemic lupus erythematosus
    _____ e. Systemic sclerosis

    1. Connective tissue changes affecting the glomerulus
    2. Diffuse and nodular glomerulosclerosis
    3. Deposition of sodium urate crystals in interstitium and tubules
    4. Vascular lesions with fibrosis
    5. Deposition of hyaline substance in kidney

25. When obtaining a nursing history from a patient with cancer of the urinary system, the nurse recognizes that a risk factor associated with cancer of both the kidney and the bladder is
    a. smoking.
    b. a family history of cancer.
    c. chronic use of phenacetin.
    d. chronic, recurrent nephrolithiasis.

26. Thirty percent of patients with kidney cancer have metastasis at the time of diagnosis. This occurs because
    a. the only treatment modalities for the disease are palliative.
    b. diagnostic tests are not available to detect tumors before they metastasize.
    c. the classic symptoms of hematuria and palpable mass do not occur until the disease is advanced.
    d. early metastasis to the brain impairs the patient's ability to recognize the seriousness of symptoms.

27. A 60-year-old man with cancer of the bladder has laser photocoagulation for treatment of the tumor. Following the procedure, the nurse plans to
    a. assess the patient for symptoms of cystitis.
    b. encourage the patient to use warm sitz baths.
    c. monitor the patient for irritative bladder symptoms.
    d. monitor urine output from the urinary catheter for hematuria.

28. Match the following characteristics with their associated types of urinary incontinence (answers may be used more than once).

    _____ a. Caused by overactivity of the detrusor muscle
    _____ b. Found following prostatectomy
    _____ c. Treated with Kegel exercises
    _____ d. Occurs with spinal cord lesions above S2
    _____ e. Involuntary urination with minimal warning
    _____ f. Common in postmenopausal women
    _____ g. Loss of urine caused by problems of mobility
    _____ h. Caused by outlet obstruction
    _____ i. Occurs without warning or stress equally during day and night
    _____ j. Bladder contracts by reflex, overriding central inhibition
    _____ k. Leakage of urine from overfull bladder
    _____ l. Involuntary urination with increased intraabdominal pressure

    1. Stress incontinence
    2. Urge incontinence
    3. Overflow incontinence
    4. Reflex incontinence
    5. Functional incontinence

29. Indicate the type of incontinence the following drugs are used to treat and the rationale for their use.
    a. Anticholinergic drugs
    b. α-Adrenergic blockers

30. To assist the patient with stress incontinence, the nurse teaches the patient to
    a. void every 2 hours to prevent leakage.
    b. use absorptive perineal pads to contain urine.
    c. perform pelvic floor muscle exercises 40 to 50 times per day.
    d. increase intraabdominal pressure during voiding to empty the bladder completely.

31. Nursing care that applies to the management of all urinary catheters in hospitalized patients includes
    a. measuring urine output every 1 to 2 hours to ensure patency.
    b. turning the patient frequently from side to side to promote drainage.
    c. using strict sterile technique during irrigation and obtaining culture specimens.
    d. daily cleaning of the catheter insertion site with soap and water and application of an antimicrobial ointment.

32. A patient has a right ureteral catheter placed following a lithotripsy for a stone in the ureter. In caring for the patient after the procedure, the nurse
    a. milks or strips the catheter every 2 hours.
    b. measures ureteral urinary drainage every 1 to 2 hours.
    c. irrigates catheter with 30-mL sterile saline every 4 hours.
    d. encourages ambulation to promote urinary peristaltic action.

33. During assessment of the patient who has a nephrectomy, the nurse would expect to find
    a. shallow, slow respirations.
    b. clear breath sounds in all lung fields.
    c. decreased breath sounds in the lower left lobe.
    d. decreased breath sounds in the right and left lower lobes.

34. Match the following urinary diversions with their descriptions.
    _____ a. Ileal conduit   1. Continent diversion created by formation of ileal pouch with stoma
    _____ b. Cutaneous ureterostomy   requiring catheterization
    _____ c. Kock pouch   2. Abdominal stoma formed from resected ileum into which ureters are
    _____ d. Orthotopic neobladder   implanted
                                  3. Stoma created from ureter(s) brought to abdominal wall
                                  4. Section of bowel reshaped and connected to ureters and urethra

35. A patient with bladder cancer undergoes cystectomy with formation of an ileal conduit. During the patient's first postoperative day, the nurse plans to
    a. measure and fit the stoma for a permanent appliance.
    b. encourage high oral intake to flush mucus from the conduit.
    c. teach the patient to self-catheterize the stoma every 4 to 6 hours.
    d. empty the drainage bag every 2 to 3 hours and measure the urinary output.

36. A teaching plan developed by the nurse for the patient with a new ileal conduit includes instructions to
    a. clean the skin around the stoma with alcohol every day.
    b. use a wick to keep the skin dry during appliance changes.
    c. use sterile supplies and technique during care of the stoma.
    d. change the appliance every day and wash it with soap and warm water.

37. ***Delegation Decision:*** Indicate which of the listed nursing interventions may be delegated to nursing assistive personnel (NAP) (select all that apply).
    a. Assess for need for catheterization.
    b. Provide perineal care with soap and water around a urinary catheter.
    c. Teach patient pelvic floor (Kegel) muscle exercises.
    d. Insert indwelling catheter for uncomplicated patient.
    e. Use bladder scanner to estimate residual urine.
    f. Assist incontinent patient to commode at regular intervals.
    g. Determine the type of incontinence the patient is experiencing.

CASE STUDY
Bladder Cancer
Patient Profile

P.G. is a 55-year-old mechanic who has been healthy all his life until he passed some blood in his urine and saw a urologist at his wife's insistence. A urine specimen for cytology revealed atypical cells, and a diagnosis of bladder cancer was made following a cystoscopy with biopsy of bladder tissue. Intravesical therapy with Bacille-Calmette-Guérin (BCG) is planned.

Subjective Data

- Has smoked a pack of cigarettes a day since he was a teenager
- Says he dreads having the chemotherapy because he has heard cancer drugs cause such severe side effects

Objective Data

- Cystoscopy and biopsy results: Moderately differentiated Jewett-Strong-Marshall stage A tumor on the left lateral bladder wall, with $T_2N_0M_0$ pathologic stage; fulguration performed during cystoscopy
- Continues to have gross hematuria

Clinical Decision-Making Questions

Using a separate sheet of paper, answer the following questions.

1. What does staging of bladder tumors indicate?
2. What information and instructions would the nurse provide for P.G. about his intravesical therapy?
3. How can P.G. help to prevent future bladder tumors from occurring?
4. How should the nurse explain the importance of follow-up cystoscopies?
5. What surgery might be indicated if the chemotherapy is not effective?
6. *Priority Decision:* Based on the assessment data presented, what are the priority nursing diagnoses? Are there any collaborative problems?

CHAPTER
47

Nursing Management: Acute Kidney Injury and Chronic Kidney Disease

1. Match the following conditions and characteristics with their associated etiologies of acute kidney injury (AKI) (answers may be used more than once).

_____ a. Decreased cardiac output
_____ b. Mechanical outflow obstruction
_____ c. Initial cause of most acute renal failure
_____ d. Prostate cancer
_____ e. Tubular obstruction by myoglobin
_____ f. Hypovolemia
_____ g. Renal stones
_____ h. Nephrotoxic drugs
_____ i. Bladder cancer
_____ j. Renal vascular obstruction
_____ k. Acute glomerulonephritis
_____ l. Anaphylaxis

1. Prerenal
2. Intrarenal
3. Postrenal

2. Complete the following statements related to acute tubular necrosis.
   a. Acute tubular necrosis is a type of acute kidney injury that results primarily from _____
      and _____.
   b. Renal ischemia leads to acute tubular necrosis by disrupting the _____ and causing
      patchy destruction of the _____
   c. Nephrotoxic agents cause necrosis of the _____ that sloughs off and blocks the
      _____.
   d. Acute tubular necrosis from nephrotoxic injury is more likely to be reversible if the _____
      is not initially destroyed.

3. AKI is staged using the acronym RIFLE. What do the initials stand for (what stage)?

                                    Stage
   R
   I
   F
   L
   E

4. The nurse determines that a patient with oliguria has prerenal oliguria when
   a. urine testing reveals a low specific gravity.
   b. the causative factor is malignant hypertension.
   c. urine testing reveals a high sodium concentration.
   d. reversal of the oliguria occurs with fluid replacement.

5. Tubular damage is indicated in the patient with AKI by a urinalysis finding of
   a. hematuria.
   b. specific gravity fixed at 1.010.
   c. urine sodium of 12 mEq/L (12 mmol/L).
   d. osmolality of 1000 mOsm/kg (1000 mmol/kg).

6. Metabolic acidosis occurs in the oliguric phase of AKI as a result of impaired
   a. ammonia synthesis.
   b. excretion of sodium.
   c. excretion of bicarbonate.
   d. conservation of potassium.

7. The nurse determines that a patient with AKI is in the recovery phase when the patient experiences
   a. a return to normal weight.
   b. a urine output of 3700 mL/day.
   c. decreasing blood urea nitrogen (BUN) and creatinine levels.
   d. decreasing sodium and potassium levels.

8. While caring for the patient in the oliguric phase of AKI, the nurse monitors the patient for associated collaborative problems, notifying the health care provider when
   a. urine output is 300 mL/day.
   b. edema occurs in the feet, legs, and sacral area.
   c. the cardiac monitor reveals a depressed T wave and a sagging ST segment.
   d. the patient experiences increasing muscle weakness and abdominal cramping.

9. Identify whether the following statements are true (*T*) or false (*F*). If a statement is false, correct the bold word(s) to make the statement true.
   _____ a. The most common cause of death in AKI is **irreversible metabolic acidosis**.
   _____ b. Serum **urea** is increased during catabolism of body protein.
   _____ c. During the oliguric phase of AKI, daily fluid intake is limited to **1000** mL plus the prior day's measurable fluid loss.
   _____ d. **Dietary sodium and potassium** during the oliguric phase of AKI are managed according to the patient's urinary output.
   _____ e. One of the most important nursing measures in managing fluid balance in the patient with AKI is taking **accurate daily weights**.

10. A 68-year-old man with a history of heart failure resulting from hypertension has AKI as a result of the effects of nephrotoxic diuretics. Currently his serum potassium is 6.2 mEq/L (6.2 mmol/L) with cardiac changes, his BUN is 108 mg/dL (38.6 mmol/L), his creatinine is 4.1 mg/dL (362 µmol/L), and his serum HCO_3^- is 14 mEq/L (14 mmol/L). He is somnolent and disoriented. What three criteria for treatment with renal replacement therapy does he meet?

    a.

    b.

    c.

11. Prevention of AKI is important because of the high mortality rate. Which of the patients below are at risk (select all that apply)?
    a. an 86-year-old female scheduled for a cardiac catheterization
    b. a 48-year-old male with multiple injuries from a motor vehicle accident
    c. a 64-year-old female with chronic heart failure admitted with bloody stools
    d. a 32-year-old female following abruptio placentae and a C-section delivery
    e. a 58-year-old male with prostate cancer undergoing preoperative workup for prostatectomy

12. *Priority Decision:* A patient on a medical unit has a potassium level of K$^+$ 6.8 mEq/L. The priority action for the nurse would be
    a. check the patient's blood pressure (BP).
    b. place the patient on a cardiac monitor.
    c. instruct the patient to avoid high potassium foods.
    d. call the lab and request a redraw of the lab to verify results.

13. A patient with AKI has a serum potassium level of 6.7 mEq/L (6.7 mmol/L) and the following arterial blood gas results: pH 7.28, $PaCO_2$ 30 mm Hg, PaO_2 86 mm Hg, HCO_3^- 18 mEq/L (18 mmol/L). The nurse recognizes that treatment of the acid-base problem with sodium bicarbonate would cause a decrease in the
    a. pH.
    b. potassium level.
    c. bicarbonate level.
    d. carbon dioxide level.

14. In replying to a patient's questions about the seriousness of her chronic kidney disease (CKD), the nurse knows that the stage of CKD is based on the
    a. total daily urine output.
    b. glomerular filtration rate.
    c. serum creatinine and urea levels.
    d. degree of altered mental status.

15. List two clinical manifestations for each body system and their pathophysiologic causes that can be noted by the nurse when performing physical assessment of the following systems on the patient with CKD.

	Findings	Cause
a. Skin		
b. Cardiovascular		
c. Respiratory		
d. GI		
e. Neurologic		

16. List the alterations that occur in at least 10 serum laboratory values in CKD.

    a.

    b.

    c.

    d.

    e.

    f.

    g.

    h.

    i.

    j.

17. The nurse identifies a nursing diagnosis of risk for injury: fracture related to alterations in calcium and phosphorus metabolism for a patient with CKD. The pathologic process directly related to the risk for fractures is
    a. loss of aluminum through the impaired kidneys.
    b. deposition of calcium phosphate in soft tissues of the body.
    c. impaired vitamin D activation resulting in decreased GI absorption of calcium.
    d. increased release of parathyroid hormone in response to decreased calcium levels.

18. The most appropriate snack for the nurse to offer the patient with CKD is
    a. raisins.
    b. ice cream.
    c. dill pickles.
    d. hard candy.

19. Match the following drugs with their use in CKD (answers may be used more than once).
    _____ a. Erythropoietin
    _____ b. IV glucose and insulin
    _____ c. nifedipine (Procardia)
    _____ d. sevelamer (Renagel)
    _____ e. sodium polystyrene sulfonate (Kayexalate)
    _____ f. cinacalcet (Sensipar)
    _____ g. furosemide (Lasix)
    _____ h. calcium acetate (PhosLo)
    _____ i. IV 10% calcium gluconate

    1. Treatment of hyperkalemia
    2. Treatment of mineral and bone disorder
    3. Treatment of anemia
    4. Treatment of hypertension

20. Identify whether the following statements are true (*T*) or false (*F*). If a statement is false, correct the bold word(s) to make the statement true.
    _____ a. A nutrient that is commonly supplemented for the patient on dialysis because it is dialyzable is **iron**.
    _____ b. The syndrome that includes all the signs and symptoms seen in the various body systems in CKD is **azotemia**.
    _____ c. The use of calcium-based phosphate binders in the patient with CKD is contraindicated when serum **calcium** levels are increased.
    _____ d. The use of **morphine** is contraindicated in the patient with CKD because accumulation of its metabolites may cause seizures.

21. During the nursing assessment of the patient with renal insufficiency, the nurse asks the patient specifically about a history of
    a. angina.
    b. asthma.
    c. hypertension.
    d. rheumatoid arthritis.

22. The patient with end-stage renal disease tells the nurse that she hates the thought of being tied to the machine but is glad to start dialysis because she will be able to eat and drink what she wants. Based on this information, the nurse identifies the nursing diagnosis of
    a. self-esteem disturbance related to dependence on dialysis.
    b. anxiety related to perceived threat to health status and role functioning.
    c. ineffective self-health management related to lack of knowledge of treatment plan.
    d. risk for imbalanced nutrition: more than body requirements related to increased dietary intake.

23. Indicate whether the following characteristics are associated with peritoneal dialysis (PD) or hemodialysis (HD).
    _____ a. Requires vascular access
    _____ b. Increased hyperlipidemia
    _____ c. Lowers serum triglycerides
    _____ d. Portable system
    _____ e. Less cardiovascular stress
    _____ f. More protein loss
    _____ g. Intensifies anemia
    _____ h. Rapid fluid and creatinine loss
    _____ i. Requires fewer dietary restrictions

24. The dialysate for PD contains
    a. electrolytes in an equal concentration to that of the blood.
    b. calcium in a lower concentration than in the blood.
    c. sodium in a higher concentration than in the blood.
    d. dextrose in a higher concentration than in the blood.

25. Complete the following statements.
    a. An exchange in PD includes the phases of _____, _____, and _____.
    b. The amount of peritoneal dialysate used for one exchange for an average individual is _____ liter(s).
    c. The patient using _____ PD usually dialyzes during sleep and leaves the fluid in the abdomen during the day.

26. To prevent the most common serious complication of PD, it is important for the nurse to
    a. infuse the dialysate slowly.
    b. use strict aseptic technique in the dialysis procedures.
    c. have the patient empty the bowel before the inflow phase.
    d. reposition the patient frequently and promote deep breathing.

27. Match the characteristics with the type of vascular access sites (answers may be used more than once).
    _____ a. 2 to 4 weeks required for healing
    _____ b. Least likely to thrombose
    _____ c. Usually used for access for continuous renal replacement therapy
    _____ d. May lead to distal ischemia
    _____ e. Most prone to infection
    _____ f. 4 to 6 weeks required for healing

    1. Temporary catheters
    2. Native AV fistula
    3. Arteriovenous (AV) graft

28. A patient on hemodialysis develops a thrombus of a subcutaneous AV graft requiring its removal. While waiting for a replacement graft or fistula, the patient is most likely to have
    a. peritoneal dialysis.
    b. a percutaneous jugular vein cannula.
    c. a percutaneous femoral vein cannula.
    d. a Silastic catheter tunneled subcutaneously to the jugular vein.

29. A patient with end-stage renal failure is scheduled for hemodialysis following healing of an AV fistula. The nurse explains that during dialysis
    a. he will be able to visit, read, sleep, or watch TV while reclining in a chair.
    b. he will be placed on a cardiac monitor to detect any adverse effects that might occur.
    c. the dialyzer will remove and hold part of his blood for 20 to 30 minutes to remove the waste products.
    d. a large catheter with two lumens will be inserted into the fistula to send blood to and return it from the dialyzer.

30. The nurse evaluates the patency of an AV graft by
    a. palpating for pulses distal to the graft site.
    b. auscultating for the presence of a bruit at the site.
    c. evaluating the color and temperature of the extremity.
    d. assessing for the presence of numbness and tingling distal to the site.

31. A patient with AKI is a candidate for continuous renal replacement therapy (CRRT). The most common indication for use of CRRT is
    a. azotemia.
    b. pericarditis.
    c. hyperkalemia.
    d. fluid overload.

32. A patient rapidly progressing toward end-stage renal disease asks about the possibility of a kidney transplant. In responding to the patient, the nurse knows that contraindications to kidney transplantation include
    a. hepatitis C infection.
    b. coronary artery disease.
    c. refractory hypertension.
    d. extensive vascular disease.

33. During the immediate postoperative care of the recipient of a kidney transplant, the nurse expects to
    a. regulate fluid intake hourly based on urine output.
    b. find urine-tinged drainage on the abdominal dressing.
    c. medicate the patient frequently for incisional flank pain.
    d. remove the urinary catheter to evaluate the ureteral implant.

34. Infection is a significant cause of morbidity and mortality in kidney transplant patients. List at least three reasons for this.

    1.

    2.

    3.

CASE STUDY
Kidney Transplant
Patient Profile

D.B. had end-stage renal disease resulting from hypertension. She underwent hemodialysis for 2 years and then received a cadaveric renal transplant 1 year ago. She had one episode of acute rejection 3 months after transplant. Her baseline creatinine has been 1.2 to 1.3 mg/dL (106-115 mmol/L). She came to the clinic complaining of decreased urinary output, fever, and tenderness at the transplant site. She is admitted to the hospital for a kidney biopsy.

Subjective Data

• Tells the nurse if she loses this kidney, she does not think she can stand to go back on dialysis

Objective Data

• Laboratory test findings
  • Serum creatinine: 3.0 mg/dL (265 μmol/L)
  • BUN: 70 mg/dL (25 mmol/L)
  • Glucose: 404 mg/dL (22.4 mmol/L)
  • K^+: 5.1 mEq/L (5.1 mmol/L)
  • HCO_3^-: 18 mEq/L (18 mmol/L)
• Blood pressure: 150/90 mm Hg

Collaborative Care

• Muromonab-CD3 (Orthoclone OKT3) therapy initiated for 10 days
• Mycophenolate mofetil (CellCept)
• Methylprednisolone (Solu-Medrol)
• Furosemide (Lasix)
• Nifedipine (Procardia)
• Sodium bicarbonate
• Tacrolimus (Prograf)
• Insulin

Clinical Decision-Making Questions

Using a separate sheet of paper, answer the following questions.

1. Explain the physiology of acute rejection.
2. Identify the abnormal diagnostic study results and why each would occur. What significance do the abnormal results have for nursing care?
3. Explain the rationale for D.B.'s collaborative care. How does each immunosuppressive medication work? (See Chapter 14.)
4. What clinical manifestations may develop as a result of immunosuppressive therapy? What nursing care is indicated?
5. Explain the long-term problems of a patient with a kidney transplant.
6. *Priority Decision:* Based on the assessment data presented, what are the priority nursing diagnoses? Are there any collaborative problems?

Nursing Assessment: Endocrine System

1. Identify the glands in the following illustration.

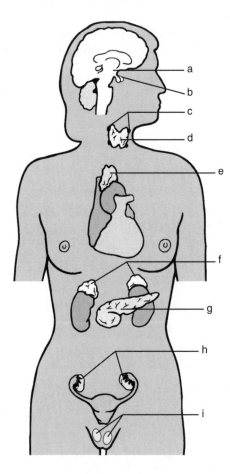

a. _____   f. _____

b. _____   g. _____

c. _____   h. _____

d. _____   i. _____

e. _____

2. Match the following hormones with their secretory gland (answers may be used more than once).

_____ a. Thyroxin (T$_4$)
_____ b. Cortisol
_____ c. Glucagon
_____ d. Prolactin
_____ e. Progesterone
_____ f. Growth hormone (GH)
_____ g. Triiodothyronine (T$_3$)
_____ h. Melanocyte-stimulating hormone
_____ i. Insulin
_____ j. Thyroid-stimulating hormone (TSH)
_____ k. Calcitonin
_____ l. Gonadotropic hormones
_____ m. Somatostatin
_____ n. Epinephrine/norepinephrine
_____ o. Adrenocorticotropic hormone (ACTH)
_____ p. Antidiuretic hormone (ADH)
_____ q. Parathormone

1. Anterior pituitary
2. Posterior pituitary
3. Thyroid
4. Parathyroid
5. β-Cells of islets of Langerhans
6. α-Cells of islets of Langerhans
7. δ-Cells of islets of Langerhans
8. Adrenal cortex
9. Adrenal medulla
10. Ovaries

3. Identify whether the following statements are true (*T*) or false (*F*). If a statement is false, correct the bold word(s) to make the statement true.

_____ a. Overproduction of the **adrenal cortex** may cause masculinization in women.
_____ b. Two hormones that have all cells as target tissue include **GH** and **TSH**.
_____ c. Epinephrine and norepinephrine are considered **hormones** when they are secreted by the adrenal medulla and are considered **neurotransmitters** when they are secreted by nerve cells.
_____ d. In a person who normally works a night shift from 11:00 PM to 7:00 AM and sleeps from 8:00 AM to 3:00 PM, a serum analysis of cortisol taken at 7:30 AM would reveal a **false-high** cortisol level.
_____ e. An example of a complex negative feedback system is the regulation of **insulin**.
_____ f. Hormones that act on the anterior pituitary gland to stimulate tropic hormone secretion are known as **releasing hormones**.
_____ g. Endocrine glands that have negative feedback systems to the hypothalamus include the **pancreas** and the **parathyroid gland**.
_____ h. **Androgens** secreted by the adrenal cortex are responsible for the sex drive in women.
_____ i. The mechanism for the action of **protein hormones** is binding to receptors inside the cell.

4. Match each hormone with the primary factor that stimulates its secretion and the primary factor that inhibits its secretion (factors may be used more than once).

Stimulate	Inhibit	Hormone	Primary Factor
_____	_____	a. TSH or thyrotropin	1. Increased stress
_____	_____	b. Corticotropin-releasing hormone	2. Increased serum thyroxin
_____	_____	c. ADH	3. Decreased serum T$_3$
_____	_____	d. Follicle-stimulating hormone (FSH)	4. Increased serum cortisol
_____	_____	e. Calcitonin	5. Increased serum estrogen
_____	_____	f. Aldosterone	6. Decreased serum estrogen
_____	_____	g. Glucagon	7. Increased serum glucose
_____	_____	h. Parathyroid hormone (PTH)	8. Decreased serum glucose
_____	_____	i. Insulin	9. Increased serum calcium
			10. Decreased serum calcium
			11. Decreased arterial blood pressure (BP)
			12. Increased arterial BP
			13. Increased plasma osmolality
			14. Decreased plasma osmolality

5. The normal response to increased serum osmolality is the release of
   a. aldosterone from the adrenal cortex, which stimulates sodium excretion by the kidney.
   b. ADH from the posterior pituitary gland, which stimulates the kidney to reabsorb water.
   c. mineralocorticoids from the adrenal gland, which stimulate the kidney to excrete potassium.
   d. calcitonin from the thyroid gland, which increases bone resorption and decreases serum calcium levels.

6. That hormones of one gland influence the function of hormones of another gland is demonstrated by the fact that
   a. increased insulin levels inhibit the secretion of glucagon.
   b. increased testosterone levels inhibit the release of estrogen.
   c. increased cortisol levels stimulate the secretion of insulin.
   d. increased atrial natriuretic peptide (ANP) levels inhibit the secretion of aldosterone.

7. Following the ingestion of a high-protein, carbohydrate-free meal
   a. both insulin and glucagon are inhibited because blood glucose levels are unchanged.
   b. insulin is released to facilitate the breakdown of amino acids into glucose, and glucagon is inhibited.
   c. insulin is inhibited by low glucose levels and glucagon is released to promote gluconeogenesis.
   d. glucagon is released to promote gluconeogenesis and insulin is released to facilitate movement of amino acids into muscle cells.

8. Two effects of hypokalemia on the endocrine system are
   a. decreased insulin and aldosterone release.
   b. decreased glucagon and increased cortisol release.
   c. decreased release of atrial natriuretic factor and increased ADH release.
   d. decreased release of parathyroid hormone and increased calcitonin release.

9. Identify one specific finding identified by the nurse during assessment of each of the patient's functional health patterns that indicates a risk factor for endocrine problems or a patient response to an actual endocrine problem.
   a. Health perception–health management
   b. Nutritional-metabolic
   c. Elimination
   d. Activity-exercise
   e. Sleep-rest
   f. Cognitive-perceptual
   g. Self-perception–self-concept
   h. Role-relationship
   i. Sexuality-reproductive
   j. Coping–stress tolerance
   k. Value-belief

10. In a patient with an elevated serum cortisol, the nurse would expect other laboratory findings to reveal
    a. hypokalemia.
    b. hyponatremia.
    c. hypoglycemia.
    d. decreased serum triglycerides.

11. Manifestations of endocrine problems in the older adult that are commonly attributed to the aging process are
    a. tremors and paresthesias.
    b. fatigue and mental impairment.
    c. fluid retention and hypertension.
    d. hyperpigmentation and oily skin.

12. Common nonspecific manifestations that may alert the nurse to endocrine dysfunction include
    a. goiter and alopecia.
    b. exophthalmos and tremors.
    c. weight loss, fatigue, and depression.
    d. polyuria, polydipsia, and polyphagia.

13. A potential adverse effect of palpation of an enlarged thyroid gland is
    a. carotid artery obstruction.
    b. damage to the cricoid cartilage.
    c. release of excessive thyroid hormone into circulation.
    d. hoarseness from pressure on the recurrent laryngeal nerve.

14. Complete the following sentences related to abnormal assessment findings of the endocrine system.
    a. Tetanic muscle spasms are associated with hypofunction of the _____ gland.
    b. Hyperpigmentation is associated with hypofunction of the _____ gland.
    c. Exophthalmos is associated with excessive secretion of the _____ gland.
    d. Moon face is associated with _____ secretion of the adrenal gland.
    e. A goiter is associated with either hyperfunction or hypofunction of the _____ gland.
    f. An increase in hand and foot size is associated with excessive secretion of _____ hormone.
    g. Striae are associated with excessive secretion of the _____ gland.
    h. Heat intolerance is associated with _____ secretion of the thyroid gland.

15. A patient has a low serum T_3 level, and the health care provider orders measurement of the TSH level. If the TSH level is elevated, this indicates that
    a. the cause of the low T_3 level is most likely primary hypothyroidism.
    b. the negative feedback system is failing to stimulate the anterior pituitary gland.
    c. the patient has an underactive thyroid gland that is not receiving TSH stimulation.
    d. there is most likely a tumor of the anterior pituitary gland that is causing increased production of TSH.

16. To ensure accurate results of a fasting blood glucose analysis, the nurse has the patient fast for at least
    a. 2 hours.
    b. 4 hours.
    c. 8 hours.
    d. 12 hours.

17. Match the following diagnostic studies with the descriptions:
    _____ a. Oral glucose tolerance test
    _____ b. Total calcium
    _____ c. Serum phosphate
    _____ d. 17-ketosteroids
    _____ e. ACTH stimulation test
    _____ f. Glycosylated hemoglobin (Hb)
    _____ g. Water deprivation test
    _____ h. ACTH (dexamethasone) suppression test

    1. Increased level may indicate primary hyperparathyroidism
    2. Normal response is decreased cortisol
    3. Normal response is increased plasma cortisol
    4. Used to diagnose diabetes mellitus
    5. Decreased level indicates hyperparathyroidism
    6. Differentiates causes of polyuria
    7. Evaluates glucose control over time
    8. Evaluates adrenocortical and gonadal function

1. In addition to promoting the transport of glucose from the blood into the cell, insulin also
   a. enhances the breakdown of adipose tissue for energy.
   b. stimulates hepatic glycogenolysis and gluconeogenesis.
   c. prevents the transport of triglycerides into adipose tissue.
   d. accelerates the transport of amino acids into cells and their synthesis into protein.

2. Complete the following statements.
   a. Tissues that require insulin for glucose transport are _____ and _____ tissues.
   b. In type 1 diabetes, the body's own _____ cells are attacked and destroyed.
   c. Four hormones released that are counter-regulatory to insulin are _____, _____, _____ and _____.
   d. The type of diabetes that is strongly related to human leukocyte antigen (HLA) types is _____.

3. Indicate whether the following mechanisms of diabetes mellitus are characteristic of the pathophysiology of type 1 (1) or type 2 (2) diabetes.
   _____ a. Insulin resistance
   _____ b. β-cell secretory exhaustion
   _____ c. Inherited defect in insulin receptors
   _____ d. Immune mediated
   _____ e. Genetic predisposition
   _____ f. Inappropriate glucose production by the liver
   _____ g. β-cell destruction
   _____ h. Altered production of adipokines
   _____ i. Compensatory increased insulin production
   _____ j. Exposure to a virus

4. Describe the process that occurs to cause the following classic diabetes symptoms.
   a. Polyuria
   b. Polydipsia
   c. Polyphagia

5. Which of the following patients would a nurse plan to teach how to prevent or delay the development of diabetes?
   a. A 62-year-old obese white man.
   b. An obese 50-year-old Hispanic woman.
   c. A child whose father has type 1 diabetes.
   d. A 34-year-old woman whose parents both have type 2 diabetes.

6. *Priority Decision:* When caring for a patient with metabolic syndrome, the nurse gives the highest priority to teaching the patient about
   a. maintaining a normal weight.
   b. performing daily aerobic exercise.
   c. eliminating red meat from the diet.
   d. monitoring the blood glucose periodically.

7. During routine health screening, a patient is found to have a fasting plasma glucose (FPG) of 132 mg/dL (7.33 mmol/L). At a follow-up visit, a diagnosis of diabetes would be made based on (select all that apply)
   a. glucosuria of 3+.
   b. an A1C of 7.5%.
   c. a FPG of ≥126 mg/dL (6.9 mmol/L).
   d. random blood glucose of 126 mg/dL (7.0 mmol/L).
   e. a 2-hour oral glucose tolerance test (OGTT) of 190 mg/dL (10.5 mmol/L).

8. The nurse determines that a patient with a 2-hour OGTT of 152 mg/dL has
   a. diabetes.
   b. impaired fasting glucose.
   c. impaired glucose tolerance.
   d. elevated glycosylated hemoglobin (Hb).

9. When teaching the patient with diabetes about insulin administration, the nurse instructs the patient to
   a. pull back on the plunger after inserting the needle to check for blood.
   b. clean the skin at the injection site with an alcohol swab before each injection.
   c. consistently use the same size of the appropriate strength insulin syringe to avoid dosing errors.
   d. rotate injection sites from arms to thighs to abdomen with each injection to prevent lipodystrophies.

10. A patient with type 1 diabetes uses 20 U of 70/30 neutral protamine Hagedorn (NPH/regular) in the morning and at 6:00 PM. When teaching the patient about this regimen, the nurse stresses that
    a. hypoglycemia is most likely to occur before the noon meal.
    b. a set meal pattern with a bedtime snack is necessary to prevent hypoglycemia.
    c. flexibility in food intake is possible because insulin is available 24 hours/day.
    d. pre-meal glucose checks are required to determine needed changes in daily dosing.

11. Lispro insulin (Humalog) with NPH insulin is ordered for a patient with newly diagnosed type 1 diabetes. The nurse knows that when lispro insulin is used, it should be administered
    a. only once a day.
    b. 1 hour before meals.
    c. 30 to 45 minutes before meals.
    d. at mealtime or within 15 minutes of meals.

12. A diabetic patient is learning to mix regular insulin and NPH insulin in the same syringe. The nurse determines that additional teaching is needed when the patient
    a. withdraws the NPH dose into the syringe first.
    b. injects air equal to the NPH dose into the NPH vial first.
    c. removes any air bubbles after withdrawing the first insulin.
    d. adds air equal to the insulin dose into the regular vial and withdraws the dose.

13. *Delegation Decision:* The following interventions are planned for a diabetic patient. Which intervention can the nurse delegate to nursing assistive personnel (NAP)?
    a. Discuss complications of diabetes.
    b. Check that the bath water is not too hot.
    c. Check the patient's technique for drawing up insulin.
    d. Teach the patient to use the glucometer for in-home glucose monitoring

14. The home care nurse should intervene to correct a patient whose insulin administration includes
    a. warming a prefilled refrigerated syringe in the hands before administration.
    b. storing syringes prefilled with NPH and regular insulin needle-up in the refrigerator.
    c. placing the insulin bottle currently in use in a small container on the bathroom countertop.
    d. mixing an evening dose of regular insulin with insulin glargine in one syringe for administration.

15. The major advantage of using an insulin pump is that
    a. tight glycemic control can be maintained.
    b. errors in insulin dosing are less likely to occur.
    c. complications of insulin therapy are prevented.
    d. frequent blood glucose monitoring is unnecessary.

16. A patient taking insulin has recorded fasting glucose levels above 200 mg/dL (11.1 mmol/L) on awakening for the last five mornings. The nurse advises the patient to
    a. increase the evening insulin dose to prevent the dawn phenomenon.
    b. use a single-dose insulin regimen with an intermediate-acting insulin.
    c. monitor the glucose level at bedtime, between 2:00 and 4:00 AM, and on arising.
    d. decrease the evening insulin dosage to prevent night hypoglycemia and the Somogyi effect.

17. Match the following oral glucose-lowering agents with their descriptions (answers may be used more than once).
    _____ a. Decreases endogenous glucose production
    _____ b. Should be taken within 30 minutes of each meal
    _____ c. Decreases glycogenolysis
    _____ d. Enhance cell sensitivity to insulin
    _____ e. Rapid- and short-acting release of insulin from the pancreas
    _____ f. Delays glucose absorption from the gastrointestinal (GI) tract
    _____ g. Stimulates production and release of insulin and enhances cellular sensitivity to insulin
    _____ h. Increases glucose uptake, especially in muscles
    _____ i. Primary effect is decreased glucose production by liver
    _____ j. Effectiveness measured by 2-hour postprandial glucose
    _____ k. Taken with the first bite of each meal
    _____ l. Not used in patients with heart failure

    1. Sulfonylurea
    2. Meglitinide
    3. Biguanide
    4. α-Glucosidase inhibitor
    5. Thiazolidinediones

18. *Priority Decision:* The nurse is assessing a newly admitted diabetic patient. Which of these observations should be addressed as a priority by the nurse?
    a. Bilateral numbness of both hands
    b. Stage II pressure ulcer on the right heel
    c. Rapid respirations with deep inspiration
    d. Areas of lumps and dents on the abdomen

19. In nutritional management of all types of diabetes, it is important for the patient to
    a. eat regular meals at regular times.
    b. restrict calories to promote moderate weight loss.
    c. eliminate sucrose and other simple sugars from the diet.
    d. limit saturated fat intake to 30% of dietary calorie intake.

20. Goals of nutritional therapy for the patient with type 2 diabetes include maintenance of
    a. ideal body weight.
    b. normal serum glucose and lipid levels.
    c. a special diabetic diet using dietetic foods.
    d. five small meals per day with a bedtime snack.

21. To prevent hyperglycemia or hypoglycemia with exercise, the nurse teaches the patient using glucose-lowering agents that exercise should be undertaken
    a. only after a 10- to 15-g carbohydrate snack is eaten.
    b. about 1 hour after eating, when blood glucose levels are rising.
    c. when glucose monitoring reveals that the blood glucose is in the normal range.
    d. when blood glucose levels are high because exercise always has a hypoglycemic effect.

22. The nurse assesses the diabetic patient's technique of self-monitoring of blood glucose (SMBG) 3 months after initial instruction. An error in the performance of SMBG noted by the nurse that requires intervention is
    a. doing the SMBG before and after exercising.
    b. puncturing the finger on the side of the finger pad.
    c. cleaning the puncture site with alcohol before the puncture.
    d. holding the hand down for a few minutes before the puncture.

23. A nurse working in an outpatient clinic plans a screening program for diabetes. Recommendations for screening would include
    a. OGTT for all minority populations every year.
    b. FPG for all individuals at age 45 and then every 3 years.
    c. testing all people under the age of 21 for islet cell antibodies.
    d. testing for type 2 diabetes only in overweight or obese individuals.

24. A patient with diabetes calls the clinic because she is experiencing nausea and flulike symptoms. The nurse advises the patient to
    a. administer the usual insulin dosage.
    b. hold fluid intake until the nausea subsides.
    c. come to the clinic immediately for evaluation and treatment.
    d. monitor the blood glucose every 1 to 2 hours and call if the glucose rises over 150 mg/dL (8.3 mmol/L).

25. Ketoacidosis occurs as a complication of diabetes when
    a. illnesses causing nausea and vomiting lead to bicarbonate loss with body fluids.
    b. the glucose level becomes so high that osmotic diuresis promotes fluid and electrolyte loss.
    c. an insulin deficit causes the body to metabolize large amounts of fatty acids rather than glucose for energy.
    d. the patient skips meals after taking insulin, leading to rapid metabolism of glucose and breakdown of fats for energy.

26. List five signs and symptoms that are present in diabetic ketoacidosis (DKA) that are not seen in hyperglycemic hyperosmolar syndrome (HHS).

    a.

    b.

    c.

    d.

    e.

27. The treatment for DKA and HHS differs primarily in that
    a. DKA requires administration of bicarbonate to correct acidosis.
    b. potassium replacement is not necessary in management of HHS.
    c. HHS requires greater fluid replacement to correct the dehydration.
    d. administration of glucose is withheld in HHS until the blood glucose reaches a normal level.

28. Indicate whether the following characteristics are associated with hypoglycemia (1), hyperglycemia (2), or both (3).
    _____ a. Slurred speech and irritability
    _____ b. Headache
    _____ c. Nausea and vomiting
    _____ d. Too much exercise without food
    _____ e. Increased dietary intake
    _____ f. Cold, clammy skin
    _____ g. Precipitated by stress
    _____ h. Changes in vision

29. A diabetic patient is found unconscious at home, and a family member calls the clinic. After determining that no glucometer is available, the nurse advises the family member to
    a. try to arouse the patient to drink some orange juice.
    b. administer 10 U of regular insulin subcutaneously.
    c. call for an ambulance to transport the patient to a medical facility.
    d. administer glucagon 1 mg intramuscularly (IM) or subcutaneously.

30. Two days following a self-managed hypoglycemic episode at home, the patient tells the nurse that his blood glucose levels since the episode have been between 80 and 90 mg/dL. The best response by the nurse is,
    a. "That is a good range for your glucose levels."
    b. "You should call your health care provider because you need to have your insulin increased."
    c. "That level is too low in view of your recent hypoglycemia, and you should increase your food intake."
    d. "You should only take half your insulin dosage for the next few days to get your glucose level back to normal."

31. In diabetes, atherosclerotic disease affecting the cerebrovascular, cardiovascular, and peripheral vascular systems
    a. can be prevented by tight glucose control.
    b. occurs with a higher frequency and earlier onset than in the nondiabetic population.
    c. is caused by the hyperinsulinemia related to insulin resistance common in type 2 diabetes.
    d. cannot be modified by reduction of risk factors such as smoking, obesity, and high fat intake.

32. Match the following characteristics as they relate to complications of diabetes (answers may be used more than once).
    _____ a. Male impotence
    _____ b. Damage to small vessels that supply the renal glomeruli.
    _____ c. Related to altered lipid metabolism of diabetes
    _____ d. Microaneurysms and destruction of retinal capillaries
    _____ e. Atrophy of small muscles of the hands and feet
    _____ f. Capillary and arteriole membrane thickening specific to diabetes
    _____ g. Pain and paresthesia of the legs
    _____ h. Ulceration and amputation of the lower extremities
    _____ i. Foot ulcers without patient feeling pain
    _____ j. Delayed gastric emptying
    _____ k. Ischemic heart disease
    _____ l. Painless myocardial infarction

    1. Microvascular
    2. Macrovascular
    3. Autonomic neuropathy
    4. Sensory neuropathy

33. Following the teaching of foot care to a diabetic patient, the nurse determines that additional instruction is needed when the patient says,
    a. "I should wash my feet daily with soap and warm water."
    b. "I should always wear shoes to protect my feet from injury."
    c. "If my feet are cold, I should wear socks instead of using a heating pad."
    d. "I'll know if I have sores or lesions on my feet because they will be painful."

34. A 72-year-old woman is diagnosed with diabetes. The nurse recognizes that management of diabetes in the older adult
    a. does not require as tight glucose control as in younger diabetics.
    b. is usually not treated unless the patient becomes severely hyperglycemic.
    c. does not include treatment with insulin because of limited dexterity and vision.
    d. usually requires that a younger family member be responsible for care of the patient.

CASE STUDY

Hypoglycemia

Patient Profile

F.W., a 24-year-old with type 1 diabetes, was brought to the first aid tent provided for participants in a charity marathon. She is well maintained on a regimen of self-monitoring of blood glucose, insulin, and diet.

Subjective Data

- States that she feels cold, she has a headache, and her fingers feel numb
- She took her usual insulin dose this morning but was unable to eat her entire breakfast because of a lack of time
- Completed the entire marathon in a personal-best time

Objective Data

- Has slurred speech and unsteady gait
- Pulse: 120 beats/min
- Appears confused
- Capillary blood glucose level: 48 mg/dL (2.7 mmol/L)

Clinical Decision-Making Questions

Using a separate sheet of paper, answer the following questions.

1. Describe what F.W. could have done to prevent this hypoglycemic event.
2. What is the etiology of the signs and symptoms displayed by F.W.?
3. How would you expect to treat F.W.'s hypoglycemia?
4. *Priority Decision:* What are the priority teaching needs for this patient once her condition has stabilized?
5. What adjustments in her diabetic regimen could F.W. make to allow her to continue with her exercise habits?
6. *Priority Decision:* Based on the assessment data presented, what are the priority nursing diagnoses? Are there any collaborative problems?

CHAPTER 50

Nursing Management: Endocrine Problems

1. A patient suspected of having acromegaly has an elevated plasma growth hormone (GH) level. In acromegaly, the nurse would also expect the patient's diagnostic results to include
   a. hyperinsulinemia.
   b. a plasma glucose of <70 mg/dL (3.9 mmol/L).
   c. decreased GH levels with an oral glucose challenge test.
   d. elevated levels of serum somatomedin C (insulin-like growth factor-1 [IGF-1]).

2. During assessment of the patient with acromegaly, the nurse would expect the patient to report
   a. infertility.
   b. dry, irritated skin.
   c. undesirable changes in appearance.
   d. an increase in height of 2 to 3 inches a year.

3. A patient with acromegaly is treated with a transsphenoidal hypophysectomy. Postoperatively the nurse
   a. ensures that any clear nasal drainage is tested for glucose.
   b. maintains the patient flat in bed to prevent cerebrospinal fluid (CSF) leakage.
   c. assists the patient with toothbrushing every 4 hours to keep the surgical area clean.
   d. encourages deep breathing, coughing, and turning to prevent respiratory complications.

4. Identify whether the following statements are true (*T*) or false (*F*). If a statement is false, correct the bold word(s) to make the statement true.
   _____ a. Octreotide (Sandostatin) is a **dopamine agonist** in primary treatment of acromegaly to **block the action** of GH.
   _____ b. A patient with diabetes mellitus who undergoes a hypophysectomy will require a **larger** dose of insulin than preoperatively.
   _____ c. Pituitary tumors causing either hyperpituitarism or hypopituitarism may cause **visual changes** and **disturbances**.
   _____ d. Early hypofunction of the pituitary gland usually results in nonspecific symptoms primarily because there are no obvious manifestations of **growth hormone** deficiencies in adults.

5. Identify five hormones that are replaced when panhypopituitarism results from radiation therapy or total hypophysectomy as treatment for pituitary tumors.
   a.

   b.

   c.

   d.

   e.

6. In the following diagram of the pathophysiology of ADH problems, indicate in the appropriate blanks whether the processes are increased (↑) or decreased (↓) in syndrome of inappropriate ADH (SIADH) and diabetes insipidus (DI).

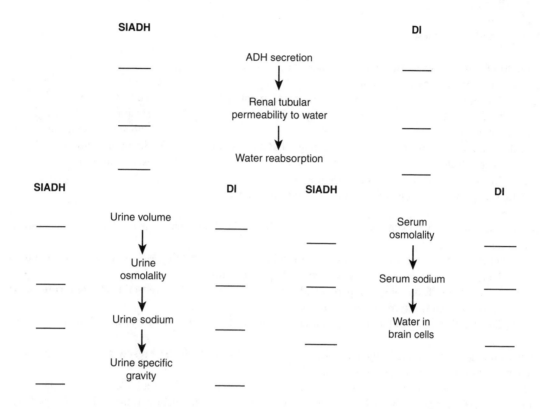

7. During care of the patient with SIADH, the nurse should
   a. monitor neurologic status at least every 2 hours.
   b. keep the head of the bed elevated to prevent ADH release.
   c. teach the patient receiving treatment with diuretics to restrict sodium intake.
   d. notify the health care provider if the patient's blood pressure (BP) decreases more than 20 mm Hg from baseline.

8. A patient with SIADH is treated with water restriction and administration of IV fluids. The nurse evaluates that treatment has been effective when the patient experiences
   a. increased urine output, decreased serum sodium, and increased urine specific gravity.
   b. increased urine output, increased serum sodium, and decreased urine specific gravity.
   c. decreased urine output, increased serum sodium, and decreased urine specific gravity.
   d. decreased urine output, decreased serum sodium, and increased urine specific gravity.

9. In a patient with central diabetes insipidus, administration of ADH during a water deprivation test will result in a(n)
   a. decrease in body weight.
   b. increase in urinary output.
   c. decrease in blood pressure.
   d. increase in urine osmolality.

10. A patient with diabetes insipidus is treated with nasal desmopressin (DDAVP). The nurse determines that the drug is not having an adequate therapeutic effect when the patient experiences
    a. headache and weight gain.
    b. nasal irritation and nausea.
    c. a urine specific gravity of 1.002.
    d. an oral intake greater than urinary output.

11. When caring for a patient with nephrogenic diabetes insipidus, the nurse would expect treatment to include
    a. fluid restriction.
    b. thiazide diuretics.
    c. a high-sodium diet.
    d. chlorpropamide (Diabinese).

12. Match the following characteristics with their related disorders.
    _____ a. Viral-induced hyperthyroidism
    _____ b. Autoimmune fibrous and lymphocytic replacement of thyroid gland
    _____ c. Enlarged thyroid gland
    _____ d. Lymphocytic infiltration of thyroid gland that may occur postpartum
    _____ e. Bacterial or fungal infection of thyroid gland
    _____ f. Malignant or benign deformity of the thyroid gland

    1. Goiter
    2. Thyroid nodules
    3. Hashimoto's thyroiditis
    4. Subacute granulomatous thyroiditis
    5. Silent thyroiditis
    6. Acute thyroiditis

13. Identify whether the following statements are true (*T*) or false (*F*). If a statement is false, correct the bold word(s) to make the statement true.
    _____ a. The two most common forms of hyperthyroidism are **Graves' disease** and **toxic nodular goiters**.
    _____ b. Exophthalmos may occur in **any form of hyperthyroidism**.
    _____ c. Clinical manifestations of hyperthyroidism occur as a result of **increased metabolic rate** and **tissue sensitivity to the sympathetic nervous system**.
    _____ d. Diagnostic testing in the patient with Graves' disease will reveal an **increased TSH level**.

14. A patient with Graves' disease asks the nurse what caused the disorder. The best response by the nurse is,
    a. "The cause of Graves' disease is not known, although it is thought to be genetic."
    b. "It is usually associated with goiter formation from an iodine deficiency over a long period of time."
    c. "Antibodies develop against thyroid tissue and destroy it, causing a deficiency of thyroid hormones."
    d. "In genetically susceptible persons, antibodies are formed that cause excessive thyroid hormone secretion."

15. A patient is admitted to the hospital in thyrotoxic crisis. On physical assessment of the patient, the nurse would expect to find
    a. hoarseness and laryngeal stridor.
    b. bulging eyeballs and dysrhythmias.
    c. elevated temperature and signs of heart failure.
    d. lethargy progressing suddenly to impairment of consciousness.

16. Match the following characteristics and rationales for the uses of the drugs used in treatment of hyperthyroidism (answers may be used more than once).
    _____ a. Treatment of choice in nonpregnant adults
    _____ b. Decreases release of thyroid hormones
    _____ c. Often used with iodine to produce euthyroid before surgery
    _____ d. Used to decrease size and vascularity of thyroid gland preoperatively
    _____ e. Used to control sympathetic symptoms
    _____ f. Blocks peripheral conversion of T_4 to T_3
    _____ g. Decreases thyroid secretion by damaging thyroid gland
    _____ h. Often causes hypothyroidism over time

    1. Propylthiouracil (PTU)
    2. Potassium iodide
    3. Propranolol (Inderal)
    4. Radioactive iodine (^{131}I)

17. Identify one nursing diagnosis that is appropriate for the patient with the following manifestations of hyperthyroidism.
    a. Exophthalmos
    b. Weight loss and hunger
    c. Hair loss and vitiligo
    d. Exhaustion and dyspnea

18. Preoperative instructions for the patient scheduled for a subtotal thyroidectomy include teaching the patient
    a. how to support the head with the hands when moving.
    b. that coughing should be avoided to prevent pressure on the incision.
    c. that the head and neck will need to remain immobile until the incision heals.
    d. that any tingling around the lips or in the fingers after surgery is expected and temporary.

19. Identify the rationale for having the following items immediately available in the patient's room following a thyroidectomy.
    a. Tracheostomy tray
    b. Calcium salts for IV administration
    c. Oxygen equipment

20. When providing discharge instructions to a patient following a subtotal thyroidectomy, the nurse advises the patient to
    a. never miss a daily dose of thyroid replacement therapy.
    b. avoid regular exercise until thyroid function is normalized.
    c. use warm saltwater gargles several times a day to relieve throat pain.
    d. reduce caloric intake by at least half the amount taken before surgery.

21. Causes of primary hypothyroidism in adults include
    a. malignant or benign thyroid nodules.
    b. surgical removal or failure of the pituitary gland.
    c. surgical removal or radiation of the thyroid gland.
    d. autoimmune-induced atrophy of the thyroid gland.

22. The nurse has identified the following nursing diagnoses for a patient who is hypothyroid. For each nursing diagnosis, identify an appropriate etiology for the diagnosis and at least two common signs or symptoms of hypothyroidism that support the diagnosis.
    a. Disturbed sleep pattern related to _____ as manifested by _____ and _____.
    b. Imbalanced nutrition: more than body requirements related to _____ as manifested by _____ and _____.
    c. Disturbed thought processes related to _____ as manifested by _____ and _____.
    d. Activity intolerance related to _____ as manifested by _____ and _____.

23. When replacement therapy is started for a patient with long-standing hypothyroidism, it is most important for the nurse to monitor the patient for
    a. insomnia.
    b. weight loss.
    c. nervousness.
    d. dysrhythmias.

24. A patient with hypothyroidism is treated with levothyroxin (Synthroid). When teaching the patient about the therapy, the nurse
    a. explains that alternate-day dosage may be used if side effects occur.
    b. provides written instruction for all information related to the medication therapy.
    c. assures the patient that a return to normal function will occur with replacement therapy.
    d. informs the patient that medications must be taken until hormone balance is reestablished.

25. Indicate whether the following clinical manifestations are characteristic of hyperparathyroidism (1) or hypoparathyroidism (2).
    _____ a. Decreased bone density
    _____ b. Muscle spasms and stiffness
    _____ c. Psychomotor retardation
    _____ d. Calcium nephrolithiasis
    _____ e. Personality changes
    _____ f. Decreased contractility of myocardium
    _____ g. Dry, scaly skin
    _____ h. Skeletal pain
    _____ i. Abdominal cramping
    _____ j. Cardiac dysrhythmias

26. An appropriate nursing intervention for the patient with hyperparathyroidism is to
    a. pad side rails as a seizure precaution.
    b. increase fluid intake to 3000 to 4000 mL daily.
    c. maintain bed rest to prevent pathologic fractures.
    d. monitor the patient for Trousseau's phenomenon and Chvostek's sign.

27. When the patient with parathyroid disease experiences symptoms of hypocalcemia, a measure that can be used to raise serum calcium levels temporarily is to
    a. administer IV normal saline.
    b. have the patient rebreathe in a paper bag.
    c. administer furosemide (Lasix) as ordered.
    d. administer oral phosphorus supplements.

28. A patient with hypoparathyroidism resulting from surgical treatment of hyperparathyroidism is preparing for discharge. The nurse teaches the patient that
    a. milk and milk products should be increased in the diet.
    b. parenteral replacement of parathyroid hormone (PTH) will be required for life.
    c. calcium supplements with vitamin D can effectively maintain calcium balance.
    d. bran and whole-grain foods should be used to prevent GI effects of replacement therapy.

29. A patient is admitted to the hospital with a diagnosis of Cushing syndrome. On physical assessment of the patient, the nurse would expect to find
    a. hypertension, peripheral edema, and petechiae.
    b. weight loss, buffalo hump, and moon face with acne.
    c. abdominal and buttock striae, truncal obesity, and hypotension.
    d. anorexia, signs of dehydration, and hyperpigmentation of the skin.

30. A patient is scheduled for a bilateral adrenalectomy. During the postoperative period, the nurse would expect administration of corticosteroids to be
    a. reduced to promote wound healing.
    b. withheld until symptoms of hypocortisolism appear.
    c. increased to promote an adequate response to the stress of surgery.
    d. reduced because excessive hormones are released during surgical manipulation of the glands.

31. A patient with Addison's disease comes to the emergency department with complaints of nausea, vomiting, diarrhea, and fever. The nurse would expect collaborative care to include
    a. parenteral injections of adrenocorticotropic hormone (ACTH).
    b. IV administration of vasopressors.
    c. IV administration of hydrocortisone.
    d. IV administration of D_5W with 20 mEq KCl.

32. During discharge teaching for the patient with Addison's disease, the nurse identifies a need for additional instruction when the patient says,
    a. "I should always call the doctor if I develop vomiting or diarrhea."
    b. "If my weight goes down, my dosage of steroid is probably too high."
    c. "I should double or triple my steroid dose if I undergo rigorous physical exercise."
    d. "I need to carry an emergency kit with injectable hydrocortisone in case I can't take my medication by mouth."

33. A patient who is on corticosteroid therapy for treatment of an autoimmune disorder has the following additional drugs ordered. How is the need for these drugs related to the effects of corticosteroids?
    a. Furosemide (Lasix)
    b. Pantoprazole (Protonix)
    c. Alendronate (Fosamax)
    d. Insulin
    e. Potassium

34. A patient with mild iatrogenic Cushing syndrome is on an alternate-day regimen of corticosteroid therapy. The nurse explains to the patient that this regimen
    a. maintains normal adrenal hormone balance.
    b. prevents ACTH release from the pituitary gland.
    c. minimizes hypothalamic-pituitary-adrenal suppression.
    d. provides a more effective therapeutic effect of the drug.

35. When caring for a patient with primary hyperaldosteronism, the nurse would question a health care provider's order for the use of
    a. furosemide (Lasix).
    b. amiloride (Midamor).
    c. spironolactone (Aldactone).
    d. aminoglutethimide (Cytadren).

36. *Priority Decision:* The priority nursing intervention during the management of the patient with a pheochromocytoma is
    a. administering IV fluids.
    b. monitoring blood pressure.
    c. administering β-adrenergic blocking agents.
    d. monitoring intake and output (I&O) and daily weights.

CASE STUDY
Cushing Syndrome
Patient Profile

T.H. is a 26-year-old elementary school teacher. He seeks the advice of his health care provider because of changes in his appearance over the past year.

Subjective Data

- Reports weight gain (particularly through his midsection), easy bruising, and edema of his feet, lower legs, and hands
- Has been having increasing insomnia

Objective Data

- Physical examination: BP 150/110; 2+ edema of lower extremities; purplish striae on abdomen; thin extremities with thin, friable skin; severe acne of the face and neck
- Blood analysis: Glucose 167 mg/dL (9.3 mmol/L); white blood cell (WBC) count 13,600/μL; lymphocytes 12%; red blood cell (RBC) count 6.6×10^6 μL; K^+ 3.2 mEq/L (3.2 mmol/L)

Clinical Decision-Making Questions

Using a separate sheet of paper, answer the following questions.

1. Discuss the probable causes of the alterations in T.H.'s blood values.
2. Explain the pathophysiology of Cushing syndrome.
3. What diagnostic testing would identify the cause of T.H.'s Cushing syndrome?
4. What is the usual treatment of Cushing syndrome?
5. What is meant by a "medical adrenalectomy"?
6. *Priority Decision:* What are the priority nursing responsibilities in the care of this patient?
7. *Priority Decision:* Based on the assessment data presented, what are the priority nursing diagnoses? Are there any collaborative problems?

Nursing Assessment: Reproductive System

1. Identify the structures in the following illustrations by filling in the blanks on the next page with the correct answers from the list of terms below (some terms will be used in both illustrations).

Terms

anus
bladder
body of uterus
cervix
Cowper's gland
ductus deferens
ejaculatory duct
epididymis
fallopian tube

fornix of vagina
fundus of uterus
glans
ovary
penis
prostate gland
rectum
round ligament
scrotum

seminal vesicle
symphysis pubis
testis
ureter
ureterosacral ligament
urethra
vagina
vaginal introitus

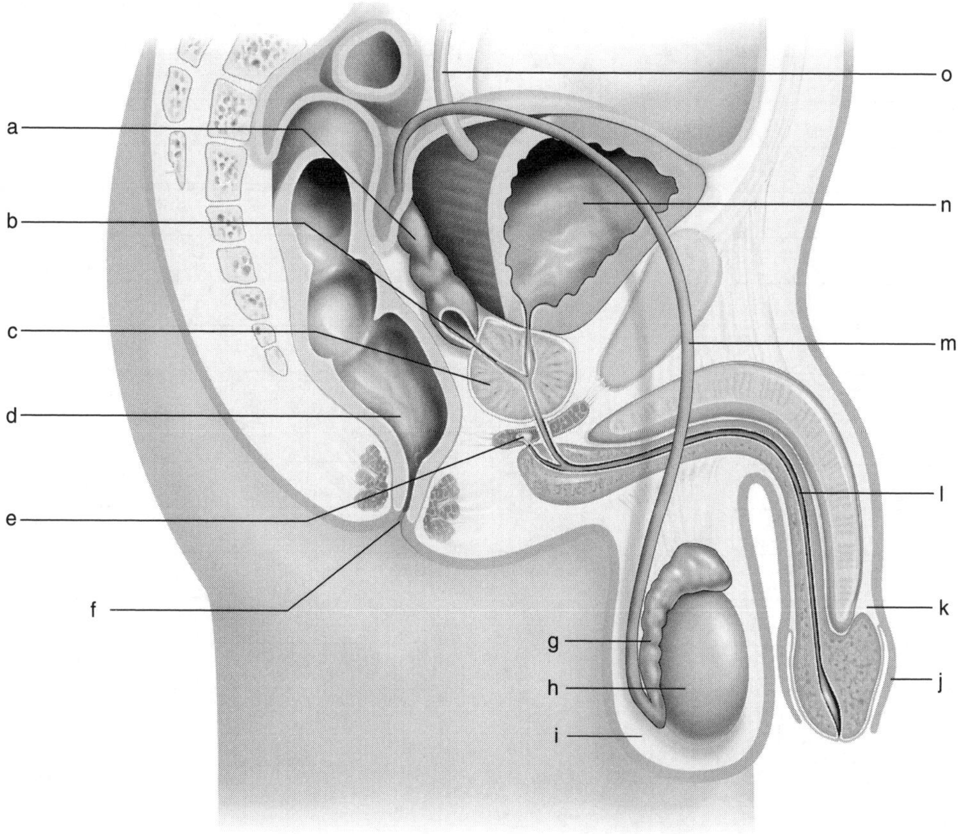

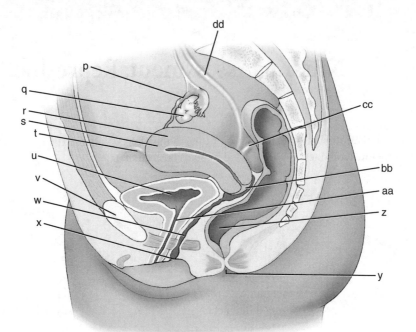

a. _____   p. _____

b. _____   q. _____

c. _____   r. _____

d. _____   s. _____

e. _____   t. _____

f. _____   u. _____

g. _____   v. _____

h. _____   w. _____

i. _____   x. _____

j. _____   y. _____

k. _____   z. _____

l. _____   aa. _____

m. _____   bb. _____

n. _____   cc. _____

o. _____   dd. _____

2. Using the list of terms below, identify the structures in the following illustrations.

Terms

alveoli

anus

areola

clitoris

labia majora

labia minora

mons pubis

nipple

pectoralis major muscle

perineum

prepuce

urethra

vaginal introitus

vestibule

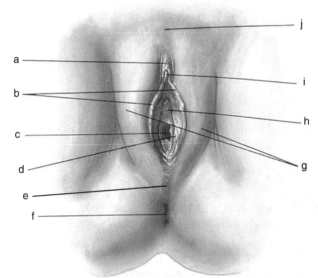

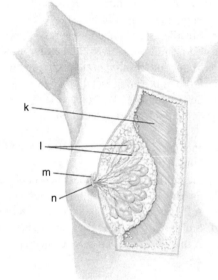

a. _____

b. _____

c. _____

d. _____

e. _____

f. _____

g. _____

h. _____

i. _____

j. _____

k. _____

l. _____

m. _____

n. _____

3. Number in sequence from 1 to 8 the passage of sperm through, and the formation of semen in, the structures of the male reproductive system.
   _____ a. Ductus deferens
   _____ b. Urethra
   _____ c. Epididymis
   _____ d. Prostate gland
   _____ e. Seminiferous tubules
   _____ f. Cowper's glands
   _____ g. Seminal vesicles
   _____ h. Ejaculatory duct

4. Match the following descriptions with the structures of the female breast.
   _____ a. Pigmented center of breast
   _____ b. Erectile tissue containing pores
   _____ c. Carry milk from alveoli to lactiferous sinuses
   _____ d. Major composition of nonlactating breast
   _____ e. Store milk during lactation
   _____ f. Sebaceous-like gland on areola
   _____ g. Secrete milk during lactation

   1. Alveoli
   2. Montgomery's tubercles
   3. Lactiferous sinuses
   4. Areola
   5. Ducts
   6. Adipose tissue
   7. Nipple

5. Identify whether the following statements are true (*T*) or false (*F*). If a statement is false, correct the bold word(s) to make the statement true.
   _____ a. The normal process of destruction of oocytes throughout the female life span is known as **atresia**.
   _____ b. Fertilization of an ovum by a sperm occurs in the **uterus**.
   _____ c. A Pap smear should include cells from the **ectocervix**.
   _____ d. Mobility of sperm into the uterus is promoted by **thin, watery cervical mucus** at the time of ovulation.
   _____ e. A middle-aged woman is considered to be in menopause when she has not had a menstrual period for **2 years**.

6. Match the descriptions with the reproductive hormones (answers may be used more than once).
   _____ a. Called interstitial cell–stimulating hormone (ICSH) in men
   _____ b. Stimulated by elevated estrogen levels
   _____ c. Produced by testes
   _____ d. Elevated at onset of menopause
   _____ e. Stimulates growth and maturity of ovarian follicles
   _____ f. Stimulates testosterone production
   _____ g. Required for female sex characteristics
   _____ h. Needed for growth of mammary glands
   _____ i. Needed for male sex characteristics
   _____ j. Increased by decreased testosterone levels
   _____ k. Responsible for ovarian follicle maturation
   _____ l. Responsible for spermatogenesis
   _____ m. Maintains implanted egg
   _____ n. Completes follicle maturation

   1. FSH
   2. Luteinizing hormone (LH)
   3. Prolactin
   4. Estrogen
   5. Progesterone
   6. Testosterone
   7. ICSH
   8. Gonadotropin-releasing hormone (GnRH)

7. A 72-year-old man asks the nurse whether it is normal for him to become impotent at his age. The best response by the nurse includes the information that
   a. most decreased sexual function in older adults is due to psychologic stress.
   b. physiologic changes of aging may require increased stimulation for an erection to occur.
   c. although the penis decreases in size in older men, there should be no change in sexual function.
   d. benign changes in the prostate gland that occur with aging can cause a decreased ability to attain an erection.

8. List one problem associated with each of the following that may be identified during assessment of the reproductive system.
   a. Rubella
   b. Mumps
   c. Diabetes mellitus
   d. Antihypertensive agents

9. A 58-year-old man has difficulty starting a urinary stream, and benign prostatic hyperplasia (BPH) is suspected. Assessment of the patient for the presence of BPH involves
   a. palpation of the scrotum and testes for a mass.
   b. palpating the base of the penis for enlargement.
   c. palpating the inguinal ring while the patient bears down.
   d. a digital rectal examination to palpate the prostate gland.

10. When assessing an aging adult man, the nurse notes as normal the finding of
   a. decreased penis size.
   b. decreased pubic hair.
   c. a decrease in scrotal color.
   d. unilateral breast enlargement.

11. Identify one specific finding identified by the nurse during assessment of each of the patient's functional health patterns that indicates a risk factor for reproductive problems or a patient response to an actual reproductive problem.
   a. Health perception–health management
   b. Nutritional-metabolic
   c. Elimination
   d. Activity-exercise
   e. Sleep-rest
   f. Cognitive-perceptual
   g. Self-perception–self-concept
   h. Role-relationship
   i. Sexuality-reproductive
   j. Coping–stress tolerance
   k. Value-belief

12. During examination of the breast, the nurse establishes the presence of nipple and skin retraction by
   a. compressing the nipple.
   b. lying the patient supine with her hand above and behind her head.
   c. systematically palpating the breast tissue in a circular or spoke pattern.
   d. asking the patient to lift her hands above her head and then press her hands on her hips while seated.

13. During examination of the female reproductive system, the nurse would note as abnormal the finding of
   a. clear vaginal discharge.
   b. perineal episiotomy scars.
   c. nonpalpable Skene's ducts.
   d. reddened base of the vulva.

14. Match the following laboratory tests with their purpose.
   _____ a. Urine human chorionic gonadotropin (hCG)
   _____ b. Serum estradiol
   _____ c. Serum FSH
   _____ d. Venereal Disease Research Laboratory (VDRL)
   _____ e. Fluorescent treponemal antibody absorption (FTAAbs)
   _____ f. Urine FSH assay
   _____ g. Rapid plasma reagin (RPR)
   _____ h. Gram stain
   _____ i. Prostate-specific antigen (PSA)

   1. Identifies secondary gonadal failure
   2. Used for rapid diagnosis of gonorrhea
   3. Specific antibody test for syphilis
   4. Measures ovarian function
   5. Quick nonspecific antibody test for syphilis
   6. Detects pregnancy
   7. Used to detect prostate cancer
   8. Nonspecific antibody test for syphilis screening
   9. Used to validate menopause

Copyright © 2011, 2007, 2004, 2000, 1996, 1992 by Mosby, Inc., an affiliate of Elsevier Inc. All rights reserved.

15. Following a dilation and curettage (D&C), it is important for the nurse to assess the patient for the complication of
    a. infection.
    b. hemorrhage.
    c. urinary retention.
    d. perforation of the bladder.

16. Diagnostic tests of the reproductive system that are operative procedures requiring surgical anesthesia include
    a. culdoscopy and conization.
    b. colposcopy and breast biopsy.
    c. laparoscopy and endometrial biopsy.
    d. dilation with curettage and contrast mammography.

17. The fertility test that requires the couple to have sexual intercourse at the time of ovulation and come for testing 2 to 8 hours after intercourse is the
    a. Huhner's test.
    b. semen analysis.
    c. endometrial biopsy.
    d. hysterosalpingogram.

CHAPTER 52

Nursing Management: Breast Disorders

1. A woman at the health clinic tells the nurse she does not do breast self-examination (BSE) because it just seems too much of a bother. The best response by the nurse is that BSE
   a. reduces mortality from breast cancer in women under the age of 50.
   b. is useful to help women learn how their breasts normally look and feel.
   c. has little value in detection of cancer and is not recommended anymore.
   d. is the most common way that malignant tumors of the breast are discovered.

2. Identify the four screening guidelines for breast cancer accepted by organizations involved with breast cancer.
   a.

   b.

   c.

   d.

3. When teaching a 24-year-old woman who desires to learn breast self-examination (BSE), the nurse knows it is important to
   a. provide time for a return demonstration.
   b. emphasize the statistics related to breast cancer survival and mortality.
   c. have the woman set a consistent monthly date for performing the examination.
   d. inform the woman that professional examinations are not necessary unless she finds an abnormality.

4. The diagnostic test that is most accurate and advantageous in terms of time and expense in diagnosing malignant breast disorders is
   a. mammography.
   b. open surgical biopsy.
   c. fine-needle aspiration.
   d. stereotactic core biopsy.

5. While examining a patient's breasts, the nurse notes multiple, bilateral mobile lumps. To assess the patient further, the most appropriate question by the nurse is,
   a. "Do you have a high caffeine intake?"
   b. "When did you last have a mammogram?"
   c. "Is there a history of breast cancer in your mother or sisters?"
   d. "Do the size and tenderness of the lumps change with your menstrual cycle?"

6. While teaching the patient with fibrocystic changes in the breast, the nurse explains to the patient that this condition is significant because fibrocystic changes
   a. commonly become malignant over time.
   b. make it more difficult to examine the breasts.
   c. will eventually cause atrophy of breast tissue.
   d. can be controlled with hormone replacement therapy (HRT).

7. Match the following descriptions with their related benign breast disorder (answers may be used more than once).

_____ a. More common in women 40–60 years of age.

_____ b. Occurs in 10% of women ages 15-40.

_____ c. Occurs most often during lactation

_____ d. Associated with increased conversion of androgens
to estrogen

_____ e. Associated with breast trauma

_____ f. Multicolored, sticky nipple discharge

_____ g. Common cause is *Staphylococcus aureus*

_____ h. Involves ducts in subareolar area

_____ i. Usually resolves in 6 to 12 months

_____ j. Wartlike growth in mammary ducts near nipple

_____ k. Well-delineated, very mobile tumors

1. Fibroadenoma
2. Mastitis
3. Intraductal papilloma
4. Ductal ectasia
5. Fat necrosis
6. Senescent gynecomastia

8. The highest frequency of breast cancer in women is in those who
   a. are obese.
   b. are over the age of 60.
   c. have fibrocystic breast changes.
   d. have an inherited alteration of the BRCA1 or BRCA2 gene.

9. The nurse would be most concerned when examination of a patient's breasts revealed
   a. a large, tender, moveable mass in the upper inner quadrant.
   b. an immobile, hard, nontender lesion in the upper outer quadrant.
   c. a 2- to 3-cm, firm, defined, mobile mass in the lower outer quadrant.
   d. a painful, immobile mass with reddened skin in the upper outer quadrant.

10. The best prognosis is indicated in the patient with breast cancer when diagnostic studies reveal
    a. negative axillary lymph nodes.
    b. aneuploid DNA tumor content.
    c. cells with high S-phase fractions.
    d. an estrogen and progesterone receptor–negative tumor.

11. Recurrence or metastasis of breast cancer occurs
    a. most often at sites distant from the breast.
    b. only through the lymphatic chains draining the breast.
    c. most commonly to the bowel and reproductive organs.
    d. in patients who have small tumors with negative axillary lymph nodes.

12. The health care provider of a patient with a positive biopsy of a 2-cm breast tumor has recommended a lumpectomy with radiation therapy or a modified radical mastectomy as treatment. The patient says she does not know how to choose and asks the female nurse what she would do if she had to make the choice. The best response by the nurse is,
    a. "It doesn't matter what I would do. It is a decision you have to make for yourself."
    b. "There are advantages and disadvantages of both procedures. What do you know about these procedures?"
    c. "I would choose the modified radical mastectomy because it would ensure that the entire tumor was removed."
    d. "The lumpectomy maintains a nearly normal breast, but the survival rate is not as good as it is with a mastectomy."

13. A patient undergoing either a mastectomy or a lumpectomy for treatment of breast cancer can also usually expect to undergo
    a. chemotherapy.
    b. radiation therapy.
    c. hormonal therapy.
    d. axillary node dissection.

14. Lymphatic mapping with sentinel lymph node dissection (SLND) is planned for a patient undergoing a modified radical mastectomy for breast cancer. The nurse understands that
    a. if one sentinel lymph node is positive for malignant cells, all of the sentinel lymph nodes will be removed.
    b. lymphatic mapping indicates which lymph nodes are most likely to have metastasis and all of those nodes are removed.
    c. if malignant cells are found in any sentinel nodes, a complete axillary lymph node dissection will be done.
    d. lymphatic mapping with sentinel lymph node dissection provides metastatic lymph nodes to test for responsiveness to chemotherapy.

15. Identify the type of radiation therapy (primary, adjuvant to surgery, high-dose brachytherapy, or palliative) related to the following situations.
    a. Used to treat possible local residual cancer cells post-mastectomy
    b. Used to reduce tumor size and stabilize metastatic lesions for pain relief
    c. Alternative to traditional radiation therapy for early stage breast cancer
    d. Follows local excision of tumor
    e. May be completed in 5 days

16. A patient with a positive breast biopsy tells the nurse that she read about tamoxifen (Nolvadex) on the Internet and asks about its use. The best response by the nurse includes the information that
    a. tamoxifen is the primary treatment for breast cancer if axillary lymph nodes are positive for cancer.
    b. tamoxifen is used only to prevent the development of new primary tumors in women with high risk for breast cancer.
    c. tamoxifen is the treatment of choice after surgery if the tumor has receptors for estrogen and progesterone on its cells.
    d. because tamoxifen has been shown to increase the risk for uterine cancer, it is used only when other treatment has not been successful.

17. During the immediate postoperative period following a mastectomy, the nurse initially institutes exercises for the affected arm by
    a. having the patient brush or comb her hair with the affected arm.
    b. performing full passive range-of-motion (ROM) exercises to the affected arm.
    c. asking the patient to flex and extend the fingers and wrist of the operative side.
    d. having the patient crawl her fingers up the wall, raising her arm above her head.

18. Following a modified radical mastectomy, a patient develops lymphedema of the affected arm. The nurse teaches the patient to
    a. avoid skin-softening agents on the arm.
    b. protect the arm from any type of trauma.
    c. abduct and adduct the arm at the shoulder hourly.
    d. keep the arm positioned so that it is in straight and dependent alignment.

19. A patient undergoing surgery and radiation for treatment of breast cancer has a nursing diagnosis of disturbed body image related to absence of the breast. An appropriate nursing intervention for the patient is to
    a. provide the patient with information about surgical breast reconstruction.
    b. restrict visitors and phone calls until the patient feels better about herself.
    c. arrange for a Reach to Recovery visitor or similar resource available in the community.
    d. encourage the patient to obtain a permanent breast prosthesis as soon as she is discharged from the hospital.

20. A 56-year-old patient is undergoing a mammoplasty for breast reconstruction following a mastectomy 1 year ago. During the preoperative preparation of the patient, it is important that the nurse
    a. determine why the patient is choosing reconstruction surgery rather than the use of an external prosthesis.
    b. ensure that the patient has realistic expectations about the outcome and possible complications of the surgery.
    c. inform the patient that implants used for breast reconstruction have been shown to cause immune-related diseases.
    d. let the patient know that although the shape will be different from the other breast, the nipple can be reconstructed from other erectile tissue.

21. A patient undergoing a modified radical mastectomy for cancer of the breast is going to use tissue expansion and an implant for breast reconstruction. The nurse knows that
    a. weekly injections of water or saline into the expander will be required.
    b. the expander cannot be placed until healing from the mastectomy is complete.
    c. this method of breast reconstruction uses the patient's own tissue to replace breast tissue.
    d. the nipple from the affected breast will be saved to be grafted onto the reconstructed breast.

CASE STUDY
Metastatic Breast Cancer
Patient Profile

P.T., a 57-year-old married lawyer, was found to have a 4 × 6-cm firm, fixed mass in the upper, outer quadrant of the right breast during a routine physical examination, and a stereotactic core biopsy indicated a malignant tumor. Although the surgeon recommended a mastectomy because of the size of the tumor, P.T. chose to have a lumpectomy. Now 3 weeks postoperative, she is scheduled for chemotherapy.

Subjective Data

• Never had a routine mammogram
• Never practiced BSE
• States she deserves to have breast cancer for being so careless about her health
• Chose to have a lumpectomy to remove the tumor despite its large size because she believes that her breasts are critical in her relationship with her husband

Objective Data

• Physical examination
  • Right breast: Healed lumpectomy breast incision and right axillary incision
  • Limited ROM of right arm
  • Groshong catheter in place on left upper chest
• Diagnostic studies
  • Pathology: Estrogen receptor–positive infiltrating ductal carcinoma; 8 of 12 lymph nodes positive for malignant cells
  • Staging: Stage IIIA carcinoma of the right breast
• Clinical course
  • Lumpectomy performed to remove tumor 3 weeks ago
  • Chemotherapy with CAF protocol planned—cyclophosphamide (Cytoxan), doxorubicin (Adriamycin), and 5-fluorouracil (5-FU)

Clinical Decision-Making Questions

Using a separate sheet of paper, answer the following questions.

1. Why is chemotherapy indicated for P.T.?
2. Compare the three chemotherapeutic agents planned for P.T. with respect to classification type, cell specificity, and common side effects.
3. What can the nurse do to help P.T. reduce or manage the common physical effects of the chemotherapy?
4. What does the finding that P.T.'s tumor is estrogen receptor–positive mean? What additional treatment modalities might this suggest?
5. How could the nurse help P.T. cope with her feelings of guilt and maintain a positive relationship with her husband?
6. What are some possible reasons that P.T. did not perform BSE or have mammography performed?
7. P.T.'s husband asks the nurse about his wife's problems concentrating during their conversations. How should the nurse respond?
8. *Priority Decision:* What are the teaching priorities for P.T. regarding follow-up care related to recurrence of the breast cancer?
9. *Priority Decision:* Based on the assessment data presented, what are the priority nursing diagnoses? Are there any collaborative problems?

CHAPTER
53

Nursing Management:
Sexually Transmitted Diseases

1. The current incidence of sexually transmitted diseases (STDs) is related in part to
   a. increased social acceptance of homosexuality.
   b. increased virulence of organisms causing STDs.
   c. the use of oral agents rather than condoms as contraceptives.
   d. development of resistance of microorganisms to common antibiotics.

2. Match the following microorganisms with the disease they cause.
   _____ a. *Treponema pallidum*   1. Gonorrhea
   _____ b. *Chlamydia trachomatis*   2. Genital herpes
   _____ c. *Neisseria gonorrhoeae*   3. Syphilis
   _____ d. Human papillomavirus (HPV)   4. Nongonococcal urethritis
   _____ e. Herpes simplex virus   5. Genital warts

3. A female patient with a purulent vaginal discharge is seen at an outpatient clinic. The nurse would expect a diagnosis of gonorrhea to
   a. be treated with benzathine penicillin G.
   b. be confirmed with a Gram stain smear of the exudate.
   c. indicate the presence of pelvic inflammatory disease (PID).
   d. be treated with cefixime (Suprax) and doxycycline (Vibramycin).

4. A 22-year-old woman with multiple sexual partners seeks care after several weeks of experiencing painful and frequent urination and vaginal discharge. Although the results of a culture of cervical secretions are not yet available, the nurse explains to the patient that she will be treated as if she has gonorrhea and chlamydia to prevent
   a. obstruction of the fallopian tubes.
   b. endocarditis and aortic aneurysms.
   c. disseminated gonococcal infection.
   d. polyarthritis and generalized adenopathy.

5. During evaluation and treatment of gonorrhea in a young man at the health clinic, it is most important that the nurse question the patient about
   a. a prior history of STDs.
   b. when the symptoms began.
   c. the date of his last sexual activity.
   d. the names of his recent sexual partners.

6. Indicate whether the following clinical manifestations of syphilis are characteristic of primary (P), secondary (S), latent (L), or tertiary (T) syphilis.
   _____ a. Condyloma lata
   _____ b. Heart failure
   _____ c. Destructive skin, bone, and soft tissue lesions
   _____ d. Chancre
   _____ e. Mental deterioration
   _____ f. Generalized adenopathy
   _____ g. Absence of symptoms with a positive FTA-ABS test
   _____ h. Tabes dorsalis
   _____ i. Generalized cutaneous rash
   _____ j. Saccular aneurysms

271

7. A premarital blood test for syphilis reveals that a woman has a positive Venereal Disease Research Laboratory (VDRL) test. The nurse advises the patient that
   a. a single dose of penicillin will cure the syphilis.
   b. she should question her fiancé about prior sexual contacts.
   c. a lumbar puncture to evaluate cerebrospinal fluid (CSF) is necessary to rule out active syphilis.
   d. additional testing to detect specific antitreponemal antibodies is necessary.

8. The nurse encourages serologic testing for the human immunodeficiency virus (HIV) in the patient with syphilis primarily because
   a. syphilis is more difficult to treat in patients with HIV infection.
   b. the presence of HIV infection increases the risk of contacting syphilis.
   c. central nervous system (CNS) involvement is more common in patients with HIV infection and syphilis.
   d. the incidence of syphilis is highest in those with high rates of sexual promiscuity and drug abuse.

9. In establishing screening programs for populations at high risk for chlamydial infections, the nurse recognizes that in women, *C. trachomatis* infection most often results in
   a. cervicitis.
   b. no symptoms.
   c. acute urethritis.
   d. liver inflammation.

10. A male patient returns to the clinic with a recurrent urethral discharge after being treated for a chlamydial infection 2 weeks ago. Which statement by the patient indicates the most likely cause of the recurrence of his infection?
   a. "I took the vibramycin twice a day for a week."
   b. "I haven't told my girlfriend about my infection yet."
   c. "I had a couple of beers while I was taking the medication."
   d. "I've only had sexual intercourse once since my medication was finished."

11. A diagnosis of chlamydial infection can be made in a male patient when
   a. cultures for chlamydial organisms are positive.
   b. direct fluorescent antibody (DFA) tests are positive.
   c. Gram stain smears and cultures are negative for gonorrhea.
   d. signs and symptoms of epididymitis or proctitis are also present.

12. Identify whether the following statements are true (*T*) or false (*F*). If a statement is false, correct the bold word(s) to make the statement true.
   _____ a. Herpes simplex virus type 2 (HSV-2) is capable of causing **only genital lesions**.
   _____ b. The primary symptoms of genital herpes include painful **vesicular lesions that rupture and ulcerate**.
   _____ c. Treatment with acyclovir can **cure** genital herpes.
   _____ d. To prevent transmission of genital herpes, **condoms should be used** when lesions are present.
   _____ e. Recurrent symptomatic genital herpes may be precipitated by **sexual activity** and **stress**.

13. During the physical assessment of a female patient with HPV infection, the nurse would expect to find
   a. purulent vaginal discharge.
   b. a painless, indurated lesion on the vulva.
   c. painful perineal vesicles and ulcerations.
   d. multiple coalescing gray warts in the perineal area.

14. It is most important for the nurse to teach the female patient with genital warts to
   a. have an annual Pap smear.
   b. apply topical acyclovir faithfully as directed.
   c. have her sexual partner treated for the condition.
   d. use a contraceptive to prevent pregnancy, which might exacerbate the disease.

15. Based on the incidence of STDs in the United States, the nurse informs individuals who have unprotected sexual activity with multiple partners that they are at highest risk for contracting
    a. syphilis.
    b. gonorrhea.
    c. chlamydia.
    d. genital warts.

16. Indicate what treatment or precautions should be taken during pregnancy or delivery when the patient has active
    a. syphilis.
    b. gonorrhea.
    c. genital herpes.
    d. genital warts.

17. Although an 18-year-old girl knows that abstinence is one way to prevent STDs, she does not consider that an alternative. She asks the nurse at the clinic if there are other measures for preventing STDs. The nurse informs her that
    a. abstinence is the only way to prevent STDs.
    b. voiding immediately after intercourse will decrease risk of infection.
    c. a vaccine can prevent genital warts and cervical cancer caused by some strains of HPV.
    d. thorough hand washing after contact with genitals can prevent oral-genital spread of STDs.

18. The patient who is most likely to have a nursing diagnosis of risk for noncompliance is the patient with
    a. syphilis.
    b. gonorrhea.
    c. genital herpes.
    d. HPV infection.

CASE STUDY
Gonorrhea
Patient Profile

C.J., a 20-year-old college student, had intercourse with a prostitute while he was on vacation. He returns home 3 days later and has intercourse with his fiancée, Ms. A. The next day he begins to experience symptoms of an STD.

Subjective Data
- Experiences pain and burning on urination
- Has a yellowish white discharge from his penis
- Expresses concern over the possibility of having gonorrhea and what this diagnosis would mean in his relationship with his fiancée

Objective Data
- Positive Gram stain for *N. gonorrhoeae*

Clinical Decision-Making Questions
Using a separate sheet of paper, answer the following questions.

1. C.J. asks the nurse's advice on how to tell his fiancée about the diagnosis. What should the nurse's advice be?
2. What symptoms will Ms. A. have if she becomes infected?
3. What physical examinations and laboratory procedures are required to establish a diagnosis of gonorrhea in C.J. and Ms. A.?
4. What measures can be used to assist the couple in coping with the psychologic implications of the infection?
5. What treatment will be prescribed for C.J. and Ms. A.?
6. What are the possible complications of untreated gonorrhea in men and in women?
7. *Priority Decision:* Based on the assessment data presented, what are the priority nursing diagnoses? Are there any collaborative problems?

CHAPTER 54

Nursing Management: Female Reproductive Problems

1. A couple seeks assistance from an infertility specialist for evaluation of their infertility. The nurse informs the couple that during the initial visit, they can expect
   a. physical and psychosocial functioning examinations.
   b. assessment of tubal patency with a hysterosalpingogram.
   c. pelvic ultrasound for the woman and semen analysis for the man.
   d. postcoital testing to evaluate sperm numbers and motility in cervical and vaginal secretions.

2. An infertile couple is instructed in at-home ovulation testing using basal body temperature. The nurse explains that this testing
   a. can identify the need for intrauterine insemination as a result of anovulation.
   b. requires that the temperature be taken by the same route every morning on awakening before any activity.
   c. is an easy, nonstressful way to determine when ovulation occurs and when to have intercourse if pregnancy is desired.
   d. indicates when ovulation occurs by revealing a sharp rise in temperature followed by a drop in basal body temperature.

3. A patient with a 10-week pregnancy is admitted to the emergency department with vaginal bleeding and abdominal cramping. The nurse recognizes that
   a. the patient will be scheduled for an immediate D&C.
   b. the patient will recover quickly when the bleeding stops.
   c. the patient is most likely experiencing a spontaneous abortion.
   d. treatment of the patient with bed rest is usually successful in preventing further bleeding.

4. Mifepristone (Mifeprex) is prescribed for a perimenopausal woman who has an unexpected and unwanted pregnancy. The nurse informs the patient that this drug
   a. is toxic to trophoblastic tissue and destroys embryonic cells.
   b. causes uterine contractions that expel the products of conception.
   c. is only effective in terminating a pregnancy during the first 4 weeks.
   d. will block the action of progesterone, which is needed to support pregnancy.

5. Premenstrual syndrome (PMS) is most likely to be diagnosed in a woman
   a. who has symptoms only when oral contraceptives are used.
   b. whose symptoms can be controlled with the use of progesterone.
   c. whose symptoms can be correlated with altered serum levels of estrogen and progesterone.
   d. who has the same symptom pattern following ovulation for two or three consecutive menstrual cycles.

6. When teaching a patient with PMS about management of the disorder, the nurse includes the need to
   a. supplement the diet with vitamins C and E.
   b. use estrogen supplements during the luteal phase.
   c. limit dietary intake of caffeine, salt, and refined sugar.
   d. limit exercise and physical activity when symptoms are present.

7. The rationale for the regular use of nonsteroidal antiinflammatory drugs (NSAIDs) during the first several days of the menstrual period for women who have primary dysmenorrhea is that these drugs
   a. suppress ovulation and the production of prostaglandins that occur with ovulation.
   b. cause uterine relaxation and small vessel constriction, preventing cramping and abdominal congestion.
   c. inhibit the production of prostaglandins believed to be responsible for menstrual pain and associated symptoms.
   d. block the release of luteinizing hormone, preventing the increase in progesterone associated with maturation of the corpus luteum.

8. Match the following characteristics with their related menstrual irregularities (answers may be used more than once).
   _____ a. Common cause is use of hormonal contraceptives
   _____ b. May be caused by strenuous exercise or severe dieting
   _____ c. Bleeding or spotting between menstrual periods
   _____ d. Associated with endometrial cancer or uterine fibroids
   _____ e. Increased duration or amount of menstrual bleeding
   _____ f. Excessive bleeding at irregular intervals
   _____ g. Absence of menses

   1. Amenorrhea
   2. Menorrhagia
   3. Metrorrhagia

9. A young woman who runs vigorously as a form of exercise has not had a menstrual period in more than 6 months. The nurse advises her that
   a. normal periods will return when she stops running.
   b. uterine balloon therapy may be necessary to promote uterine sloughing of the overgrown endometrium.
   c. progesterone or birth control pills should be used to prevent persistent overgrowth of the endometrium.
   d. unopposed progesterone production causes an overgrowth of the endometrium that increases her risk for endometrial cancer.

10. A patient with abdominal pain and irregular vaginal bleeding is admitted to the hospital with a suspected ectopic pregnancy. The most appropriate action by the nurse is to
    a. provide analgesics for pain relief.
    b. monitor her vital signs and pain frequently.
    c. explain the need for frequent blood samples for β-hCG monitoring.
    d. offer support for the patient's emotional response to the loss of the pregnancy.

11. Identify whether the following statements are true (*T*) or false (*F*). If a statement is false, correct the bold word(s) to make the statement true.
    _____ a. During the **perimenopausal** period, a woman experiences cessation of menses.
    _____ b. Menopause occurs in response to decreasing levels of **FSH**.
    _____ c. Physical responses directly related to decreased estrogen during menopause include **hot flashes** and **atrophic vaginitis**.
    _____ d. If estrogen replacement is used by a postmenopausal woman with a uterus, it is important that progesterone be taken to decrease the risk for **endometrial cancer**.
    _____ e. Research contributing to evidence-based practice indicates that hormone replacement with estrogen and progesterone increases the risk for **cardiovascular disease**.

12. Identify four beneficial effects and four potential risks related to HRT that should be discussed with a woman during perimenopause.

    Benefits
    a.
    b.
    c.
    d.

    Risks
    e.
    f.
    g.
    h.

13. Match the following characteristics with the related infections (answers may be used more than once).
    _____ a. Pruritic, frothy greenish or gray discharge
    _____ b. May be treated with over-the-counter (OTC) antifungal agents
    _____ c. Thick, white, cottage cheese–like discharge
    _____ d. Treated with regimens for chlamydia
    _____ e. Fishy-smelling watery discharge
    _____ f. Intense itching and dysuria
    _____ g. Hemorrhagic cervix and vagina
    _____ h. Severe recurrent infections associated with HIV infection
    _____ i. Mucopurulent discharge and postcoital spotting

    1. Vulvovaginal candidiasis
    2. Trichomoniasis
    3. Bacterial vaginosis
    4. Cervicitis

14. A patient is diagnosed and treated for a *Gardnerella vaginalis* infection at a clinic. For her treatment to be effective, the nurse tells the patient that
    a. her sexual partner must also be examined and treated.
    b. her sexual partner must use a condom during intercourse.
    c. she should wear minipads to prevent reinfection as long as she has vaginal drainage.
    d. the vaginal cream must be used at bedtime when she lies down to prevent loss from the vagina.

15. A young woman is admitted to the hospital with acute pelvic inflammatory disease (PID). During the nursing history, the nurse notes as a significant risk factor the patient's
    a. lack of any method of birth control.
    b. sexual activity with multiple partners.
    c. use of a vaginal sponge for contraception.
    d. recent antibiotic-induced monilial vaginitis.

16. In implementing care for the patient with acute PID, the nurse
    a. performs vaginal irrigations every 4 hours.
    b. promotes bed rest in semi-Fowler's position.
    c. instructs the patient to use tampons to control vaginal drainage.
    d. ambulates the patient frequently to promote drainage of exudate.

17. A 20-year-old patient with PID is crying and tells the nurse that she is afraid she will not be able to have children as a result of the infection. The nurse's best response to the patient is,
    a. "I would not worry about that right now. Our immediate concern is to cure the infection you have."
    b. "The possibility of infertility following PID is high. Would you like to talk about what it means to you?"
    c. "Sterility following PID is possible, but not common, and it is too soon to know what the effects will be."
    d. "The infection can cause more serious complications such as abscesses and shock that you should be more concerned about."

18. Identify whether the following statements are true (*T*) or false (*F*). If a statement is false, correct the bold word(s) to make the statement true.
    _____ a. The presence of ectopic uterine tissue that bleeds and causes pelvic and abdominal adhesions and cysts is known as **uterine leiomyoma**.
    _____ b. Two gynecologic conditions that subside with the onset of menopause are **endometriosis** and **cervical polyps**.
    _____ c. Polycystic ovary syndrome results in benign cysts forming on the ovaries as a result of **estrogen and testosterone** production but not progesterone.
    _____ d. Treatment of endometriosis and leiomyomas depends on the severity of **the symptoms and the woman's desire to maintain fertility**.
    _____ e. Danazol (Danacrine) and Lupron (GnRH analog) are used to treat endometriosis and leiomyomas to create a **pseudopregnancy**.
    _____ f. The most common symptom of cervical polyps is **menorrhagia**.
    _____ g. An **ovarian cyst** may cause severe pain if twisting of the pedicle occurs.

19. A patient with a stage 0 cervical cancer identified from a Pap smear asks the nurse what this finding means. The nurse's response includes the information that
    a. malignant cells have extended beyond the cervix but not to the pelvic wall.
    b. abnormal cells are present but are confined to the epithelial layer of the cervix.
    c. atypical cells characteristic of inflammation, but not necessarily malignancy, are present.
    d. this is a common finding on Pap testing and she will be examined frequently to see whether the abnormal cells spread beyond the cervix.

20. Fertility and normal reproductive function can be maintained when a cancer of the cervix is treated with
    a. external radiation therapy.
    b. internal radiation implants.
    c. conization or laser surgery.
    d. cryotherapy or subtotal hysterectomy.

21. A woman who is postmenopausal for 10 years calls the clinic because of vaginal bleeding. The nurse schedules a visit for the patient and informs her to expect to have
    a. an endometrial biopsy.
    b. abdominal radiography.
    c. a laser treatment to the cervix.
    d. only a routine pelvic examination and Pap smear.

22. A patient has been diagnosed with cancer of the ovary. In planning care for the patient, the nurse recognizes that treatment indicated for the patient depends on
    a. results of a direct-needle biopsy of the ovary.
    b. results of a laparoscopy with multiple biopsies.
    c. whether the patient desires to maintain fertility.
    d. the findings of metastasis by ultrasound or CT scan.

23. Indicate whether the following factors are associated with an increased risk for cervical cancer (C), endometrial cancer (E), ovarian cancer (O), or vaginal cancer (V).
    _____ a. Obesity
    _____ b. BRCA gene mutations
    _____ c. Smoking
    _____ d. Early sexual activity
    _____ e. Intrauterine exposure to diethylstilbestrol (DES)
    _____ f. Unopposed estrogen-only replacement therapy
    _____ g. HPV infection
    _____ h. Early menarche and late menopause
    _____ i. Low socioeconomic status
    _____ j. Family history

24. During assessment of the patient with vulvar cancer, the nurse would expect to find
    a. soreness and itching of the vulva.
    b. labial lesions with purulent exudate.
    c. severe excoriation of the labia and perineum.
    d. painless, firm nodules embedded in the labia.

25. A 44-year-old woman undergoing a total abdominal hysterectomy asks whether she will need to take estrogen until she reaches the age of menopause. The best response by the nurse is,
    a. "You are close enough to normal menopause that you probably won't need additional estrogen."
    b. "Yes, it will help prevent the more intense symptoms caused by surgically induced menopause."
    c. "Because your ovaries won't be removed, they will continue to secrete estrogen until your normal menopause."
    d. "There are so many risks associated with estrogen replacement therapy that it is best to begin menopause now."

26. A nursing diagnosis of disturbed body image is likely to be most appropriate for the patient undergoing a
    a. vaginectomy
    b. hemivulvectomy.
    c. pelvic exenteration.
    d. radical hysterectomy.

27. During treatment with an intrauterine radioactive implant, the patient
    a. may ambulate in the room as desired.
    b. should have all care provided by the same nurse.
    c. can have unlimited duration and number of visitors.
    d. is restricted to bed rest with turning from side to side.

28. When teaching a patient with problems of pelvic support to perform Kegel exercises, the nurse tells the patient to
    a. contract her muscles as if trying to stop the flow of urine.
    b. tighten the lower abdominal muscles over the bladder area.
    c. squeeze all the perineal muscles as if trying to close the vagina.
    d. lie on the floor and do leg lifts to strengthen the abdominal muscles.

29. Match the following uterine structure abnormalities with their descriptions.

_____ a. Uterine prolapse   1. Opening between vagina and bladder
_____ b. Cystocele   2. Protrusion of rectum through vaginal wall
_____ c. Rectocele   3. Protrusion of bladder through vaginal wall
_____ d. Vesicovaginal fistula   4. Opening between rectum and vagina
_____ e. Rectovaginal fistula   5. Displacement of uterus through vagina

30. An appropriate outcome for a patient who undergoes an anterior colporrhaphy is that the patient will
    a. maintain normal bowel patterns.
    b. adjust to temporary ileal conduit.
    c. urinate within 8 hours postoperatively.
    d. experience healing of excoriated vaginal and vulvar tissue.

31. *Priority Decision:* On admission of a victim of sexual assault to the emergency department, the first priority of the nurse is to
    a. contact a rape support person for the patient.
    b. assess the patient for urgent medical problems.
    c. question the patient about the details of the assault.
    d. inform the patient what procedures and treatments will be performed.

32. To prepare a woman who has been raped for physical examination, the nurse first
    a. administers prophylaxis for STDs and tetanus.
    b. ensures that a signed informed consent is obtained from the patient.
    c. provides a private place for the patient to talk about what happened to her.
    d. instructs the patient not to wash, eat, drink, or urinate before the examination.

CASE STUDY
Acute Pelvic Inflammatory Disease
Patient Profile

A.R., a 23-year-old unmarried woman, has a recent history of gonorrhea. For the past 2 weeks, she has had a heavy purulent vaginal discharge and general malaise. Concerned that her symptoms appear to be worsening, A.R. makes an appointment at the gynecologic clinic.

Subjective Data

• Experiences an increase in lower abdominal pain during vaginal examination
• Expresses concern over worsening of her condition and the effect this will have on future childbearing ability

Objective Data

• Vital signs: T 101° F (38.3° C), HR 90, RR 18, BP 110/58
• Physical examination: Heavy, purulent vaginal discharge
• Diagnostic studies: Vaginal discharge positive for *N. gonorrhoeae*
• Admitted to the hospital for monitoring, IV fluids, and antibiotic therapy

---

Clinical Decision-Making Questions

Using a separate sheet of paper, answer the following questions.

1. What route does the gonococcus take in the development of PID?
2. What are the clinical manifestations of acute PID?
3. How would A.R.'s infection be managed if it was decided to treat her as an outpatient? What instructions should she receive?
4. How does chronic PID compare with acute PID?
5. *Priority Decision:* What priority measures should the nurse take to prevent extension of the infection?
6. How should the nurse respond to A.R.'s concern over the effect of this infection on her future childbearing ability?
7. *Priority Decision:* Based on the assessment data presented, what are the priority nursing diagnoses? Are there any collaborative problems?

CHAPTER
55

Nursing Management:
Male Reproductive Problems

1. A patient asks the nurse what the difference between benign prostatic hyperplasia (BPH) and cancer of the prostate is. The best response by the nurse includes the information that BPH is
   a. a benign tumor that does not spread beyond the prostate gland.
   b. a precursor to prostate cancer but does not yet show any malignant changes.
   c. an enlargement of the gland caused by an increase in the size of existing cells.
   d. a benign enlargement of the gland caused by an increase in the number of normal cells.

2. When taking a nursing history from a patient with BPH, the nurse would expect the patient to report
   a. nocturia, dysuria, and bladder spasms.
   b. urinary frequency, hematuria, and perineal pain.
   c. urinary hesitancy, postvoid dribbling, and weak urinary stream.
   d. urinary urgency with a forceful urinary stream and cloudy urine.

3. The extent of urinary obstruction caused by BPH can be determined by
   a. a cystometrogram.
   b. transrectal ultrasound.
   c. urodynamic flow studies.
   d. postvoiding catheterization.

4. The effect of finasteride (Proscar) in the treatment of BPH is
   a. a reduction in the size of the prostate gland.
   b. relaxation of the smooth muscle of the urethra.
   c. increased bladder tone that promotes bladder emptying.
   d. relaxation of the bladder detrusor musculature promoting urine flow.

5. On admission to the ambulatory surgical center, a patient with BPH informs the nurse that he is going to have a laser treatment of his enlarged prostate. The nurse plans patient teaching with the knowledge that the patient will need
   a. monitoring for postoperative urinary retention.
   b. teaching about the effects of general anesthesia.
   c. to be informed of the possibility of short-term incontinence.
   d. instruction about home management of an indwelling catheter.

6. The most common screening intervention for detecting BPH in men over age 50 is an annual
   a. urinalysis.
   b. PSA level.
   c. cystoscopy.
   d. digital rectal examination.

7. Match the following therapies used for BPH with their characteristics (answers may be used more than once).

    _____ a. Involves an external incision prostatectomy

    _____ b. Results in delayed sloughing of tissue

    _____ c. Most common surgical procedure to treat BPH

    _____ d. Use of low-wave radiofrequency to precisely destroy prostate tissue

    _____ e. Used with patients who are poor surgical candidates

    _____ f. Resectoscopic excision and cauterization of prostate tissue

    _____ g. Indicated when there is very little prostatic enlargement

    _____ h. Most effective long-term treatment of BPH

    _____ i. Use of microwave heat to destroy prostate tissue

    _____ j. Relieves symptoms of obstruction.

    _____ k. Can be used on patients taking anticoagulants

    _____ l. Indicated for very large prostate gland

    _____ m. Temporary solution to obstructive problems

    _____ n. Inappropriate for men with rectal problems

1. Transurethral resection of prostate (TURP)
2. Transurethral incision of the prostate (TUIP)
3. Simple open prostatectomy
4. Transurethral microwave thermotherapy (TUMT)
5. Laser prostatectomy
6. Transurethral needle ablation (TUNA)
7. Intraprostatic urethral stents

8. Before undergoing TURP, the patient should be informed that
    a. some degree of urinary incontinence is likely to occur.
    b. this surgery results in some degree of retrograde ejaculation.
    c. erectile dysfunction is a common complication of this prostate surgery.
    d. an indwelling catheter will be used to maintain urinary output until healing is complete.

9. Following a TURP, a patient has a continuous bladder irrigation. Four hours after surgery, the catheter is draining thick, bright red clots and tissue. The nurse should
    a. release the traction on the catheter.
    b. manually irrigate the catheter until the drainage is clear.
    c. increase the rate of the irrigation and take the patient's vital signs.
    d. clamp the drainage tube and notify the patient's health care provider.

10. A patient with continuous bladder irrigation following a prostatectomy tells the nurse he has bladder spasms and leaking of urine around the catheter. The nurse should first
    a. slow the rate of the irrigation.
    b. assess the patency of the catheter.
    c. encourage the patient to try to urinate around the catheter.
    d. administer a belladonna and opium (B&O) suppository as prescribed.

11. The nurse provides discharge teaching to a patient following a TURP and determines that the patient understands the instructions when he says,
    a. "I should use daily enemas to avoid straining until healing is complete."
    b. "At least I don't have to worry about developing cancer of the prostate now."
    c. "I should avoid heavy lifting, climbing, and driving until my follow-up visit."
    d. "Every day I should drink 10 to 12 glasses of liquids such as coffee, tea, or soft drinks."

12. Identify three findings in the following areas that are present in the patient with prostatic cancer that differ from findings in BPH.
    a. Prostatic palpation
    b. Blood tests
    c. Extraurinary symptoms

13. A 55-year-old man asks the nurse what he can do to decrease the risk of prostate cancer. The nurse explains that
    a. treatment of any enlargement of the prostate gland will help prevent prostate cancer.
    b. nothing can decrease the risk because prostate cancer is primarily a disease of aging.
    c. substituting fresh fruits and vegetables for high-fat foods in the diet may lower the risk of prostate cancer.
    d. using a natural herb, saw palmetto, has been found to be an effective protection against prostate cancer.

14. When caring for a patient following a radical prostatectomy with a perineal approach, an appropriate nursing diagnosis for the nurse to identify is risk for infection related to
    a. urinary retention.
    b. wound contamination.
    c. altered bowel function.
    d. chemotherapeutic agents.

15. Identify whether the following statements are true (*T*) or false (*F*). If a statement is false, correct the bold word(s) to make the statement true.
    _____ a. A **radical prostatectomy** is a treatment option for all patients with prostatic cancer except those with stage D tumors.
    _____ b. The preferred hormonal therapy for treatment of prostate cancer includes **estrogen** and **androgen-receptor blockers**.
    _____ c. Early detection of cancer of the prostate is increased with annual rectal examinations and **serum prostatic acid phosphatase (PAP) measurements**.
    _____ d. Because of the variety of treatment options available for cancer of the prostate, it is common for a patient to have a nursing diagnosis of **decisional conflict**.
    _____ e. An annual prostate examination is recommended starting at **age 45** for **Hispanic** men because of the increased mortality rate from prostatic cancer in this population.
    _____ f. **Chronic bacterial prostatitis** manifests with symptoms of a urinary tract infection with a swollen, very tender prostate gland.
    _____ g. Drainage of the prostate through intercourse, masturbation, and prostatic massage is indicated for management of **chronic prostatitis**.

16. Word Search. Find the words that are described by the clues on the next page. The words may be located horizontally, vertically, or diagonally and may be reversed.

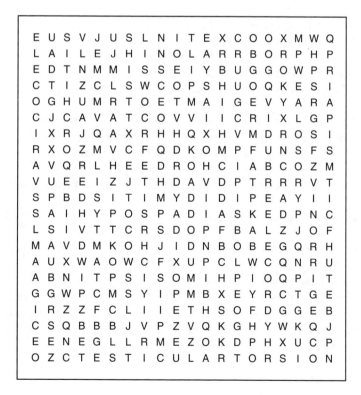

```
E U S V J U S L N I T E X C O O X M W Q
L A I L E J H I N O L A R R B O R P H P
E D T N M M I S S E I Y B U G G O W P R
C T I Z C L S W C O P S H U O Q K E S I
O G H U M R T O E T M A I G E V Y A R A
C J C A V A T C O V V I I C R I X L G P
I X R J Q A X R H H Q X H V M D R O S I
R X O Z M V C F Q D K O M P F U N S F S
A V Q R L H E E D R O H C I A B C O Z M
V U E E I Z J T H D A V D P T R R R V T
S P B D S I T I M Y D I D I P E A Y I I
S A I H Y P O S P A D I A S K E D P N C
L S I V T T C R S D O P F B A L Z J O F
M A V D M K O H J I D N B O B E G Q R H
A U X W A O W C F X U P C L W C Q N R U
A B N I T P S I S O M I H P I O Q P I T
G G W P C M S Y I P M B X E Y R C T G E
I R Z Z F C L I I E T H S O F D G G E B
C S Q B B B J V P Z V Q K G H Y W K Q J
E E N E G L L R M E Z O K D P H X U C P
O Z C T E S T I C U L A R T O R S I O N
```

Clues

a. Painful, prolonged erection
b. Ventral urinary meatus
c. Complication of mumps
d. Painful downward curvature of an erect penis
e. Twisted spermatic cord
f. Removal of penile foreskin
g. Inflammation of the prepuce
h. Sperm-filled cyst of epididymis
i. Retracted tight foreskin preventing return over glans
j. Scrotal lymphedema
k. Inflammation of the epididymis
l. Dorsal urinary meatus
m. Testicular vein dilation
n. Undescended testicle

17. Serum tumor markers that may be elevated on diagnosis of cancer of the testicle and used to monitor the response to therapy include
    a. tumor necrosis factor (TNF) and C-reactive protein (CRP).
    b. α-fetoprotein (AFP) and human chorionic gonadotropin (hCG).
    c. prostate-specific antigen (PSA) and prostate acid phosphatase (PAP).
    d. carcinoembryonic antigens (CEAs) and antinuclear antibodies (ANAs).

18. When teaching a patient testicular self-examination, the nurse instructs the patient to report a finding of
    a. an irregular-feeling epididymis.
    b. one testis larger than the other.
    c. the spermatic cord within the testicle.
    d. a firm, nontender nodule on the testis.

19. The nurse teaches the patient having a vasectomy that following the procedure
    a. the amount of ejaculate will be noticeably decreased.
    b. he may have difficulty maintaining an erection for several months.
    c. an alternative form of contraception must be used for 6 to 8 weeks.
    d. the testes will gradually decrease production of sperm and testosterone.

20. A patient seeking medical intervention for erectile dysfunction should be thoroughly evaluated primarily because
    a. treatment of erectile dysfunction is based on the cause of the problem.
    b. psychologic counseling can reverse the problem in 80% to 90% of the cases.
    c. new invasive and experimental techniques currently used have unknown risks.
    d. most treatments for erectile dysfunction are contraindicated in patients with systemic diseases.

21. Match the following treatment modalities for erectile dysfunction with their characteristics (answers may be used more than once).

    _____ a. Blood drawn into corporeal bodies and held with a ring
    _____ b. Indicated for hypogonadism
    _____ c. Relaxes smooth muscle in the penis
    _____ d. Direct application of drugs that increases blood flow in penis
    _____ e. Devices implanted into corporeal bodies to firm the penis
    _____ f. Should be avoided in patients using nitrates

    1. Androgen replacement therapy
    2. Intracavernosal self-injection of vasoactive drugs
    3. Vacuum constriction device (VCD)
    4. Penile implants
    5. Sildenafil (Viagra)

CASE STUDY

Testicular Cancer

Patient Profile

Following a shower last evening, 19-year-old C.E. was performing his routine testicular self-examination when he discovered a firm lump on his left testis. After a medical examination, he was admitted to the hospital for a left orchiectomy and lymph node resection.

Subjective Data

- Has a history of an undescended left testis, which was surgically corrected at age 4
- Expresses concern about surgery and how it will affect him
- Asks about his prognosis and chances for recovery after the surgery
- Denies back pain

Objective Data

- Very firm, nontender nodule on left testis
- Local lymph node enlargement
- No gynecomastia noted
- Biopsy revealed seminoma germ cell tumor

Clinical Decision-Making Questions

Using a separate sheet of paper, answer the following questions.

1. Explain the development and risk factors for cancer of the testis.
2. How does cancer of the testis differ from a spermatocele on examination?
3. What is C.E.'s prognosis if the malignancy is in early stages?
4. What blood tests for tumor markers should be done preoperatively and are indicated for long-term follow-up care and why?
5. How can the nurse help C.E. deal with the psychological components of his illness?
6. What effect will this surgery have on C.E.'s sexual functioning?
7. **Priority Decision:** Based on the assessment data presented, what are the priority nursing diagnoses? Are there any collaborative problems?

Nursing Assessment: Nervous System

1. Using the list of terms below, identify the structures in the following illustration.

Terms

axon
axon hillock
collateral axon
dendrites
Golgi apparatus

mitochondrion
myelin sheath
neuron cell body
Nissl bodies
node of Ranvier

nucleolus
nucleus
Schwann cell
synaptic knobs
telodendria

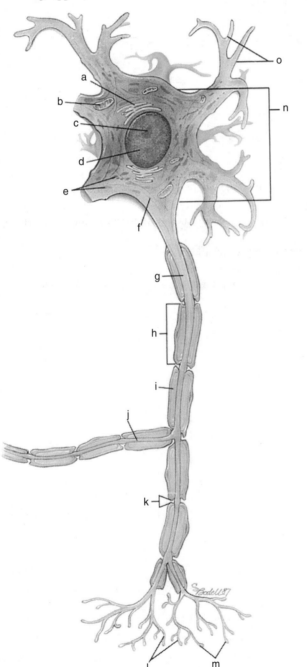

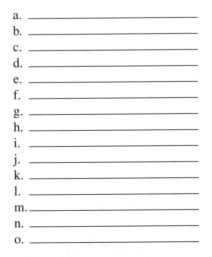

a. _____

b. _____

c. _____

d. _____

e. _____

f. _____

g. _____

h. _____

i. _____

j. _____

k. _____

l. _____

m. _____

n. _____

o. _____

2. Using the following list of terms, identify the structures in the illustration below.

Terms

arachnoid

body of vertebra

central canal

dorsal horn

dorsal root

dura mater

lateral horn

pia mater

spinal cord

spinal ganglia

spinal nerves

substantia gelatinosa

sympathetic ganglion

transverse process of vertebra

ventral horn

ventral root

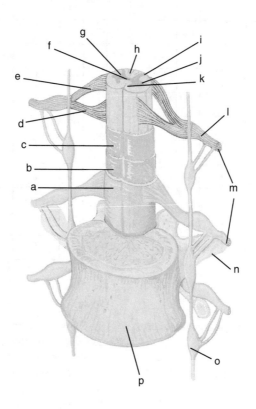

3. Crossword Puzzle

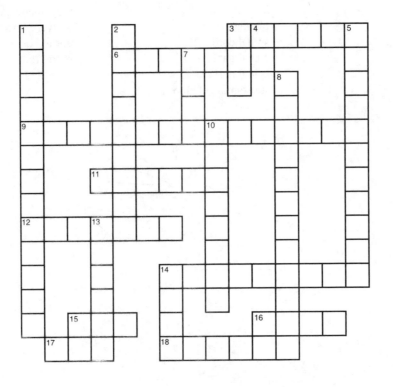

Across

3. Synaptic _____: spaces where neurotransmitters cross from neuron to neuron
6. Junction between two neurons
9. Produces myelin sheath of nerve fibers in CNS
11. Component of white matter
12. Part of the cell body of a neuron
14. Action _____: an event that causes depolarization
15. Innermost meningeal mater
16. Site where cranial nerve V (CN-V) arises
17. Assessed in part with orientation and memory (abbr.)
18. Basic unit of the nervous system

Down

1. Gaps in peripheral nerve axons
2. Help form blood-brain barrier
3. Protective fluid of CNS (abbr.)
4. Lower extremity (abbr.)
5. Produces myelin sheath of peripheral nerves
7. Carries impulses from nerve cell body
8. May occur with damage to peripheral axons
10. Carries impulses to nerve cell body
13. Area of brain concerned with emotions and aggression
14. Common symptom of disease
15. By mouth
16. Orally

4. Identify whether the following statements are true (*T*) or false (*F*). If a statement is false, correct the bold word(s) to make the statement true.

_____ a. Neuroglial cells that line the ventricles and assist in production of CSF are called **microglia**.

_____ b. During depolarization of a nerve cell **sodium** moves into the cell, creating a **positive** intracellular environment relative to the outside.

_____ c. An action potential traveling down an axon hopping from node to node travels much **slower** than it would on unmyelinated fiber.

_____ d. **Oligodendrocytes** provide structural support to neurons and form the blood-brain barrier.

_____ e. The transmission of an action potential at a synapse depends on the **number** of presynaptic cells releasing neurotransmitters.

5. A patient has a lesion involving the fasciculus gracilis/cuneatus of the spinal cord. The nurse would expect the patient to experience loss of
   a. pain and temperature sensations.
   b. touch, deep pressure, vibration, and position sense.
   c. unconscious information about body position and muscle tension.
   d. voluntary muscle control from the cerebral cortex to the peripheral nerves.

6. Lower motor neurons differ from upper motor neurons primarily in that lesions of the lower motor neurons
   a. cause hyporeflexia and flaccidity.
   b. affect motor control of the lower body.
   c. arise in structures above the spinal cord.
   d. interfere with reflex arcs in the spinal cord.

7. Match the following functions with the associated area of the brain.
   _____ a. Major relay center for sensory and motor input to cerebrum
   _____ b. Responsible for arousal
   _____ c. Controls initiation, execution, and completion of voluntary and automatic movements
   _____ d. Controls judgment, insight, and reasoning
   _____ e. Regulates respiratory, vasomotor, and cardiac function
   _____ f. Sound and visual interpretation
   _____ g. Maintains trunk stability and equilibrium
   _____ h. Registers visual images
   _____ i. Integrates somatic and special sensory inputs
   _____ j. Related to emotion and sexual response
   _____ k. Regulates endocrine and autonomic functions
   _____ l. Responsible for verbal expression

   1. Anterior frontal lobe
   2. Temporal lobe
   3. Parietal lobe
   4. Occipital lobe
   5. Limbic system
   6. Broca's area
   7. Basal ganglia
   8. Thalamus
   9. Hypothalamus
   10. Reticular activating system
   11. Medulla
   12. Cerebellum

8. Spinal nerves of the peripheral nervous system differ from cranial nerves in that
   a. only spinal nerves occur in pairs.
   b. cranial nerves affect only the sensory and motor functions of the head and neck.
   c. the cell bodies of all cranial nerves are located in the brain, whereas cell bodies of spinal nerves are located in the spinal cord.
   d. all spinal nerves contain both afferent sensory and efferent motor fibers, whereas cranial nerves contain one or the other or both.

9. Indicate whether the following descriptions are characteristic of the sympathetic nervous system (S) or the parasympathetic nervous system (P).
   _____ a. Preganglionic cell bodies are located in spinal segments T1-L2
   _____ b. Norepinephrine released by most postganglionic fibers
   _____ c. Responsible for conservation and restoration of energy stores
   _____ d. Cause pupillary constriction and accommodation for near vision
   _____ e. Necessary for male ejaculation
   _____ f. Acetylcholine released at both preganglionic and postganglionic nerve endings
   _____ g. Increase heart rate (HR) and dilate coronary arteries
   _____ h. Relax sphincters of the gastrointestinal (GI) and genitourinary (GU) tract
   _____ i. Necessary for male erection
   _____ j. Preganglionic cell bodies located in brainstem and sacral spinal segment
   _____ k. Responsible for some effects of CN-III and CN-X

10. A patient has an atherosclerotic plaque in the middle cerebral artery. The nurse recognizes that
    a. assessment will reveal distended jugular veins.
    b. cerebral circulation may be maintained through the circle of Willis.
    c. the patient will develop a loss of temporal and parietal lobe function.
    d. increased pressure in the middle cerebral artery will back up into the vertebral arteries.

11. Match the supportive and protective structures of the nervous system with their characteristics.

    _____ a. Skull
    _____ b. Vertebral column
    _____ c. Dura mater
    _____ d. Blood-brain barrier
    _____ e. Ventricles
    _____ f. Falx cerebri
    _____ g. Arachnoid layer
    _____ h. Pia mater
    _____ i. Tentorium cerebelli

    1. Produce and circulate CSF
    2. Forms a space with pia mater through which blood vessels and nerves pass
    3. Separates cerebrum from the posterior fossa
    4. Provides for flexibility while protecting spinal barrier
    5. Inner layer of meninges
    6. Protects brain from external trauma
    7. Protects against harmful blood-borne agents
    8. Prevents expansion of brain tissue into adjacent hemisphere
    9. Outer layer of meninges

12. During neurologic assessment of the older adult, the nurse would expect to find
    a. absent deep tendon reflexes.
    b. below-average intelligence score.
    c. decreased sensation of touch and temperature.
    d. decreased frequency of spontaneous awakening.

13. Identify three factors that should be considered when taking the history of a patient with a neurologic problem.
    a.

    b.

    c.

14. Identify one specific finding identified by the nurse during assessment of each of the patient's functional health patterns that indicates a risk factor for neurologic problems or a patient response to an actual neurologic problem.
    a. Health perception–health management
    b. Nutritional-metabolic
    c. Elimination
    d. Activity-exercise
    e. Sleep-rest
    f. Cognitive-perceptual
    g. Self-perception–self-concept
    h. Role-relationship
    i. Sexuality-reproductive
    j. Coping–stress tolerance
    k. Value-belief

15. Match the following cranial nerves (CN) with their methods of evaluation (evaluation methods may be used more than once, and some nerves may be tested with more than one method).

    _____ a. Olfactory (I)
    _____ b. Optic (II)
    _____ c. Oculomotor (III)
    _____ d. Trochlear (IV)
    _____ e. Trigeminal (V)
    _____ f. Abducens (VI)
    _____ g. Facial (VII)
    _____ h. Cochlear branch of acoustic (VIII)
    _____ i. Glossopharyngeal (IX)
    _____ j. Vagus (X)
    _____ k. Spinal accessory (XI)
    _____ l. Hypoglossal (XII)

    1. Resistive shoulder shrug
    2. Smile, frown, and close eyes
    3. Light touch to the face
    4. Confrontation
    5. Tongue protrusion
    6. Corneal reflex test
    7. Identify odors
    8. Pupillary response
    9. Oblique eye movement
    10. Salt and sugar discrimination
    11. Gag reflex
    12. Lateral eye movement
    13. Ticking watch

16. During an assessment of the motor system, the nurse finds that the patient has a staggering gait and an abnormal arm swing. The nurse uses this information to
    a. assist the patient to cope with the disability.
    b. plan a rehabilitation program for the patient.
    c. protect the patient from injury caused by falls.
    d. help establish a diagnosis of cerebellar dysfunction.

17. Match the assessment methods that may elicit the following abnormal findings.

    _____ a. Cotton wisp
    _____ b. Plantar stimulation
    _____ c. Sharp end of a pin
    _____ d. Heel-to-shin test
    _____ e. Hold arms forward at shoulder with palms up
    _____ f. Passive ROM to limbs
    _____ g. Applying dual stimulus a few millimeters
    apart on the tips of fingers
    _____ h. Simultaneously stimulating opposite sides
    of the body
    _____ i. Have the patient stand with feet close together
    and close the eyes
    _____ j. Tuning fork to bony prominences

    1. Hypertonia
    2. Loss of position sense
    3. Lack of vibratory sense
    4. Absence of two-point discrimination
    5. Analgesia
    6. Absence of light touch
    7. Sensory extinction
    8. Extension of the toes
    9. Lack of coordination
    10. Pronator drift

18. The normal response to striking the triceps tendon with a reflex hammer is
    a. forearm pronation.
    b. extension of the arm.
    c. flexion of the arm at the elbow.
    d. flexion and supination of the elbow.

19. Normal deep-tendon reflexes are graded as
    a. 1/5.
    b. 2/5.
    c. 3/5.
    d. 4/5.

20. To prepare a patient for a lumbar puncture, the nurse
    a. sedates the patient with medication before the test.
    b. withholds beverages containing caffeine for 8 hours.
    c. has the patient sit on the side of the bed, leaning on a padded over-the-bed table.
    d. positions the patient in a lateral recumbent position with the hips, knees, and neck flexed.

21. Following a lumbar puncture, the nurse assesses the patient for
    a. headache.
    b. lower limb paralysis.
    c. allergic reactions to the dye.
    d. hemorrhage from the puncture site.

22. Nursing care of the patient following a myelogram includes
    a. restricting fluids until the patient is ambulatory.
    b. keeping the patient positioned flat in bed for at least several hours.
    c. positioning the patient with the head of the bed elevated 30 degrees.
    d. providing mild analgesics for pain associated with the insertion of needles.

23. The neurologic diagnostic test that has the highest risk of complications and requires frequent monitoring of neurologic and vital signs following the procedure is
    a. a myelogram.
    b. cerebral angiography.
    c. an electroencephalogram.
    d. transcranial Doppler sonography.

24. In noting the results of an analysis of CSF, the nurse identifies as an abnormal finding a
    a. pH of 7.35.
    b. WBC count of 5/μL (0.005/L).
    c. clear, colorless appearance.
    d. glucose level of 30 mg/dL (1.7 mmol/L).

Nursing Management:
Acute Intracranial Problems

1. Identify two ways the following three-volume components of intracranial pressure (ICP) can be changed to adapt to small increases in intracranial pressure.
   a. Cerebrospinal fluid (CSF)
   b. Brain tissue
   c. Blood tissue

2. Complete the following statements related to ICP.
   a. Normal ICP ranges from _____ to _____ mm Hg.
   b. Autoregulation to maintain constant blood flow to the brain becomes ineffective when the MAP is below

   _____ mm Hg, and the brain becomes _____. Autoregulation also becomes ineffective when MAP

   is greater than _____ mm Hg because the vessels are maximally _____.
   c. The CPP is the pressure needed to ensure blood flow to the brain. Normal CPP is _____ mm Hg. Calculate

   the CPP of a patient whose blood pressure (BP) is 106/52 and ICP is 14 mm Hg: _____ mm Hg.
   d. A patient with an ICP of 34 mm Hg and a systemic BP of 108/64 has a CPP of _____ mm Hg.
   e. Cerebral ischemia and neuronal death occur when CPP is less than _____ mm Hg. A CPP less than

   _____ mm Hg is incompatible with life.

3. Indicate whether the following factors increase (I) or decrease (D) cerebral blood flow.
   _____ a. $PaCO_2$ of 30 mm Hg
   _____ b. PaO_2 of 45 mm Hg
   _____ c. Decreased MAP
   _____ d. Increased ICP
   _____ e. Arterial blood pH of 7.3

4. Match the common causes of cerebral edema with their related types (answers may be used more than once).
   _____ a. Destructive lesions or trauma   1. Vasogenic
   _____ b. Increased permeability of blood-brain barrier   2. Cytotoxic
   _____ c. Local disruption of cell membranes   3. Interstitial
   _____ d. Ingested toxins
   _____ e. Hydrocephalus

5. In the following events that occur in the progression of increased ICP, indicate whether the event is directly **caused by** (CB) increased ICP or is a **cause of** (CO) increased ICP (see Figure 57-3).
   _____ a. Tissue edema from initial insult
   _____ b. Edema of necrotic tissue
   _____ c. Compression of blood vessels
   _____ d. Vasodilation
   _____ e. Brainstem compression and herniation

6. The earliest signs of increased ICP the nurse should assess for include
   a. Cushing's triad.
   b. unexpected vomiting.
   c. decreasing level of consciousness (LOC).
   d. dilated pupil with sluggish response to light.

7. The nurse recognizes the presence of Cushing's triad in the patient with
   a. increased pulse, irregular respiration, increased BP.
   b. decreased pulse, irregular respiration, increased pulse pressure.
   c. increased pulse, decreased respiration, increased pulse pressure.
   d. decreased pulse, increased respiration, decreased systolic BP.

8. Increased ICP in the left cerebral cortex caused by intracranial bleeding causes displacement of brain tissue to the right hemisphere beneath the falx cerebri. The nurse knows that this is referred to as
   a. uncal herniation.
   b. tentorial herniation.
   c. cingulate herniation.
   d. temporal lobe herniation.

9. *Priority Decision:* A patient has ICP monitoring with an intraventricular catheter. A priority nursing intervention for the patient is
   a. aseptic technique to prevent infection.
   b. constant monitoring of ICP waveforms.
   c. removal of CSF to maintain normal ICP.
   d. sampling CSF to determine abnormalities.

10. Identify whether the following statements are true (*T*) or false (*F*). If a statement is false, correct the bold word(s) to make the statement true.
    _____ a. During ICP monitoring, the patient may be at risk for development of increased ICP when the height of the **P2 wave** is higher than the **P1 wave**.
    _____ b. The transducer of an ICP monitor should be level to the **phlebostatic axis**.
    _____ c. When ICP is measured using a CSF drainage device, the drain must be closed for at least **6 minutes** to get an accurate reading.
    _____ d. A complication of removal of CSF during ICP monitoring to control ICP is **ventricular collapse**.
    _____ e. The **jugular venous bulb catheter** provides direct measurement of brain oxygenation and temperature.
    _____ f. The normal range for the pressure of oxygen in brain tissue (PbtO$_2$) is **20-40 mm Hg**.

11. Match the following treatments used to manage increased ICP with their effects.
    _____ a. Oxygen administration   1. Decreased cerebral metabolism
    _____ b. Hypertonic saline   2. Prevention of hypoxia
    _____ c. Osmotic diuretics   3. Decreased volume of brain water
    _____ d. Dexamethasone (Decadron)   4. Increased osmolality of brain ECF
    _____ e. Barbiturates   5. Decreased lesion edema

12. Metabolic and nutritional needs of the patient with increased ICP are best met with
    a. enteral feedings that are low in sodium.
    b. the simple glucose available in D$_5$W IV solutions.
    c. a fluid restriction that promotes a moderate dehydration.
    d. balanced, essential nutrition in a form that the patient can tolerate.

13. The three criteria assessed by the Glasgow Coma Scale (GCS) are
    a.

    b.

    c.

14. A patient with an intracranial problem does not open his eyes to any stimulus, has no verbal response except moaning and muttering when stimulated, and flexes his arm in response to painful stimuli. The nurse records the patient's GCS score as
    a. 6.
    b. 7.
    c. 9.
    d. 11.

15. When assessing the body functions of a patient with increased ICP, the nurse should initially assess
    a. corneal reflex testing.
    b. extremity strength testing.
    c. pupillary reaction to light.
    d. circulatory and respiratory status.

16. CN III originating in the midbrain is assessed by the nurse for an early indication of pressure on the brainstem by
    a. assessing for nystagmus.
    b. testing the corneal reflex.
    c. testing pupillary reaction to light.
    d. testing for oculocephalic (doll's eyes) reflex.

17. A patient has a nursing diagnosis of risk for ineffective cerebral tissue perfusion related to cerebral edema. An appropriate nursing intervention for the patient is
    a. avoiding positioning the patient with neck and hip flexion.
    b. maintaining hyperventilation to a $PaCO_2$ of 15 to 20 mm Hg.
    c. clustering nursing activities to provide periods of uninterrupted rest.
    d. routine suctioning to prevent accumulation of respiratory secretions.

18. An unconscious patient with increased ICP is on ventilatory support. The nurse notifies the health care provider when arterial blood gas (ABG) measurement results reveal a
    a. pH of 7.43.
    b. SaO_2 of 94%.
    c. PaO_2 of 50 mm Hg.
    d. $PaCO_2$ of 30 mm Hg.

19. The nurse is monitoring a patient for increased ICP following a head injury. Which of the following manifestations indicate an increased ICP (select all that apply)?
    a. fever
    b. oriented to name only
    c. narrowing pulse pressure
    d. dilated right pupil > left pupil
    e. decorticate posturing to painful stimulus

20. While the nurse performs ROM on an unconscious patient with increased ICP, the patient experiences severe decerebrate posturing reflexes. The nurse should
    a. use restraints to protect the patient from injury.
    b. administer CNS depressants to lightly sedate the patient.
    c. perform the exercises less frequently because posturing can increase ICP.
    d. continue the exercises because they are necessary to maintain musculoskeletal function.

21. Match the following types of head injury with their descriptions.
    _____ a. Linear skull fracture
    _____ b. Depressed skull fracture
    _____ c. Compound skull fracture
    _____ d. Comminuted skull fracture
    _____ e. Basilar skull fracture
    _____ f. Posterior fossa fracture
    _____ g. Frontal lobe skull fracture
    _____ h. Orbital skull fracture
    _____ i. Parietal skull fracture
    _____ j. Temporal skull fracture
    _____ k. Cerebral concussion
    _____ l. Cerebral contusion

    1. Depressed skull fracture and scalp lacerations with communication to intracranial cavity
    2. Temporary, minor injury with transient reduction in neural activity and level of consciousness (LOC)
    3. Possible pneumocranium, CSF rhinorrhea
    4. Fractured skull without alteration in fragments
    5. Bruising of brain, often associated with coup-contrecoup injury
    6. May involve dural tear with CSF otorrhea, vertigo, and Battles' sign
    7. Multiple linear fracture with fragmentation of bone
    8. Causes periorbital ecchymosis
    9. Inward indentation of the skull with possible pressure on brain
    10. Cortical blindness or visual-field defects
    11. Boggy temporal muscle because of extravasation of blood
    12. May cause deafness, loss of taste, and CSF otorrhea

22. A patient with a head injury has bloody drainage from the ear. To determine whether CSF is present in the drainage, the nurse
    a. examines the tympanic membrane for a tear.
    b. tests the fluid for a halo sign on a white dressing.
    c. tests the fluid with a glucose-identifying strip or stick.
    d. collects 5 mL of fluid in a test tube and sends it to the laboratory for analysis.

23. The nurse suspects the presence of an arterial epidural hematoma in the patient who experiences
    a. failure to regain consciousness following a head injury.
    b. a rapid deterioration of neurologic function within 24 to 48 hours following a head injury.
    c. nonspecific, nonlocalizing progression of alteration in LOC occurring over weeks or months.
    d. unconsciousness at the time of a head injury with a brief period of consciousness followed by a decrease in LOC.

24. Skull radiographs and a computed tomography (CT) scan provide evidence of a depressed parietal fracture with a subdural hematoma in a patient admitted to the emergency department following an automobile accident. In planning care for the patient, the nurse anticipates that
    a. the patient will receive life-support measures until the condition stabilizes.
    b. immediate burr holes will be made to rapidly decompress the intracranial cavity.
    c. the patient will be treated conservatively with close monitoring for changes in neurologic status.
    d. the patient will be taken to surgery for a craniotomy for evacuation of blood and decompression of the cranium.

25. *Priority Decision:* When a patient is admitted to the emergency department following a head injury, the nurse's first priority in management of the patient once a patent airway is confirmed is
    a. maintaining cervical spine precautions.
    b. determining the presence of increased ICP.
    c. monitoring for changes in neurologic status.
    d. establishing IV access with a large-bore catheter.

26. A 54-year-old man is recovering from a skull fracture with a subacute subdural hematoma. He has return of motor control and orientation but appears apathetic and has reduced awareness of his environment. When planning discharge of the patient, the nurse explains to the patient and the family that
    a. continuous improvement in the patient's condition should occur until he has returned to pretrauma status.
    b. the patient's complete recovery may take years, and the family should plan for his long-term dependent care.
    c. the patient is likely to have long-term emotional and mental changes that may require continued professional help.
    d. role changes in family members will be necessary because the patient will be dependent on his family for care and support.

27. Identify whether the following statements are true (*T*) or false (*F*). If a statement is false, correct the bold word(s) to make the statement true.
    _____ a. Without treatment, **only malignant** brain tumors will cause death as a result of increased growth leading to increased ICP and compression of vital brain centers.
    _____ b. Symptoms of visual disturbances and seizures may indicate a tumor of the **temporal** lobe.
    _____ c. The most common malignant brain tumor is **an astrocytoma**.
    _____ d. Tumors that are considered inoperable are those located in the upper brainstem or **deep in the dominant hemisphere**.
    _____ e. Radiation therapy for brain tumors may cause serious **increases in ICP**.

28. Assisting the family to understand what is happening to the patient is an especially important role of the nurse when the patient has a tumor of the
    a. ventricles.
    b. frontal lobe.
    c. parietal lobe.
    d. occipital lobe.

29. Match the following types of cranial surgery with their descriptions.
    _____ a. Burr holes
    _____ b. Craniotomy
    _____ c. Craniectomy
    _____ d. Cranioplasty
    _____ e. Sterotactic surgery
    _____ f. Shunt procedures

    1. Excision of cranial bone without replacement
    2. Three-dimensional targeting of cranial tissue
    3. Placement of tubes to redirect CSF from one area to another
    4. Opening into cranium with a drill to remove blood and fluid
    5. Replacement of part of the cranium with an artificial plate
    6. Opening into cranium with removal of bone flap to open dura

30. For the patient undergoing a craniotomy, the nurse provides information about the use of wigs and hairpieces or other methods to disguise hair loss
    a. during preoperative teaching.
    b. if the patient asks about their use.
    c. in the immediate postoperative period.
    d. when the patient expresses negative feelings about his or her appearance.

31. Successful achievement of patient outcomes for the patient with cranial surgery would best be indicated by the
    a. ability to return home in 6 days.
    b. ability to meet all self-care needs.
    c. acceptance of residual neurologic deficits.
    d. absence of signs and symptoms of increased ICP.

32. Indicate whether the following descriptions are characteristic of meningitis (M) or encephalitis (E).
    _____ a. Most frequently caused by bacteria
    _____ b. Is an inflammation of the brain
    _____ c. May be transmitted by insect vectors
    _____ d. CSF production is increased
    _____ e. Almost always has a viral cause
    _____ f. Involves an inflammation of pia mater and arachnoid layer
    _____ g. Has a rapid onset of symptoms
    _____ h. Cerebral edema is a major problem
    _____ i. Exudate may impair normal CSF flow and absorption

33. A patient is admitted to the hospital with possible bacterial meningitis. During the initial assessment, the nurse questions the patient about a recent history of
    a. mosquito or tick bites.
    b. chickenpox or measles.
    c. cold sores or fever blisters.
    d. an upper respiratory infection.

34. Classic symptoms of bacterial meningitis include
    a. papilledema and psychomotor seizures.
    b. high fever, nuchal rigidity, and severe headache.
    c. behavioral changes with memory loss and lethargy.
    d. positive Kernig's and Brudzinski's signs and hemiparesis.

35. Vigorous control of fever in the patient with meningitis is required to prevent complications. Identify four undesirable effects of fever in the patient with meningitis.
    a.

    b.

    c.

    d.

36. On physical examination of a patient with headache and fever, the nurse would suspect a brain abscess when the patient has
    a. seizures.
    b. nuchal rigidity.
    c. focal symptoms.
    d. signs of increased ICP.

CASE STUDY

Neurologic Complications

Patient Profile

J.K., a 16-year-old unrestrained driver, suffered a compound fracture of the skull and facial fractures in a motor vehicle accident. On admission to the hospital, he was immediately taken to surgery for evacuation of a right subdural hematoma in the temporal region and repair of facial fractures. On the fourth postoperative day, the nurse discovers the following findings during assessment of J.K.

Subjective Data

• Increasingly difficult to arouse

Objective Data

• GCS decreased from 10 to 5
• Signs of nuchal rigidity
• Vital signs: T 102.2° F (39° C); BP 110/60; HR 114
• ICP ranges between 20 and 30 mm Hg despite CSF drainage and mannitol

---

Clinical Decision-Making Questions

Using a separate sheet of paper, answer the following questions.

1. What is the probable cause of J.K.'s change in neurologic status?
2. What were the contributing factors that put J.K. at risk for complications after a head injury and surgery?
3. Discuss the pathophysiologic basis for the symptoms exhibited by J.K.
4. *Priority Decision:* On the basis of the nursing assessment, what are the priority interventions?
5. Discuss the possible areas for organisms to gain access to the meninges in the case of J.K.
6. *Priority Decision:* Based on the assessment data presented, what are the priority nursing diagnoses? Are there any collaborative problems?

Nursing Management: Stroke

1. In promoting health maintenance for prevention of strokes, the nurse understands that the highest risk for the most common type of stroke is present in
   a. African Americans.
   b. women who smoke.
   c. individuals with hypertension and diabetes.
   d. those who are obese with high dietary-fat intake.

2. A thrombus that develops in a cerebral artery does not always cause a loss of neurologic function because
   a. the body can dissolve atherosclerotic plaques as they form.
   b. some tissues of the brain do not require constant blood supply to prevent damage.
   c. circulation through the circle of Willis may provide blood supply to the affected area of the brain.
   d. neurologic deficits occur only when major arteries are occluded by thrombus formation around an atherosclerotic plaque.

3. A patient comes to the emergency department immediately after experiencing numbness of the face and an inability to speak, but while the patient awaits examination, the symptoms disappear and the patient requests discharge. The nurse stresses that it is important for the patient to be evaluated primarily because
   a. the patient has probably experienced an asymptomatic lacunar stroke.
   b. the symptoms are likely to return and progress to worsening neurologic deficit in the next 24 hours.
   c. neurologic deficits that are transient occur most often as a result of small hemorrhages that clot off.
   d. the patient has probably experienced a transient ischemic attack (TIA), which is a sign of progressive cerebral vascular disease.

4. Match the characteristics with their related type of stroke (answers may be used more than once).
   _____ a. Onset unrelated to activity
   _____ b. Rupture of atherosclerotic vessels
   _____ c. Carries the poorest prognosis
   _____ d. Type most often signaled by TIAs
   _____ e. High initial mortality
   _____ f. Creates mass that compresses brain
   _____ g. Symptoms of meningeal irritation
   _____ h. Commonly occurs during or after sleep
   _____ i. Quick onset and resolution
   _____ j. Caused by rupture of intracranial aneurysm
   _____ k. Strong association with hypertension
   _____ l. Associated with sudden, severe headache
   _____ m. Associated with endocardial disorders

   1. Thrombotic
   2. Embolic
   3. Intracerebral hemorrhage
   4. Subarachnoid hemorrhage

5. The neurologic functions that are affected by a stroke are primarily related to
   a. the amount of tissue area involved.
   b. the rapidity of the onset of symptoms.
   c. the brain area perfused by the affected artery.
   d. the presence or absence of collateral circulation.

6. Indicate whether the following manifestations of a stroke are more likely to occur with right brain damage (R) or left brain damage (L).
   _____ a. Aphasia
   _____ b. Left homonymous hemianopsia
   _____ c. Agnosia
   _____ d. Quick, impulsive behavior
   _____ e. Inability to remember words
   _____ f. Neglect of the left side of the body

7. Identify whether the following statements are true (*T*) or false (*F*). If a statement is false, correct the bold word(s) to make the statement true.
   _____ a. **Receptive** aphasia is characterized by a lack of comprehension of both verbal and written language.
   _____ b. **Dysarthria** results from a disturbance in Broca's area and is an impairment in speaking and writing.
   _____ c. A lesion that affects both Wernicke's area and Broca's area is most likely to cause **global** aphasia.
   _____ d. A **nonfluent dysphasia** is characterized by the presence of speech that contains little meaningful communication.
   _____ e. The long-term effect of paralysis of an extremity resulting from a stroke is **flaccidity**.

8. A patient is admitted to the hospital with a left hemiplegia. To determine the size and location and to ascertain whether a stroke is ischemic or hemorrhagic, the nurse anticipates that the health care provider will request a
   a. CT scan.
   b. lumbar puncture.
   c. cerebral arteriogram.
   d. positron emission tomography (PET).

9. A carotid endarterectomy is being considered as treatment for a patient who has had several TIAs. The nurse explains to the patient that this surgery
   a. is used to restore blood circulation to the brain following an obstruction of a cerebral artery.
   b. involves intracranial surgery to join a superficial extracranial artery to an intracranial artery.
   c. involves removing an atherosclerotic plaque in the carotid artery to prevent an impending stroke.
   d. is used to open a stenosis in a carotid artery with a balloon and stent to restore cerebral circulation.

10. The incidence of ischemic stroke in patients with TIAs and other risk factors is reduced with the administration of
    a. furosemide (Lasix).
    b. lovastatin (Mevacor).
    c. daily low-dose aspirin.
    d. nimodipine (Nimotop).

11. *Priority Decision:* The priority intervention in the emergency department for the patient with a stroke is
    a. intravenous fluid replacement.
    b. administration of osmotic diuretics to reduce cerebral edema.
    c. initiation of hypothermia to decrease the oxygen needs of the brain.
    d. maintenance of respiratory function with a patent airway and oxygen administration.

12. A diagnosis of a ruptured cerebral aneurysm has been made in a patient with manifestations of a stroke. The nurse anticipates that treatment options that would be evaluated for the patient include
    a. hyperventilation therapy.
    b. surgical clipping of the aneurysm.
    c. administration of hyperosmotic agents.
    d. administration of thrombolytic therapy.

13. During the acute phase of a stroke, the nurse assesses the patient's vital signs and neurologic status every 4 hours. A cardiovascular sign that the nurse would see as the body attempts to increase cerebral blood flow is
    a. hypertension.
    b. fluid overload.
    c. cardiac dysrhythmias.
    d. S_3 and S_4 heart sounds.

14. Identify four nursing diagnoses in which impaired neuromotor function can be an etiologic factor.

a.

b.

c.

d.

15. A nursing intervention that is indicated for the patient with hemiplegia is
    a. the use of a footboard to prevent plantar flexion.
    b. immobilization of the affected arm against the chest with a sling.
    c. positioning the patient in bed with each joint lower than the joint proximal to it.
    d. having the patient perform passive ROM of the affected limb with the unaffected limb.

16. A newly admitted patient who has suffered a right-sided brain stroke has a nursing diagnosis of disturbed visual sensory perception related to homonymous hemianopsia. Early in the care of the patient, the nurse should
    a. place objects on the right side within the patient's field of vision.
    b. approach the patient from the left side to encourage the patient to turn the head.
    c. place objects on the patient's left side to assess the patient's ability to compensate.
    d. patch the affected eye to encourage the patient to turn the head to scan the environment.

17. Four days following a stroke, a patient is to start oral fluids and feedings. Before feeding the patient, the nurse should first
    a. check the patient's gag reflex.
    b. order a soft diet for the patient.
    c. raise the head of the bed to a sitting position.
    d. evaluate the patient's ability to swallow small sips of ice water.

18. An appropriate food for a patient with a stroke who has mild dysphagia is
    a. fruit juices.
    b. pureed meat.
    c. scrambled eggs.
    d. fortified milkshakes.

19. A patient's wife asks the nurse why her husband did not receive the clot busting medication (tPA) she has been reading about. Her husband is diagnosed with a hemorrhagic stroke. What should the nurse respond?
    a. "He didn't arrive within the time frame for that therapy."
    b. "Not everyone is eligible for this drug. Has he had surgery lately?"
    c. "You should discuss the treatment of your husband with his doctor."
    d. "The medication you are talking about dissolves clots and could cause more bleeding in your husband's head."

20. To promote communication during rehabilitation of the patient with aphasia, an appropriate nursing intervention is to
    a. use gestures, pictures, and music to stimulate patient responses.
    b. talk about activities of daily living (ADLs) that are familiar to the patient.
    c. structure statements so that the patient does not have to respond verbally.
    d. use flashcards with simple words and pictures to promote language recall.

21. A patient with a right hemisphere stroke has a nursing diagnosis of unilateral neglect related to sensory-perceptual deficits. During the patient's rehabilitation, it is important for the nurse to
    a. avoid positioning the patient on the affected side.
    b. place all objects for care on the patient's unaffected side.
    c. teach the patient to care consciously for the affected side.
    d. protect the affected side from injury with pillows and supports.

22. A patient with a stroke has a right-sided hemiplegia. The nurse prepares family members to help control behavior changes seen with this type of stroke by teaching them to
    a. ignore undesirable behaviors manifested by the patient.
    b. provide directions to the patient verbally in small steps.
    c. distract the patient from inappropriate emotional responses.
    d. supervise all activities before allowing the patient to pursue them independently.

23. The nurse can assist the patient and the family in coping with the long-term effects of a stroke by
    a. informing family members that the patient will need assistance with almost all ADLs.
    b. explaining that the patient's prestroke behavior will return as improvement progresses.
    c. encouraging the patient and family members to seek assistance from family therapy or stroke support groups.
    d. helping the patient and family understand the significance of residual stroke damage to promote problem-solving and planning.

24. *Delegation Decision:* Which intervention should the nurse delegate to the LPN when caring for a patient following an acute stroke?
    a. assess the patient's neurologic status
    b. assess patient's gag reflex before beginning feeding
    c. administer ordered antihypertensives and platelet inhibitors
    d. teach the patient's caregivers strategies to minimize unilateral neglect

---

CASE STUDY

Stroke

Patient Profile

R.C., a 38-year-old married woman, was admitted unconscious to the hospital after her family could not rouse her in the morning. She was accompanied by her husband and three daughters, ages 10, 13, and 15.

Subjective Data

- Has no history of hypertension or other health problems
- Had complained of a headache the day before she developed unconsciousness

Objective Data

- Diagnostic tests reveal a subarachnoid hemorrhage
- Vital signs: BP 150/82; RR 16; HR 56; T 101° F (38.3° C)
- Glasgow Coma Scale score: 5

Clinical Decision-Making Questions

Using a separate sheet of paper, answer the following questions.

1. What diagnostic tests would be indicated to determine the cause of R.C.'s unconsciousness?
2. What signs of increased intracranial pressure are present in R.C.?
3. What should the family be told to expect in terms of R.C.'s condition?
4. *Priority Decision:* What nursing interventions have the highest priority for R.C. at this stage of her illness?
5. What treatment modalities indicated for thrombotic strokes are contraindicated for R.C.?
6. What therapeutic options are available for the patient with a hemorrhagic stroke resulting from a ruptured aneurysm?
7. *Priority Decision:* Based on the assessment data presented, what are the priority nursing diagnoses? Are there any collaborative problems?

Nursing Management:
Chronic Neurologic Problems

1. Match the following characteristics with their related type of headache (answers may be used more than once).
   _____ a. Alcohol is the only dietary trigger
   _____ b. Chronic, dull, persisting intermittently over months or years
   _____ c. Strong family history
   _____ d. Bilateral pressure or tightness sensation
   _____ e. Commonly recurs several times a day for several weeks
   _____ f. May occur with or between migraine headaches
   _____ g. Severe, sharp, penetrating head pain
   _____ h. May be accompanied by unilateral ptosis or lacrimation
   _____ i. May be accompanied by nausea, vomiting, and irritability.
   _____ j. Abrupt onset lasting 5-180 minutes
   _____ k. Unilateral or bilateral throbbing pain
   _____ l. May be preceded by prodrome

   1. Tension-type
   2. Migraine
   3. Cluster

2. The most important method of diagnosing functional headaches is
   a. EMG.
   b. CT scan.
   c. cerebral blood flow studies.
   d. a thorough history of the headache.

3. Drug therapy for acute migraine and cluster headaches that appears to alter the pathophysiologic process includes
   a. β-adrenergic blockers such as propranolol (Inderal).
   b. serotonin antagonists such as methysergide (Sansert).
   c. tricyclic antidepressants such as amitriptyline (Elavil).
   d. specific serotonin receptor agonists such as sumatriptan (Imitrex).

4. A nursing intervention that is appropriate for the patient with a nursing diagnosis of anxiety related to lack of knowledge of etiology and treatment of headache is to
   a. help the patient examine lifestyle patterns and precipitating factors.
   b. administer medications as ordered to relieve pain and promote relaxation.
   c. provide a quiet, dimly lit environment to reduce stimuli that increase muscle tension and anxiety.
   d. support the patient's use of counseling or psychotherapy to enhance conflict resolution and stress reduction.

5. *Delegation Decision:* The nurse is preparing to admit a newly diagnosed patient experiencing tonic-clonic seizures. Which of the actions could the nurse delegate to nursing assistive personnel (NAP)?
   a. complete the admission assessment
   b. explain the call system to the patient
   c. obtain the suction equipment from the supply cabinet
   d. place a padded tongue blade on the wall above the patient's bed

6. Generalized seizures differ from partial seizures in that
   a. partial seizures are confined to one side of the brain and remain focal in nature.
   b. generalized seizures result in loss of consciousness whereas partial seizures do not.
   c. generalized seizures result in temporary residual deficits during the postictal phase.
   d. generalized seizures have no warning because the entire brain is affected at the onset.

7. Match the following characteristics with their related types of seizures (answers may be used more than once).

_____ a. Also known as petit mal seizure

_____ b. Sudden, excessive jerk of body that may hurl the person to the ground

_____ c. Often involve behavioral, emotional, and cognitive functions with altered consciousness

_____ d. Often accompanied by incontinence or tongue or cheek biting

_____ e. Brief staring spell accompanied by peculiar behavior during seizure or postictal confusion

_____ f. Focal motor, sensory, or autonomic symptoms without loss of consciousness

_____ g. Formerly known as grand mal seizure

_____ h. Falling spell from loss of muscle tone accompanied by brief unconsciousness

_____ i. Staring spell lasting a few seconds

_____ j. Psychomotor seizures with repetitive behaviors and lip smacking

_____ k. Alterations in memory, sexual sensations, and distortions of visual or auditory sensations

_____ l. Loss of consciousness, stiffening of the body with subsequent jerking of extremities

_____ m. Known as temporal lobe seizures

_____ n. Very brief and may occur in clusters

1. Generalized tonic-clonic
2. Typical absence
3. Atypical absence
4. Myoclonic
5. Atonic
6. Simple partial
7. Complex partial

8. Identify whether the following statements are true (*T*) or false (*F*). If a statement is false, correct the bold word(s) to make the statement true.

_____ a. Status epilepticus is most serious in **tonic-clonic seizures** because it can cause ventilatory insufficiency and hypoxemia.

_____ b. Permanent brain damage may occur from status epilepticus of **any type of** seizure.

_____ c. The most useful tool for diagnosing epilepsy is **the EEG**.

_____ d. Immediate medical care should be sought for **all** seizures.

_____ e. A tonic-clonic seizure with loss of consciousness that is preceded by an aura is a **partial** seizure that generalizes.

9. A patient admitted to the hospital following a generalized tonic-clonic seizure asks the nurse what caused the seizure. The best response by the nurse is,
   a. "So many factors can cause epilepsy that it is impossible to say what caused your seizure."
   b. "Epilepsy is an inherited disorder. Does anyone else in your family have a seizure disorder?"
   c. "In seizures, some type of trigger causes sudden, abnormal bursts of electrical brain activity."
   d. "Scar tissue in the brain alters the chemical balance, creating uncontrolled electrical discharges."

10. A patient with a seizure disorder is being evaluated for surgical treatment of the seizures. The nurse recognizes that one of the requirements for surgical treatment is
    a. identification of scar tissue that is able to be removed.
    b. an adequate trial of drug therapy that had unsatisfactory results.
    c. development of toxic syndromes from long-term use of antiseizure drugs.
    d. the presence of symptoms of cerebral degeneration from repeated seizures.

11. The nurse teaches the patient taking antiseizure drugs that the method most commonly used to measure compliance and to monitor for toxicity is
    a. monthly EEGs.
    b. a daily seizure log.
    c. urine testing for drug levels.
    d. blood testing for drug levels.

12. When teaching a patient with a seizure disorder about the medication regimen, it is most important for the nurse to stress that
    a. the patient should increase the dosage of the medication if stress is increased.
    b. most over-the-counter and prescription drugs are safe to take with antiseizure drugs.
    c. stopping the medication abruptly may increase the intensity and frequency of seizures.
    d. if gingival hypertrophy occurs, the drug should be stopped and the health care provider notified.

13. The nurse finds a patient in bed having a generalized tonic-clonic seizure. During the seizure activity, the nurse should take the following actions (select all that apply)
    a. loosen restrictive clothing.
    b. turn the patient to the side.
    c. protect the patient's head from injury.
    d. place a padded tongue blade between the patient's teeth.
    e. restrain the patient's extremities to prevent soft tissue and bone injury.

14. Following a generalized tonic-clonic seizure, the patient is tired and sleepy. The nurse should
    a. suction the patient before allowing him to rest.
    b. allow the patient to sleep as long as he feels sleepy.
    c. stimulate the patient to increase his level of consciousness.
    d. check the patient's level of consciousness every 15 minutes for an hour.

15. During the diagnosis and long-term management of a seizure disorder, the nurse recognizes that one of the major needs of the patient is assistance to
    a. manage the complicated drug regimen of seizure control.
    b. cope with the effects of negative social attitudes toward epilepsy.
    c. adjust to the very restricted lifestyle required by a diagnosis of epilepsy.
    d. learn to minimize the effect of the condition in order to obtain employment.

16. Match the chronic neurologic disorders with their pathophysiologic descriptions.
    _____ a. Multiple sclerosis (MS)
    _____ b. Parkinson's disease
    _____ c. Myasthenia gravis
    _____ d. Huntington's disease
    _____ e. Amyotrophic lateral sclerosis (ALS)

    1. Degeneration of motor neurons in brainstem and spinal cord
    2. Deficiency of acetylcholine and GABA in basal ganglia and extrapyramidal system
    3. Immune-mediated inflammatory destruction of myelin and replacement with glial scar tissue
    4. Autoimmune antibody destruction of cholinergic receptors at the neuromuscular junction
    5. Degeneration of dopamine-producing neurons in substantia nigra of midbrain and basal ganglia

17. A 38-year-old woman has newly diagnosed MS and asks the nurse what is going to happen to her. The best response by the nurse is,
    a. "You need to plan for a continuous loss of movement, sensory functions, and mental capabilities."
    b. "Most people with MS have periods of attacks and remissions, with progressively more nerve damage over time."
    c. "You will most likely have a steady course of chronic progressive nerve damage that will change your personality."
    d. "It is common for people with MS to have an acute attack of weakness and then not have any other symptoms for years."

18. During assessment of a patient admitted to the hospital with an acute exacerbation of MS, the nurse would expect to find
    a. tremors, dysphasia, and ptosis.
    b. bowel and bladder incontinence and loss of memory.
    c. motor impairment, visual disturbances, and paresthesias.
    d. excessive involuntary movements, hearing loss, and ataxia.

19. The nurse explains to a patient newly diagnosed with MS that the diagnosis is made primarily by
    a. T-cell analysis of the blood.
    b. analysis of cerebrospinal fluid.
    c. history and clinical manifestations.
    d. magnetic resonance imaging (MRI) findings.

20. Mitoxantrone (Novantrone) is being considered as treatment for a patient with progressive-relapsing MS. The nurse explains that a disadvantage of this drug compared with other drugs used for MS is that it
    a. must be given subcutaneously every day.
    b. has a lifetime dose limit because of cardiac toxicity.
    c. is an anticholinergic agent that causes urinary incontinence.
    d. is an immunosuppressant agent that increases the risk for infection.

21. A patient with MS has a nursing diagnosis of self-care deficit related to muscle spasticity and neuromuscular deficits. In providing care for the patient, it is most important for the nurse to
    a. perform all ADLs for the patient to conserve the patient's energy.
    b. teach the family members how to care adequately for the patient's needs.
    c. encourage the patient to maintain social interactions to prevent social isolation.
    d. promote the use of assistive devices so the patient can participate in self-care activities.

22. A patient with newly diagnosed MS has been hospitalized for evaluation and initial treatment of the disease. Following discharge teaching, the nurse realizes that additional instruction is needed when the patient says,
    a. "It is important for me to avoid exposure to people with upper respiratory infections."
    b. "When I begin to feel better, I should stop taking the prednisone to prevent side effects."
    c. "I plan to use vitamin supplements and a high-protein diet to help manage my condition."
    d. "I must plan with my family how we are going to manage my care if I become more incapacitated."

23. List the classic triad of signs associated with Parkinson's disease, and identify one consequence in patient function for each of the signs.
    a.

    b.

    c.

24. A patient with a tremor is evaluated for Parkinson's disease. The nurse explains to the patient that Parkinson's disease can be confirmed by
    a. CT and MRI scans.
    b. relief of symptoms with administration of dopaminergic agents.
    c. the presence of tremors that increase during voluntary movement.
    d. a cerebral angiogram that reveals the presence of cerebral atherosclerosis.

25. An observation of the patient made by the nurse that is most indicative of Parkinson's disease is
    a. large, embellished handwriting.
    b. weakness of one leg resulting in a limping walk.
    c. difficulty arising from a chair and beginning to walk.
    d. the onset of muscle spasms occurring with voluntary movement.

26. A patient with Parkinson's disease is started on levodopa. The nurse explains that this drug
    a. stimulates dopamine receptors in the basal ganglia.
    b. promotes the release of dopamine from brain neurons.
    c. is a precursor of dopamine that is converted into dopamine in the brain.
    d. prevents the excessive breakdown of dopamine in the peripheral tissues.

27. To reduce the risk for falls in the patient with Parkinson's disease, the nurse teaches the patient to
    a. use an elevated toilet seat.
    b. use a walker or cane for support.
    c. consciously lift the toes when stepping.
    d. rock side to side to initiate leg movements.

28. A patient with myasthenia gravis is admitted to the hospital with respiratory insufficiency and severe weakness. A diagnosis of cholinergic crisis is made when
    a. the patient's respiration is impaired because of muscle weakness.
    b. administration of edrophonium (Tensilon) increases muscle weakness.
    c. the edrophonium (Tensilon) test results in improved muscle contractility.
    d. electromyography reveals decreased response to repeated stimulation of muscles.

29. ***Priority Decision:*** During care of a patient in myasthenic crisis, the nurse's first priority for the patient is maintenance of
    a. mobility.
    b. nutrition.
    c. respiratory function.
    d. verbal communication.

30. A patient at the clinic for a routine health examination mentions that she is exhausted because her legs bother her so much at night that she cannot sleep. The nurse questions the patient further about her leg symptoms with the knowledge that if she has "restless legs syndrome,"
    a. the condition can be readily diagnosed with electromyography.
    b. other more serious nervous system dysfunctions may be present.
    c. dopaminergic agents are often effective in managing the symptoms.
    d. the symptoms can be controlled by vigorous exercise of the legs during the day.

31. When providing care for a patient with amyotrophic lateral sclerosis (ALS), the nurse recognizes that one of the most distressing problems experienced by the patient is
    a. painful spasticity of the face and extremities.
    b. retention of cognitive function with total degeneration of motor function.
    c. uncontrollable writhing and twisting movements of the face, limbs, and body.
    d. the knowledge that there is a 50% chance the disease has been passed to any offspring.

32. In providing care for patients with chronic, progressive neurologic disease, the major goal of treatment that the nurse works toward is to
    a. meet the patient's personal care needs.
    b. return the patient to normal neurologic function.
    c. maximize neurologic functioning as long as possible.
    d. prevent the development of additional chronic diseases.

CASE STUDY
Multiple Sclerosis
Patient Profile

D.S., a 32-year-old white woman, born and raised in Minneapolis, is diagnosed with MS after an episode of numbness and tingling on the left side of her body that started several months ago. Two years ago she had an episode of optic neuritis in the right eye.

Subjective Data

- Difficulty seeing out of the right eye
- Numbness and tingling on the left side that worsens in hot weather
- Tires easily
- Used all sick days at work; concerned about losing her job and her ability to care for her 3-year-old son

Objective Data

- Crying softly during the interview
- Appears tense and anxious
- Prolonged visual evoked response in right eye
- MRI scan of head shows several plaques in white matter

Clinical Decision-Making Questions

Using a separate sheet of paper, answer the following questions.

1. What is the pathophysiology of MS?
2. What precipitating factors for MS are present in D.S.'s life?
3. Why did it take so long for a definitive diagnosis to be made for D.S.?
4. *Priority Decision:* What are the priority teaching needs for D.S.?
5. What treatment would be appropriate for D.S.?
6. *Priority Decision:* Based on the assessment data presented, what are the priority nursing diagnoses? Are there any collaborative problems?

CHAPTER 60

Nursing Management: Alzheimer's Disease, Dementia, and Delirium

1. Identify the following manifestations of cognitive impairment as primarily characteristic of delirium (DL) or dementia (DM).
   _____ a. Reduced awareness
   _____ b. Impaired judgments
   _____ c. Sleep-wake cycle reversed
   _____ d. Distorted thinking and perception
   _____ e. Words difficult to find
   _____ f. Course fluctuates; lucid intervals
   _____ g. Insidious onset with prolonged course and duration
   _____ h. Struggles to perform well with mental status testing
   _____ i. Orientation fluctuates in severity
   _____ j. Generally normal alertness

2. Identify whether the following statements are true (*T*) or false (*F*). If a statement is false, correct the bold word(s) to make the statement true.
   _____ a. The two major causes of dementia are **neurodegenerative conditions** and **multi-infarction**.
   _____ b. **Neurodegenerative** dementia can be diagnosed by brain lesions identified with neuroimaging.
   _____ c. Dementia caused by hepatic or renal **encephalopathy** is potentially reversible.
   _____ d. Dementia resulting from **vascular** causes can be prevented.
   _____ e. A genetic mutation that has been found in some patients with Alzheimer's disease (AD) causes overproduction of **tau proteins**.

3. A patient with dementia has manifestations of depression. The nurse knows that treatment of the patient with antidepressants will most likely
   a. improve cognitive function.
   b. not alter the course of either condition.
   c. cause interactions with the drugs used to treat the dementia.
   d. be contraindicated because of the CNS-depressant effect of antidepressants.

4. The nurse uses the Mini-Mental State Examination to evaluate a patient with cognitive impairment primarily because this test
   a. is a good tool to evaluate mood and thought processes.
   b. is a good tool to determine the etiology of dementia.
   c. can help document the degree of cognitive impairment in delirium and dementia.
   d. is useful for initial evaluation of mental status, but additional tools are needed to evaluate cognition changes over time.

5. During assessment of a patient with dementia, the nurse determines that the condition is potentially reversible on finding that the patient
   a. has long-standing abuse of alcohol.
   b. has a history of Parkinson's disease.
   c. was infected with the HIV 10 years ago.
   d. recently developed symptoms of hypothyroidism.

6. The wife of a patient who is manifesting deterioration in memory asks the nurse whether her husband has AD. The nurse explains that a diagnosis of AD is usually made when
   a. a CT scan of the brain indicates brain atrophy.
   b. a urine test indicates elevated levels of isoprostanes.
   c. all other possible causes of dementia have been eliminated.
   d. blood analysis reveals increased amounts of β-amyloid protein.

7. Collaborative care of patients with AD focuses on
   a. replacement of deficient acetylcholine in the brain.
   b. drug therapy to enhance cognition and control undesirable behaviors.
   c. the use of memory-enhancing techniques to delay disease progression.
   d. prevention of other chronic diseases that hasten the progression of AD.

8. Match each of the following medications used in the management of AD with its classification and use.

Medication	Classification	Use
a. amitriptyline (Elavil)	1. Cholinesterase inhibitors	8. Improved cognition
b. haloperidol (Haldol)	2. Selective serotonin reuptake inhibitors	9. Behavior management
c. donepezil (Aricept)	3. Tricyclic antidepressants	10. Treatment of depression
d. lorazepam (Ativan)	4. Conventional antipsychotics	11. Treatment of sleep disturbances
e. risperidone (Risperdal)	5. Atypical antipsychotics	
f. memantine (Namenda)	6. Benzodiazepines	
g. doxepin (Sinequan)	7. N-methyl-D-aspartate receptor agonist	
h. fluoxetine (Prozac)		
i. olanzapine (Zyprexa)		
j. rivastigmine (Exelon)		
k. sertraline (Zoloft)		

9. A patient with AD in a long-term care facility is wandering the halls very agitated, asking for her family and crying. The best action by the nurse is to
   a. ask the patient, "Why are you behaving this way?"
   b. tell the patient, "Let's go get a snack in the kitchen."
   c. ask the patient, "Wouldn't you like to lie down now?"
   d. tell the patient, "Just take some deep breaths and calm down."

10. The sister of a patient with early-onset AD asks the nurse whether prevention of the disease is possible. In responding, the nurse explains that there is no known way to prevent Alzheimer's, but some theories being studied include (select all that apply)
   a. a clear pattern of inheritance of early-onset AD is indicated in some families.
   b. the management of CV risk factors may help avoid or delay cognitive decline.
   c. the use of alcohol, especially wine, is associated with the development of AD.
   d. individuals that do information processing activities have a lower risk for AD.
   e. the relationship of AD and inflammation and the effect of free radicals on neurons exist.

11. A patient with moderate AD has a nursing diagnosis of impaired memory related to effects of dementia. An appropriate nursing intervention for the patient is
   a. posting clocks and calendars in the patient's environment.
   b. monitoring the patient's activity to maintain a safe patient environment.
   c. establishing and consistently following a daily schedule with the patient.
   d. stimulating thought processes by asking the patient questions about recent activities.

12. The caregiver for a patient with AD expresses an inability to make decisions, concentrate, or sleep. The nurse determines that the caregiver
   a. is also developing signs of AD.
   b. is manifesting symptoms of caregiver-role strain.
   c. needs a period of respite from the care of the patient.
   d. should ask other family members to participate in the patient's care.

13. The wife of a man with moderate AD has a nursing diagnosis of social isolation related to diminishing social relationships and behavioral problems of the patient with AD. A nursing intervention that would be appropriate to provide respite care and allow the wife to have satisfactory contact with significant others is to
    a. help the wife arrange for adult day care for the patient.
    b. encourage permanent placement of the patient in an Alzheimer's unit of a long-term care facility.
    c. refer the wife to a home health agency to arrange daily home nursing visits to assist with the patient's care.
    d. arrange for hospitalization of the patient for 3 or 4 days so that the wife can visit out-of-town friends and relatives.

14. The nurse assesses a postoperative patient who has Parkinson's disease for early signs of delirium based on the knowledge that
    a. anticholinergic medications used to treat Parkinson's disease can precipitate delirium in older adults.
    b. older patients are more likely to develop delirium, and most patients with Parkinson's disease are older adults.
    c. decreased levels of dopamine in the CNS found in Parkinson's disease have also been shown to be related to the onset of delirium.
    d. the decreased production of acetylcholine in patients with Parkinson's disease may also be responsible for development of delirium.

15. ***Delegation Decision:*** The RN in charge at a long-term care facility could delegate which of the following activities to nursing assistive personnel (NAP) (select all that apply)?
    a. Assist the patient with eating.
    b. Provide personal hygiene and skin care.
    c. Check the environment for safety hazards.
    d. Assist the patient to the bathroom at regular intervals.
    e. Monitor for skin breakdown and swallowing difficulties.

16. A 72-year-old woman is hospitalized in the intensive care unit (ICU) with pneumonia resulting from chronic obstructive pulmonary disease (COPD). She has a fever, productive cough, and adventitious breath sounds throughout her lungs. In the past 24 hours, her fluid intake was 1000 mL and her urine output 700 mL. She was diagnosed with early-stage AD 6 months ago but has been able to maintain her ADLs with supervision. Identify at least six risk factors for the development of delirium in this patient.
    a.

    b.

    c.

    d.

    e.

    f.

17. A 68-year-old man is admitted to the emergency department with multiple blunt traumas following a one-vehicle car accident. He is restless; disoriented to person, place, and time; and agitated. He resists attempts at examination and calls out the name "Janice." The nurse suspects delirium rather than dementia in this patient based on
    a. the fact that he wouldn't have been allowed to drive if he had dementia.
    b. his hyperactive behavior, which differentiates his condition from the hypoactive behavior of dementia.
    c. the report of emergency personnel that he was noncommunicative when they arrived at the accident scene.
    d. the report of his family that, although he has heart disease and is "very hard of hearing," this behavior is unlike him.

18. The management of a patient with delirium includes
    a. the use of restraints to protect the patient from injury.
    b. the use of short-acting benzodiazepines to sedate the patient.
    c. identification and treatment of underlying causes when possible.
    d. administration of high doses of an antipsychotic drug such as haloperidol (Haldol).

CASE STUDY
Alzheimer's Disease
Patient Profile

G.D. is a 79-year-old man whose wife noticed that he has become increasingly forgetful over the past 3 years. Recently he was diagnosed with AD.

Subjective Data

- Wanders out of the house at night
- States that he "sees things that aren't there"
- Is able to dress, bathe, and feed himself
- Has trouble figuring out how to use his electric razor
- His wife is distressed about his cognitive decline
- His wife says she is depressed and cannot watch him at night and get rest herself

Objective Data

- CT scan: Moderate cerebral atrophy

Clinical Decision-Making Questions

Using a separate sheet of paper, answer the following questions

1. What pathophysiologic changes are associated with AD?
2. How is a diagnosis of AD made?
3. What progression of symptoms should G.D.'s wife be told to expect over the course of the disease?
4. What suggestions can the nurse make to relieve some of the stress on the wife?
5. What community resources might be available to G.D. and his wife?
6. *Priority Decision:* Based on the assessment data presented, what are the priority nursing diagnoses for G.D.? Are there any collaborative problems?
7. *Priority Decision:* Based on the assessment data presented, what are the priority nursing diagnoses for G.D.'s wife? Are there any collaborative problems?

CHAPTER

61

Nursing Management: Peripheral Nerve and Spinal Cord Problems

1. Identify whether the following statements are true (*T*) or false (*F*). If a statement is false, correct the bold word(s) to make the statement true.

_____ a. Trigeminal neuralgia affects the **sensory branches of the trigeminal nerve**, whereas Bell's palsy affects the **motor branches of the facial nerve**.

_____ b. Herpes simplex virus infection is strongly associated as a precipitating factor in the development of **trigeminal neuralgia**.

_____ c. **Antiseizure drugs** are the drugs of choice for treatment of Bell's palsy.

_____ d. Gentle upward massage of the face may be indicated to maintain circulation in the patient with **trigeminal neuralgia**.

_____ e. A special need of patients with both trigeminal neuralgia and Bell's palsy is **oral hygiene**.

_____ f. Severe withdrawal behavior and suicidal tendencies may be seen in patients with **trigeminal neuralgia**.

2. ***Priority Decision:*** When planning care for the patient with trigeminal neuralgia, the nurse sets the highest priority on the patient outcome of
   a. relief of pain.
   b. protection of the cornea.
   c. maintenance of nutrition.
   d. maintenance of positive body image.

3. Surgical intervention is being considered for a patient with trigeminal neuralgia. The nurse recognizes that the procedure that has the least residual effects with a positive outcome is
   a. glycerol rhizotomy.
   b. gamma knife radiosurgery.
   c. microvascular decompression.
   d. percutaneous radiofrequency rhizotomy.

4. When providing care for a patient with an acute attack of trigeminal neuralgia, the nurse should
   a. carry out all hygiene and oral care for the patient.
   b. use conversation to distract the patient from pain.
   c. maintain a quiet, comfortable, draft-free environment.
   d. have the patient examine the mouth after each meal for residual food.

5. A patient is admitted to the hospital with Guillain-Barré syndrome. She had a weakness in her feet and ankles that has progressed to weakness with numbness and tingling in both legs. During the acute phase of her illness, the nurse recognizes that
   a. the most important aspect of care is to monitor the patient's respiratory rate and depth and vital capacity.
   b. early treatment with corticosteroids can suppress the immune response and prevent ascending nerve damage.
   c. although voluntary motor neurons are damaged by the inflammatory response, the autonomic nervous system is unaffected by the disease.
   d. the most serious complication of this condition is ascending demyelination of the peripheral nerves of the lower brainstem and cranial nerves.

6. A patient with Guillain-Barré syndrome asks whether he is going to die as the paralysis spreads toward his chest. In responding to the patient, the nurse knows that
   a. patients who require ventilatory support almost always die.
   b. death occurs when nerve damage affects the brain and meninges.
   c. most patients with Guillain-Barré syndrome make a complete recovery.
   d. if death can be prevented, residual paralysis and sensory impairment are usually permanent.

7. Match the following characteristics with their related condition (answers may be used more than once).

   _____ a. Results from dormant infection   1. Botulism

   _____ b. Inhibits transmission of acetylcholine at myoneural junction   2. Tetanus

   _____ c. Transmitted through wound contamination   3. Neurosyphilis

   _____ d. Initially manifests with GI symptoms with subsequent absorption of neurotoxin

   _____ e. Primary prevention is immunization

   _____ f. Infection of any part of the nervous system

   _____ g. Blocks inhibitory transmitters in the spinal cord and brain

   _____ h. Prevented by boiling food for 10 minutes

   _____ i. Generalized tonic spasms, stiff jaw and neck

   _____ j. Degenerative changes in spinal cord and brainstem

   _____ k. Descending paralysis with cranial nerve involvement

8. In planning community education for prevention of spinal cord injuries, the nurse targets
   a. elderly men.
   b. teenage girls.
   c. elementary school-age children.
   d. adolescent and young adult men.

9. A patient is admitted with a spinal cord injury at the C7 level. During assessment the nurse identifies the presence of spinal shock on finding
   a. paraplegia with a flaccid paralysis.
   b. tetraplegia with total sensory loss.
   c. total hemiplegia with sensory and motor loss.
   d. spastic tetraplegia with loss of pressure sensation.

10. Match the syndromes of incomplete spinal cord lesions with their descriptions.

   _____ a. Central cord syndrome

   _____ b. Anterior cord syndrome

   _____ c. Brown-Séquard syndrome

   _____ d. Posterior cord syndrome

   _____ e. Cauda equina syndrome/conus medullaris syndrome

1. Spinal cord damage resulting in ipsilateral motor paralysis and contralateral loss of pain and sensation below the level of the lesion
2. Damage to the most distal cord and nerve roots, resulting in flaccid paralysis of the lower limbs and areflexic bowel and bladder
3. Rare cord damage resulting in loss of proprioception below the lesion level with retention of motor control and temperature and pain sensation
4. Often caused by flexion injury with acute compression of cord resulting in complete motor paralysis and loss of pain and temperature sensation below the level of injury
5. Cord damage common in cervical region resulting in greater weakness in upper extremities than lower

11. An initial incomplete spinal cord injury often results in complete cord damage because of
    a. edematous compression of the cord above the level of the injury.
    b. continued trauma to the cord resulting from damage to stabilizing ligaments.
    c. infarction and necrosis of the cord caused by edema, hemorrhage, and metabolites.
    d. mechanical transection of the cord by sharp vertebral bone fragments after the initial injury.

12. A patient with a spinal cord injury has spinal shock. The nurse plans care for the patient based on the knowledge that
    a. rehabilitation measures cannot be initiated until spinal shock has resolved.
    b. the patient will need continuous monitoring for hypotension, tachycardia, and hypoxemia.
    c. resolution of spinal shock is manifested by spasticity, hyperreflexia, and reflex emptying of the bladder.
    d. the patient will have complete loss of motor and sensory functions below the level of the injury, but autonomic functions are not affected.

13. Two days following a spinal cord injury, a patient asks continually about the extent of impairment that will result from the injury. The best response by the nurse is,
    a. "You will have more normal function when spinal shock resolves and the reflex arc returns."
    b. "The extent of your injury cannot be determined until the secondary injury to the cord is resolved."
    c. "When your condition is more stable, an MRI will be done that can reveal the extent of the cord damage."
    d. "Because long-term rehabilitation can affect the return of function, it will be years before we can tell what the complete effect will be."

14. Indicate the lowest level of acute spinal cord injury at which the following effects occur.
    a. GI hypomotility with paralytic ileus and gastric distention
    b. Loss of all respiratory muscle function
    c. Respiratory diaphragmatic breathing
    d. Decreased response of the sympathetic nervous system

15. A patient is admitted to the emergency department with a spinal cord injury at the level of T2. Which of the following findings is of most concern to the nurse?
    a. SpO_2 of 92%
    b. HR of 42 beats/min
    c. Blood pressure of 88/60
    d. Loss of motor and sensory function in arms and legs

16. Match the following activities with the highest level of spinal cord injury that the activity can be expected (not all answers will be used).

    _____ a. Ambulate with crutches and leg braces
    _____ b. Indoor mobility in manual wheelchair
    _____ c. Completely independent ambulation with short
    leg braces and canes
    _____ d. Have normal respiratory function
    _____ e. Drive electric wheelchair with chin control
    _____ f. Be independent in self-care and wheelchair use

    1. C1-3
    2. C4
    3. C5
    4. C6
    5. C7-8
    6. T1-6
    7. T6-12
    8. L1-2
    9. L3-4

17. One indication for surgical therapy of the patient with a spinal cord injury is when
    a. there is incomplete cord lesion involvement.
    b. the ligaments that support the spine are torn.
    c. a high cervical injury causes loss of respiratory function.
    d. evidence of continued compression of the cord is apparent.

18. *Priority Decision:* A patient is admitted to the emergency department with a possible cervical spinal cord injury following an automobile crash. During the admission of the patient, the nurse places the highest priority on
    a. maintaining a patent airway.
    b. assessing the patient for head and other injuries.
    c. maintaining immobilization of the cervical spine.
    d. assessing the patient's motor and sensory function.

19. Without surgical stabilization, immobilization and traction of the patient with a cervical spinal cord injury most frequently requires the use of
    a. kinetic beds.
    b. hard cervical collars.
    c. skeletal traction with skull tongs.
    d. sternal-occipital-mandibular immobilizer (SOMI) brace.

20. The health care provider has ordered IV dopamine (Intropin) for a patient in the emergency department with a spinal cord injury. The nurse determines that the drug is having the desired effect when assessment findings include
    a. pulse rate of 68.
    b. respiratory rate of 24.
    c. blood pressure of 106/82.
    d. temperature of 96.8° F (36.0° C).

21. *Priority Decision:* During assessment of a patient with a spinal cord injury, the nurse determines that the patient has a poor cough with diaphragmatic breathing. Based on this finding, the nurse's first action should be to
    a. institute frequent turning and repositioning.
    b. use tracheal suctioning to remove secretions.
    c. assess lung sounds and respiratory rate and depth.
    d. prepare the patient for endotracheal intubation and mechanical ventilation.

22. Following a T2 spinal cord injury, the patient develops paralytic ileus. While this condition is present, the nurse anticipates that the patient will need
    a. IV fluids.
    b. tube feedings.
    c. parenteral nutrition.
    d. nasogastric suctioning.

23. Urinary function during the acute phase of spinal cord injury is maintained with
    a. an indwelling catheter.
    b. intermittent catheterization.
    c. insertion of a suprapubic catheter.
    d. use of incontinent pads to protect the skin.

24. A week following a spinal cord injury at T2, a patient experiences movement in his leg and tells the nurse he is recovering some function. The nurse's best response to the patient is,
    a. "It is really still too soon to know if you will have a return of function."
    b. "That could be a really positive finding. Can you show me the movement?"
    c. "That's wonderful. We will start exercising your legs more frequently now."
    d. "I'm sorry, but the movement is only a reflex and does not indicate normal function."

25. *Priority Decision:* A patient with a spinal cord injury suddenly experiences a throbbing headache, flushed skin, and diaphoresis above the level of injury. After checking the patient's vital signs and finding a systolic BP of 210 and a HR of 58, number the list of nursing actions in order of priority from highest priority to lowest (begin with number 1 as first priority).
    _____ Administer ordered prn nifedipine (Procardia)
    _____ Check for bladder distention
    _____ Document the occurrence, treatment, and response.
    _____ Place call to physician
    _____ Raise the head of bed (HOB) to ≥45 degrees
    _____ Loosen tight clothing on the patient

26. A patient with paraplegia has developed an irritable bladder with reflex emptying. The nurse teaches the patient
    a. hygiene care for an indwelling urinary catheter.
    b. how to perform intermittent self-catheterization.
    c. to empty the bladder with manual pelvic pressure in coordination with reflex voiding patterns.
    d. that a urinary diversion, such as an ileal conduit, is the easiest way to handle urinary elimination.

27. In counseling patients with spinal cord lesions regarding sexual function, the nurse advises a male patient with a complete lower motor neuron lesion that he
    a. is most likely to have reflexogenic erections and may experience orgasm if ejaculation occurs.
    b. may have uncontrolled reflex erections, but that orgasm and ejaculation are usually not possible.
    c. has a lesion with the greatest possibility of successful psychogenic erection with ejaculation and orgasm.
    d. will probably be unable to have either psychogenic or reflexogenic erections with no ejaculation or orgasm.

28. During the patient's process of grieving for the losses resulting from spinal cord injury, the nurse
    a. helps the patient understand that working through the grief will be a lifelong process.
    b. should assist the patient to move through all stages of the mourning process to acceptance.
    c. lets the patient know that anger directed at the staff or the family is not a positive coping mechanism.
    d. facilitates the grieving process so that it is completed by the time the patient is discharged from rehabilitation.

29. A patient with a metastatic tumor of the spinal cord is scheduled for removal of the tumor by a laminectomy. In planning postoperative care for the patient, the nurse recognizes that
    a. most cord tumors cause autodestruction of the cord as in traumatic injuries.
    b. metastatic tumors are commonly extradural lesions that can be removed completely.
    c. radiation therapy is routinely administered following surgery for all malignant spinal cord tumors.
    d. because complete removal of intramedullary tumors is not possible, the surgery is considered palliative.

CASE STUDY
Spinal Cord Injury
Patient Profile

S.M. is an 18-year-old high school student who sustained a C7 spinal cord injury when she dove into a lake while swimming with her friends. S.M. is admitted directly to the ICU.

Subjective Data

• Has patchy sensation in her upper extremities

Objective Data

• Very weak bicep and tricep strength bilaterally
• Moderate strength in both of her lower extremities
• Bowel and bladder control present
• Radiographs show no fracture dislocation of the spine
• Placed on bed rest with a hard cervical collar
• Methylprednisolone administered per protocol

Clinical Decision-Making Questions

Using a separate sheet of paper, answer the following questions.

1. What spinal cord syndrome is S.M. experiencing?
2. What is the physiologic reason that S.M. can move her lower extremities better than her upper extremities?
3. Why does S.M. have a spinal cord injury without having sustained any spinal fracture?
4. What is the rationale for the use of the methylprednisolone?
5. What psychologic problems are anticipated?
6. What can be done to begin long-term plans for S.M.?
7. *Priority Decision:* Based on the assessment data presented, what are the priority nursing diagnoses? Are there any collaborative problems?

Nursing Assessment:
Musculoskeletal System

1. Using the list of terms below, identify the structures in the following illustration.

Terms

Articular cartilage
Compact bone
Diaphysis
Endosteum

Epiphyseal line
Epiphysis
Medullary cavity
Periosteum

Red marrow cavities
Spongy bone
Yellow marrow

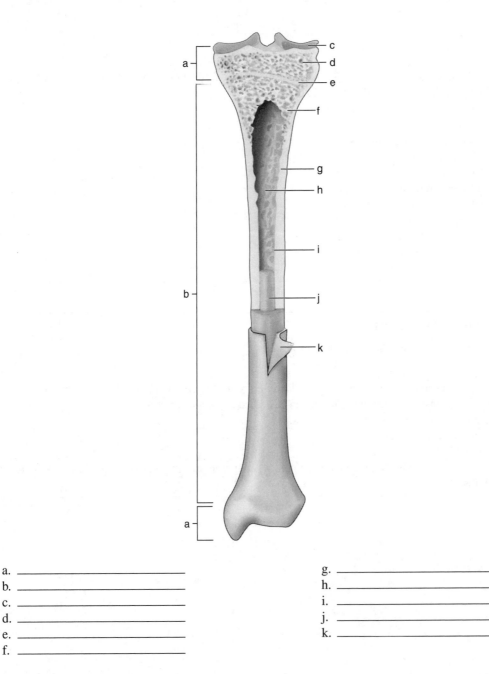

a. _____
b. _____
c. _____
d. _____
e. _____
f. _____

g. _____
h. _____
i. _____
j. _____
k. _____

2. Using the terms below, identify the structures in the following illustration.

Terms
blood vessels
canaliculi
osteon (haversian system)
periosteum

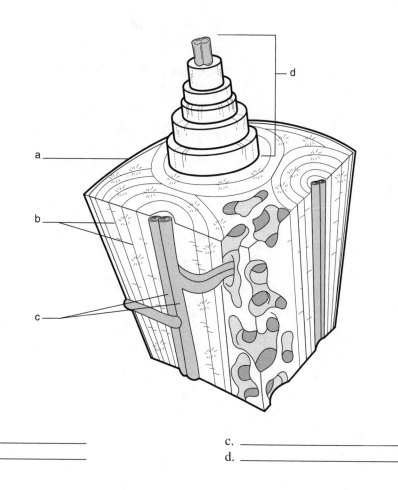

a. _____   c. _____
b. _____   d. _____

3. Using the terms below, identify the structures in the following illustration.

Terms

articular cartilage   bursa   nerve
blood vessel   joint capsule   periosteum
bone   joint cavity   synovial membrane

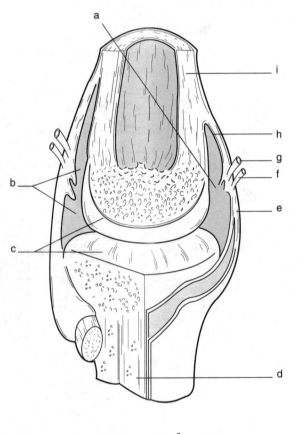

a. _____   f. _____
b. _____   g. _____
c. _____   h. _____
d. _____   i. _____
e. _____

4. Word Search. Find the words that are described by the clues given below. The words may be located horizontally, vertically, or diagonally and may be reversed.

```
M  I  T  I  S  O  M  E  T  R  I  C  E  T
P  N  A  E  S  R  E  V  A  H  T  P  E  O
R  A  D  E  T  A  I  R  T  S  I  E  R  L
S  T  B  U  R  S  A  E  A  P  U  M  E  I
O  R  A  R  S  N  I  L  H  V  D  U  M  G
S  O  S  T  E  O  C  Y  T  E  L  G  O  A
S  P  E  R  I  O  S  T  E  U  M  A  C  M
C  H  E  L  E  I  A  E  N  M  A  H  R  E
A  Y  R  T  S  F  F  W  D  A  L  Y  A  N
L  U  S  B  O  S  T  E  O  B  L  A  S  T
C  O  W  A  A  C  T  I  N  E  O  L  U  X
I  M  C  A  N  A  L  I  C  U  L  I  S  T
U  L  Y  T  A  M  M  U  I  V  O  N  Y  S
M  S  E  G  A  L  I  T  R  A  C  E  N  S
```

Clues

a. System of structural unit of compact bone
b. Contractile unit of myofibrils
c. Cancellous bone at end of long bones
d. Mature bone cell
e. Attaches muscles to bone
f. Connective tissue covering bone
g. Lining of joint capsule
h. Muscle contraction that produces hypertrophy
i. Mineral responsible for muscle contraction
j. Canals extending from lacunae to connect osteocytes
k. Bone cell responsible for resorption of bone
l. Decrease in size of muscle
m. Thin myofibril filaments
n. Small sacs of connective tissue lined with synovium and synovial fluid
o. Bone cell responsible for the formation of bone
p. Lack of blood supply makes this tissue slow healing
q. Connects bone to bone at the joint
r. Connective tissue surrounding muscle
s. Most common type of cartilage tissue
t. Characteristic of skeletal muscle

5. In performing range of motion (ROM) with a patient, the nurse puts each joint through its full movement. Match the type of movements that can be performed on the following joints (answers may be used more than once, and joints may have more than one movement).

    _____ a. Knee   1. Flexion/extension
    _____ b. Hip   2. Abduction/adduction
    _____ c. Thumb   3. Circumduction
    _____ d. Radioulnar joint   4. Rotation
    _____ e. Shoulder
    _____ f. Elbow
    _____ g. Wrist

6. While having his height measured during a routine health examination, a 79-year-old man asks the nurse why he is "shrinking." The nurse explains that decreased height occurs with aging because
   a. decreased muscle mass results in a stooped posture.
   b. loss of cartilage in the knees and hip joints cause a loss of height.
   c. long bones become less dense and shorten as bone tissue compacts.
   d. vertebrae become more compressed with thinning of intervertebral disks.

7. A 78-year-old woman has a physiologic change related to aging in her joints. An appropriate nursing diagnosis related to common changes of aging in the musculoskeletal system is
   a. fatigue.
   b. risk for falls.
   c. self-care deficit.
   d. risk for impaired skin integrity.

8. When obtaining information about the patient's use of medications, the nurse recognizes that both bone and muscle function may be impaired when the patient reports taking
   a. corticosteroids.
   b. oral hypoglycemic agents.
   c. potassium-depleting diuretics.
   d. nonsteroidal antiinflammatory drugs.

9. Identify one specific finding noted by the nurse during assessment of each of the patient's functional health patterns that indicates a risk factor for musculoskeletal problems or a patient response to an actual musculoskeletal problem.
   a. Health perception–health management
   b. Nutritional-metabolic
   c. Elimination
   d. Activity-exercise
   e. Sleep-rest
   f. Cognitive-perceptual
   g. Self-perception–self-concept
   h. Role-relationship
   i. Sexuality-reproductive
   j. Coping–stress tolerance

10. During muscle-strength testing, the patient has active movement against gravity and some resistance to pressure. The nurse scores this finding as
    a. 2.
    b. 3.
    c. 4.
    d. 5.

11. On observation of the patient, the nurse notes the presence of a gait disturbance. To evaluate the patient further, the nurse should
    a. palpate the hips for crepitation.
    b. measure the length of the limbs.
    c. evaluate the degree of leg movement.
    d. compare the muscle mass of one leg with the other.

12. A patient with severe joint immobility is receiving physical and exercise therapy. To evaluate the effect of the treatment, the nurse may assess joint range of motion with a(n)
    a. myometer.
    b. ergometer.
    c. goniometer.
    d. arthrometer.

13. Match the following assessment abnormalities with their descriptions.
    _____ a. Lordosis
    _____ b. Myalgia
    _____ c. Valgum deformity (knock knees)
    _____ d. Ankylosis
    _____ e. Subluxation
    _____ f. Ganglion
    _____ g. Atrophy
    _____ h. Scoliosis
    _____ i. Torticollis
    _____ j. Crepitation
    _____ k. Contracture
    _____ l. Varum deformity (bowlegs)
    _____ m. Kyphosis

    1. Partial joint dislocation
    2. Shortening of muscle or ligament
    3. Knees together, >1 inch between medial malleoli
    4. Convex curve of the spine
    5. Grating sensation between bones
    6. Generalized muscle pain
    7. Fluid-filled cyst
    8. Knees apart, medial malleoli together
    9. Lateral twisting of the neck
    10. Lateral curvature of the spine
    11. Flabby appearance of muscle
    12. Fixed joint
    13. Concave curve of the spine

14. Complete the following statements.
    a. The most common diagnostic test used to assess musculoskeletal disorders is _____.
    b. Insertion of a needle into a joint for aspiration and analysis of synovial fluid is known as a(n) _____.
    c. A test that is specific for visualization of intervertebral disk abnormalities is a(n) _____.
    d. A fast, precise measurement of the bone mass of the spine, forearm, and total body calcium to evaluate osteoporosis can be obtained with the use of _____.
    e. The study in which needles are inserted into muscles to measure electrical activity of muscles is a(n) _____.
    f. The enzyme that is most predominant in skeletal muscle is _____.

15. Identify three serologic tests that may be positive or elevated in rheumatic arthritis.
    a.

    b.

    c.

Nursing Management: Musculoskeletal Trauma and Orthopedic Surgery

1. A 72-year-old man tells the nurse that he cannot perform most of the physical activities he could do 5 years ago because of overall joint aches and pains. To prevent further deconditioning and the risk for developing musculoskeletal problems, the nurse can advise the patient to
   a. avoid the use of canes and walkers because they increase dependence on ambulation aids.
   b. limit weight-bearing exercise to prevent stress on fragile bones and possible hip fractures.
   c. increase his activity by more frequently climbing stairs in buildings and environments with steps.
   d. use enteric-coated aspirin or ibuprofen to decrease inflammation and pain so that exercise can be maintained.

2. The nurse teaches individuals that one of the best ways to prevent musculoskeletal injuries during physical exercise is to
   a. increase muscle strength with daily isometric exercises.
   b. avoid exercising on concrete or hard pavement surfaces.
   c. perform stretching and warm-up exercises before exercise.
   d. wrap susceptible joints with elastic bandages or adhesive tape before exercise.

3. Word Search: Find the words that are described by the clues on the next page. The words may be located horizontally, vertically, or diagonally, and may be reversed.

```
V R M Q A I T N Q C T B Z A X W E N N D
Y E E X X D C E I L A R I P S T E W I D
Q P N S J Q G M O A R E A N P P R S A Y
K E I B I R A O R X R C Q N O M L T R A
L T S U K C T R G J J P U Z S O X U T Z
K I C R N D U D R W L A S L C V J I S Z
C T U S X M H N E M U M H A C N E J W G
I I S I I L K Y N F E O T G I L I R T W
T V I T F M C S P Z I I J F Q Q F E S Y
S E N I A V U L S I O N F R A C T U R E
N S J S D Y I E V N D U Y X Q T O V O X
E T U Q O E C N N F C L M E X V O U W S
E R R O W S T N K R L W A Q H W S R Z L
R A Y E D H S U O N O I T A X U L B U S
G I Y H X Y O T N P A T H O L O G I C K
Q N Y Z B B A L O I S G S L Q W C Y J Z
R I L L L T P A U T M T D X I Q Z F I C
M N M I O I C P X C V M L E M P T Y O P
K J Q R D P T R H O J Q O J R L K N X Q
E U B X D N W A G F F F H C X D V I G V
E R Y B K Q S C B P W D V J L V W J K F
A Y A I D G O E K K O E V J I D J O T D
```

Clues
a. Inflammation of synovial membrane sac at friction sites
b. Incomplete separation of articular surfaces of joint caused by ligament injury
c. Compression of median nerve in wrist
d. Tear within muscles or ligaments of shoulder
e. Complete separation of articular surface of joint caused by ligament injury
f. Cartilage compression and tearing associated with rotational stress
g. Tearing of a ligament
h. Tendon and muscle strain with inflammation and decreased circulation
i. Stretching of muscle and fascia sheath
j. One side splintered and other side bent
k. Line of fracture twists along shaft of bone
l. Fracture with communication with external environment
m. Slanted fracture line
n. Fracture with more than two fragments
o. Spontaneous fracture at site of bone disease
p. Line of fracture at right angle to longitudinal axis
q. Ligament pulls a bone fragment loose

4. Application of RICE (rest, ice, cold, compression, and elevation) is indicated for initial management of
   a. muscle spasms.
   b. sprains and strains.
   c. repetitive strain injury.
   d. dislocations and subluxations.

5. Management during the first 48 hours after an acute soft-tissue injury of the ankle includes (select all that apply)
   a. use of elastic wrap.
   b. initial immobilization and rest.
   c. elevation of ankle above the heart.
   d. alternating the use of heat and cold.
   e. administration of antiinflammatory drugs.

6. Match the characteristics of the fracture healing process with their stages (answers may be used more than once).
   _____ a. Unorganized network of bone woven about fracture parts   1. Hematoma
   _____ b. Closure of space between bone fragments   2. Granulation
   _____ c. Semisolid blood clot at the ends of fragments   3. Callus formation
   _____ d. Absorption of excess cells   4. Ossification
   _____ e. Hematoma converts to granulation   5. Consolidation
   _____ f. Deposition and absorption of bone in response to stress   6. Remodeling
   _____ g. Active phagocytosis absorbs products of local necrosis
   _____ h. Radiologic union
   _____ i. First stage to prevent movement at fracture site
   _____ j. Return to preinjury strength and shape
   _____ k. Composed of cartilage, osteoblasts, calcium, and phosphorus
   _____ l. Formation of osteoid
   _____ m. Stage at which radiographic union first apparent
   _____ n. Clinical union

7. A patient is brought to the emergency department following a fall while rock climbing that injured his lower left leg. The nurse identifies the presence of a fracture based on the cardinal sign of
   a. muscle spasms.
   b. obvious deformity.
   c. edema and swelling.
   d. pain and tenderness.

8. A patient with a fractured femur experiences the complication of malunion. The nurse recognizes that with this complication
   a. the fracture heals in an unsatisfactory position.
   b. the fracture fails to heal properly despite treatment.
   c. fracture healing progresses more slowly than expected.
   d. loss of bone substances occurs as a result of immobilization.

9. Identify whether the following statements are true (*T*) or false (*F*). If a statement is false, correct the bold word(s) to make the statement true.
   _____ a. Realignment of bone fragments into anatomic position is known as **fixation**.
   _____ b. **Traction** may be used to both reduce a fracture and immobilize a fracture.
   _____ c. The disadvantage of open reduction and internal fixation of a fracture is that the patient has an increased risk for **complications related to immobility**.
   _____ d. Pressure causing circulatory, nerve, and skin impairment is most likely to occur with the use of **skeletal** traction.
   _____ e. A cast or splint is a type of **external fixation**.

10. A patient with a fractured femur has a hip spica cast applied. While the cast is drying, the nurse should
    a. elevate the legs above the level of the heart for 24 hours.
    b. turn the patient to both sides and prone to supine every 2 hours.
    c. cover the cast with a light blanket to avoid chilling from evaporation.
    d. assess the patient frequently for abdominal pain, nausea, and vomiting.

11. A patient is admitted with an open fracture of the tibia following a bicycle accident. During assessment of the patient, the nurse questions the patient specifically about
    a. any previous injuries to the leg.
    b. the status of tetanus immunization.
    c. the use of antibiotics in the last month.
    d. whether the injury was exposed to dirt or gravel.

12. *Priority Decision:* A patient has fallen in the bathroom of the hospital room and complains of pain in the upper right arm and elbow. Before splinting the injury, the nurse knows that the priority management of a possible fracture should include
    a. elevation of the arm.
    b. application of ice to the site.
    c. notification of the health care provider.
    d. neurovascular checks below the site of the injury.

13. To assess for neurologic status in a patient with a fractured humerus, the nurse asks the patient to
    a. evert, invert, dorsiflex, and plantar flex the foot.
    b. abduct, adduct, and oppose the fingers, and pronate and supinate the hand.
    c. assess the location, quality, and intensity of pain below the site of the injury.
    d. assess the color, temperature, capillary refill, peripheral pulses, and presence of edema in the extremity.

14. A patient is discharged from the outpatient clinic following application of a synthetic fiberglass long-arm cast for a fractured ulna. Before discharge, the nurse instructs the patient to
    a. never get the cast wet.
    b. move the shoulder and fingers frequently.
    c. place tape petals around the edges of the cast when it is dry.
    d. use a sling to support the arm at waist level for the first 48 hours.

15. A patient with a long leg cast is allowed to ambulate with crutches with no weight bearing on the affected leg. The nurse teaches the patient to use a
    a. swing-to gait.
    b. two-point gait.
    c. four-point gait.
    d. swing-through gait.

16. A patient with a fractured tibia accompanied by extensive soft-tissue damage initially has a splint applied and held in place with an elastic bandage. An early sign that would alert the nurse that the patient is developing compartment syndrome is
    a. paralysis of the toes.
    b. absence of peripheral pulses.
    c. progressive pain unrelieved by usual analgesics.
    d. the skin over the injury site is blanched when the bandage is removed.

17. Identify the problems that are indicated by each of the six Ps characteristic of an impending compartment syndrome.
    a.

    b.

    c.

    d.

    e.

    f.

18. Surgical treatment that is indicated for compartment syndrome is
    a. fasciotomy.
    b. amputation.
    c. internal fixation.
    d. release of tendons.

19. Match the following characteristics with the related type of fracture (answers may be used more than once).
    _____ a. Possible radial nerve and brachial artery damage
    _____ b. Moving the patient may cause serious injury from bone fragments
    _____ c. Often occurs when breaking a fall with an outstretched hand
    _____ d. Airway patency is a major concern
    _____ e. Deformity, shortening of extremity, and inability to move hip and knee occur
    _____ f. Hanging arm cast may be used to reduce the fracture
    _____ g. High incidence in patients with osteoporosis
    _____ h. Stress fracture more common
    _____ i. Drastic change in appearance requiring supportive care
    _____ j. Fractured distal radius and possible styloid process of ulna
    _____ k. Most serious complication is displacement of fracture
    _____ l. May be accompanied by intraabdominal lacerations and hemorrhage
    _____ m. Vulnerable site because of lack of anterior muscle covering
    _____ n. Internal fixation with intermedullary rod or compression plates preferred
    _____ o. Halo apparatus may be used for immobilization with cervical injury

    1. Colles' fracture
    2. Fractured humerus
    3. Fractured pelvis
    4. Femoral shaft fracture
    5. Fractured tibia
    6. Stable vertebral fracture
    7. Facial fractures

20. A fat embolism is most likely to occur
    a. 24 to 48 hours following a fractured tibia.
    b. 36 to 72 hours following a skull fracture.
    c. 4 to 5 days following a fractured femur.
    d. 5 to 6 days following a pelvic fracture.

21. The nurse suspects a fat embolism rather than a pulmonary embolism from a venous thrombosis in the patient with a fracture who develops
    a. tachycardia and dyspnea.
    b. a sudden onset of chest pain.
    c. ECG changes and decreased PaO_2.
    d. petechiae around the neck and upper chest.

22. Identify whether the following statements are true (*T*) or false (*F*). If a statement is false, correct the bold word(s) to make the statement true.

    _____ a. **Extracapsular** hip fractures often occur in individuals with osteoporosis and minor injury.

    _____ b. An **intertrochanteric** fracture of the hip occurs between the greater and lesser trochanter.

    _____ c. Avascular necrosis is a serious complication of displaced **subtrochanteric** fractures.

    _____ d. The preferred treatment of extracapsular fractures is **sliding hip screws or intermedullary devices,** whereas intracapsular fractures are usually repaired with **hip prostheses**.

    _____ e. **Intracapsular** hip fractures are also known as fractures of the neck of the femur.

23. An older adult woman is admitted to the emergency department after falling at home. The nurse cautions the patient not to put weight on the leg after finding
    a. inability to move the toes and ankle.
    b. edema of the thigh extending to the knee.
    c. internal rotation of the leg with groin pain.
    d. shortening and external rotation of the leg.

24. A patient with an extracapsular hip fracture is admitted to the orthopedic unit and placed in Buck's traction. The nurse explains to the patient that the purpose of the traction is to
    a. pull bone fragments back into alignment.
    b. immobilize the leg until healing is complete.
    c. reduce pain and muscle spasms before surgery.
    d. prevent damage to the blood vessels at the fracture site.

25. A patient with a fractured right hip has an open reduction and internal fixation of the fracture. Postoperatively the nurse plans to
    a. get the patient up to the chair the first postoperative day.
    b. position the patient only on the back and unoperative side.
    c. keep leg abductor splints on the patient except when bathing.
    d. ambulate the patient with partial weight bearing by discharge.

26. Discharge instructions for the patient following a hip prosthesis include
    a. restricting walking for 2 to 3 months.
    b. taking a bath rather than a shower to prevent falling.
    c. keeping the leg internally rotated while sitting and standing.
    d. having a family member put on the patient's shoes and socks.

27. When preparing a patient for discharge following fixation of a mandibular fracture, the nurse determines that teaching has been successful when the patient says,
    a. "I can keep my mouth moist by sucking on hard candy."
    b. "I should cut the wires with scissors if I begin to vomit."
    c. "I may use a bulk-forming laxative if my liquid diet causes constipation."
    d. "I should use a moist swab to clean my mouth every time I eat something."

28. A patient 24 hours after a below-the-knee amputation uses the call system to tell the nurse his dressing (a compression bandage) has fallen off. What action should the nurse take?
    a. apply ice to the site
    b. cover the incision with dry gauze
    c. reapply the compression dressing
    d. elevate the extremity on a couple of pillows

29. A patient who suffered a traumatic below-the-elbow amputation in a boating accident is withdrawn, does not look at the arm, and asks to be left alone. An appropriate nursing diagnosis of the patient includes
    a. impaired adjustment.
    b. disturbed body image.
    c. impaired social interaction.
    d. ineffective individual coping.

30. A patient complains of pain in the foot of a leg that was recently amputated. The nurse recognizes that the pain
    a. is caused by swelling at the incision.
    b. should be treated with ordered analgesics.
    c. will become worse with the use of a prosthesis.
    d. can be managed with diversion because it is psychologic.

31. ***Priority Decision:*** An immediate prosthetic fitting during surgery is used for a patient with a traumatic below-the-knee amputation. During the immediate postoperative period, a priority nursing intervention is to
    a. assess the site for hemorrhage.
    b. monitor the patient's vital signs.
    c. elevate the residual limb on pillows.
    d. have the patient flex and extend the knee every hour.

32. The nurse positions a patient with an above-the-knee amputation with a delayed prosthetic fitting prone several times a day to
    a. prevent flexion contractures.
    b. assess the posterior skin flap.
    c. reduce edema in the residual limb.
    d. relieve pressure on the incision site.

33. A patient who had a below-the-knee amputation is to be fitted with a temporary prosthesis. It is most important for the nurse to teach the patient to
    a. inspect the residual limb daily for irritation.
    b. apply an elastic shrinker before applying the prosthesis.
    c. perform ROM exercises to the affected leg four times a day.
    d. apply alcohol to the residual limb every morning and evening to toughen the skin.

34. Match the following joint surgeries with their uses.

    _____ a. Synovectomy
    _____ b. Osteotomy
    _____ c. Debridement
    _____ d. Arthroplasty
    _____ e. Arthrodesis

    1. Reconstruction or replacement of a joint to relieve pain and correct deformity
    2. Surgical fusion of a joint to relieve pain
    3. Used in rheumatoid arthritis to remove the tissue involved in joint destruction
    4. Correction of bone deformity by removal of a wedge or slice of bone
    5. Arthroscopic removal of degenerative tissue in joints

35. A 65-year-old patient has undergone a right total hip arthroplasty with a cemented prosthesis for treatment of severe osteoarthritis of the hip. Patient activity that the nurse anticipates on the patient's first or second postoperative day includes
    a. transfer from bed to chair twice a day only.
    b. turning from the back to the unaffected side q2hr only.
    c. crutch walking with non–weight bearing on the operative leg.
    d. ambulation and weight bearing on the right leg with a walker.

36. When positioning the patient with a total hip arthroplasty, it is important that the nurse maintain the affected extremity in
    a. adduction and flexion.
    b. extension and abduction.
    c. abduction and internal rotation.
    d. adduction and external rotation.

37. Following a knee arthroplasty, a patient has a continuous passive-motion machine for the affected joint. The nurse explains to the patient that this device is used to
    a. relieve edema and pain at the incision site.
    b. promote early joint mobility and increase knee flexion.
    c. prevent venous stasis and the formation of a deep venous thrombosis.
    d. improve arterial circulation to the affected extremity to promote healing.

38. A patient with severe ulnar deviation of the hands undergoes an arthroplasty with reconstruction and replacement of finger joints. Postoperatively it is most important for the nurse to
    a. position the fingers lower than the elbow.
    b. perform neurovascular assessments of the fingers q2-4hr.
    c. encourage the patient to gently flex, extend, abduct, and adduct the fingers q4hr.
    d. remind the patient that function of the hands is more important than their cosmetic appearance.

39. *Priority Decision:* Following change-of-shift handoff, which patient should the nurse assess first?
    a. a 58-year-old male experiencing phantom pain and requesting analgesic
    b. a 72-year-old male being transferred to a skilled nursing unit following repair of a hip fracture
    c. a 25-year-old female in left leg skeletal traction asking for the weights to be lifted for a few minutes
    d. a 68-year-old male with a new lower leg cast complaining that the cast is too tight and he can't feel his toes

---

CASE STUDY
Fracture
Patient Profile

H.A., a 30-year-old telephone lineman, was seen in the emergency department after falling from a pole. His right lower extremity was splinted with a cardboard splint and a large, bulky dressing.

Subjective Data

- Complains of severe pain in the right leg
- Expresses concern about notifying his wife about the accident and his whereabouts
- Asks how long he will be off work

Objective Data

- Avulsion of soft tissue on the anterolateral aspect of the tibia
- Obvious deformity, marked swelling, and ecchymosis in region of injury

---

Clinical Decision-Making Questions
Using a separate sheet of paper, answer the following questions.

1. Was the immobilization of the fracture at the scene of the accident appropriate?
2. What is the appropriate nursing neurovascular assessment of the injured extremity?
3. *Priority Decision:* What are the priority therapeutic and nursing interventions to prevent infection?
4. What specific nursing actions should the nurse implement to alleviate H.A.'s pain?
5. How would the nurse answer H.A.'s question about time off from work based on the stages of fracture healing?
6. How should the nurse notify Mrs. A. about her husband's accident?
7. *Priority Decision:* Based on the assessment data presented, what are the priority nursing diagnoses? Are there any collaborative problems?

Nursing Management:
Musculoskeletal Problems

1. A patient with chronic osteomyelitis has been hospitalized for a surgical debridement procedure. The nurse explains to the patient that surgical treatment is necessary because
   a. removal of the infection prevents the need for bone and skin grafting.
   b. formation of scar tissue has led to a protected area of bacterial growth.
   c. the process of depositing new bone blocks the vascular supply to the bone.
   d. antibiotics are not effective against microorganisms that cause chronic osteomyelitis.

2. A patient with osteomyelitis has a nursing diagnosis of risk for injury. An appropriate nursing intervention is
   a. providing ROM exercise q4hr to the involved extremity.
   b. using careful and appropriate disposal of soiled dressings.
   c. gently handling the involved extremity during movement.
   d. measuring the circumference of the affected extremity daily.

3. A patient who experienced an open fracture of the humerus 2 weeks ago is having increased pain at the fracture site. To identify a possible causative agent of osteomyelitis at the site, the nurse would expect testing to include
   a. x-rays.
   b. a CT scan.
   c. a bone biopsy.
   d. white blood cell (WBC) count and erythrocyte sedimentation rate (ESR).

4. Following 2 weeks of IV antibiotic therapy, a patient with acute osteomyelitis of the tibia is prepared for discharge from the hospital. The nurse determines that additional instruction is needed when the patient says,
   a. "I will need to continue antibiotic therapy for 4 to 6 weeks."
   b. "I shouldn't bear weight on my affected leg until healing is complete."
   c. "I can use a heating pad to my lower leg for comfort and to promote healing."
   d. "I should notify the health care provider if the pain in my leg becomes worse."

5. During a follow-up visit to a patient with acute osteomyelitis treated with IV antibiotics, the home care nurse is told by the patient's wife that she can hardly get the patient to eat because his mouth is so sore. In checking the patient's mouth, the nurse would expect to find
   a. a dry, cracked tongue with a central furrow.
   b. white, curdlike membranous lesions of the mucosa.
   c. ulcers of the mouth and lips surrounded by a reddened base.
   d. single or clustered vesicles on the tongue and buccal mucosa.

6. Match the following characteristics with their related types of bone tumors (answers may be used more than once).
   _____ a. May transform into a malignant form
   _____ b. Arises in cancellous ends of long bones
   _____ c. Benign overgrowth of bone and cartilage
   _____ d. Often brought to attention by injury
   _____ e. Extremely malignant and metastasizes early
   _____ f. High rate of local recurrence

   1. Osteochondroma
   2. Osteosarcoma
   3. Osteoclastoma

7. A 24-year-old patient with a 12-year history of Becker's muscular dystrophy is hospitalized with heart failure. An appropriate nursing intervention for this patient is
   a. to feed and bathe the patient to avoid exhausting the muscles.
   b. frequent repositioning to avoid skin and respiratory complications.
   c. to provide hand weights for the patient to exercise the upper extremities.
   d. using orthopedic braces to promote ambulation to prevent muscle wasting.

8. Identify whether the following statements are true (*T*) or false (*F*). If a statement is false, correct the bold word(s) to make the statement true.
   _____ a. **Chemotherapy** may be used in the management of all primary bone cancer.
   _____ b. The most common cause of acute low back pain is **herniation of an intervertebral disk**.
   _____ c. Use of **NSAIDs** for chronic low back pain is important in being able to maintain exercise and activity throughout the day.
   _____ d. Low back pain that radiates down the buttock along the distribution of the sciatic nerve generally indicates **acute lumbosacral strain**.
   _____ e. **Degenerative disk disease** is a major factor in the development of herniated intervertebral disks.

9. The nurse teaches the patient recovering from an episode of acute low back pain to
   a. perform daily exercise as a lifelong routine.
   b. sit in a chair with the hips higher than the knees.
   c. avoid occupations in which the use of the body is required.
   d. sleep on the abdomen or on the back with the legs extended.

10. A laminectomy and spinal fusion are performed on a patient with a herniated lumbar intervertebral disk. During the postoperative period, which of the following patient findings is of most concern to the nurse?
    a. Paralytic ileus
    b. Urinary incontinence
    c. Greater pain at the graft site than at the lumbar incision site
    d. Leg and arm movement and sensation unchanged from preoperative status

11. Before repositioning the patient to the side after a lumbar laminectomy, the nurse
    a. raises the head of the bed 30 degrees.
    b. has the patient flex the knees and hips.
    c. places a pillow between the patient's legs.
    d. has the patient grasp the side rail on the opposite side of the bed.

12. Match the following foot problems with their characteristics (answers may be used more than once).
    _____ a. Breakdown of metatarsal arch
    _____ b. Papilloma growth on sole of foot
    _____ c. Local thickening of skin caused by pressure on bony prominences
    _____ d. Deformity of second toe with callus on dorsum of proximal interphalangeal joint
    _____ e. Tumor on nerve tissue between third and fourth metatarsal heads
    _____ f. Lateral angulation of large toe toward second toe
    _____ g. Metatarsal arch support used in conservative treatment
    _____ h. May be trimmed with razor or scalpel after softening
    _____ i. Surgical treatment is removal of bursal sac and bony enlargement
    _____ j. Thickening of skin on weight-bearing part of foot

    1. Hallux valgus (bunion)
    2. Hammertoe
    3. Morton's neuroma
    4. Pes planus
    5. Corn
    6. Callus
    7. Plantar wart

13. In promoting healthy feet, the nurse recognizes the factor that is associated with most foot problems is
    a. poor foot hygiene.
    b. congenital deformities.
    c. improperly fitting shoes.
    d. peripheral vascular disease.

14. Match the following metabolic bone diseases with their characteristics (answers may be used more than once).

_____ a. Loss of total bone mass and substance   1. Osteomalacia
_____ b. Results from vitamin D deficiency   2. Paget's disease
_____ c. Replacement of normal marrow with vascular connective tissue   3. Osteoporosis
_____ d. Generalized bone decalcification with bone deformity
_____ e. Most common in bones of spine, hips, and wrists
_____ f. Abnormal remodeling and resorption of bone
_____ g. Bowed legs and cranial enlargement

15. Which of the following female patients are at risk for developing osteoporosis (select all that apply)?
    a. 60-year-old white aerobics instructor
    b. 55-year-old Asian American cigarette smoker
    c. 68-year-old white who is underweight and inactive
    d. 62-year-old African American on estrogen therapy
    e. 58-year-old Native American who started menopause prematurely

16. Identify three methods of preventing osteoporosis in postmenopausal women.
    a.

    b.

    c.

17. A patient is started on alendronate (Fosamax) once weekly for the treatment of osteoporosis. The nurse determines that further instruction about the drug is needed when the patient says,
    a. "I should take the drug with a meal to prevent stomach irritation."
    b. "This drug will reverse my bone loss and increase my bone density."
    c. "I need to sit or stand upright for at least 30 minutes after taking the drug."
    d. "I will still need to take my calcium supplements while taking this new drug."

CASE STUDY
Herniated Intervertebral Disk
Patient Profile

- G.B. is a 38-year-old truck driver who slipped on a wet floor at work and landed on his buttocks.

Subjective Data

- Experienced immediate, severe lower back pain, with pain radiating into his right buttock
- Had worsening of pain in 3 days, with pain radiating down his entire leg into his foot
- Experienced tingling of his toes
- Rested at home for 2 weeks without relief
- Smokes a pack of cigarettes a day

Objective Data

- Height: 5 ft 8 in; weight: 253 lb
- Diagnostic studies: MRI revealed a large herniated disk at L4-5 level.

Collaborative Care

- Underwent microdiskectomy at L4-5
- Expected discharge 2 days after surgery

Clinical Decision-Making Questions

Using a separate sheet of paper, answer the following questions.

1. What risk factors for low back pain does G.B. have?
2. What preoperative teaching is indicated for G.B.?
3. What postoperative activity restrictions will G.B. need to follow?
4. What postoperative nursing assessments should be made?
5. *Priority Decision:* What are the priority needs to include in the discharge teaching for G.B.?
6. *Priority Decision:* Based on the assessment data presented, what are the priority nursing diagnoses? Are there any collaborative problems?

Nursing Management: Arthritis and Connective Tissue Diseases

1. A 60-year-old woman has pain on motion in her fingers and asks the nurse whether this is just a result of aging. The best response by the nurse includes the information that
   a. joint pain with functional limitation is a normal change that affects all people to some extent.
   b. joint pain that develops with age is usually related to previous trauma or infection of the joints.
   c. this is a symptom of a systemic arthritis that eventually affects all joints as the disease progresses.
   d. changes in the cartilage and bones of joints may cause symptoms of pain and loss of function in some people as they age.

2. Number in sequence from 1 to 6 the pathophysiologic processes that occur in osteoarthritis (OA).
   _____ a. Erosion of articular surfaces
   _____ b. Joint space narrows
   _____ c. Incongruity in joint surfaces leads to reduction in motion
   _____ d. Joint cartilage becomes yellow and granular
   _____ e. Osteophytes form at joint margins
   _____ f. Cartilage becomes softer and less elastic

3. Indicate whether the following statements are true (*T*) or false (*F*). If a statement is false, correct the bold word(s) to make the statement true.
   _____ a. **Bouchard's** nodes are reddened, tender protuberances found at the distal interphalangeal (DIP) joints in some patients with OA.
   _____ b. The pain of later OA is most commonly caused by **swelling and stretching of soft tissue around the joint**.
   _____ c. Joint stiffness in OA can be caused by **crepitation**.
   _____ d. First-line drug therapy used in the management of osteoarthritis is **aspirin**.
   _____ e. Pain and immobility of osteoarthritis may be aggravated by **falling barometric pressure**.

4. To preserve function and the ability to perform activities of daily living, the nurse teaches the patient with OA to
   a. avoid exercise that involves the affected joints.
   b. plan and organize less stressful ways to perform tasks.
   c. maintain normal activities during an acute episode to prevent loss of function.
   d. use mild analgesics to control symptoms when performing tasks that cause pain.

5. A patient with OA uses NSAIDs to decrease pain and inflammation. The nurse teaches the patient that common side effects of these drugs include
   a. allergic reactions, fever, and oral lesions.
   b. fluid retention, hypertension, and bruising.
   c. skin rashes, gastric irritation, and headache.
   d. prolonged bleeding time, blood dyscrasias, and hepatic damage.

6. A patient with OA asks the nurse whether he could try glucosamine and chondroitin for control of his symptoms. The best response by the nurse includes the information that
   a. some patients find these supplements helpful for relieving arthritis knee pain and improving mobility.
   b. although these substances may not help, there is no evidence that they can cause any untoward effects.
   c. these supplements are a fad that has not been shown to reduce pain or increase joint mobility in patients with OA.
   d. only dosages of these supplements available by prescription are high enough to provide any benefit in treatment of OA.

7. A patient taking ibuprofen (Motrin) for treatment of OA has good pain relief but is experiencing increased dyspepsia and nausea with the drug's use. The nurse consults the patient's primary care provider about
   a. adding misoprostol (Cytotec) to the patient's drug regimen.
   b. substituting naproxen (Naprosyn) for the ibuprofen (Motrin).
   c. administering the ibuprofen with antacids to decrease the GI irritation.
   d. returning to the use of acetaminophen, but at a dose of 5 g/day instead of 4 g/day.

8. The basic pathophysiologic process of rheumatoid arthritis (RA) is
   a. destruction of joint cartilage and bones by an autoimmune process.
   b. initiated by a viral infection that destroys the synovial membranes of joints.
   c. the presence of HLA-DR4 antigen that causes inflammatory responses throughout the body.
   d. an immune response that activates complement and produces inflammation of joints and other organ systems.

9. Indicate whether the following descriptions are most characteristic of osteoarthritis (OA), rheumatoid arthritis (RA), or both (B).
   _____ a. Most commonly occurs in women
   _____ b. Affects knees, hips, and spine (weight-bearing joints)
   _____ c. Asymmetric involvement of joints
   _____ d. Joint pain, stiffness, and limitation of motion
   _____ e. Inflammatory synovial fluid
   _____ f. Joint stiffness after periods of inactivity
   _____ g. Firm, subcutaneous, nontender nodules
   _____ h. RF negative
   _____ i. Fatigue, anorexia, and weight loss
   _____ j. Joint stiffness in the morning resolves in about 30 minutes
   _____ k. Associated with autoantibodies to abnormal immunoglobulin G (IgG)

10. During the physical assessment of the patient with moderate RA, the nurse would expect to find
    a. hepatomegaly.
    b. Heberden's nodes.
    c. spindle-shaped fingers.
    d. crepitus on joint movement.

11. Laboratory findings that the nurse would expect to be present in the patient with RA include
    a. polycythemia.
    b. increased IgG.
    c. decreased WBC.
    d. increased C-reactive protein (CRP).

12. Describe the three most common extraarticular manifestations of RA.
    a.

    b.

    c.

13. Match the following drugs used in the management of rheumatoid arthritis with their characteristics (answers may be used more than once).

_____ a. Requires monitoring for bone marrow depression

_____ b. Binds to TNF, blocking its effect

_____ c. Causes orange-yellow urine

_____ d. Antimalarial agent often used initially for mild RA

_____ e. Immunosuppresive agent that inhibits DNA and RNA synthesis

_____ f. Used intraarticularly for acute flare of one or two joints

_____ g. Blocks action of interleukin-1, decreasing the inflammatory response

_____ h. Use requires periodic eye examination for retinal damage

_____ i. First drug of choice for patients with moderate to severe RA

_____ j. Systemic use limited to life-threatening exacerbations

_____ k. Sulfonamide with antiinflammatory effects by blocking prostaglandin synthesis

_____ l. Antirheumatic agent that may take 3 to 6 months to have effect

_____ m. Used with disease-modifying antirheumatic drugs (DMARDs) for additional antiinflammatory effect

_____ n. Systemic doses must be tapered to prevent exacerbation of symptoms

_____ o. Blocks action of interleukin-6, a proinflammatory cytokine

1. hydroxychloroquine (Plaquenil)
2. corticosteroids
3. anakinra (Kineret)
4. parenteral gold
5. sulfazalazine (Azulfidine)
6. etanercept (Enbrel)
7. methotrexate (Rheumatrex)
8. NSAIDs and aspirin
9. azathioprine (Imuran)
10. tocilizumab (Actemra)

14. A 70-year-old patient is being evaluated for symptoms of RA. The nurse recognizes that a major problem in the management of RA in the older adult is that
   a. RA is usually more severe in older adults.
   b. older patients are not as likely to comply with treatment regimens.
   c. drug interactions and toxicity are more likely to occur with multidrug therapy.
   d. laboratory and other diagnostic tests are not effective in identifying RA in older adults.

15. After teaching a patient with RA about the prescribed therapeutic regimen, the nurse determines that further instruction is needed when the patient says,
   a. "It is important for me to perform my prescribed exercises every day."
   b. "I should perform most of my daily chores in the morning when my energy level is highest."
   c. "An ice pack to a joint for 10 minutes may help relieve pain and inflammation when I have an acute flare."
   d. "I can use assistive devices such as padded utensils, electric can openers, and elevated toilet seats to protect my joints."

16. A patient recovering from an acute exacerbation of RA tells the nurse she is too tired to bathe. The nurse should
   a. give the patient a bed bath to conserve her energy.
   b. allow the patient a rest period before showering with the nurse's help.
   c. tell the patient that she can skip bathing if she will walk in the hall later.
   d. inform the patient that it is important for her to maintain self-care activities.

17. After teaching a patient with RA to use heat and cold therapy to relieve symptoms, the nurse determines that teaching has been effective when the patient says,
   a. "Heat treatments should not be used if muscle spasms are present."
   b. "Cold applications can be applied for 15 to 20 minutes to relieve joint stiffness."
   c. "I should use heat applications for 20 minutes to relieve the symptoms of an acute flare."
   d. "When my joints are painful, I can use a bag of frozen corn for 10 to 15 minutes to relieve the pain."

18. The nurse teaches the patient with RA that one of the most effective methods of aerobic exercise is
   a. ballet dancing.
   b. casual walking.
   c. aquatic exercises.
   d. low-impact aerobic exercises.

19. Characteristics of spondyloarthritides associated with the HLA-B27 antigen include
    a. symmetric polyarticular arthritis.
    b. an absence of extraarticular disease.
    c. presence of rheumatoid factor and autoantibodies.
    d. high level of involvement of sacroiliac joints and the spine.

20. An important nursing intervention for the patient with ankylosing spondylitis is to teach the patient to
    a. wear roomy shoes with good orthotic support.
    b. sleep on the side with the knees and hips flexed.
    c. keep the spine slightly flexed while sitting, standing, or walking.
    d. perform back, neck, and chest stretches and deep breathing exercises.

21. Match the following characteristics with their related rheumatic disorders (answers may be used more than once).
    _____ a. Associated with nonrestorative sleep, irritable   1. Psoriatic arthritis
                   bowel syndrome, and anxiety   2. Reactive arthritis
    _____ b. Characteristic symptom of erythema migrans   3. Septic arthritis
    _____ c. Methotrexate is a treatment of choice   4. Lyme disease
    _____ d. Symptoms include urethritis and conjunctivitis   5. Sjögren syndrome
    _____ e. Infection of a joint often caused by hematogenous route   6. Fibromyalgia
    _____ f. Inflammation and dysfunction of salivary and lacrimal glands
    _____ g. Diagnosed by finding of hypersensitive tender points
    _____ h. An inflammatory polyarthritis associated with psoriasis
    _____ i. Increased risk in persons with decreased host resistance
    _____ j. Lymph nodes, bone marrow, and visceral organs may
                   become involved
    _____ k. Systemic infection with migratory polyarthritis that may
                   involve cardiac and neurologic function
    _____ l. Self-limiting arthritis following GI (enteral) or sexually
                   transmitted infections

22. A patient is seen at the outpatient clinic for a sudden onset of inflammation and severe pain in the great toe.
    A diagnosis of gout is made on the basis of
    a. a family history of gout.
    b. elevated urine uric acid levels.
    c. elevated serum uric acid levels.
    d. the presence of sodium urate crystals in synovial fluid.

23. During treatment of the patient with an acute attack of gout, the nurse would expect to administer
    a. aspirin.
    b. colchicine.
    c. allopurinol (Zyloprim).
    d. probenecid (Benemid).

24. A patient with gout is treated with drug therapy to prevent future attacks. The nurse teaches the patient that it is most
    important to
    a. avoid all foods high in purine, such as organ meats.
    b. have periodic determination of serum uric acid levels.
    c. perform active ROM of all joints that have been affected by gout.
    d. increase the dosage of medication with the onset of an acute attack.

25. The pathophysiology of systemic lupus erythematosus (SLE) is characterized by
    a. destruction of nucleic acids and other self-proteins by autoantibodies.
    b. overproduction of collagen that disrupts the functioning of internal organs.
    c. formation of abnormal IgG that attaches to cellular antigens, activating complement.
    d. increased activity of T-suppressor cells with B-cell hypoactivity, resulting in an immunodeficiency.

26. Identify the most common clinical manifestations of SLE that may occur in each of the following organ systems.
    a. Dermatologic
    b. Musculoskeletal
    c. Cardiac
    d. Pulmonary
    e. Renal
    f. Central nervous
    g. Hematologic

27. A patient with newly diagnosed SLE asks the nurse how the disease will affect her life. The best response by the nurse is,
    a. "You can plan to have a near-normal life since SLE rarely causes death."
    b. "It is difficult to tell because the disease is so variable in its severity and progression."
    c. "Life span is shortened somewhat in people with SLE, but the disease can be controlled with long-term use of corticosteroids."
    d. "Most people with SLE have alternating periods of remissions and exacerbations with rapid progression to permanent organ damage."

28. During an acute exacerbation, a patient with SLE is treated with corticosteroids. The nurse would expect the steroids to begin to be tapered when serum laboratory results indicate
    a. increased RBC.
    b. decreased ESR.
    c. decreased anti-DNA.
    d. increased complement.

29. Teaching that the nurse will plan for the patient with SLE includes
    a. ways to avoid exposure to sunlight.
    b. increasing dietary protein and carbohydrate intake.
    c. the necessity of genetic counseling before planning a family.
    d. the use of nonpharmacologic pain interventions instead of analgesics.

30. During assessment of the patient with systemic sclerosis, the nurse would expect to find
    a. thickening of the skin of the fingers and hands.
    b. cool, cyanotic fingers with thinning skin over the joints.
    c. swan-neck deformity or ulnar drift deformity of the hands.
    d. low back pain, stiffness, and limitation of spine movement.

31. When caring for the patient with CREST syndrome (calcinosis, Raynaud's phenomenon, esophageal dysfunction, sclerodactyly, and telangiectasis) associated with systemic sclerosis, the nurse teaches the patient to
    a. monitor and keep a log of daily BP.
    b. maintain a fluid intake of at least 3000 mL/day.
    c. avoid exposure to the sun or other ultraviolet light.
    d. protect the hands and feet from cold exposure and injury.

32. During the acute phase of dermatomyositis, an appropriate patient outcome is when he or she
    a. relates improvement in pain.
    b. does not experience aspiration.
    c. performs active ROM four times daily.
    d. maintains absolute rest of affected joints.

33. During assessment of the patient diagnosed with fibromyalgia syndrome (FMS), the nurse would expect the patient to report
    a. generalized muscle twitching and spasms.
    b. nonrestorative sleep with resulting fatigue.
    c. profound and progressive muscle weakness that limits ADLs.
    d. widespread musculoskeletal pain that is accompanied by inflammation and fever.

34. One criterion for a diagnosis of FMS is
    a. fiber atrophy found on muscle biopsy.
    b. elimination of all other causes of musculoskeletal pain.
    c. the presence of the manifestations of chronic fatigue syndrome.
    d. the elicitation of pain on palpation of at least 11 of 18 identified tender points.

35. One important nursing intervention for the patient with FMS is to teach the patient to
    a. rest the muscles as much as possible to avoid triggering pain.
    b. plan nighttime sleep and naps to obtain 12 to 14 hours of sleep a day.
    c. try the use of food supplements such as glucosamine and chondroitin for relief of pain.
    d. use stress-management techniques such as biofeedback, guided imagery, or autogenic training.

36. A patient with debilitating fatigue has been diagnosed with chronic fatigue syndrome. List the four major criteria that must be present for this diagnosis to be made.
    a.

    b.

    c.

    d.

CASE STUDY
Rheumatoid Arthritis
Patient Profile

N.M. is a 36-year-old obese white woman who has RA. When her symptoms began to interfere with her daily activities, she sought medical help.

Subjective Data

- Has painful, stiff hands and feet
- Feels tired all of the time
- Reports an intermittent low-grade fever
- Takes naproxen (Naprosyn) 500 mg twice daily
- Wears a copper bracelet on the advice of a neighbor

Objective Data

- Hands show mild ulnar drift and puffiness
- Temperature: 100° F (37.8° C)
- Admitted to the hospital for examination and comprehensive treatment plan
- Methotrexate (Rheumatrex) therapy is to be initiated

Clinical Decision-Making Questions

Using a separate sheet of paper, answer the following questions.

1. How might the nurse explain the pathophysiology of rheumatoid arthritis to N.M.?
2. What manifestations does N.M. have that suggest the diagnosis of RA?
3. What results may be expected from methotrexate therapy? What are the nursing responsibilities related to methotrexate therapy?
4. What are some suggestions that may be offered to N.M. concerning home management and joint protection?
5. How can the nurse help N.M. recognize ineffective, unproved methods of treatment?
6. What other sources of information regarding arthritis might the nurse suggest to N.M.?
7. *Priority Decision:* Based on the assessment data presented, what are the priority nursing diagnoses? Are there any collaborative problems?

CHAPTER 66

Nursing Management: Critical Care

1. A primary difference in the skills of a certified critical care nurse compared with nurses certified in medical-surgical nursing is an ability to
   a. diagnose and treat life-threatening diseases.
   b. detect and manage early complications of health problems.
   c. provide intensive psychologic support to the patient and family.
   d. use advanced technology to assess and maintain physiologic function.

2. Identify which of the common three reasons patients are admitted to the ICU apply in the following situations.
   a. Patient with diabetic ketoacidosis
   b. Patient with nondisplaced skull fracture who is alert and oriented
   c. Postoperative patient with mitral valve replacement
   d. Comatose patient who had an anaphylactic reaction with cardiopulmonary arrest at home with reestablishment of cardiac function

3. A nursing intervention indicated for the patient in the ICU who has a nursing diagnosis of anxiety related to ICU environment and sensory overload is
   a. providing flexible visiting schedules for caregivers.
   b. eliminating unnecessary alarms and overhead paging.
   c. administering sedatives or psychotropic drugs to promote rest.
   d. allowing the patient to do as many self-care activities as possible.

4. The critical care nurse includes caregivers of the patient in the ICU as part of the health care team primarily because
   a. the costs of critical care will affect the entire family.
   b. caregivers are responsible for making health care decisions for the patient.
   c. the extent of the caregivers' involvement affects the patient's clinical course.
   d. caregivers who are ignored are more likely to question the patient's quality of care.

5. Review the concepts of cardiac output (CO), preload, and afterload by indicating whether the following conditions cause an increase or a decrease in the parameters under normal conditions.
   a. If HR is decreased, CO is _____.
   b. If stroke volume (SV) is increased, CO is _____.
   c. A decrease in preload will _____ SV.
   d. An increase in fluid administration will _____ preload.
   e. A decrease in afterload causes _____ CO.
   f. Increased systemic vascular resistance (SVR) _____ afterload.

6. During hemodynamic monitoring, the nurse finds that the patient has a decreased CO with unchanged pulmonary artery wedge pressure (PAWP), HR, and SVR. The nurse identifies that the patient has a decrease in
   a. SV.
   b. preload.
   c. afterload.
   d. contractility.

7. Before taking hemodynamic measurements, the monitoring equipment must be referenced by
   a. confirming that when pressure in the system is zero, the equipment reads zero.
   b. positioning the stopcock nearest the transducer level with the phlebostatic axis.
   c. placing the transducer on the left side of the chest at the fourth intercostal space.
   d. placing the patient in a left lateral position with the transducer level with the top surface of the mattress.

8. Identify whether the following statements are true (*T*) or false (*F*). If a statement is false, correct the bold word(s) to make the statement true.
   _____ a. When a patient has an arterial catheter placed for arterial blood gas (ABG) sampling, the low pressure alarm must be activated to detect **disconnection** of the line.
   _____ b. A pulmonary artery flow–directed catheter has a balloon at the distal tip that floats into the **left atrium**.
   _____ c. The pressure obtained when the balloon of the pulmonary artery catheter is inflated reflects the preload of the **right ventricle**.
   _____ d. In the absence of mitral valve impairment, the left ventricular end-diastolic pressure is reflected by the **PAWP**.
   _____ e. A decrease in SVO_2 (mixed venous blood) when arterial oxygenation, hemoglobin, and tissue perfusion are unchanged indicates **increased oxygen consumption**.

9. In preparing the patient for insertion of a pulmonary artery catheter, the nurse
   a. obtains informed consent from the patient.
   b. places the patient in high Fowler's position.
   c. ensures that the patient has continuous ECG monitoring.
   d. performs an Allen test to confirm adequate ulnar artery perfusion.

10. Describe the techniques the nurse uses to obtain the following data from the pulmonary artery catheter.
    a. PAWP
    b. Thermodilution CO (TDCO)

11. A patient in the ICU with hemodynamic monitoring has the following values.
    BP: 90/68 mm Hg
    HR: 124
    PAWP: 22 mm Hg
    CO: 3.2 L/min
    RAP (CVP): 14 mm Hg
    Pulmonary artery pressure: 38/20 mm Hg

    a. Calculate the additional values that can be determined from these findings.
       MAP _____
       PAMP _____
       SV _____
       SVR _____

    b. What interpretation can the nurse make about the patient's circulatory status and cardiac function from these values?

12. A patient has SvO_2 of 52%, CO of 4.8 L/min, SpO_2 of 95%, and unchanged hemoglobin level. The nurse should assess the patient for
    a. dysrhythmias.
    b. pain on movement.
    c. pulmonary edema.
    d. signs of septic shock.

13. The nurse observes a PAWP waveform on the monitor when the balloon of the patient's pulmonary artery catheter is deflated. The nurse recognizes that
    a. the patient is at risk for embolism because of occlusion of the catheter with a thrombus.
    b. the patient is developing pulmonary edema that has increased the pulmonary artery pressure.
    c. the patient is at risk for an air embolus because the injected air cannot be withdrawn into the syringe.
    d. the catheter must be immediately repositioned to prevent pulmonary infarction or pulmonary artery rupture.

14. The use of the intraaortic balloon pump (IABP) would be indicated for the patient with
    a. an insufficient aortic valve.
    b. a dissecting thoracic aortic aneurysm.
    c. generalized peripheral vascular disease.
    d. acute myocardial infarction with heart failure.

15. Identify whether the following statements are true (*T*) or false (*F*). If a statement is false, correct the bold word to make the statement true.
    _____ a. The rapid deflation of the intraaortic balloon causes a decreased **preload**.
    _____ b. During intraaortic counterpulsation, the balloon is **inflated** during diastole.
    _____ c. A primary effect of the intraaortic balloon pump is increased **systolic** pressure.

16. To prevent arterial trauma during the use of the IABP, the nurse should
    a. reposition the patient every 2 hours.
    b. check the site for bleeding every hour.
    c. prevent hip flexion of the cannulated leg.
    d. cover the insertion site with an occlusive dressing.

17. A patient who is hemodynamically stable has an order to wean the IABP. The nurse should
    a. decrease the augmentation pressure to zero.
    b. stop the machine since hemodynamic parameters are satisfactory.
    c. stop the infusion flow through the catheter when weaning is initiated.
    d. change the pumping ratio from 1:1 to 1:2 or 1:3 until the balloon is removed.

18. Ventricular assist devices are designed to
    a. provide permanent, total circulatory support when the left ventricle fails.
    b. temporarily partially or totally support circulation until a donor heart can be obtained.
    c. support circulation only when patients cannot be weaned from cardiopulmonary bypass.
    d. reverse the effects of circulatory failure in patients with acute myocardial infarction (MI) in cardiogenic shock.

19. A comatose patient with a possible cervical spine injury is intubated with a nasal endotracheal tube. The nurse recognizes that in comparison with an oral endotracheal tube, a nasal tube
    a. requires the placement of a bite block.
    b. is more likely to cause laryngeal trauma.
    c. requires greater respiratory effort in breathing.
    d. provides for easier suctioning and secretion removal.

20. In preparing a patient in the ICU for oral endotracheal intubation, the nurse
    a. places the patient supine with the head extended and neck flexed.
    b. tells the patient that the tongue must be extruded while the tube is inserted.
    c. positions the patient supine with the head hanging over the edge of the bed to align the mouth and trachea.
    d. informs the patient that while it will not be possible to talk during insertion of the tube, speech will be possible after it is correctly placed.

21. A patient has an oral endotracheal (ET) tube inserted to relieve an upper airway obstruction and to facilitate secretion removal. The first responsibility of the nurse immediately following placement of the tube is to
    a. suction the tube to remove secretions.
    b. secure the tube to the face with adhesive tape.
    c. place an end tidal CO_2 detector on the ET tube.
    d. assess for bilateral breath sounds and symmetric chest movement.

22. The nurse uses the minimal occluding volume to inflate the cuff on an endotracheal tube to minimize the incidence of
    a. infection.
    b. hypoxemia.
    c. tracheal necrosis.
    d. accidental extubation.

23. Complete the following statements related to the patient with an endotracheal tube.
    a. After inflating an endotracheal (ET) tube cuff, the nurse monitors the cuff pressure every _____ hours with a manometer to verify that the cuff pressure is _____ mm Hg.
    b. Equipment that should be at the bedside for all patients undergoing endotracheal intubation includes _____ equipment and a _____.
    c. A catheter used to suction an ET tube should be no larger than _____ the diameter of the ET tube.
    d. When suctioning an ET tube, the nurse uses a suction pressure of _____ mm Hg.
    e. During ET tube suctioning, each suction pass should be no longer than _____ seconds.
    f. To prevent hypoxemia during ET tube suctioning, the nurse always _____ the patient before and after suctioning.

24. The nurse suctions the patient's ET tube when the patient
    a. has peripheral crackles in all lobes.
    b. has not been suctioned for 2 hours.
    c. has coarse rhonchi over central airways.
    d. needs stimulation to cough and deep-breathe.

25. While suctioning the ET tube of a spontaneously breathing patient, the nurse notes that the patient develops bradycardia with premature ventricular contractions. The nurse should
    a. stop the suctioning and assess the patient for spontaneous respirations.
    b. attempt to resuction the patient with reduced suction pressure and pass time.
    c. stop the suctioning and ventilate the patient with slow, small-volume breaths using a bag-valve-mask (BVM) device.
    d. stop suctioning and ventilate the patient with a BVM device with 100% oxygen until the HR returns to baseline.

26. Identify two precautions the nurse should take during mouth care and repositioning of an oral ET tube to prevent and detect tube dislodgement.
    a.

    b.

27. A patient with an oral ET tube has a nursing diagnosis of risk for aspiration related to presence of artificial airway. Appropriate nursing interventions for this patient are to (select all that apply)
    a. assess gag reflex.
    b. ensure the cuff is properly inflated.
    c. suction the patient's mouth frequently.
    d. raise the head of the bed 30 to 45 degrees unless the patient is unstable.
    e. keep the ventilator tubing cleared of condensed water.

28. Although his oxygen saturation is above 92%, an orally intubated, mechanically ventilated patient is restless and very anxious. What intervention should be used first to decrease the risk of accidental extubation?
    a. Obtain an order and apply soft wrist restraints.
    b. Remind the patient that he needs the tube inserted to breathe.
    c. Administer sedatives and have a caregiver stay with the patient.
    d. Move the patient to an area close to the nurses' station for closer observation.

29. Identify four indications for mechanical ventilation.
    a.

    b.

    c.

    d.

30. Indicate whether the following are characteristic of negative-pressure ventilators (N), positive-pressure ventilators (P), or both (B).

    _____ a. Reduce intrathoracic pressure causing air to be pulled into lungs

    _____ b. Require an artificial airway

    _____ c. Expiration is passive

    _____ d. Most similar to physiologic ventilation

    _____ e. Applied to outside of the body

    _____ f. Most frequently used with acutely ill patients

    _____ g. Frequently used in the home for neuromuscular or nervous system disorders

31. Match the following types of positive-pressure ventilators with their descriptions (answers may be used more than once).

    _____ a. Peak inspiratory pressure predetermined

    _____ b. Preset volume of gas delivered with variable pressure based on compliance

    _____ c. Risk for hyperventilation and hypoventilation

    _____ d. Volume delivered varies based on selected pressure and patient lung compliance

    _____ e. Consistent volume delivered with each breath.

    1. Volume ventilator
    2. Pressure ventilator

32. Identify the ventilatory settings and modes described below.

    a. Positive pressure applied throughout the entire respiratory cycle of spontaneously breathing patient

    _____

    b. Patient self-regulates the rate and depth of spontaneous respirations, but may also receive preset volume and frequency breaths by ventilator _____

    c. Positive pressure applied only during inspiration that supplies a rapid flow of gas _____

    d. Preset tidal volume delivered at set frequency and more frequently when the patient attempts to inhale

    _____

    e. Positive pressure applied to airway during exhalation _____

    f. Delivery of small tidal volumes at a rapid respiratory rate _____

    g. Prolonged inspiration and shortened expiration set to promote alveolar expansion and prevent collapse

    _____

33. A patient in acute respiratory failure is receiving assist-control mechanical ventilation with a peak end-expiratory pressure (PEEP) of 10 cm H_2O. A sign that alerts the nurse to undesirable effects of increased airway and thoracic pressure is

    a. decreased BP.

    b. decreased PaO_2.

    c. increased crackles.

    d. decreased spontaneous respirations.

34. The nurse recognizes that a factor commonly responsible for sodium and fluid retention in the patient on mechanical ventilation is

    a. increased ADH release.

    b. increased release of atrial natriuretic factor.

    c. increased insensible water loss via the airway.

    d. decreased renal perfusion with release of renin.

35. ***Delegation Decision:*** The RN caring for a stable patient on mechanical ventilation in a long-term acute care facility plans the following interventions. Indicate whether the intervention must be done by the RN (*RN*) or if the intervention could be delegated to the LPN (*LPN*) or nursing assistive personnel (*NAP*) who would report back to the RN.

    _____ a. administer routinely scheduled medications

    _____ b. administer sedatives, analgesics, and paralytic medications

    _____ c. administer enteral nutrition

    _____ d. obtain vital signs and measure urine output

    _____ e. educate the patient and caregiver about mechanical ventilation and weaning

    _____ f. assist the respiratory therapist with repositioning and securing the ET tube

    _____ g. auscultate breath sounds and respiratory effort

    _____ h. perform passive or assisted range-of-motion exercises

    _____ i. maintain appropriate cuff inflation on the ET tube

    _____ j. provide personal hygiene and skin care

36. A patient receiving mechanical ventilation is very anxious and agitated, and neuromuscular blocking agents are used to promote ventilation. The nurse recognizes that
    a. the patient will be too sedated to be aware of the details of care.
    b. caregivers should be encouraged to provide stimulation and diversion.
    c. the patient should always be addressed and explanations of care given.
    d. communication will not be possible with the use of neuromuscular blocking agents.

37. Identify five problems associated with inadequate nutrition in the patient receiving prolonged mechanical ventilation.
    a.

    b.

    c.

    d.

    e.

38. The nurse determines that alveolar hypoventilation is occurring in a patient on a ventilator when
    a. the patient develops cardiac dysrhythmias.
    b. auscultation reveals an air leak around the ET cuff.
    c. ABG results show a $PaCO_2$ of 32 mm Hg and a pH of 7.47.
    d. the patient tries to breathe faster than the ventilator setting.

39. When weaning a patient from a ventilator, the nurse plans
    a. to decrease the delivered FIO_2 concentration.
    b. intermittent trials of spontaneous ventilation followed by ventilatory support to provide rest.
    c. substitution of ventilator support with a manual resuscitation bag if the patient becomes hypoxemic.
    d. to implement weaning procedures around the clock until the patient does not experience ventilatory fatigue.

40. A patient is to be discharged home with mechanical ventilation. Before discharge, it is most important for the nurse to
    a. teach the caregiver to care for the patient with a home ventilator.
    b. help the caregiver plan for placement of the patient in a long-term care facility.
    c. stress the advantages for the patient in being cared for in the home environment.
    d. have the caregiver arrange for around-the-clock home health nurses for the first several weeks.

CASE STUDY
Critically Ill Patient
Patient Profile

D.V., age 42, has a history of HIV infection with the development of manifestations of AIDS 2 years ago. He has been hospitalized and treated twice for *Pneumocystis jiroveci* pneumonia and is now admitted to ICU with a suspected cryptococcal meningitis. ICP monitoring is instituted, and an arterial line and flow-directed pulmonary artery catheter are inserted. Endotracheal intubation with assist-control mechanical ventilation at 12 breaths/min, 15 cm H_2O PEEP, and FIO_2 of 50% is established. (Note: This patient is very critically ill and requires you to review ICP, septic shock, multiple organ dysfunction syndrome [MODS], and respiratory failure.)

Subjective Data

- Friend relates that D.V. had two generalized tonic-clonic seizures in the 2 hours before admission.

Objective Data

- GCS score: 6
- ICP: 22 mm Hg
- Vital signs: T 102.2° F (39° C); HR 80; RR 26/min; BP 100/46 mm Hg
- ABGs: PaO_2 65 mm Hg; $PaCO_2$ 32 mm Hg; HCO_3-16 mEq/L; pH 7.26
- Other laboratory results: Glucose 228 mg/dL (12.6 mmol/L); lactate 3 mEq/L (3 mmol/L); WBC 18,500/μL
- Hemodynamic monitoring values: CO 6 L/min; PAP 8 mm Hg; PAWP 15 mm Hg; SVR 530 dyne sec/cm⁵; SvO_2 90%; SaO_2 92%
- Skin warm and dry
- Foley catheter inserted with 30 mL urine return

Clinical Decision-Making Questions

Using a separate sheet of paper, answer the following questions.

1. What are the best indicators to use in D.V.'s case to monitor his hemodynamic status?
2. What effect might the use of PEEP have on D.V.'s intracranial pressure?
3. What is D.V.'s MAP? What MAP would be necessary to promote tissue and cerebral perfusion and yet not increase ICP?
4. What drugs and fluids would be indicated for D.V.'s treatment?
5. How may D.V.'s condition be complicated by gastrointestinal ischemia?
6. Explain the processes that account for the abnormal assessment findings in D.V.
7. **Priority Decision:** Based on the assessment data presented, what are the priority nursing diagnoses? Are there any collaborative problems?

Nursing Management: Shock, Systemic Inflammatory Response Syndrome, and Multiple Organ Dysfunction Syndrome

1. The key factor in describing any type of shock is
   a. hypoxemia.
   b. hypotension.
   c. vascular collapse.
   d. inadequate tissue perfusion.

2. Match the following precipitating factors with their related types of shock (answers may be used more than once).

   _____ a. Acute myocardial infarction
   _____ b. Insect bites
   _____ c. Burns
   _____ d. Severe pain
   _____ e. Ventricular dysrhythmias
   _____ f. Abdominal compartment syndrome
   _____ g. Hemorrhage
   _____ h. Urinary tract infection
   _____ i. Spinal cord injury
   _____ j. Ruptured spleen
   _____ k. Pneumonia
   _____ l. Severe vomiting and diarrhea
   _____ m. Ascites
   _____ n. Pulmonary embolism
   _____ o. Epidural block
   _____ p. Vaccines

   1. Neurogenic
   2. Cardiogenic
   3. Anaphylactic
   4. Septic
   5. Hypovolemic
   6. Obstructive

3. Identify whether the following statements are true (*T*) or false (*F*). If a statement is false, correct the bold word(s) to make the statement true.
   _____ a. **Cardiogenic** shock is characterized by increased systemic vascular resistance (SVR), decreased CO, and decreased pulmonary artery wedge pressure (PAWP).
   _____ b. In septic shock, bacterial endotoxins cause vascular changes that result in **decreased systemic vascular resistance** with **increased cardiac output**.
   _____ c. Bradycardia with hypotension is characteristic of **neurogenic shock**.
   _____ d. In anaphylactic shock, death may occur as a result of **respiratory** failure.
   _____ e. Hypovolemic shock from **relative** hypovolemia may occur with diabetes insipidus.
   _____ f. Hemodynamic monitoring in the patient with cardiogenic shock will reveal an **increased** PAWP and a **decreased** cardiac output.

4. Complete the following pathophysiologic mechanisms that occur in the compensated stage of hypovolemic shock. Fill in the blanks below with the following words or phrases (see Figure 67-7).

Aldosterone secretion
α-Adrenergic stimulation
β-Adrenergic stimulation
Decreased capillary hydrostatic pressure
Increased BP
Increased heart strength and rate

Increased serum osmolality
Increased venous return to heart
Release of ADH
Renal water reabsorption
Renin release

a. Decreased BP → _____ → Fluid movement into intravascular space.

b. Decreased BP → Activation of sympathetic nervous system → _____ → Decreased blood flow to kidneys, skin, and GI tract.

c. Decreased BP → Activation of sympathetic nervous system → _____ coronary vasodilation and _____.

d. Decreased kidney perfusion → _____ → Increased angiotensin I.

e. Increased angiotensin II → _____ → Increased renal sodium reabsorption.

f. Increased angiotensin II → Venous and arterial vasoconstriction → _____ and _____.

g. Increased renal sodium reabsorption → _____ → _____.

h. Increased ADH → _____ → Increased blood volume.

5. From the data presented in question 4, identify six clinical manifestations that may be evident in a patient in the compensated stage of shock.
   a.

   b.

   c.

   d.

   e.

   f.

6. The nurse suspects sepsis as a cause when the laboratory test results of a patient in shock include
   a. hypokalemia.
   b. increased BUN.
   c. thrombocytopenia.
   d. decreased hemoglobin.

7. Progressive tissue hypoxia leading to anaerobic metabolism and metabolic acidosis is characteristic of the progressive stage of shock. Identify what changes occur in the following tissues to cause this increasing tissue hypoxia.
   a. Renal
   b. Lung
   c. Capillaries
   d. Cardiac

8. A patient with severe trauma has been treated for hypovolemic shock. The nurse recognizes that the patient is in the irreversible stage of shock when assessment findings include
   a. a lactic acidosis with a pH of 3.32.
   b. marked hypotension and refractory hypoxemia.
   c. unresponsiveness that responds only to painful stimuli.
   d. profound vasoconstriction with absent peripheral pulses.

9. *Priority Decision:* A patient with acute pancreatitis is experiencing hypovolemic shock. Which of the following initial orders for the patient will the nurse implement first?
   a. Start 1000 mL of normal saline at 500 mL/hr.
   b. Obtain blood cultures before starting IV antibiotics.
   c. Draw blood for hematology and coagulation factors.
   d. Administer high flow oxygen (100%) with a nonrebreather bag.

10. An abnormal finding that the nurse would expect to find in early, compensated shock is
    a. metabolic acidosis.
    b. increased serum sodium.
    c. decreased blood glucose.
    d. increased serum potassium.

11. In late, irreversible shock in a patient with massive thermal burns, the nurse would expect the patient's laboratory results to reveal
    a. respiratory alkalosis.
    b. decreased potassium.
    c. increased blood glucose.
    d. increased ammonia (NH_3) levels.

12. A patient with hypovolemic shock is receiving lactated Ringer's for fluid replacement therapy. During this therapy, it is most important for the nurse to monitor the patient's
    a. serum pH.
    b. serum sodium.
    c. serum potassium.
    d. hemoglobin and Hct.

13. The nurse determines that a large amount of crystalloid fluids administered to a patient in septic shock is effective when hemodynamic monitoring reveals
    a. CO of 2.6 L/min.
    b. CVP of 15 mm Hg.
    c. PAWP of 4 mm Hg.
    d. HR of 106 beats/min.

14. When caring for a patient in cardiogenic shock, the nurse recognizes that the metabolic demands of turning and moving the patient exceed the oxygen supply when hemodynamic monitoring reveals a change in
    a. SvO_2 from 62% to 54%.
    b. SV from 52 to 68 mL/beat.
    c. CO from 4.2 L/min to 4.8 L/min.
    d. SVR from 1300 dyne/sec/cm^5 to 1120 dyne/sec/cm^5.

15. During administration of IV norepinephrine (Levophed), the nurse should assess the patient for
    a. hypotension.
    b. marked diuresis.
    c. metabolic alkalosis.
    d. decreased tissue perfusion.

16. When administering any vasoactive drug during the treatment of shock, the nurse knows that the goal of the therapy is to
    a. constrict vessels to maintain BP.
    b. increase urine output to 50 mL/hr.
    c. maintain a MAP of at least 60 mm Hg.
    d. dilate vessels to improve tissue perfusion.

17. Identify two medical therapies that are specific to each of the following types of shock.
    a. Cardiogenic
    b. Hypovolemic
    c. Septic
    d. Anaphylactic

18. Identify four drugs and their actions that are used in treatment of cardiogenic shock that are not generally used for other types of shock.

    Drug   **Actions**

    a.

    b.

    c.

    d.

19. *Priority Decision:* The priority nursing responsibility in the prevention of shock is
    a. frequently monitoring all patients' vital signs.
    b. using aseptic technique for all invasive procedures.
    c. being aware of the potential for shock in all patients at risk.
    d. teaching patients health promotion activities to prevent shock.

20. Five indicators of tissue perfusion that should be monitored in critically ill patients are

    a.

    b.

    c.

    d.

    e.

21. Match each assessment area with the frequency with which the nurse should monitor its status when caring for an unstable patient in the acute phases of shock (some answers may not be used).
    _____ a. Renal function   1. Continuously
    _____ b. HR, BP, CVP, and PAP   2. q15min
    _____ c. Neurologic function   3. q1hr
    _____ d. GI function   4. q2hr
    _____ e. Respiratory rate and rhythm   5. q4hr
    _____ f. Oxygen saturation   6. q8hr
    _____ g. Breath sounds
    _____ h. ECG
    _____ i. Response to medication and fluid
                administration
    _____ j. Normal body temperature

22. A patient in the progressive stage of shock has rapid, deep respirations. The nurse determines that the patient's hyperventilation is compensating for a metabolic acidosis when the patient's arterial blood gas results include
    a. pH 7.42, PaO_2 80 mm Hg.
    b. pH 7.48, PaO_2 69 mm Hg.
    c. pH 7.38, $PaCO_2$ 30 mm Hg.
    d. pH 7.32, $PaCO_2$ 48 mm Hg.

23. On the table below, indicate (with an X) which collaborative interventions would be appropriate for the type of shock.

	O₂ Supplement	Volume Expansion— Crystalloid	Volume Expansion— Colloid	Circulatory Assist Device	Anti-biotics	Anti-histamine	Vaso-dilator	Vaso-pressor	Inotropes	Anti-Inflammatory
Anaphylactic										
Cardiogenic										
Hypovolemic										
Neurogenic										
Obstructive										
Septic										

24. A patient in shock has a nursing diagnosis of fear related to severity of condition and perceived threat of death as manifested by verbalization of anxiety about condition and fear of death. An appropriate nursing intervention for the patient is to
    a. administer antianxiety agents.
    b. allow caregivers to visit as much as possible.
    c. call a member of the clergy to visit the patient.
    d. inform the patient of the current plan of care and its rationale.

25. Identify whether the following statements are true (*T*) or false (*F*). If a statement is false, correct the bold word(s) to make the statement true.
    _____ a. Systemic inflammatory response syndrome (SIRS) is always present in a patient with **sepsis**.
    _____ b. Multiple organ dysfunction syndrome (MODS) **may occur independently** from SIRS.
    _____ c. All patients with septic shock develop **MODS**.
    _____ d. The **respiratory** system is often the first to show evidence of dysfunction in SIRS and MODS.
    _____ e. A common initial mediator that causes endothelial damage leading to SIRS and MODS is **endotoxin**.

26. Match the mechanism that can trigger SIRS with the injury/event to which it relates (answers may be used more than once).
    a. Burns
    b. Fungi
    c. Gram-negative bacteria
    d. Myocardial infarction
    e. Pancreatitis
    f. Post-cardiac resuscitation
    g. Surgical procedure
    h. Viruses

    1. Mechanical tissue trauma
    2. Global perfusion defect
    3. Ischemic/necrotic tissue
    4. Microbial invasion
    5. Endotoxin release

27. An intervention that may prevent GI bacterial and endotoxin translocation in a critically ill patient with SIRS is
    a. early enteral feedings.
    b. surgical removal of necrotic tissue.
    c. aggressive, multiple antibiotic therapy.
    d. strict aseptic technique in all procedures.

28. A patient with a gunshot wound to the abdomen is being treated for hypovolemic and septic shock. To monitor the patient for early organ damage associated with MODS, it is most important for the nurse to assess
    a. urine output.
    b. lung sounds.
    c. peripheral circulation.
    d. central venous pressure.

29. The development of MODS is confirmed in a patient who manifests
    a. a urine output of 30 mL/hr, a BUN of 65 mg/dL, and a WBC of 1120/µL.
    b. upper GI bleeding, Glasgow Coma Scale (GCS) score of 7, and an Hct of 25%.
    c. respiratory rate of 45/min, a $PaCO_2$ of 60, and a chest x-ray with bilateral diffuse patchy infiltrates.
    d. an elevated serum amylase and lipase, a serum creatinine of 3.8 mg/dL, and a platelet count of 15,000/µL.

CASE STUDY
Septic Shock
Patient Profile

A.M. is an 81-year-old man who was brought to the emergency department via an ambulance from a local nursing home. He was found by the nurses on their 6:00 AM rounds to be very confused, restless, and hypotensive.

Past Health History

A.M. is a type 1 diabetic with a history of prostate cancer, myocardial infarction, and heart failure. He has been a resident of the nursing home for 3 years. He has had an indwelling urinary catheter in place for 5 days because of difficulty voiding. Until today, A.M. has been very oriented and cooperative. His current medications are metoprolol (Lopressor), lisinopril (Zestril), hydrochlorothiazide (HydroDiuril), isosorbide (Isordil), and insulin.

Subjective Data

• Denies any pain or discomfort (but patient is confused and this information may be unreliable)

Objective Data

• Neurologic: Lethargic, confused to place and time, easily aroused, does not follow commands; moves all extremities in response to stimuli
• Cardiovascular: BP 80/60; HR 112 and regular; T 104° F (40° C) rectal; heart sounds normal without murmurs or S3, S4; peripheral pulses weak and thready
• Skin: Warm, dry, flushed
• Respiratory: RR 34 and shallow; breath sounds audible in all lobes with crackles bilaterally in the bases
• GI/GU: Abdomen soft with hypoactive bowel sounds; urinary catheter in place draining scant, purulent urine
In the emergency department, two 16-gauge IVs were inserted, and 700 mL of normal saline were given over the first hour. The patient was placed on 40% oxygen via face mask. The urinary catheter was removed and cultured, and blood cultures were drawn at two intervals. A new catheter was inserted. The patient was started on IV antibiotics and transferred to the ICU with the diagnosis of septic shock resulting from gram-negative sepsis.
• In the ICU, a pulmonary catheter was inserted in addition to an arterial line.
• ABG results were pH 7.25; PaO_2 60 mm Hg; $PaCO_2$ 28 mm Hg; HCO_3^- 12 mEq/L; and SaO_2 82%
• Hemodynamic pressures taken were right atrial pressure (CVP), PAP, PAWP, cardiac output, and SVR
• Laboratory test results were WBC 21,000/µL; Na^+ 133 mEq/L; K^+ 4.5 mEq/L; Cl^- 96 mEq/L; glucose 230 mg/dL; creatinine 1.7 mg/dL; hemoglobin 12 g/dL; Hct 36%
A.M.'s BP continued to drop despite several liters of crystalloids. Dopamine was started and titrated up as needed to try to maintain the patient's BP, in addition to more fluid administration. Despite all efforts, including intubation and mechanical ventilation, A.M. died on the sixth hospital day. The cause was multiple-organ dysfunction syndrome caused by gram-negative sepsis.

Clinical Decision-Making Questions

Using a separate sheet of paper, answer the following questions.

1. What risk factors for septic shock were present in A.M.?
2. What preventive measures could have been taken by the nursing home staff in regard to A.M.?
3. What are the major pathophysiologic changes associated with sepsis?
4. Discuss the mechanism for hypotension in the patient with septic shock.
5. Explain the physiologic reasons for the following assessment parameters found in this patient.
   - Decreased LOC
   - Warm, dry, and flushed skin
   - Tachycardia
   - Tachypnea
   - Fever
   - Decreased SVR
   - Increased CO
   - Oliguria
   - Hyperglycemia
6. Why was a pulmonary artery catheter indicated for A.M.?
7. Analyze the results of the ABGs.
8. Describe the changes in the hemodynamic pressure that would be expected in A.M.
9. Explain the rationale for fluid therapy and the use of dopamine.
10. *Priority Decision:* Based on the assessment data provided, what are the priority nursing diagnoses? What collaborative problems are present?

CHAPTER

68 Nursing Management: Respiratory Failure and Acute Respiratory Distress Syndrome

1. Respiratory failure can be defined as
   a. the absence of ventilation.
   b. any episode in which part of the airway is obstructed.
   c. inadequate gas exchange to meet the metabolic needs of the body.
   d. an episode of acute hypoxemia caused by a pulmonary dysfunction.

2. Indicate whether the following descriptions are characteristic of hypoxemic respiratory failure (HO) or hypercapnic respiratory failure (HC).
   _____ a. Primary problem is inadequate oxygen transfer
   _____ b. Most often caused by V/Q mismatch and shunt
   _____ c. Referred to as ventilatory failure
   _____ d. Exists when PaO_2 is 60 mm Hg or less, even when oxygen is administered at 60%
   _____ e. Risk of inadequate oxygen saturation of hemoglobin exists
   _____ f. The body is unable to compensate for acidemia of increased $PaCO_2$
   _____ g. Primary problem is insufficient carbon dioxide removal
   _____ h. Referred to as oxygenation failure
   _____ i. Results from an imbalance between ventilatory supply and ventilatory demand

3. Indicate whether the following statements are true (*T*) or false (*F*). If a statement is false, correct the bold word(s) to make the statement true.
   _____ a. A V/Q ratio of 1:1 (V/Q = 1) reflects an **alveolar ventilation** of 4 to 5 L that is matched by 4 to 5 L of **blood flow** to the lungs each minute.
   _____ b. The V/Q ratio is **1 or greater** when there is less ventilation to an area of the lung than perfusion.
   _____ c. An extreme V/Q imbalance resulting from blood leaving the heart without being exposed to ventilated areas of the lung is known as **a shunt**.
   _____ d. An intrapulmonary shunt occurs when an obstruction impairs the flow of **blood to ventilated areas of the lung**.
   _____ e. In differentiating between a V/Q mismatch and an intrapulmonary shunt, an increase in PaO_2 on oxygen administration occurs in the patient with **an intrapulmonary shunt**.
   _____ f. Gas transport is slowed in **shunt**, resulting in exertional hypoxemia that is not present at rest.

4. Match the following physiologic mechanisms of hypoxemia with their common causes.
   _____ a. V/Q mismatch 1 or greater   1. Pulmonary fibrosis
   _____ b. V/Q mismatch 1 or less   2. Ventricular septal defect
   _____ c. Anatomic shunt   3. Pulmonary embolism
   _____ d. Intrapulmonary shunt   4. Atelectasis
   _____ e. Diffusion limitation   5. Pulmonary edema

5. Match the mechanisms of hypoxemic respiratory failure that may occur in the patient with pneumonia with the responsible factors.
   _____ a. V/Q mismatch   1. Thickening of alveolar-capillary membrane from secretions and fluid accumulation
   _____ b. Diffusion limitation   2. Consolidation of lung lobules with exudate and alveolar collapse
   _____ c. Shunt   3. Decreased alveolar ventilation from obstruction of bronchioles and terminal respiratory units
   _____ d. Alveolar hypoventilation   4. Pleuritic pain and inflammation

6. Hypercapnic respiratory failure is most likely to occur in the patient who has
   a. rapid, deep respirations in response to pneumonia.
   b. slow, shallow respirations as a result of sedative overdose.
   c. large airway resistance as a result of severe bronchospasm.
   d. poorly ventilated areas of the lung caused by pulmonary edema.

7. Acute respiratory failure in a patient with chronic lung disease would most likely be indicated by ABG results of
   a. PaO_2 52 mm Hg, $PaCO_2$ 56 mm Hg, pH 7.4.
   b. PaO_2 46 mm Hg, $PaCO_2$ 52 mm Hg, pH 7.36.
   c. PaO_2 48 mm Hg, $PaCO_2$ 54 mm Hg, pH 7.38.
   d. PaO_2 50 mm Hg, $PaCO_2$ 54 mm Hg, pH 7.28.

8. Indicate whether the following manifestations are primarily characteristic of hypoxemic (HO) or hypercapnic (HC) respiratory failure.
   _____ a. Cyanosis
   _____ b. Morning headache
   _____ c. Rapid, shallow respirations
   _____ d. Metabolic acidosis
   _____ e. "Three-word" dyspnea
   _____ f. Use of tripod position
   _____ g. Respiratory acidosis

9. The nurse detects the early onset of hypoxemia in the patient who experiences
   a. restlessness.
   b. hypotension.
   c. central cyanosis.
   d. cardiac dysrhythmias.

10. The nurse assesses that a patient in respiratory distress is developing respiratory fatigue and the risk of respiratory arrest when the patient
    a. cannot breathe unless he is sitting upright.
    b. uses the abdominal muscles during expiration.
    c. has an increased inspiratory/expiratory (I/E) ratio.
    d. has a change in respiratory rate from rapid to slow.

11. A patient has a PaO_2 of 50 mm Hg and a $PaCO_2$ of 42 mm Hg because of an intrapulmonary shunt. The patient is most likely to respond best to
    a. positive pressure ventilation.
    b. oxygen administration at a FiO_2 of 100%.
    c. administration of oxygen per nasal cannula at 1 to 3 L/min.
    d. clearance of airway secretions with coughing and suctioning.

12. A patient with a massive hemothorax and pneumothorax has absent breath sounds in the right lung. To promote improved V/Q matching, the nurse positions the patient
    a. on the left side.
    b. on the right side.
    c. in a reclining chair bed.
    d. supine with the head of the bed elevated.

13. A patient in hypercapnic respiratory failure has a nursing diagnosis of ineffective airway clearance related to increasing exhaustion. An appropriate nursing intervention for the patient includes
    a. inserting an oral airway.
    b. performing augmented coughing.
    c. teaching the patient "huff" coughing.
    d. teaching the patient slow pursed-lip breathing.

14. After endotracheal intubation and mechanical ventilation have been started, a patient in respiratory failure becomes very agitated and is breathing asynchronously with the ventilator. It is most important for the nurse to first
    a. evaluate the patient's pain level, ABGs, and electrolyte values.
    b. sedate the patient to unconsciousness to eliminate patient awareness.
    c. administer the PRN vecuronium (Norcuron) to promote synchronous ventilations.
    d. slow the rate of ventilations provided by the ventilator to allow for spontaneous breathing by the patient.

15. Hemodynamic monitoring is instituted in severe respiratory failure primarily to
    a. detect V/Q mismatches.
    b. continuously measure the arterial BP.
    c. evaluate oxygenation and ventilation status.
    d. evaluate cardiac status and blood flow to tissues.

16. Identify an example of a drug that is used for the patient in acute respiratory failure (ARF) that
    a. relieves bronchospasm
    b. reduces airway inflammation
    c. reduces pulmonary congestion
    d. treats pulmonary infections

17. In caring for a patient in ARF, the nurse recognizes that noninvasive positive-pressure ventilation (NIPPV) may be indicated for a patient who
    a. is comatose and has high oxygen requirements.
    b. has copious secretions that require frequent suctioning.
    c. responds to hourly bronchodilator nebulization treatments.
    d. is alert and cooperative but has increasing respiratory exhaustion.

18. Although acute respiratory distress syndrome (ARDS) may result from direct lung injury or indirect lung injury as a result of systemic inflammatory response syndrome (SIRS), the nurse is aware that ARDS is most likely to occur in the patient with a host insult resulting from
    a. septic shock.
    b. oxygen toxicity.
    c. multiple trauma.
    d. prolonged hypotension.

19. Identify the three primary changes that occur in the injury or exudative phase of ARDS.
    a.

    b.

    c.

20. Patients with ARDS who survive the acute phase of lung injury and who progress to the fibrotic stage manifest
    a. chronic pulmonary edema and atelectasis.
    b. resolution of edema and healing of lung tissue.
    c. continued hypoxemia because of diffusion limitation.
    d. increased lung compliance caused by the breakdown of fibrotic tissue.

21. In caring for the patient with ARDS, the most characteristic sign the nurse would expect the patient to exhibit is
    a. increased PAWP.
    b. refractory hypoxemia.
    c. bronchial breath sounds.
    d. progressive hypercapnia.

22. The nurse suspects the early stage of ARDS in any seriously ill patient who
    a. develops respiratory acidosis.
    b. has diffuse crackles and rhonchi.
    c. exhibits dyspnea and restlessness.
    d. has a decreased PaO_2 and an increased $PaCO_2$.

23. A patient with ARDS has a nursing diagnosis of risk for infection. To detect the presence of infections commonly associated with ARDS, the nurse monitors
    a. gastric aspirate for pH and blood.
    b. the quality, quantity, and consistency of sputum.
    c. for subcutaneous emphysema of the face, neck, and chest.
    d. the mucous membranes of the oral cavity for open lesions.

24. The best patient response to treatment of ARDS occurs when initial management includes
    a. treatment of the underlying condition.
    b. administration of prophylactic antibiotics.
    c. treatment with diuretics and mild fluid restriction.
    d. endotracheal intubation and mechanical ventilation.

25. When mechanical ventilation is used for the patient with ARDS, PEEP is often applied to
    a. prevent alveolar collapse and open up collapsed alveoli.
    b. permit smaller tidal volumes with permissive hypercapnia.
    c. promote complete emptying of the lungs during exhalation.
    d. permit extracorporeal oxygenation and carbon dioxide removal outside the body.

26. The nurse suspects that a patient with PEEP is experiencing negative effects of this ventilatory maneuver upon finding a(n)
    a. increasing PaO_2.
    b. decreasing HR.
    c. decreasing blood pressure.
    d. increasing central venous pressure (CVP).

27. Prone positioning is considered for a patient with ARDS who has not responded to other measures to increase PaO_2. The nurse knows that this strategy
    a. increases the mobilization of pulmonary secretions.
    b. decreases the workload of the diaphragm and intercostal muscles.
    c. promotes opening of atelectatic alveoli in the upper portion of the lung.
    d. promotes perfusion of nonatelectatic alveoli in the anterior portion of the lung.

CASE STUDY
Acute Respiratory Failure
Patient Profile

P.C. is a 75-year-old married woman with severe oxygen- and corticosteroid-dependent COPD. She is admitted to the medical ICU with ARF and pneumonia.

Subjective Data

• Complains of increasing shortness of breath and difficulty breathing on minimal exertion

Objective Data

• ABGs on 2 L O_2/min: pH 7.3; $PaCO_2$ 55 mm Hg; PaO_2 60 mm Hg; SaO_2 84%
• Awake, alert, and oriented
• Sitting in tripod position and using pursed-lip breathing

Collaborative Care

• O_2 at 2 L/min per noninvasive positive-pressure ventilation
• Albuterol (Ventolin, Proventil) nebulization every hour PRN
• IV aminophylline
• IV antibiotics
• IV corticosteroids

Clinical Decision-Making Questions

Using a separate sheet of paper, answer the following questions.

1. What type of respiratory failure is P.C. primarily experiencing? Briefly describe how this situation illustrates the concept of acute chronic respiratory failure.
2. What factors contributed to the development of respiratory failure in P.C.?
3. What are the pathophysiologic effects and clinical manifestations of P.C.'s respiratory failure?
4. How do the tripod position and pursed-lip breathing contribute to respiratory function?
5. What is NIPPV? When is it contraindicated?
6. *Priority Decision:* Which of the treatments instituted for P.C. is the most important in returning her to her usual level of respiratory function?
7. *Priority Decision:* Based on the assessment data presented, what are the priority nursing diagnoses? Are there any collaborative problems?

1. **Priority Decision:** Triage the following patient situations that may be present in an emergency department as 1, 2, 3, 4, or 5 of the Emergency Severity Index.
   _____ a. A 6-year-old child with a temperature of 103.2° F (39.6° C)
   _____ b. A 22-year-old woman with asthma in acute respiratory distress
   _____ c. An infant who has been vomiting for 2 days
   _____ d. A 50-year-old man with low back pain and spasms
   _____ e. A 32-year-old woman who is unconscious following an automobile accident
   _____ f. A 40-year-old woman with rhinitis and a cough
   _____ g. A 58-year-old man with midsternal chest pain
   _____ h. A teenager with an angulated forearm following a sports injury

2. The nurse performing a primary survey in the emergency department is assessing
   a. the acuity of the patient's condition to determine priority of care.
   b. whether the patient is responsive enough to provide needed information.
   c. whether the resources of the emergency department are adequate to treat the patient.
   d. the status of airway, breathing, circulation, disability, and exposure/environmental control.

3. Identify two life-threatening conditions that the nurse may identify during each step of the primary survey and one appropriate intervention for the conditions that may be performed during the assessment.

	Conditions	Interventions
Airway with Cervical Spine Stabilization and/or Immobilization		
Breathing		
Circulation		
Disability		

4. During the secondary survey of a trauma patient in the emergency department, it is important that the nurse obtain details of the incident primarily because
   a. the mechanism of injury can indicate specific injuries.
   b. important facts may be forgotten when needed later for legal actions.
   c. alcohol use associated with many accidents can affect treatment of injuries.
   d. many types of accidents or trauma must be reported to government agencies.

5. Identify five interventions that are performed during the "F" step of the secondary survey.
   a.

   b.

   c.

   d.

   e.

6. Placement of a nasogastric tube is contraindicated during emergency care when the patient has a possible
   a. inhalation injury.
   b. head or facial trauma.
   c. intraabdominal bleed.
   d. cervical spine fracture.

7. In assessing the emergency patient's health history, what information is obtained with the use of the mnemonic AMPLE?
   a. A
   b. M
   c. P
   d. L
   e. E

8. A trauma patient has open wounds and the nurse questions the patient regarding her tetanus immunization status. Tetanus immunoglobulin would be administered if the patient has
   a. had only three doses of tetanus toxoid.
   b. had less than three doses of tetanus toxoid.
   c. not had a dose of tetanus toxoid in the past 5 years.
   d. not had a dose of tetanus toxoid in the past 10 years.

9. In which of the following situations would therapeutic hypothermia be instituted in the ED?
   a. 48-year-old male found unconscious by neighbors. On ED arrival, he is moaning and moving all extremities.
   b. 62-year-old man defibrillated by EMTs. On ED arrival, he is not responsive although his heart rhythm and BP are stable.
   c. 30-year-old female who suffered heat exhaustion following a marathon. On ED arrival, she is hypotensive and extremely diaphoretic with a temperature of 102.6° F.
   d. 38-year-old female found face down in her bathtub. She has a history of seizures. On ED arrival, she is responsive to pain only, and she was intubated by paramedics with evidence of pulmonary edema. Her pulse oximetry is >90%.

10. Following the death in the emergency department of a 36-year-old man from a massive head injury, it would be appropriate for the nurse to
    a. ask the family members to consider donating their loved one's organs.
    b. notify an organ-procurement agency that a death has occurred that could result in organ donation.
    c. explain to the family what a generous act it would be to donate the patient's organs to another patient who needs them.
    d. ask the family to check the patient's driver's license to determine whether he had designated approval of donation of his organs in case of death.

11. Match the heat-related emergencies with their characteristics (answers may be used more than once).
    _____ a. Rectal temperature of 99.6°–104° F (37.5°–40° C)   1. Heat edema
    _____ b. Treated with rapid cooling methods   2. Heat cramps
    _____ c. Related to salt deficiency following heavy work   3. Heat exhaustion
                without adequate fluids   4. Heat stroke
    _____ d. High risk of mortality and morbidity
    _____ e. Volume and electrolyte depletion
    _____ f. Elevated core temperature without sweating
    _____ g. Oxygen administration necessary
    _____ h. Causes mild confusion, headache, and dilation of pupils
    _____ i. Extremity swelling is only symptom

12. During rewarming of a patient's toes that have suffered deep frostbite, the nurse
    a. applies sterile dressings to blisters.
    b. places the feet in a cool water bath.
    c. ensures that analgesics are administered.
    d. massages the digits to increase circulation.

13. ***Priority Decision:*** A patient is brought to the emergency department following a skiing accident in which he was not found for several hours. He is rigid and has slowed respiratory and heart rates. During the initial assessment of the patient, the nurse should
   a. manage and maintain ABCs (airway, breathing, circulation).
   b. initiate active core-rewarming interventions.
   c. monitor the core temperature via the axillary route.
   d. expose the patient to check for areas of frostbite and other injuries.

14. A homeless man is brought to the emergency department in profound hypothermia with a temperature of 85° F (29.4° C). On initial assessment, the nurse would expect to find
   a. shivering and lethargy.
   b. fixed and dilated pupils.
   c. respirations of 6–8/min.
   d. BP obtainable only by Doppler.

15. Indicate whether each of the following conditions occurs with freshwater near-drowning (F), saltwater near-drowning (S), or both (B).
   _____ a. Water leaks from alveoli to capillary bed and circulation
   _____ b. Noncardiogenic pulmonary edema
   _____ c. Destruction of surfactant
   _____ d. Fluid is drawn into the alveoli from the pulmonary capillaries
   _____ e. Destruction of alveolar-capillary membrane

16. ***Priority Decision:*** The priority of management of the near-drowning patient is
   a. correction of hypoxia.
   b. correction of acidosis.
   c. maintenance of fluid balance.
   d. prevention of cerebral edema.

17. The ascending paralysis caused by exposure to the wood tick or dog tick may cause respiratory arrest unless
   a. the tick is removed.
   b. antibiotics are administered.
   c. an antidote for the neurotoxin is administered.
   d. hemodialysis is instituted to remove the neurotoxin.

18. Identify whether the following statements are true (*T*) or false (*F*). If a statement is false, correct the bold word(s) to make the statement true.
   _____ a. The bite of a cat carries a risk of infection from ***Staphylococcus aureus***.
   _____ b. Rabies vaccination is always indicated when a bite is caused by a **carnivorous wild animal**.
   _____ c. Emergency management of surface exposure to most toxins is **application of topical steroids**.
   _____ d. Treatment of ingested toxic alkali substances includes administration of **activated charcoal**.
   _____ e. Elimination of poisons that cause severe acidosis would include the use of **cathartics**.

19. For the following ingested poisons, identify all those for which gastric lavage may be considered.
   _____ a. Aspirin
   _____ b. Lorazepam (Ativan)
   _____ c. Iron supplements
   _____ d. Bleach
   _____ e. Acetaminophen (Tylenol)
   _____ f. Drain cleaner

20. A patient is admitted unconscious to the emergency department by his family, who brought an empty container of Elavil found near the patient. A large oral-gastric tube is inserted and the nurse prepares to administer
   a. cathartics.
   b. syrup of ipecac.
   c. a gastric lavage.
   d. activated charcoal.

21. In the following diagram, mark the columns that apply to each of the biologic agents of terrorism.

Agent	Bacterial	Viral	Person-to-Person Spread	Antibiotic Treatment	Vaccine
Botulism					
Anthrax					
Plague					
Hemorrhagic fever					
Tularemia					
Smallpox					

22. Match the following biologic agents of terrorism with their characteristics (answers may be used more than once).
_____ a. No established treatment for most forms.
_____ b. The septicemic form is most lethal
_____ c. Toxins cause hemorrhage and destruction of lung tissue (inhaled form)
_____ d. Neurotoxins that cause paralysis and respiratory failure
_____ e. Spread by flea bites
_____ f. Hemorrhage of tissues with organ failure
_____ g. Lesions are pustular vesicles
_____ h. Skin lesions are most common form
_____ i. Primarily an infection of rabbits
_____ j. Disease was eradicated in 1980
_____ k. Death may occur within 24 hours of exposure

1. Botulism
2. Anthrax
3. Smallpox
4. Plague
5. Tularemia
6. Hemorrhagic fever

23. A victim of a sublethal dose (<600 rad) of whole-body ionizing radiation exposure is admitted to the emergency department several hours after exposure. On assessment the nurse would expect the patient to report
a. hair loss.
b. nausea and vomiting.
c. bleeding from the gums and nose.
d. bruises on skin not covered by clothing.

24. As a member of a volunteer disaster medical assistance team, the nurse would be expected to
a. triage casualties of a tornado that hit the local community.
b. assist with implementing the hospital's emergency response plan.
c. train citizens of communities how to respond to mass casualty incidents.
d. deploy to local or other communities with disasters to provide medical assistance.

CASE STUDY
Heat Stroke
Patient Profile

M.M., age 72, was taking a short break from nailing new shingles on his roof during the summer when he lost consciousness and collapsed in his yard. Accompanied by his wife, he was brought by ambulance to the emergency department.

Subjective Data

• Wife states he has been working all week on the roof even though he has not felt well the last day or two

Objective Data

• Vital signs: T 106.6° F (41.4° C); HR 124 and weak and thready; RR 36 and shallow; BP 82/40
• Skin hot, dry, and pale

Clinical Decision-Making Questions

Using a separate sheet of paper, answer the following questions.

1. What factors in M.M.'s history place him at risk for heat stroke?
2. What laboratory tests would the nurse anticipate to be ordered, and what alterations in these tests would be indications of heat stroke?
3. How would cooling for M.M. be carried out?
4. What supportive treatment is indicated for M.M.?
5. What should Mrs. M. be told about M.M.'s condition?
6. *Priority Decision:* Based on the assessment data presented, what are the priority nursing diagnoses? Are there any collaborative problems?

CHAPTER 1

1. a, b, d, f, g, i
2. Required educational preparation may be an associate, baccalaureate, or master's degree; or the only specified requirement may be that a nurse is a registered nurse regardless of educational preparation. Other requirements may include a specific number of years of work in the specialized area or an examination.
3. a, b, c. Rationale: Certification usually requires an exam to verify a certain knowledge base and experience in the specialty area to develop the expertise. Certification is a voluntary process that provides recognition of one's expertise.
4. b. Rationale: CNLs are educated to be generalists who apply EBP to patient care, and manage and provide care for a group of patients on a specific unit or setting. Nursing research is a focus of many advanced nursing degrees; terminal degrees in nursing are doctorates (DNP), and CNS and NPs specialize.
5. a. F, complexity; b. T; c. T; d. F, The Joint Commission (TJC)
6. QSEN six competencies are (1) Patient-centered care, (2) Teamwork and collaboration, (3) EBP, (4) Quality improvement, (5) Safety, and (6) Informatics.
7. In order:
   4 Make recommendations for practice or generate data
   1 Ask a clinical question
   3 Critically analyze the evidence
   2 Find and collect the evidence
   5 Evaluate the outcomes in the clinical setting
8. P = Patient/population
   I = Intervention
   C = Comparison
   O = Outcome
   T = Time period
9. d. Rationale: Evidence-based clinical practice guidelines are developed from summaries of research results and reflect the best known state of practice at the time. Use of these guidelines leads to more positive outcomes of care and would be best to use in planning care or programs.
10. (1) NANDA International Nursing Diagnoses, (2) NOC, (3) NIC.
11. d. Rationale: The use of a standardized electronic health record for each citizen is being promoted primarily to provide all care providers ready access to patient information to coordinate care and to prevent duplication of information and erratic delivery of care.

12. b. nurse informatists deal specifically with nursing informatics (the process and development). The other roles use nursing informatics.
13. a. 2; b. 3; c. 4; d. 1; e. 2; f. 5; g. 3; h. 2; i. 5; j. 4
14. a. Independent: assessment of physical and psychologic status, evaluation of response to medications, and dietary teaching
    b. Collaborative: Communication with the health care provider regarding assessment findings and laboratory results and communication with the dietitian about dietary orders and patient status
    c. Dependent: Administration of medication
15. a. CP; b. ND; c. ND; d. ND; e. ND; f. ND; g. ND; h. CP; i. ND; j. CP
16. Activity intolerance related to prolonged bed rest as evidenced by shortness of breath on exertion, weakness and fatigue, failure of pulse to return to preactivity level after 3 minutes.
17. a. Life-threatening problems. b. Physiologic needs. c. Psychosocial needs. d. Patient's preference may at times be a priority. Should determine what the patient priorities are.
18. For anorexia, nursing measures would include mouth care, odor control, presentation of foods, offering favorite foods, etc. These measures differ from those for difficulty swallowing, which would include checking gag reflex, positioning, offering small bites of formed foods, avoiding free liquids in the mouth, etc. The differences show how important it is to determine the correct etiology of a nursing diagnosis.
19. a. I: Not measurable or behavioral, nor does it ensure that he will take medications; b. C; c. I: not measurable, no criteria, and no time designation; d. I: not measurable, not behavioral; e. C
20. Many answers may be correct. Examples include the following:
    a. Turn the patient every 2 hours using the following schedule: L side → back → R side → L side → back; inspect and document all at-risk areas for blanching and erythema at each position change.
    b. Provide 8 oz. of fluids every 2 hours (even hours) while the patient is awake (the patient prefers cold liquids); assist the patient in choosing five fresh fruits or vegetables from the menu each day.
21. a. The mistake was made during assessment when the nurse did not ask why the patient had not taken her medication regularly, and the appropriate etiology for the nursing diagnosis was not validated.

b. The nursing diagnosis should be changed in this case to reflect an etiology of lack of financial resources, and nursing interventions would not be teaching about the medications but rather consulting with the health care provider regarding the use of generic medications or a change in prescription and perhaps providing the patient with a list of discount drug sources. The patient outcome would remain the same.

22. (1) Right task, (2) right circumstances, (3) right person, (4) right direction and communication, and (5) right supervision and evaluation.

23. a, c, d, f, g. Rationale: These are actions or interventions that require judgment and clinical decision-making, therefore they should be performed by an RN.

24. 3 a plan that directs an entire health care team
    1 used as guides for routine nursing care
    1, 2 used in nursing education to teach the nursing process and care planning
    3 a description of patient care required at specific times during treatment
    1 should be personalized and specific to each patient
    2 a visual diagram representing relationships between patient problems, interventions, and data.
    3 used for high volume and highly predictable case types

CHAPTER 2

1. b. Rationale: The determinants of health are factors that influence the health of individuals and groups; today the major determinant of health is behavior. Although the other factors could influence this patient's health, the smoking behavior is the most important causative factor in this situation.

2. a. rural setting; b. low income; c. gender; d. age

3. a. 2; b. 5; c. 7; d. 1; e. 3; f. 6; g. 4

4. a. 5; b. 4; c. 11; d. 2; e. 9; f. 1; g. 6; h. 10; i. 3; j. 8; k. 7

5. a. *Dynamic* and ever-changing, b. *Shared* by all members of the same cultural group, c. *Adapted* to specific conditions such as environmental factors, and d. *Learned* through oral and written histories as well as socialization

6. a. cultural knowledge; b. cultural awareness; c. cultural encounter; d. cultural skills

7. Examples may include any instances of the following:
   a. Patients may be late for appointments, skip appointments entirely, or delay seeing a health care provider because social events are more important to them.

   b. Lack of health insurance, limited financial resources, or undocumented immigrant status may deter patients from using the health care system.
   c. Ethnic foods may be high in sodium and fat or low in calcium and protein. If dietary changes required by health problems are not made within the context of the patient's normal diet, chances are high that the patient will not make the changes.
   d. Personal space zones are a strong cultural trait. A patient may move closer to the nurse, causing a feeling of discomfort for the nurse; or, if the nurse increases the personal space, the patient might be offended.
   e. Religious beliefs or practices, faith in folk medicine, or negative experiences with culturally insensitive health care may delay or prevent patients from seeking health care.

8. d. Rationale: As a Jehovah's Witness, the administration of blood or blood products is prohibited. She may also experience some distress related to the loss of her child. Pork or pork-derived products are prohibited in Islam and in strict Judaism, and strict relationships between men and women are characteristic of Islam.

9. b. Rationale: Traditional Native American rituals may include healing ceremonies used in addition to conventional therapy to promote a balance of physical, spiritual, and emotional wholeness believed to be necessary for wellness. These rituals may or may not be part of formal religious beliefs and may positively alter the progression of physical illnesses.

10. b. Rationale: In some cultural groups, especially Asian, Hispanic, and Native American, there is an emphasis on interdependence rather than independence. The nurse should be aware that in other cultures, decisions for the patient may be made by other family members or may be made collectively by the patient and his or her family. All the other options reflect insensitive assumptions that the patient should make an autonomous decision.

11. b. Rationale: In the Arabic culture, male-female roles are strictly observed. A woman should not be touched by a man other than her husband, nor should she be alone with another man. An Arabic woman would be very uncomfortable being cared for by a male nurse or would be put in the position of having to refuse the care.

12. From Table 2-7. a. benzodiazepines; b. tricyclic antidepressants; c. antipsychotics; d. analgesics; e. antihypertensive agents such as β-adrenergic

blockers, angiotensin-converting enzyme (ACE) inhibitors.

13. a. Rationale: Empacho causes abdominal pain and cramping from food balls forming in the stomach or intestinal tract. Susto is a culture-bound syndrome also known as "fright sickness." Ghost sickness causes nightmares, weakness, and a sense of suffocation; and bilis brought on by strong anger causes headaches, stomach disturbances, and loss of consciousness.

14. b, d

15. a. T; b. T

CHAPTER 3

1. Yes. Although some of the information contained in the medical history might be useful to nursing, the medical history focuses on the diagnosis of patients' health problems, whereas the nursing history is used to gather data that will provide a health profile for comprehensive health care, including patients' potential and actual health problems and health promotion.

2. Subjective: Short of breath, pain in chest upon breathing, coughing makes head hurt, aches all over. Objective: Respiratory rate of 28/min, coughing yellow sputum, skin hot and moist, temperature 102.2° F (39° C).

3. Examples: Many answers could be correct. It is helpful to preface the question with the reason it is being asked.
   a. "Many patients taking drugs for hypertension have problems with sexual function. Have you experienced any problems?"
   b. "Alcohol may interact dangerously with drugs you receive, or it may cause withdrawal problems in the hospital. Can you describe your recent alcohol intake?"
   c. "It is important to contact and treat others who might have the same infection you do. Would you please tell me with whom you have been sexually intimate in the last 6 weeks?"
   d. "Today medications are so expensive that some people must choose between eating and taking their medications. Are you able to get and take all the medications prescribed for you?"

4. d. Rationale: Data are required regarding the immediate problem, but gathering additional information can be delayed. The patient should not receive pain medication before pertinent information related to allergies or the nature of the problem is obtained. Questions that require brief answers do not elicit adequate information for a health profile. A friend or family member might not be present or adequately informed, and the patient might not achieve a pain-free state.

5. c. Rationale: When a patient describes a feeling, the nurse should ask about the factors surrounding the situation to clarify the etiology of the problem. An incorrect nursing diagnosis may be made if the statement is taken literally and if the meaning is not explored with the patient. A sense of "tired and being unable to function" does not necessarily indicate a need for rest or sleep, and there is no way to know that treatment will relieve the problem.

6. There may be many correct answers. Examples include the following:
   a. "Can you tell me how you are feeling?"
   b. "Describe your relationship with your spouse."
   c. "Can you describe your experience with this illness?"
   d. "What is your usual activity during the day?"

7. a. Areas addressed: partial location, quality, chronology, aggravating factors.
   b. Areas not addressed: quality, setting, associated manifestations, meaning of symptom

8. a. 1; b. 10; c. 10; d. 8; e. 4; f. 4, 6; g. 2, 3; h. 6; i. 6; j. 6; k. 7; l. 5; m. 3, 9; n. 2; o. 4; p. 12; q. 11; r. 2; s. 10; t. 13

9. d. Rationale: Abnormal lung sounds are usually associated with chronic bronchitis, and their absence is a negative finding. Chest pain is a positive finding, and radiation is not expected for all chest pain. Elevated blood pressure in hypertension is a positive finding, and pupils that are equal and react to light and accommodation are normal findings.

10. a. 2; b. 4; c. 3; d. 2; e. 1; f. 4; g. 1; h. 2

11. d. Rationale: The usual sequence of physical assessment techniques is inspection, palpation, percussion, and auscultation; however, because palpation and percussion can alter bowel sounds, in abdominal assessment the sequence should be inspection, auscultation, percussion, and palpation.

12. b. Rationale: A nurse should use the same efficient sequence in each examination to avoid forgetting a procedure, a step in the sequence, or a body part; but a specific method is not required. Patient safety, comfort, and privacy are considerations but are not the priorities. The nursing history data should be collected in an interview to avoid prolonging the examination.

13. Place the patient in a position of comfort and avoid unnecessary changes in position.

14. b, e. Rationale: These are situations in which an initial and thorough baseline assessment needs to be completed. a. and d. would be focused assessments; c. would be an emergency assessment.

15. Word Search. a. palpation; b. subjective; c. inspection; d. otoscope; e. focused; f. auscultation; g. objective; h. percussion; i. location.

```
E  O  N  T  E  D  L  N  O  R  C  E  S
N  A  O  F  B  I  U  Q  A  R  Q  P  E
N  O  I  T  A  T  L  U  C  S  U  A  T
O  N  T  I  L  C  F  O  C  U  S  E  D
I  G  A  N  P  I  O  N  U  B  H  O  L
T  O  C  E  V  I  T  C  E  J  B  O  N
A  F  O  T  O  S  C  O  P  E  T  M  E
P  I  L  N  O  I  S  S  U  C  R  E  P
L  O  A  O  N  M  T  I  Q  T  E  N  A
A  D  I  N  S  P  E  C  T  I  O  N  S
P  A  J  A  L  O  D  M  O  V  I  A  T
L  O  A  P  T  R  O  O  N  E  N  Y  O
```

CHAPTER 4

1. a. Maintenance of health. b. Management of illness.
   c. Appropriate selection and use of treatment options.
   d. Prevention of disease.
2. In your own words, something like this: Use every opportunity (interaction [e.g., administering medications]) to assess patients for educational needs, to provide the education needed, and/or to reinforce the education that has already occurred. The time for patient teaching is limited and every opportunity needs to be used efficiently.
3. a, b, e. Rationale: Learning is acquiring a skill or knowledge and may occur from experience rather than teaching, planned teaching using a variety of methods may increase the learning, and teaching that is planned helps organize to make learning more efficient. Teaching may occur as an incidental experience without prior planning. One hopes that the learner's behavior will change as a result of teaching; however, it is the choice of the learner to either change behavior or not.
4. a. 5; b. 1, 2, 4, 7; c. 2, 4; d. 5, 6; e. 2, 7; f. 6; g. 3
5. c. Rationale: This patient is in the precontemplation stage of behavior change—he is not considering a change, nor is he ready to learn. During this stage, the best intervention by the nurse is simply to describe the benefits of change and the risks of not changing. The consequences of not changing should not be presented as threats, but rather as a disadvantage of the current behavior. Describing what is involved in behavior change and setting priorities are recommended for later stages of change.
6. a. Example: A sudden episode *(acute)* where the heart muscle *(myocardium)* is damaged from a lack of blood supply *(infarction)*

b. Example: The intravenous *(IV)* injection of a dye to visually record *(gram)* the kidneys *(pyelo)*
   c. Example: Damage *(pathy)* to the retina *(retino)* of the eye as a complication of diabetes
7. a. Rationale: An empathetic approach to teaching requires that the nurse discover and understand the patient's world and teach according to the individual patient's needs. The other options are important but are not directly related to empathy.
8. Lack of Time: set learning priorities with the patient and use every encounter. Let the patient know how much time you have for each session.
   Feeling as a Teacher: prepare ahead of time; use available written materials; respect the patient's response to the health problem.
   Patient Circumstances: know your resources; anticipate each contact with your patient and use it to teach throughout the day; provide the patient with written materials and contact numbers if clarification is needed.
9. b. Rationale: To promote self-efficacy, it is important that the person is successful in new endeavors to strengthen the belief in his or her ability to manage a situation. To avoid early failure, the nurse should work with the patient to present simple concepts related to knowledge and skills the person already has. Motivation and relevancy are important factors in adult learning but are more often a result of self-efficacy, not a method of promoting it.
10. a. Use supplementary illustrations and written materials; provide audiotapes or audiovisual presentations with headphones that block environmental noise and promote auditory function.

b. Support the patient during this time, and do not argue about the need for change in behavior; wait until the patient is ready to learn to begin teaching.

c. Evaluate the medication schedule and change, if possible, to increase alertness; if sedation is the objective of the medication, consider teaching family members or other caregivers.

d. Provide only brief explanations, and wait to present more detailed instruction until the pain has been controlled.

e. Be sure that educational materials are written at an eighth-grade level; use audiovisual materials with simple, lay language.

f. Provide a variety of written educational materials; refer the patient to appropriate Internet resources for information.

g. Use translators and translation software programs; obtain patient teaching materials in patient's primary language.

11. b. Rationale: The nursing diagnosis should specify the exact nature of the knowledge deficit so that the objectives, strategies, implementation, and evaluation relate to the identified problem. The problem is deficient knowledge, and a nursing diagnosis stating that the knowledge deficit is related to a lack of interest is in error. The statement "potential for cardiac dysrhythmias" is a collaborative problem rather than a nursing diagnosis.

12. Example: The patient will select foods high in potassium from a given list of common foods by the time of discharge.

13. a. 3; b. 4; c. 1, 7; d. 2, 7; e. 2; f. 2; g. 6, 7; h. 2, 6, 7; i. 5; j. 3; k. 4; l. 6, 7; m. 5

14. c. Rationale: If audiovisual and written materials do not help the patient meet the learning goals, they are a waste of time and expense. The nurse should ensure that these materials are accurate and appropriate for each patient. Audiovisual materials are often supplementary either before or after other presentation of information and do not need to include all the information the patient needs to learn in order to be of value. Patients with auditory and visual limitations may find these materials useful because they can adjust the volume and size of the images.

15. Example
Action: This medicine, atorvastatin, keeps the liver from making so much cholesterol.
Uses: The medicine is used to lower cholesterol and fats in the blood. It helps to prevent heart attacks and strokes.
Side effects: Overall, this medicine does not cause many side effects. Stomach upset or intestinal gas may occur. Other effects can include liver and pancreas problems, skin rashes and itching, hair loss, muscle pain, eye changes, and headache.
Call your doctor if these problems occur or worsen.
Precautions: Tell your doctor if you get any yellowing of your eyes or skin or have vomiting. Tell your doctor if you have any liver disease in the past, alcoholism, low blood pressure, serious infections, seizure disorders, diabetes or thyroid problems, physical injuries, or blood imbalances. Drink very little or no alcohol because it can damage your liver and cause more side effects. If you have other effects not listed above, call your doctor.
Interactions: This medicine will interact with many other medicines to cause problems. Give your doctor a list of all the medicines you take. Do not start any new medicine while you are taking atorvastatin without checking with your doctor.

16. a, e. Rationale: The Internet is a valuable source of health information, but it is also unregulated, and much information is unreliable or inaccurate. As a result, both nurses and patients should learn to evaluate sources and identify accurate information. Reliable sources include universities, government health agencies, and reputable health care organizations.

17. a. direct observation
b. ask a direct question or use a written measurement tool (ask the patient to write down the serious side effects that need to be reported to the doctor)
c. direct observation with observation of verbal and nonverbal cues
d. direct observation

18. b. Rationale: A statement that documents what the patient does as a result of teaching indicates whether the learning objective has been met and provides the best documentation of patient instruction. "Understand" is not a measurable behavior and does not validate that learning has occurred. The content and strategies of patient education are documented in the teaching plan and would not be repeated in charting related to the outcome of instruction.

19. c. Millennials (1981–2000)

CHAPTER 5

1. b, d, e, g

2. a. preventing and managing crisis, carrying out prescribed regimens, adjusting to changes in the course of the disease, controlling symptoms
b. preventing social isolation, attempting to normalize interactions with others
c. carrying out prescribed regimens, controlling symptoms, preventing and managing a crisis
d. preventing social isolation, attempting to normalize interactions with others
e. preventing and managing crisis, reordering time, adjusting to changes in the course of the disease, attempting to normalize interactions with others

f. controlling symptoms, reordering time, adjusting to changes in the course of the disease, preventing social isolation

g. reordering time, preventing and managing crisis

3. a. Secondary
   b. Primary

4. Crossword Puzzle
   Across: 4. unstable; 6. stroke; 7. comeback; 13. obesity; 14. coronary artery disease
   Down: 1. stable; 2. onset; 3. cancer; 5. crisis; 8. arthritis; 9. diabetes; 10. downward; 11. acute; 12. dying

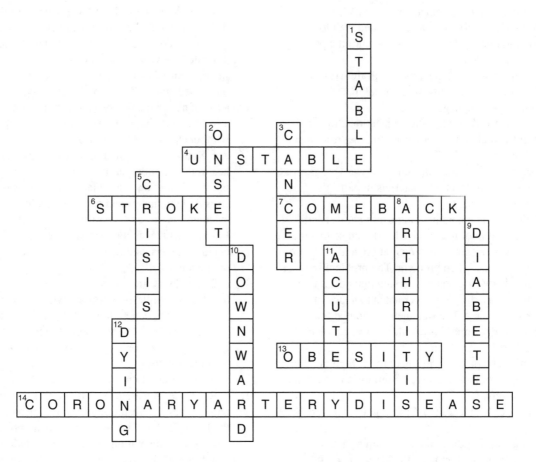

5. There are many correct responses. Examples include the following:
   a. Older people cannot learn new skills as well as younger people can ("can't teach an old dog new tricks").
   b. Most old people are ill.
   Also:
   • Old people are not (or should not be) sexually active.
   • Old people are terrible drivers.
   • Forgetfulness is a sign of senility.

6. There may be other correct responses, but examples include the following:
   a. decreased intestinal villae, decreased digestive enzyme production and secretion, decreased dentine and gingival retraction, decreased taste threshold for salt and sugar
   b. decreased force of cardiac contraction, decreased cardiac muscle mass, increased fat and collagen

c. decreased skeletal muscle mass, decreased joint flexion, stiffening of tendons and ligament, decreased cortical and trabecular bone, changes in eyes and ears that impair vision and hearing

d. decreased bladder smooth muscle and elastic tissue, decreased sphincter control

e. decreased ciliary action, decreased respiratory muscle strength, decreased elastic recoil, decreased cough force

f. decreased muscle and subcutaneous fat, collagen stiffening, decreased sebaceous gland activity, decreased sensory receptors, decreased tissue fluid, increased capillary fragility

g. decreased vessel elastin and smooth muscle, increased arterial rigidity

h. decreased blood flow to colon, decreased intestinal motility, decreased sensation to defecate, decreased muscle mass

7. c. Rationale: Age-associated memory impairment is characterized by a memory lapse or benign

forgetfulness that is not the same as a decline in cognitive functioning. Forgetting a name, date, or recent event is not serious, but the other examples indicate abnormal functioning.

8. a. S—sadness (mood); b. C—cholesterol (high); c. A—albumin (low); d. L—loss (or gain of weight); e. E—eating problems; f. S—shopping (and preparation problems).

9. d. Rationale: Older adults with an ethnic identity often have disproportionately low incomes and might not be able to afford Medicare deductibles or medications to treat health problems. Although they often live in older urban neighborhoods with extended families, they are not isolated. Ethnic diets have adequate nutrition, but health could be impaired if money is not available for food.

10. b. Rationale: This statement indicates that this patient does not understand the importance of having the test every week and that the test results will determine ongoing dosing. The other two statements indicate the patient is thinking about ways to get into town weekly.

11. Any three of the following: unplanned weight loss ($\geq$10 lb in last year), weakness, poor endurance and energy, slowness and low activity

12. a. Psychologic abuse, psychologic neglect, physical neglect, and perhaps violation of personal rights.
    b. Perform a very careful medical history and screening for mistreatment; interview the mother alone; use an assessment tool designed specifically for elder mistreatment; specifically assess for dehydration, malnutrition, pressure ulcers, and poor personal hygiene; evaluate explanations about physical findings that are not consistent with what is seen or contradictory statements between the daughter and the mother.
    c. Caregiver role strain.
    d. Community caregiver support group, formal support system for respite care

13. a. Part A
    b. Daily documentation of improvement in function
    c. Only for a limited number of days and only if the patient improves in functioning
    d. None
    e. Adult day-care programs

14. a. Rapid patient deterioration
    b. Caregiver exhaustion
    c. Alteration in or loss of family support system

15. b. Rationale: During an initial contact with an older adult, the nurse should perform a comprehensive nursing assessment that includes a history using a functional health pattern format, physical assessment, assessment of activities of daily living (ADLs) and instrumental activities of daily living (IADLs), mental status evaluation, and a social-environmental assessment. If available, a comprehensive interdisciplinary geriatric assessment may then be done to maintain and enhance the functional abilities of the older adult. The older adult and the caregiver should be interviewed separately, and the older adult should identify his or her own needs.

16. a. Rationale: The results of mental status evaluation often determine whether the patient is able to manage independent living, a major issue in older adulthood. Other elements of comprehensive assessment could determine eligibility for special problems, determination of frailty, and total service and placement needs.

17 a. Rationale: Exercise for all older adults is important to prevent deconditioning and subsequent functional decline from many different causes. Walkers and canes may improve mobility but can also decrease mobility if they are too difficult for the patient to use. Nutrition is important for muscles, but muscle strength is primarily dependent on use. Risk appraisals are usually performed for specific health problems.

18. a. Absorption of enalapril may be more complete because of delayed gastric emptying and slowed gastrointestinal (GI) motility; however, less of the drug may be metabolized to active enalaprilat because of decreased liver function. The drug is not highly plasma protein bound, but decreases in serum albumin and total body water may make more active drug available. Decreased kidney function lengthens the half-life of the drug, prolonging its action. Overall, there is likely to be an increased effect of the drug, with marked hypotension and development of side effects.
    b. When digoxin is added to the regimen for the patient, consideration must be made of not only the effect of digoxin, but also its possible interaction with enalapril. Digoxin toxicity is much more likely to occur in the older patient because of increased absorption caused by decreased GI motility and decreased kidney elimination. The half-life of digoxin may be much prolonged beyond the normally long 36 hours. Although digoxin is not highly plasma protein bound, decreased serum albumin, decreased total body water, and competition between digoxin and enalapril for plasma proteins could increase the free (active) amount of both drugs.
    c. The nurse should monitor the patient's blood pressure and apical pulse for hypotension, bradycardia, or marked tachycardia before administration of the drugs; because digoxin has such a long half-life, vital signs should also be routinely monitored throughout the day. Periodic measurement of serum digoxin levels is also advised in the older adult because of the many physiologic changes that can affect the drug's pharmacokinetics.

19. a. Emphasize medications that are essential while attempting to reduce medication use that is not essential for minor symptoms. Encourage use of medication reminder system.
    b. Use a standard assessment tool to screen medication use that includes over-the-counter (OTC) medications, eye and ear medications, cough medications, and alcohol as well as prescription drugs.
    c. Monitor medication dosage strength; normally the strength should be 30% to 50% less than that of a younger person.
    d. Encourage the use of one pharmacy, and work with health care providers and pharmacists to establish routine drug profiles for all older adult patients.
20. a, c, d. Rationale: These actions are alternatives to restraints that may help to reduce falls and keep the patient safe. A jacket vest and a seat belt are forms of restraint and require an order and frequent reassessment and order renewal.

CHAPTER 6

1. c. Rationale: The focus of community-based nursing is illness-oriented care of individuals and families in the community and home settings. Public health nurses improve health through a population focus and provide primary prevention as a focus of care.
2. b. Rationale: A prospective payment system, such as Medicare reimbursement, pays for health care services at a predetermined flat rate. If a health care provider can provide quality care at a lesser amount, the difference is profit to the provider; if not, the difference is a loss to the provider. Thus, providers are instituting systems to provide quality care in a more cost-effective manner to maintain financial balance.
3. a. socioeconomic conditions resulting in a demand for less expensive health care
   b. increasing older population with complex medical and health care needs
   c. increase in chronic illnesses that are better prevented and managed in the community
   d. increased technology available in outpatient and home settings
   e. consumer input into health care and patient preference for community-based care
4. c. Rationale: The case manager is critical in managed care to coordinate and link health care services to the patient and family during an entire illness episode across all patient care settings. Most case management is performed when patients belong to managed health care organizations where all settings for health care services are provided. Case managers do not determine when hospitalization is required, nor do they set limits on health care expenses; rather, they coordinate patient needs with cost-effective health services.

5. a. 4 (possibly with special care unit); b. 8; c. 7; d. 2; e. 6; f. 1; g. 3; h. 4; i. 5
6. Ambulatory care center
7. Home health care
8. a. F; b. F; c. T; d. F
9. b. Rationale: Medicare stipulates that registered nurses are the coordinators of patient care in the home and that they are accountable for the supervision of personal care services by home health aides and for case management services, including all aspects of care in the home. Care delivered in the home may be provided by any member of the home health care team, and the frequency is determined by the patient's and family's needs.
10. Any of the following are appropriate: Caregiver role strain, interrupted family processes, decisional conflict, stress overload, ineffective role performance
11. Specific interventions will depend on the nursing diagnoses selected. However, in general, the nurse should focus on helping family members understand and cope with the changes in roles, responsibilities, and stresses. Referral to support groups in the community or on the Internet is often helpful.

CHAPTER 7

1. a. 5, 11; b. 2, 7; c. 1, 14; d. 3, 8; e. 1, 10; f, 2, 12; g. 4, 13; h. 1, 15; i. 4, 16; j. 2, 18; k. 3, 17; l. 1, 6; m. 1, 9
2. a. T; b. T; c. T
3. b. Rationale: Complementary and alternative therapies are harmonious with the values of nursing that include a view of humans as holistic beings, an emphasis on healing and partnership relationships with patients, and a focus on health promotion and illness prevention.
4. a. Rationale: The basic concept of disease in Chinese medicine is that the opposing phenomena of yin and yang are out of balance, and this imbalance alters the movement of the vital energy of the body, known as Qi, that influences physiologic functions of the body. Acupoints are holes in the Qi meridians where the flow of Qi can be influenced but not released. Harmony with nature is necessary for health in Native American beliefs, and spiritualism and mysticism are frequently a part of Hispanic health care.
5. b. Rationale: Acupuncture is used to regulate the flow of Qi with the insertion of needles at acupoints, areas where needles may be inserted to unblock obstruction of energy and reestablish the flow of Qi. Counterirritation and inflammation are not consistent with the theory of Qi, and although electrical stimulation may be applied to the needles in electroacupuncture, this procedure releases neuropeptides within the central nervous system.

6. c. Rationale: If the nurse knows enough acupressure to suggest its use to a patient, it is appropriate to use with the patient's permission. The PRN medication for postoperative pain is not usually appropriate for a headache, nor would biofeedback training be for this situation. To simply reassure the patient that the headache will go away is not helpful.

7. b. Rationale: Massage therapy is one of the body-based methods commonly used by nurses for many different effects. Nurses can use specific massage techniques as part of nursing care that are not as comprehensive as those of massage therapists. It would be quite appropriate for the nurse to massage the patient's back.

8. b. Clinical studies have indicated that acupuncture is clearly effective in treating adult postoperative and chemotherapy-associated nausea and vomiting as well as postoperative dental pain. Reiki is an energy therapy used to heal disease, aromatherapy uses essential plant oils to promote and maintain overall health, and magnetic therapy is useful for relieving pain and promoting tissue healing.

9. a. Rationale: Because of a lack of governmental control for clinical testing of herbs or standardization of ingredient concentration or acceptable levels of contamination of pesticides, solvents, bacteria, and heavy metals, the safety and efficacy of herbal preparations are based on the manufacturer's standards. As such, the reputation and history of the manufacturer must be the major criteria for purchasing herbs. Herbs indeed can be toxic and are contraindicated or should be used with caution in certain persons.

10. b. Rationale: To serve as a resource for patients regarding complementary and alternative therapies, nurses must first develop their own knowledge base. To teach patients about their use, monitor for adverse effects and interactions with conventional therapies, and assist patients to use the therapies knowledgeably and safely, nurses themselves must be informed.

11. a. Rationale: Encourage the patient to seek the guidance of the physician regarding the safety and efficiency of using the herbal therapy rather than the medical therapy. See no. 12 below for further clarification.

12. a, b, c, e, f. Rationale: Suggesting specific herbs is "prescribing" and is outside the scope of nursing. Professional nurses should be knowledgeable about the various complementary and alternative therapies, assess their use in patients, and promote their safety.

13. Crossword Puzzle
    Across: 4. ginger; 6. Echinacea; 8. black cohosh; 11. evening primrose; 13. milk thistle; 14. aloe; 15. kava
    Down: 1. feverfew; 2. garlic; 3. saw palmetto; 5. ginkgo biloba; 7. St. John's wort; 9. hawthorn; 10. valerian; 12. ginseng

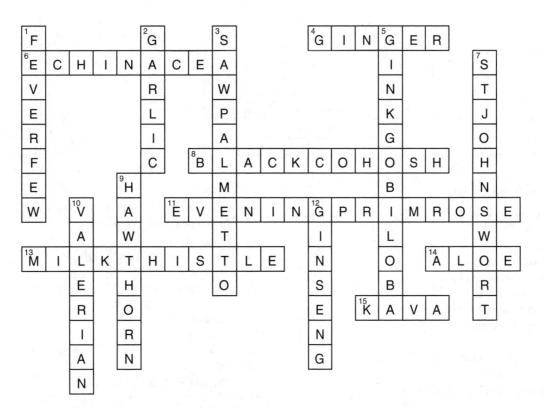

CHAPTER 8

1. b. Rationale: When individuals do not become stressed with a situation or an event, it is because the event is not perceived by them as a demand that is being made on them or as a threat to their well-being. Perceptions of stressors have great variability, and, for whatever reasons, this patient does not perceive this diagnosis as stressful.

2. Stage of resistance
3. Stage of exhaustion
4. Hardiness, resilience, attitude. Other factors that could have been selected are age, health status, personality characteristics, prior experience with stress, nutritional status, sleep status, and genetic background. These are all factors that are internal to the individual and may affect the response to stress.

5. See chart below.

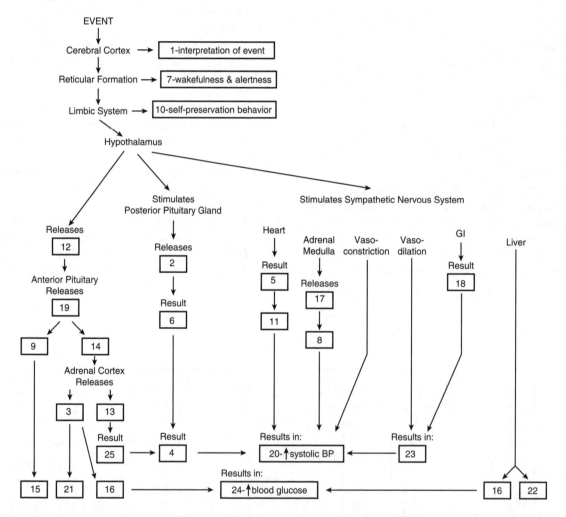

Word and Phrase List

1. interpretation of event
2. ↑ ADH
3. cortisol
4. ↑ blood volume
5. ↑ HR and stroke volume
6. ↑ water retention
7. wakefulness and alertness
8. ↑ sympathetic response
9. β-endorphin
10. self-preservation behaviors
11. ↑ cardiac output
12. corticotropin-releasing hormone
13. aldosterone
14. ACTH (adrenocorticotropic hormone)
15. blunted pain perception
16. ↑ gluconeogenesis
17. ↑ epinephrine and norepinephrine
18. ↓ digestion
19. pro-opiomelanocortin (POMC) release
20. ↑ systolic blood pressure
21. ↓ inflammatory response
22. glycogenolysis
23. ↑ blood to vital organs and large muscles
24. ↑ blood glucose
25. ↑ Na and H_2O reabsorption

6. *Objective manifestations:*
Increased heart rate
Increased blood pressure
Cool, clammy skin
Decreased bowel sounds
Hyperglycemia
Decreased lymphocytes
Decreased eosinophils
Decreased urinary output
Subjective findings:
Anxiety, fear
Decreased perception of pain
Verbalization of stress
Wakefulness, restlessness
7. b. Rationale: One of the many physiologic changes that occur as a result of prolonged, increased stress is damage to the hippocampus, resulting in long-term memory impairment and possible hippocampal atrophy. The other options here are not valid explanations for the memory loss.
8. a. P; b. N; c. P; d. N; e. P
9. *Problem-focused:*
• Attending cardiac rehabilitation program
• Planning dietary changes
• Starting an exercise program
Emotion-focused:
• Sharing feelings with spouse or other family members
• Using meditation
• Setting aside private time
• Doing favorite escape activities
10. a. Rationale: Because it is almost impossible to maintain muscle tension while breathing slowly and deeply, relaxation breathing is a component of all relaxation therapies. Progressive muscle relaxation and meditation first require relaxed breathing, and although soft music can decrease stress, it should be used with other therapies.
11. a. Peptic ulcer disease is one of several disorders with a known stress component. Although many patients have stress related to a health problem, stress-relieving interventions are always indicated for patients with diseases in which stress contributes to the problem.
12. c. Rationale: The coping behavior described is not adaptive, and the patient tells the nurse that she does not have the resources to cope with the demands of her illness. There is no evidence that emotional bonds with her family are disrupted, and her behavior does not match definitions of ineffective denial or impaired adjustment.
13. a, c, d. Rationale: Humor, journaling, and relaxation activities are realistic strategies that can be used during hospitalization in a patient with an acute episode of a chronic disease. Exercise would not be appropriate for an exacerbation of Crohn's disease.

Case Study

1. Physiologic: fever, pain, anemia, the inflammatory disease itself
Psychologic: no income, no insurance, the duration and chronicity of the disease, frequent hospital admissions, lack of social support systems
Effects: Prolonged healing of illness, progression of the inflammatory disease
2. Her refusal to seek support from boyfriend
Her depression, weakness
Her experience with the illness and hospitalizations
Her lack of financial resources
3. Increased weight, hemoglobin and hematocrit levels, strength
Decreased body temperature, number of stools
4. One approach might be using a hospital stress-rating scale to clarify the patient's perception of the situation. The nurse and the patient might not rate the stressors as being the same in intensity. Specific questions may include the following:
"What is the most stressful thing to you about being in the hospital?"
"Can you tell me what having this illness means to you?"
5. Reduce additional stressors, such as sleep deprivation, environmental stimuli.
Set short-term outcomes to achieve success.
Provide pain relief, measures for comfort, rest.
Provide stress-reducing interventions, such as relaxation and guided imagery.
6. *Nursing diagnoses:*
• Ineffective coping related to inadequate resources as manifested by crying, depression
• Stress overload related to excessive amounts of demands
• Ineffective role performance related to lack of employment
• Acute pain related to inflammatory process
• Risk for impaired skin integrity related to frequent stools and emaciation
• Imbalanced nutrition: less than body requirements related to nausea and frequent watery stools
• Risk for deficient fluid volume related to frequent watery stools and low-grade fever
Collaborative problems:
Potential complications: fluid-electrolyte imbalances, intestinal obstruction, fistula-fissure-abscess
7. Acute pain. Rationale: A physiologic need that takes priority over other physiologic and psychosocial problems.

CHAPTER 9

1. a. T; b. F, 7 hours; c. T; d. F, Nearly 50% of adults.
2. Crossword Puzzle
Across: 2. postprandial sleepiness; 5. parasomnias; 7. circadian rhythm; 9. hypopnea; 10. onset latency; 15. cataplexy; 16. nonrestorative; 17. narcolepsy; 18. efficiency; 19. apnea

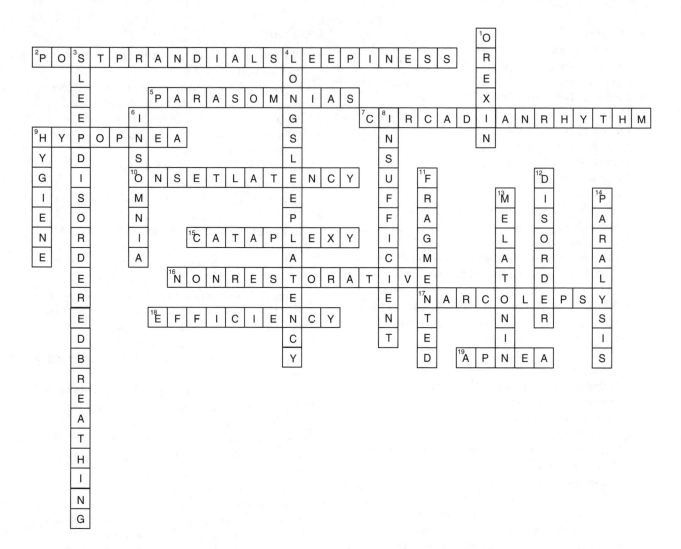

Down: 1. Orexin; 3. sleep-disordered breathing;
4. long sleep latency; 6. insomnia; 8. insufficient;
9. hygiene; 11. fragmented; 12. disorder; 13. melatonin;
14. paralysis

3. c. Rationale: The nervous system controls the cyclic changes of wake/sleep through a complex arrangement of structures with key nuclei in the brainstem, hypothalamus, and thalamus. Melatonin is an endogenous hormone that increases sleep efficiency and is released in the evening; the light–dark cycles influence our circadian rhythms, and neuropeptides influence wake behavior. These all play a role in the wake/sleep cycle and are components of the nervous system.

4. a. 4; b. 3; c. 4; d. 3; e. 4; f. 1; g. 1; h. 1; i. 2; j. 2

5. Any three of these:
a. Consumption of stimulants close to bedtime (caffeine, nicotine, methamphetamine, other drugs of abuse)
b. Side effect to medications (antidepressants, antihypertensives, corticosteroids, psychostimulants, and analgesics)
c. Drinking alcohol as a sleep aid
d. Long naps in the afternoon

e. Sleeping in late
f. Exercise near bedtime
g. Jet lag
h. Nightmares
i. Stressful life event
j. Medical conditions
k. Irregular sleep–wake schedules
l. Worry about getting enough sleep

6. b, d, e, f, g, h, i, j

7. b. Rationale: Cognitive behavior therapies are effective therapies for insomnia and should be tried first. These include relaxation training, guided imagery, education about good sleep hygiene, and regular exercise several hours before bedtime. The other therapies are used to treat insomnia with the benzodiazepine-receptor-like agents being the first choice for drug therapy. Many patients will try over-the-counter medications such as diphenhydramine (Benadryl), but tolerance develops rapidly. Complementary therapies such as melatonin have been found to be useful to help individuals fall asleep, but it is not first line therapy.

8. b. Rationale: It is not recommended that a person lie in bed awake. Alcohol should not be consumed within 6 hours of bedtime. The other statements represent strategies that may help the individual go to sleep. Exercise is good but not within 6 hours of bedtime; a light snack may help relax the person.

9. d. Rationale: Ben & Jerry's nonfat coffee fudge frozen yogurt contains 85 mg of caffeine as compared to brewed nonherbal tea with 50 mg, a Hershey bar with 10 mg, and a diet Coke with 47 mg.

10. a. Rationale: 7-Up has 0 mg of caffeine as compared with decaffeinated coffee with 5 mg, hot chocolate with 5 mg, and Dannon's coffee yogurt with 45 mg.

11. a. Rationale: Reducing the light and noise levels in the ICU can help promote opportunities for sleep. Having the TV on at all times will only add to the noise level; analgesics given for actual pain may help a patient sleep or rest but they may also alter sleep; the alarms should not be silenced except for short periods to deal with why they were alarming. Silencing them to prevent them from making noise puts the patient at risk because the nurse may not be alerted to patient changes on the monitor or problems with the infusion device.

12. a. Rationale: Desipramine and protriptyline are both tricyclic antidepressants used to treat cataplexy, and methylphenidate is an amphetamine.

13. Any of these responses:
    a. Start to get in harmony with the Moscow time zone several days before you travel.
    b. Be sure to expose yourself to daytime daylight, which will assist with synchronizing your body's clock to environmental time.
    c. Melatonin has been shown to be an effective sleep aid to help synchronize the body's rhythm.
    d. Resynchronization of the body's clock will occur at a rate of 1 hr/day if he travels eastward.

14. a. 4; b. 7; c. 6; d. 5; e. 3; f. 1; g. 8; h. 2

15. c. Rationale: CPAP is continuous positive airway pressure and is the treatment of choice for more serious sleep apnea. BiPAP is the therapy that delivers a higher inspiratory pressure and a lower expiratory pressure to prevent airway collapse. CPAP is not well tolerated and compliance is low. Compliance may be improved by involving the patient in the selection of the device and mask, showing the CPAP before therapy begins, and teaching troubleshooting to reduce anxiety. An oral appliance is used to prevent airway occlusion from the relaxed mandible and tongue.

16. d. Rationale: Most common complications in the immediate postoperative period are airway obstruction and hemorrhage. The patient may experience a sore throat, foul-smelling breath, and snoring during the recovery but they will resolve. Infection is always a potential complication of any surgery but is not common with this procedure.

Voice loss and electrolyte imbalance are generally not complications of this procedure.

17. d. Rationale: Assess the patient to determine what the problem is and then offer sleep hygiene instruction and collaborate with the physician to improve the patient's sleep behavior. Disturbed sleep is not a normal result of aging, and people need about the same amount of sleep throughout the life span. OTC and prescription sleep aids need to be used very cautiously in the elderly, and patient response monitored closely.

18. Any three of these:
    a. Nurse is too sleepy to be fully awake at work
    b. Nurse is too alert to sleep soundly the next day
    c. Increased morbidity/mortality related to cardiovascular problems
    d. Mood disorders are higher
    e. GI disturbances are more common.

19. All apply (a through e)

CHAPTER 10

1. c. Rationale: Because the patient's self-report is the most valid means of pain assessment, patients who have decreased cognitive function, such as those who are comatose, have dementia, or are mentally disabled, might not be able to report pain. In these cases, nonverbal information and behaviors are necessary considerations in pain assessment.

2. c. Rationale: Administering the smallest prescribed analgesic dose when given a choice is not consistent with current pain management guidelines and leads to undertreatment of pain and inadequate pain control. Unnecessary suffering, impaired recovery from acute illness, and increased morbidity as a result of respiratory dysfunction, increased heart rate and cardiac workload, and other physical dysfunction can occur.

3. a. Physiologic—the anatomic and physical determinants of pain
   b. Affective—the emotional response to pain
   c. Behavioral—observable actions that express or control pain
   d. Cognitive—the beliefs, attitudes, and meanings attributed to the pain
   e. Sociocultural—the demographics, support systems, social roles, and culture that influence the pain experience

4. a. Rationale: Although a peripheral nerve is one cell that carries an impulse directly from the periphery to the dorsal horn of the spinal cord with no synapses, transmission of the impulse can be interrupted by drugs known as membrane stabilizers or sodium-channel inhibitors, such as local anesthetics and some antiseizure drugs. The nerve fiber produces neurotransmitters only at synapses, not during transmission of the action potential.

5. a. Rationale: The neck and right flank are common areas of referred pain from liver damage, and examination of the liver should be considered when pain occurs without other findings in these areas. Other common areas are midscapular and left arm for cardiac pain, inner legs for bladder pain, and shoulders for gallbladder pain.

6. b. Rationale: It is known that the brain is necessary for pain perception, but because it is not clearly understood where in the brain pain is perceived, pain may be perceived even in a comatose patient who may not respond behaviorally to noxious stimuli. Any noxious stimulus should be treated as potentially painful.

7. a. 4; b. 2; c. 1; d. 3

8. a. 1, 3; b. 1, 4; c. 2, 6; d. 2, 7; e. 2, 8/9; f. 2, 8; g. 1, 5.

9. c. Rationale: Several antidepressants affect the modulatory systems by inhibiting the reuptake of serotonin and norepinephrine in descending modulatory fibers, thereby increasing their availability to inhibit afferent transmission of pain impulses. Although chronic pain is often accompanied by anxiety and depression, the antidepressants that affect the physiologic process of pain modulation are used for pain control whether depression is present or not.

10. b. Rationale: Damage to peripheral or cranial nerves causes neuropathic pain that is not well controlled by opioid analgesics alone and often includes the adjuvant use of tricyclic antidepressants or antiseizure drugs to help inhibit pain transmission. Salicylates and nonsteroidal antiinflammatory drugs (NSAIDs) are not effective for the intensity of neuropathic pain.

11. a. Onset: About 4 hours ago
    b. Duration and pattern of the pain: Continuously for about 4 hours. Similar episodes in the past month but only lasted 2 hours.
    c. Location: Right upper quadrant
    d. Intensity: Severe, 10/10
    e. Quality: Severe cramping, radiates to back
    f. Associated symptoms: Nausea
    g. Factors that increase or relieve the pain: pain better walking bent forward, more intense lying in bed

12. a. Follow the principles of pain assessment.
    b. Every patient deserves adequate pain management.
    c. Base treatment on the patient's goals.
    d. Use both drug and nondrug therapies.
    e. When appropriate, use a multimodal approach to analgesic therapy.
    f. Address pain using a multidisciplinary approach.
    g. Evaluate the effectiveness of all therapies to ensure that they are meeting the patient's goals.
    h. Prevent or manage medication side effects.
    i. Incorporate patient and caregiver teaching throughout assessment and teaching.

13. a. Rationale: Analgesics should be scheduled around the clock for patients with constant pain to prevent pain from escalating and becoming difficult to relieve. If pain control is not adequate, the analgesic dose may be increased, or an adjunctive drug may be added to the treatment plan.

14. a. Rationale: As cancer pain increases, stronger drugs are added to the regimen. This patient is using an NSAID and an antidepressant. A stronger preparation would be an opioid, but because an NSAID is already being used, a combination NSAID/opioid would not be indicated. An appropriate stronger drug would be an oral opioid, in this case oral oxycodone, but would still leave stronger drugs for expected increasing pain. Propoxyphene is not recommended in analgesic guidelines because of its limited efficacy and toxicities.

15. c. Rationale: Although tolerance to many of the side effects of opioids (nausea, sedation, respiratory depression, pruritus) develops within days, tolerance to opioid-induced constipation does not occur. A bowel regimen that includes a gentle-stimulant laxative and a stool softener should be started at the beginning of opioid therapy and continue as long as the drug is taken.

16. The addition of a basal rate does not improve pain control, reduce the number of demand doses, or improve sleep. Use of a basal rate may increase the risk of serious respiratory events in opioid-naïve patients and those at risk for respiratory difficulties (older age, existing pulmonary disease, etc.).

17. a. 2; b. 1; c. 1, 2; d. 3; e. 4; f. 1; g. 2; h. 1, 3; i. 3

18. a, b, c, d, e, f, g, h. Rationale: The major complications of epidural analgesia are catheter displacement and migration, accidental infusions of neurotoxic agents, and infection. These actions will help reduce those risks. An intrathecal catheter placement can be checked by aspirating cerebrospinal fluid (CSF); however, the individual who does this must be competent in the procedure and covered by a written policy. In many facilities, aspiration of CSF is done by the physician or advanced practice nurse.

19. b. Rationale: When a patient desires to be stoic about pain, it is important that he or she understand that pain itself can have harmful physiologic effects and that failure to report pain and participate in its control can result in severe unrelieved pain. No evidence is present in this situation that indicates fear of taking the medication.

Case Study

1. Assess the location, quality, and specifics of the pattern of the pain. Also assess the patient's prior medication use, experience with opioids, and any addictions.

2. Affective: Worried about worsening of disease, afraid of opioids

   Behavioral: Posturing, slow gait, stays in bed with severe pain

   Cognitive: Uses emptying mind to block pain

3. The symptoms he has in the mornings are related to withdrawal because of physical dependence and the long interval during the night when the opioid is not used. An adjuvant drug should be added to his regimen, and it and the Percocet should be taken around the clock. If the pain is not controlled with this measure, a stronger, sustained-release opioid such as MS Contin should be substituted for the Percocet.

4. Teach the patient to evaluate the dose required to control his pain, and see that he knows the range and frequency of his dose.

5. Explain that tolerance and physical dependence are expected with long-term opiate use and should not be confused with addiction. Addiction is a psychologic condition characterized by a drive to obtain and take substances for other than their prescribed therapeutic value. Fewer than 0.1% of patients receiving analgesics become addicted.

6. Dermal stimulation, such as massage and pressure, and additional cognitive-behavioral therapies, such as relaxation and imagery. He has a potential for using cognitive-behavioral therapies successfully because he can already mentally block the pain somewhat.

7. *Nursing diagnoses:*
   - Chronic pain related to ineffective pain management
   - Anxiety related to effects of disease process and inadequate relief from pain-relief measures
   - Activity intolerance related to pain, fatigue

   Collaborative problems:

   Potential complications: Drug-induced constipation, respiratory depression, negative nitrogen balance, opioid toxicity

CHAPTER 11

1. b, c, e, f, g, i. Table 11-1 lists the goals. Overall, goals of palliative care are to prevent and relieve suffering and to improve the quality of life for the patient.

2. a. Rationale: The family may not understand what hospice care is and may need information. Some cultures/ethnic groups may underutilize hospice because of a lack of awareness of the services offered, a desire to continue with potentially curative therapies, and concerns about a lack of minority hospice workers.

3. 1. Patient must desire services and agree in writing that only hospice care can be used to treat the terminal illness (palliative care).

   2. Patient must meet eligibility, which is less than 6 months to live, certified initially by two physicians.

4. **Respiratory**
   a. Cheyne-Stokes respiration
   b. death rattle (inability to cough and clear secretions)
   c. increased, then slowing, respiratory rate
   (Also: irregular breathing; terminal gasping)

   Skin
   a. mottling on hands, feet, and legs that progresses to the torso
   b. cold, clammy skin
   c. cyanosis on nose, nail beds, and knees
   (Also: waxlike skin when very near death)

   Gastrointestinal
   a. slowing of the GI tract with accumulation of gas and abdominal distention
   b. loss of sphincter control with incontinence
   c. bowel movement before imminent death or at time of death

   Musculoskeletal
   a. loss of muscle tone with sagging jaw
   b. difficulty speaking
   c. difficulty swallowing
   (Also: a loss of ability to move or maintain body position; loss of gag reflex)

5. b. Rationale: Hearing is often the last sense to disappear with declining consciousness, and conversations can distress patients even when they appear unresponsive. Conversation around unresponsive patients should never be other than that which one would maintain if the patients were alert.

6. a. coma
   b. absent brainstem reflexes
   c. apnea

7. b. Rationale: Bargaining is demonstrated by "if-then" grief behavior that is described by Kübler-Ross and corresponds to Rando's confrontation. Avoidance is Rando's description of denial and shock that occur early in the grief process, and Martocchio's anguish, disorganization, and despair correspond to Kübler-Ross's depression. Reorganization and restoration are Martocchio's acceptance and accommodation phase of grieving.

8. a. Rationale: Spiritual distress may surface when an individual is faced with a terminal illness, and it is characterized by verbalization about inner conflicts about beliefs and questioning the meaning of one's own existence. Individuals in spiritual distress may be able to resolve the problem and die peacefully with effective grief work, but referral to spiritual leaders should be the patient's choice.

9. a. living will
   b. durable power of attorney for health care or medical power of attorney
   c. directive to physicians
   d. natural death acts
   e. Patient Self-Determination Act (Omnibus Reconciliation Act of 1990)

f. advance directives

g. DNR (do not resuscitate)

10. b. Rationale: Palliative care is aimed at symptom management rather than curative treatment for diseases that no longer respond to treatment and is focused on caring interventions rather than on curative treatments. Palliative care and hospice are frequently used interchangeably.

11. d. Rationale: There are currently no clinical practice guidelines to relieve the shortness of breath and air hunger that often occur at the end of life. Any of the options may be tried, but whatever gives the patient the most relief should be used.

12. d. Rationale: In assisting patients with dying, end-of-life care promotes the grieving process, which involves saying goodbye. Physical care is very important for physical comfort, but assessments should be limited to essential data related to the patient's symptoms. Analgesics should be administered for pain, but patients who are sedated cannot participate in the grieving process.

13. a. DNR (do not resuscitate)

b. Full code

c. Chemical code

d. Allow natural death (AND) or Comfort code

Case Study

1. Additional assessment data should include Mr. and Mrs. J.'s reasons for not discussing her illness and impending death with their children, an assessment of their spiritual needs, what decisions, if any, they have made about where and how S.J. prefers to die, and what resources they have used or could use to assist them through the dying process. In addition, assessment and evaluation of their coping skills are necessary. A functional assessment of S.J.'s activities of daily living (ADLs) should also be made.

2. Maladaptive or dysfunctional grief is demonstrated in this family. S.J. appears to have some degree of acceptance of her impending death but feels rejected by her children. The children may be experiencing fear, guilt, anger, powerlessness, and other emotions that they cope with by withdrawing from the family. Mr. J. is also feeling guilt from wishing the ordeal would be over. Healthy grieving is blocked in this family because communication has not occurred.

3. Pain patterns should be assessed and dosages and frequencies increased to provide pain relief that is acceptable to S.J. without unnecessary sedation. Institute complementary therapies to enhance the effect of pain medication. As opioids are increased, constipation and abdominal distention could become a problem, and stool softeners may be needed. Although she is underweight, patients tend to take in less food and fluid as death approaches, and maintaining food and fluid intake is not a high priority. Because she spends most of her time in

bed and she is very thin, measures to prevent skin breakdown are essential. Oxygen therapy should be considered as a measure to relieve her shortness of breath.

4. Arrange for family meetings to discuss S.J.'s condition and the feelings of the patient and the family. The hospice nurse or a grief counselor can help all members of the family express and acknowledge their feelings of anger, fear, or guilt. The patient and family need to know that the grief reaction is normal, and they should be taught what to expect and how each individual's needs can be met as S.J.'s death approaches.

5. A multidisciplinary team of nurses, health care providers, pharmacists, dietitians, nursing assistants, social workers, clergy, and volunteers is available to this family to provide care and support to the patient and family through hospice care.

6. *Nursing diagnoses:*
   - Compromised family coping related to inadequate coping mechanisms
   - Dysfunctional grieving related to blocked communication and guilt
   - Chronic pain related to ineffective pain management
   - Risk for impaired skin integrity related to immobility and emaciation
   - Risk for constipation related to decreased oral intake and effects of drugs
   - Ineffective breathing pattern related to weakness
   - Impaired physical mobility related to pain

CHAPTER 12

1. a. 10; b. 6; c. 9; d. 1; e. 8; f. 2; g. 7; h. 3; i. 4; j. 5.

2. a. Ask; b. Advise; c. Assess; d. Assist; e. Arrange

3. c. Rationale: Nurses have a professional responsibility to help individuals stop smoking. The advice and motivation of health care professionals can be very helpful to the individual. Nurses should encourage, provide information, and work with physicians to identify ways to assist patients with quitting.

4. **Nicotine**
   a. chronic obstructive pulmonary disease (COPD)
   b. cancers: lung, mouth, esophagus, larynx, stomach, bladder, pancreas
   Others: coronary artery disease, peptic ulcer disease, GERD (see Table 12-2).
   Alcohol
   a. Dementia
   b. Cirrhosis
   Others: peripheral neuropathy, increased risk of several cancers, anemia, CAD, hypertension, GERD (see Table 12-9).
   Cocaine and Amphetamines
   a. Cardiac dysrhythmias
   b. Psychosis
   Others: nasal sores, MI, stroke (see Table 12-2).

Opioids
a. Gastric ulcer
b. Glomerulonephritis
Other: sexual dysfunction (see Table 12-2).
Cannabis
a. Bronchitis
b. Memory impairment
Other: impaired immune system, reproductive dysfunction (see Table 12-2).
5. a. 3; b. 1; c. 4; d. 1, 5; e. 3; f. 2; g. 1; h. 2; i. 4; j. 2; k. 1, 5
6. a. stimulant; sedative-hypnotic
b. opioid
c. hallucinogens
d. stimulants
e. sedative-hypnotics
f. opioid; sedative-hypnotic
7. d. Rationale: Nicotine replacement contains the same nicotine as that in tobacco but with slower absorption. The nicotine will help to prevent withdrawal symptoms because its use is reduced gradually. While the addiction is treated, the carcinogens and gases associated with tobacco smoke are eliminated.
8. a. 2; b. 3; c. 4; d. 1; e. 3; f. 4; g. 3
9. a. Rationale: Headache is a common symptom of caffeine withdrawal and often occurs in heavy caffeine users who are NPO for diagnostic tests and surgery. Nervousness, tremors, anxiety, and bronchial dilation are physiologic effects of caffeine.
10. a. gross tremors
b. seizures
c. hallucinations
d. alcohol withdrawal delirium
11. c. Rationale: Open-ended questions indicating that substance use is normal or at least understandable are helpful in eliciting information from patients who are reluctant to disclose substance use.
12. b. Rationale: This behavior is typical of ineffective denial—unable to admit the impact of the disease or event on life patterns as manifested by minimizing symptoms or events and selectively integrating information and not meeting the definitions or defining characteristics of the other nursing diagnoses.
13. b. Rationale: Smoking is the single most preventable cause of death, and most smokers start smoking by age 16. If smoking in preadolescents and adolescents could be prevented, it is unlikely that they would start smoking at a later age. Health problems associated with smoking and future use of other addictive substances would be significantly reduced.
14. a. Naloxone (Narcan) is given in case opioids are the cause of the central nervous system (CNS) depression.

b. Flumazenil (Romazicon) is given in case benzodiazepines are the cause of the CNS depression.
15. a. Rationale: The knowledge of when the patient last had alcohol intake will help the nurse anticipate the onset of withdrawal symptoms. In patients with alcohol tolerance, the amount of alcohol and the blood alcohol concentration do not reflect impairment as consistently as in the nondrinker. The type of alcohol ingested is not important because in the body it is all alcohol.
16. c. Rationale: An extreme autonomic nervous system response may be life threatening and requires immediate intervention. A quiet room is recommended, but it should be well lighted to prevent misinterpretation of the environment and visual hallucinations. Cessation of alcohol intake causes low blood alcohol levels leading to withdrawal symptoms, and fluids should be carefully administered to prevent dysrhythmias. Patients should not be restrained if at all possible because injury and exhaustion can occur as patients struggle against restraint.
17. a. Anesthesia requirements may be decreased as a result of the synergistic effect of alcohol.
b. Closely monitor VS, including temperature, because of increased risk of infection from malnutrition.
c. Postoperative care will require close monitoring for signs of withdrawal and respiratory and cardiac problems.
d. Increased pain medications may be needed postoperatively if the patient is cross-tolerant to opiates.
18. a. Rationale: Because Wernicke's encephalopathy resulting from a thiamine deficiency is a possibility in chronic alcoholism, IV thiamine is often administered to intoxicated patients to prevent the development of Korsakoff's psychosis. Thiamine should be given before any glucose solutions are administered because glucose can precipitate Wernicke's encephalopathy. Benzodiazepines may be used for sedation and to minimize withdrawal symptoms but would not be given before thiamine, and haloperidol could be used if hallucinations occur.
19. c. Rationale: This patient is demonstrating behavior characteristic of the precontemplation stage of behavior change. During this stage, the nurse should help the patient to increase her awareness of the risks and problems related to alcohol use by asking the patient what she thinks could happen if the behavior continues, providing evidence of the problem and offering factual information about the risks of the substance use.
20. d. Rationale: Elderly patients have the highest use of OTC and prescription drugs, and simultaneous use of these drugs with alcohol is a major problem. Illegal drug use is minimal in older patients except for long-term addicts.

Case Study

1. Because there is a tendency among substance abusers to take a variety of drugs simultaneously or in a sequence to obtain specific effects, as shown by N.C.'s history, he should be assessed for his pattern of abuse. Regular alcohol use in addition to other drug use or the common use of cocaine in combination with heroin or phencyclidine hydrochloride could cause withdrawal symptoms and additional manifestations that would complicate his condition and direct his care. Information about all the drugs he uses, including both OTC and prescription drugs, is necessary to avoid withdrawal syndromes, acute intoxication, overdose, or drug interactions that might be life-threatening.

2. The nurse should be aware that common behaviors that are likely to influence history taking from N.C. include manipulation, denial, avoidance, underreporting or minimizing substance abuse, giving inaccurate information, and inaccurate self-reporting. To obtain reliable information about N.C.'s drug abuse patterns, the nurse should first explain that information about his drug use is essential in the monitoring for and prevention of serious effects of the drugs while he already is very ill. Providing a need for the information and explaining how the information will be used may facilitate more honest responses by N.C. The nurse should question him without judgment about his pattern of abuse with open-ended questions, such as, "How much or how often do you use alcohol?" or "Can you describe how you use cocaine with other drugs?"

3. Physical effects of drug use that provide clues to drug abuse include collapsed and scarred veins used to inject drugs, nasal septum and mucosa damage, brown or black sputum production, and wound abscesses and cellulitis.

4. Continuous monitoring of N.C.'s vital signs, cardiac activity, level of consciousness, respiratory status, temperature, fluid and electrolyte balance, liver function, and renal function is necessary. Complications of cocaine toxicity that may occur and can be detected by monitoring include myocardial ischemia or infarction, heart failure, cardiopulmonary arrest, rhabdomyolysis with acute renal failure, stroke, respiratory distress or arrest, seizures, agitated delirium and hallucinations, electrolyte imbalances, and fever. In severe intoxication, the patient may progress rapidly through stages of stimulation and depression, which may result in death. N.C.'s use of cocaine with alcohol also increases his risk of liver injury and sudden death.

5. Assessment for neurologic, cardiovascular, and respiratory problems as described above is a critical nursing intervention in the patient with cocaine toxicity. In addition, the nurse should institute seizure precautions, provide airway management, keep open IV lines, administer medications aggressively as prescribed, and use cardiac life-support measures as indicated. Nursing interventions that are indicated for N.C.'s anxiety, nervousness, and irritability include explaining procedures using short, simple, clear statements in a calm manner; providing a safe, secure environment; decreasing environmental stimuli; reinforcing reality orientation; and encouraging participation in relaxation exercises if possible.

6. Engaging an individual who is addicted to cocaine in treatment is difficult because of the intense craving for the drug and a strong denial that cocaine is addicting or that the individual cannot control it. Motivational interviewing is indicated in even this initial encounter with N.C. The nurse should help N.C. increase his awareness of risks and problems related to his current behavior and create doubt about the use of substances. Asking him what he thinks could happen if the behavior continues, pointing out the physical symptoms he is experiencing, and offering factual information about the risks of substance abuse are indicated. Often the only motivation for a patient with a cocaine addiction to enter a treatment program is family threats, loss of job or professional license, legal action, or major health consequences; but a treatment program is indicated to provide him with new skills and an ability to deal with his addictive behavior.

7. *Nursing diagnoses:*
   - Ineffective health maintenance
   - Risk-prone health behavior
   - Impaired memory
   - Ineffective denial
   - Ineffective coping

   Collaborative problems:
   Potential complications: cardiopulmonary arrest, seizures, sudden death, cerebrovascular accident, acute renal failure

CHAPTER 13

1. Mediators/physiologic change:
   a. Interleukin-1 (IL-1) released from mononuclear phagocytic cells and prostaglandin E_2 (PGE_2) synthesis/increases the hypothalamic thermostatic set point.
   b. histamine, kinins, prostaglandins/vasodilation and hyperemia
   c. histamine, kinins, prostaglandins/increased capillary permeability and fluid shift to tissues
   d. release of chemotactic factors at site of injury/ increased release of neutrophils and monocytes from bone marrow

2. d. Rationale: A *shift to the left* is the term used to describe the presence of immature, banded nuclei neutrophils in the blood in response to an increased demand for neutrophils during tissue injury. Monocytes are increased in leukocytosis but are mature cells.

3. c. Rationale: Chemotaxis involves the release of chemicals at the site of tissue injury that attract neutrophils and monocytes to the site of injury. The attraction is chemotaxis, and when monocytes move from the blood into tissue, they are transformed into macrophages. The complement system is a pathway of chemical processes that results in cellular lysis, and vasodilation and increased capillary permeability cause the slowing of blood flow at the area.

4. d. Rationale: The processes that are stimulated by the complement system include enhanced phagocytosis, increased vascular permeability, chemotaxis, and cellular lysis. Prostaglandins and leukotrienes are released by damaged cells, and body temperature is increased by the action of prostaglandins and interleukins. All chemical mediators of inflammation increase the inflammatory response and, as a result, increase pain.

5. R = rest. Helps body use nutrients and oxygen to heal. Prevents wound healing from being disrupted.
   I = Ice. Cold causes vasoconstriction, which will help decrease swelling, pain, and congestion of the tissues. Heat may be applied after 24 to 48 hours to promote healing by increasing circulation to the area.
   C = Compression and Immobilization. Compression counters vasodilation, reduces edema, and stops bleeding. Immobilization promotes healing by decreasing metabolic needs of tissues. May prevent further tissue injury. Be sure to evaluate circulation.
   E = Elevation. Decreases edema from the inflammation and decreases pain.

6. b. Rationale: Labile cells of the skin, lymphoid organs, bone marrow, and mucous membranes divide constantly and regenerate rapidly following injury. Stable cells, such as those in bone, liver, pancreas, and kidney, regenerate only if they are injured, and permanent cells found in neurons and cardiac muscle do not regenerate when damaged.

7. a. 9; b. 5; c. 2; d. 8; e. 6; f. 1; g. 4; h. 10; i. 7; j. 3

8. c. Rationale: The process of healing by secondary intention is essentially the same as primary healing. With the greater defect and gaping wound edges of an open wound, healing and granulation take place from the edges inward and from the bottom of the wound up, resulting in more granulation tissue and a much larger scar. Tertiary healing involves suturing two layers of granulation tissue together and may require debridement of necrotic tissue.

9. a. 5; b. 2; c. 7; d. 1; e. 3.

10. a. synthesis of immune factors, blood cells, fibroblasts, collagen
    b. provide metabolic energy for inflammation; protect protein from being used for energy
    c. synthesis of fatty acids and triglycerides used for cellular membranes
    d. capillary and collagen synthesis
    e. coenzymes for fat, protein, and carbohydrate metabolism
    f. epithelial synthesis, increasing collagen synthesis and tensile strength of healing wound

11. a. 2; b. 4; c. 1; d. 3; e. 4; f. 1; g. 3; h. 2; i. 4

12. d. Rationale: Hand washing is the most important factor in preventing infection transmission and is recommended by the Centers for Disease Control and Prevention for all types of isolation precautions in health care facilities.

13. d. Rationale: Although obesity, hyperglycemia, mental deterioration, malnutrition, old age, and incontinence contribute to development of pressure ulcers, the immobility of the comatose patient presents the greatest risk for tissue damage related to pressure.

14. c. Rationale: Relief of pressure on tissues is critical to prevention and treatment of pressure ulcers, and although pressure-reduction devices may relieve some pressure and lift sheets and trapeze bars prevent skin shear, they are no substitute for frequent repositioning of the patient.

15. a. 3; b. 4; c. 2; d. 1

16. d. Rationale: Stage III is full-thickness tissue loss; subcutaneous fat may be visible, but bone, tendon, and muscle are not exposed. Answer a. describes a Stage II, b. a Stage I, and c. a stage IV.

17. d. Rationale: Repositioning does not require judgment, patient teaching, or evaluation of care. The other interventions listed are related to assessment, judgment, and teaching, all responsibilities of the RN.

Case Study

1. pain, redness of leg, edema of leg, fever
2. purulent; yellow wound
3. The WBC count is increased, indicating a pronounced leukocytosis that would be seen in acute inflammation. Neutrophils are normally 50% to 70% of the white cells, and hers are increased to 80%, indicating an early response of neutrophils to tissue damage. She also has a "shift to the left" in that normally only 0% to 8% of the neutrophils in the blood are immature, banded-nucleus cells, and she has 12% bands. All these findings are consistent with an acute inflammatory process.
4. History of diabetes, with possible circulatory impairment to lower extremities and altered blood glucose levels; increased weight; inadequate nutrients for healing possible because of confinement

to bed; has no one to help with meals; and the presence of infection in the wound.

5. Aspirin interferes with the synthesis and release of prostaglandins (PGs), which are responsible in part for fever and also act on the heat-regulating center in the hypothalamus, resulting in peripheral dilation and heat loss. Mild to moderate fevers (up to 103°F) are not usually harmful and may benefit defense mechanisms. Antipyretics are often prescribed only to control higher temperatures. To prevent acute swings in temperature and cycles of chilling/perspiring, antipyretics should be given regularly at 2- to 4-hour intervals as ordered.

6. The wound should be kept moist with continuous cleansing to remove nonviable tissue and to absorb excessive drainage. Moist gauze or absorption dressings would be the best choice in the wound that is infected.

7. Hand washing—Before application of clean gloves and immediately after gloves are removed

Clean gloves—When in contact with infectious material, such as dressings or linens with exudate
Biohazard disposal—Of dressings, gloves

8. *Nursing diagnoses:*
   - Acute pain related to inflammation of left leg
   - Hyperthermia related to inflammatory process
   - Risk for deficient fluid volume related to an increased metabolic rate
   - Risk for imbalanced nutrition: less than body requirements related to decreased intake of essential nutrients

   Collaborative problems:
   Potential complication: septicemia

CHAPTER 14

1. Crossword Puzzle
   Across: 2. gene; 3. allele; 4. mutation; 5. trait; 9. dominant allele; 10. phenotype; 12. chromosome; 13. genome; 14. locus
   Down: 1. DNA; 2. genotype; 6. autosomes; 7. RNA; 8. heterozygous; 10. pedigree; 11. carrier

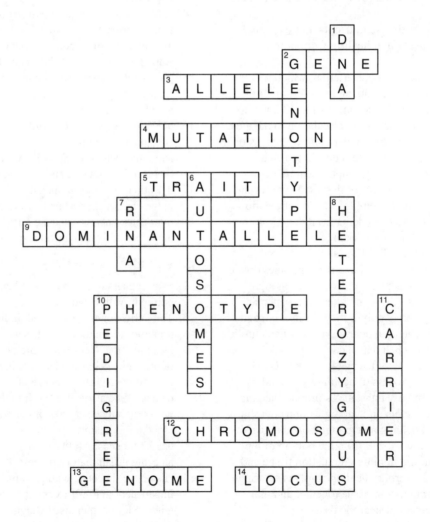

2. c. Rationale: Failure of the two chromosomes to separate during meiosis is known as nondisjunction, which causes an abnormal number of chromosomes, as in Down syndrome and Turner's syndrome. The result is two copies of the same chromosome, or sometimes a copy of a chromosome is missing. When genetic material is exchanged between the two chromosomes in a cell, crossing-over occurs, creating a greater amount of diversity in the genetic makeup of oocytes and sperm.

3. a. 50%
   b. 50%

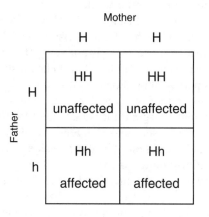

4. a. F, newborn testing for phenylketonuria; b. T; c. T; d. F, embryos; e. F, stem cell therapy.

5. a. 3; b. 1; c. 4; d. 1; e. 2; f. 3, 4; g. 2; h. 4

6. a. bone marrow, thymus gland; b. T lymphocytes, B lymphocytes, monocytes or macrophages; c. spleen; d. bone marrow, thymus gland

7. a. Rationale: Both B and T lymphocytes must be sensitized by a processed antigen to activate the immune response. Processing involves the taking up of an antigen by macrophages and expression of the antigen on the macrophage cell membrane. Antigens need not be protein, and a few antigens may combine with larger molecules that are antigenic.

8. d. Rationale: T-cytotoxic cells directly attack antigens on the cell membrane of foreign pathogens and release cytolytic substances that destroy pathogens. CD4 cells (T-helper cells) are involved in the regulation of humoral antibody response and cell-mediated immunity. Natural killer cells are involved in nonspecific killing of cells but are not considered T lymphocytes. Dendritic cells primarily capture antigens at sites of contact with the external environment and then transport the antigen to a T cell with specificity for the antigen.

9. c. Rationale: Interferon produces an antiviral effect in cells by reacting with viruses and inducing the formation of an antiviral protein that prevents new viruses from becoming assembled. Most cytokines are immunomodulatory and do not directly affect antigens, and cytokines such as interleukins may stimulate activation of immune cells.

10. b. Rationale: Production of immunoglobulins by B lymphocytes is the essential component in humoral immunity. Tumor surveillance and the production of cytokines are functions of T lymphocytes in cellular immunity, and B lymphocytes do not directly attack antigens.

11. a. Rationale: B lymphocytes activated by the presentation of an antigen differentiate into many plasma cells that secrete immunoglobulins and only a few memory cells that retain recognition of the antigen as foreign. Helper cells are T lymphocytes, and natural killer cells are large, granular lymphocytes that are neither B nor T lymphocytes.

12. a. 4; b. 5; c. 4; d. 3; e. 2; f. 1; g. 5; h. 1; i. 3

13. a. immunity against pathogens that survive inside cells; b. fungal infections; c. rejection of foreign tissue; d. contact hypersensitivity reactions; e. tumor immunity

14. d. Rationale: Aging has a pronounced effect on the thymus, which decreases in size and activity, leading to a decline in T cells. T-cell reduction is responsible for decreased tumor surveillance, resulting in an increase in cancer. B-cell activity also declines with advancing age, but the bone marrow is relatively unaffected by increasing age. Circulating autoantibodies increase and are a factor in autoimmune diseases, which increase in persons over the age of 50.

15. a. 2; b. 1; c. 4; d. 3

16. a. 2; b. 1; c. 1; d. 4; e. 3; f. 1; g. 4; h. 2; i. 1; j. 3; k. 1; l. 1; m. 4

17. a. 1. Edema and itching at injection site
    2. Rapid, weak pulse
    3. Hypotension
    4. Laryngeal spasm
    5. Dilated pupils
    b. 1. Maintain airway and provide oxygen
    2. Start IV for fluid and medication access
    3. Prepare to administer epinephrine
    4. Position flat with the legs elevated
    5. Have diphenhydramine (Benadryl) and aminophylline available

18. c. Rationale: Allergic individuals have elevated levels of IgE that react with allergens to produce symptoms of allergy. Immunotherapy involves injecting allergen extracts that will stimulate increased IgG that combines more readily with allergens without releasing histamine. The goal is to keep a "blocking" level of IgG high.

19. d. Rationale: Because there is always a possibility of an anaphylactic reaction when allergens are injected, a health care provider, emergency equipment, and essential drugs should always be available whenever injections are given. The allergen should always be administered in an extremity away from a joint so that a tourniquet can be applied for a severe reaction,

and sites should be rotated. The patient should be carefully observed for a reaction for 20 minutes after an injection.

20. d. Rationale: Two types of latex allergies can occur: A type IV allergic contact dermatitis that is caused by chemicals used in the manufacturing process of latex gloves, and a type I allergic reaction that is a response to the natural rubber latex proteins occurs within minutes of contact with the proteins and may manifest with reactions ranging from skin redness to full-blown anaphylactic shock. Powder-free gloves and avoidance of oil-based hand creams when wearing gloves help to prevent allergic reactions to latex.

21. genetic susceptibility and initiation of autoreactivity (a trigger)

22. c. Rationale: Plasmapheresis is the removal of plasma from the blood, and in autoimmune disorders is used to remove pathogenic substances found in plasma, such as autoantibodies, complexes of antibodies and antigens, and inflammatory mediators. Circulating blood cells are not affected by plasmapheresis.

23. b. Rationale: At the current time, HLA typing is used to determine paternity and to match tissue for transplantation. As more knowledge is gained, there is a strong possibility that HLA associations with certain diseases can be specified and an individual's risk for disease identified.

24. drug-induced immunosuppression with antineoplastic agents and corticosteroids

25. graft-versus-host disease

26. a. 1; b. 1; c. 3; d. 3; e. 2; f. 2; g. 1; h. 2; i. 3.

27. c. Rationale: Standard immunotherapy involves the use of three different immunosuppressants that act in different ways: a calcineurin inhibitor (cyclosporin, tacrolimus), a corticosteroid, and the antimetabolite mycophenolate mofetil. Although cyclosporin is still used, tacrolimus is the most frequently prescribed calcineurin inhibitor.

Case Study

1. IgE is the immunoglobulin involved in most allergic reactions. Chemical mediators that would be active in the patient's allergic rhinitis include histamine, serotonin, slow-releasing substance of anaphylaxis (SRS-A), eosinophil chemotactic factor-anaphylaxis (ECF-A), and complement anaphylatoxins.

2. The procedure would involve either the scratch test or prick test technique. Intradermal allergy testing is not used unless other methods do not result in conclusive reactions. A positive result is manifested by a local wheal-and-flare response that occurs within minutes after insertion of the extract and may last for 8 to 12 hours.

3. Precautions to prevent or treat severe allergic reactions are important:
   - Never leave the patient alone during the testing period.
   - Always have the following available:
     ○ Emergency equipment (oral airway, laryngoscope, endotracheal tubes, oxygen, tourniquet, IV therapy equipment, cardiac monitor with defibrillator)
     ○ Essential drugs (epinephrine, antihistamines, corticosteroids, and vasopressors)
   - Severe local reactions should be treated with removal of the extract and application of antiinflammatory topical cream to the site.

4. Antihistamines relieve allergic symptoms by competing with histamine for H_1 receptor sites and thus block the effect of histamine. The action of most antihistamines is not very effective against histamine-induced bronchoconstriction. This patient should be taught to take antihistamines on a regular basis because he has perennial allergic rhinitis that is not limited to contact with seasonal allergens. He must also be cautioned about the common side effects of antihistamines: drowsiness and impaired coordination, dry mouth, GI upset, urinary retention, blurred vision, and dizziness.

5. Household dust is controlled with air conditioners and air filtration systems in the home as well as daily damp dusting and frequent vacuuming with high-filtration vacuum bags.

6. Precautions:
   - Always have the following available:
     ○ Health care provider
     ○ Emergency equipment (oral airway, laryngoscope, endotracheal tubes, oxygen, tourniquet, IV therapy equipment, cardiac monitor with defibrillator)
     ○ Emergency drugs (epinephrine, antihistamines, corticosteroids, and vasopressors)
     ○ Administer the extract in an extremity away from a joint so that a tourniquet can be applied for a severe reaction.
     ○ Always aspirate for blood before injection of the allergen extract.
     ○ Assess for systemic reactions manifested by pruritus, urticaria, sneezing, laryngeal edema, and hypotension.
     ○ Observe patient for systemic reactions for 20 minutes following the injection.

7. *Nursing diagnoses:*
   - Ineffective health maintenance related to insufficient knowledge of medications, methods of decreasing exposure to allergens
   - Risk for injury related to effects of antihistamines
   Collaborative problems:
   Potential complication: anaphylaxis

CHAPTER 15

1. a, b, c, e. Rationale: Infectious agents, such as the human immunodeficiency virus (HIV) and the Hantavirus, have evolved to affect humans by closer association with animals as human populations push into wild animal habitats. The transfer of infectious agents from animals to humans has also resulted in West Nile virus and avian flu. Bacterial agents have also become untreatable as the result of genetic and biochemical changes stimulated by unnecessary or inadequate exposure to antibiotics.

2. methicillin-resistant *Staphylococcus aureus* (MRSA), vancomycin-resistant enterococci (VRE), penicillin-resistant *Streptococcus pneumoniae* (PRSP).

3. c. Rationale: One of the most important factors in the development of antibiotic-resistant strains of organisms has been inappropriate use of antibiotics, and patients and their families should be taught to take full courses of prescribed antibiotics without skipping doses, not to request antibiotics for viral infections, not to take antibiotics prophylactically unless specifically prescribed, and not to take leftover antibiotics. Hand washing and avoiding others with infection are general measures to prevent transmission of infections.

4. Hand washing or alcohol-based sanitizers and use of personal protective equipment (e.g., gloves).

5. a. women; b. vascular access; c. anal intercourse; d. whole blood; e. first 2 to 6 months of infection; f. HIV-infected mothers using no therapy; g. needle-stick exposure to HIV-infected blood

6. a. 3; b. 5; c. 1; d. 6; e. 2; f. 7; g. 4

7. a. reverse transcriptase inhibitors: inhibit conversion of viral RNA to single-strand viral DNA with assistance of the enzyme reverse transcriptase (step 3 from question 6).
   b. protease inhibitors: inhibit cutting of the long strands of viral RNA in the presence of the enzyme protease (step 7 from question 6).
   c. entry inhibitors: inhibit entry into cell (step 2 from question 6).
   d. Integrase inhibitors (step 5 from question 6)

8. a. Rationale: Activated CD4$^+$ T cells are an ideal target for HIV because these cells are attracted to the site of concentrated HIV in the lymph nodes, where they become infected through viral contact with CD4 receptors. CD4$^+$ T cells normally are a major component of the immune system, and their infection renders the immune system ineffective against HIV and other agents. The virus does not affect natural killer cells, and B lymphocytes are functional early in the disease, as evidenced by positive antibody titers against HIV. Monocytes do ingest infected cells and may become sites of HIV replication and spread the virus to other tissue, but this does not make the immune response ineffective.

9. a. 3; b. 1; c. 2; d. 1; e. 3; f. 2; g. 1; h. 3; i. 4; j. 3

10. a. 3; b. 6; c. 8; d. 2; e. 5; f. 7; g. 1; h. 4

11. d. Rationale: Organisms that are nonvirulent or that cause limited or localized diseases in an immunocompetent person can cause severe, debilitating, and life-threatening infections in persons with impaired immune function.

12. b. Rationale: Because there is a median delay of 2 months after infection before antibodies can be detected, testing during this "window" may result in false-negative results. Risky behaviors that may expose a person to HIV should be discussed and possible scheduling for repeated testing done. Positive results on initial testing will be verified by additional testing. Identification of sexual partners and prevention practices are important but do not relate immediately to the testing situation.

13. c. Although the "rapid" test is highly reliable and results are available in about 20 minutes, if results are positive from any testing, blood will be drawn for more specific enzyme-linked immunosorbent assay (ELISA) or Western blot testing, and another visit will be necessary to obtain the results of the additional testing. CD4$^+$ counts are not used for screening but rather are used to monitor the progression of HIV infection, and new assay tests measure resistance of the virus to antiviral drugs.

14. b. Rationale: The use of potent combination antiretroviral therapy limits the potential for selection of antiretroviral-resistant HIV variants, the major factor limiting the ability of antiretroviral drugs to inhibit virus replication and delay disease progression. The drugs selected should be ones with which the patient has not been previously treated and that are not cross-resistant with antiretroviral agents previously used by the patient.

15. c. Rationale: Guidelines for initiating antiretroviral therapy (ART) are currently in a state of flux because of the development of alternative drugs and problems with long-term side effects and compliance with regimens. In the past, ART was always recommended at the time of HIV infection diagnosis, but today new guidelines suggest that treatment can be delayed until higher levels of immune suppression are observed. Whenever treatment is started, an important consideration is the patient's readiness to initiate ART because adherence to drug regimens is a critical component of the therapy.

16. b. Rationale: An undetectable viral load in the blood does not mean that the virus is gone—it is still present in lymph nodes and other organs. Transmission is still possible, and use of protective measures must be continued.

17. c. Rationale: Pneumococcal, influenza, and hepatitis A and B vaccines should be given as early as possible in HIV infection while there is still immunologic function. Isoniazid (INH) is used

for 9 to 12 months only if a patient has reactive purified protein derivative (PPD) >5 mm, has had high-risk exposure, or has prior untreated positive PPD. Trimethoprim-sulfamethoxazole (TMP-SMX) is initiated when CD4$^+$ T cells are <200/µL or when there is a history of PCP, and varicella-zoster immune globulin (VZIG) is indicated only after significant exposure to chickenpox or shingles in patients with no history of disease or a negative varicella-zoster virus (VZV) antibody test.

18. d. Rationale: After a patient has positive HIV-antibody testing and is in early disease, the overriding goal is to keep the viral load as low as possible and to maintain a functioning immune system. The nurse should provide education regarding ways to enhance immune function to prevent the onset of opportunistic diseases in addition to teaching about the spectrum of the infection, options for care, signs and symptoms to watch for, and ways to adhere to treatment regimens.

19. *Sexual intercourse:*
    - Abstain from sexual activity
    - Noncontact sexual activities (outercourse)
    - Use of barriers during sexual activity
    Drug use:
    - Abstain from drug use
    - Do not share equipment
    - Use alternative routes to injecting
    - Do not have sexual intercourse while under the influence of drugs

20. d. Rationale: The nursing diagnosis of risk for impaired skin integrity addresses a nursing problem that occurs as a result of the diarrhea and wasting and is a problem that nursing can treat.

21. a. Rationale: All the nursing interventions are appropriate for a patient with impaired memory, but the priority is the safety of the patient when cognitive and behavioral problems impair the ability to maintain a safe environment.

Case Study

1. Post-test counseling should include the following:
   - Provide resources for medical and emotional support, with immediate assistance.
   - Evaluate suicide risk.
   - Determine the need to test others who have had risky contact with patient.
   - Discuss retesting to verify results.
   - Encourage optimism: Treatment is available, health habits can improve immune function, the patient can visit HIV-infected people, and the patient is infected with HIV but does not have AIDS.

2. Vague symptoms of fatigue, headaches, lymphadenopathy, and night sweats are characteristic of early chronic infection. CD4$^+$ T cell counts are usually >500/µL in early chronic infection. This patient experienced what could have been acute retroviral syndrome only 2 weeks ago, and it would be unlikely that he would be at a later stage than early chronic infection.

3. Additional testing at this visit should include the following:
   - Complete blood cell count (CBC)
   - Another CD4$^+$ T cell count
   - Viral load assessment (bDNA or PCR)
   - Hepatitis B serology
   - PPD skin test by Mantoux method

4. Pneumococcal, influenza, and hepatitis A and B vaccine
   INH if PPD is >5 mm reactive or, if the patient has had high-risk exposure, nutritional support and education

5. The drug therapy is not curative but has resulted in dramatic improvements in many HIV-infected patients by maintaining immune function and decreasing viral load. It is critical to take the drug combination specifically as prescribed to prevent the development of resistance by the virus. If the drugs cannot be taken for any reason, the health care provider or nurse practitioner should be notified. There are many side effects of the drugs, some of which can be controlled and are not serious but some of which can prevent use of the drugs. It is important to report any changes in the patient's condition or symptoms that develop. The patient will be closely monitored, and viral loads will be assessed 2 to 4 weeks after therapy is started and periodically after that.

6. Genotype and phenotype testing can be done to test for resistance to antiretroviral drugs. The genotype assay detects drug-resistant viral mutations that are present in the reverse transcriptase and protease genes. The phenotype assay measures the growth of the virus in various concentrations of antiretroviral drugs (similar to bacteria-antibiotic sensitivity tests).

7. *Nursing diagnoses:*
   - Anxiety
   - Fear
   - Ineffective denial
   - Anticipatory grieving
   - Deficient knowledge
   - Fatigue
   Collaborative problems:
   Potential complications: Opportunistic infections; opportunistic malignancies; myelosuppression

CHAPTER 16

1. a. Rationale: Lung cancer is the leading cause of cancer deaths in the United States for both women and men, and smoking cessation is one of the most important cancer-prevention behaviors. Cancers of the reproductive organs are the second leading cause of cancer deaths.

2. d. Rationale: Malignant cells proliferate indiscriminately and continuously and also lose the characteristic of contact inhibition, growth on top of and in between other cells. Cancer cells do not

usually proliferate at a faster rate than do normal cells, nor can cell cycles be skipped in proliferation; however, malignant proliferation is continuous, unlike normal cells.

3. a. Rationale: Cancer cells become more fetal and embryonic (undifferentiated) in appearance and function, and some produce new proteins, such as carcinoembryonic antigen (CEA) and α-fetoprotein (AFP), on cell membranes that reflect a return to more immature functioning.

4. c. Rationale: The major difference between benign and malignant cells is the ability of malignant tumor cells to invade and metastasize. Benign tumors are more often encapsulated and often grow at the same rate as malignant tumors. Benign tumors can cause death by expansion into normal tissues and organs.

5. a. 4; b. 1; c. 2; d. 6; e. 3; f. 5

6. a. T; b. T; c. F, reversible; d. T; e. F, initiation and promotion; f. T; g. T; h. F, heterogenous

7. a. rapid proliferation that causes mechanical pressure, leading to penetration of surrounding tissues
   b. decreased cell-to-cell adhesion, allowing cell movement to exterior of primary tumor and within other organ structures
   c. production of metalloproteinase enzymes capable of destroying the basement membrane of the tumor but also of lymph and blood vessels and other tissues

8. a. 5; b. 8; c. 1; d. 7; e. 4; f. 3; g. 6; h. 2

9.

	Meningioma	Meningeal sarcoma
Tissue of origin	embryonal mesoderm	embryonal mesoderm
Anatomic site	meninges	meninges
Behavior	benign	malignant

10. a. arose from epithelial tissue of the breast
    b. moderate differentiation as compared with slight differentiation or very abnormal
    c. small tumor size with a small number of lymph nodes involved, with no evidence of distant metastases

11. a. Men: annual digital rectal examination for prostate evaluation
    b. Men: annual prostate-specific antigen (PSA) blood test
    c. Women: If three normal Pap tests in a row, Pap test every 2 to 3 years; stop after age 70 if test results have been negative for past 10 years.
    d. Women: Annual professional clinical breast examination
    e. Women: Annual mammogram
    f. Annual fecal occult blood test, or flexible sigmoidoscopy every 5 years or annual fecal occult blood test and flexible sigmoidoscopy every 5 years,

or double-contrast barium enema every 5-10 years, or colonoscopy every 10 years

12. b. Rationale: Although other tests may be used in diagnosing the presence and extent of cancer, biopsy is the only method by which cells can be determined to be malignant.

13. a., c., d. A simple mastectomy can be done to prevent breast cancer in women with high risk and can be used to control, cure, or provide palliative care to breasts ulcerative with tumors. A mastectomy would not be used for biopsy or otherwise establishing a diagnosis of cancer.

14. a. 3; b. 1; c. 4; d. 1; e. 2; f. 3; g. 2

15. d. Rationale: Positive response of cancer cells to chemotherapy is most likely in tumors that arise from tissue that has a rapid rate of cellular proliferation, have a small number of cancer cells, are young tumors that have a greater percentage of proliferating cells, are not in a protected anatomic site, and have no resistant tumor cells. A state of optimum health and a positive attitude of the patient will also promote chemotherapy success.

16. a. 2; b. 1; c. 4; d. 3; e. 5

17. b. Rationale: One of the major concerns with the IV administration of chemotherapeutic agents is infiltration of drugs into tissue surrounding the infusion site. Many of these drugs are vesicants— drugs that, when infiltrated into the skin, cause severe local breakdown and necrosis. Specific measures to ensure adequate dilution, patency, and early detection of injury are important.

18. a. 4; b. 2; c. 5; d. 1; e. 3

19. b. Rationale: Patients should always be taught what to expect during a course of chemotherapy, including side effects and expected outcome. Side effects of chemotherapy are serious and may cause death, but it is important that patients be informed about what measures can be taken to help them cope with the side effects of therapy. Hair loss related to chemotherapy is usually reversible, and short-term use of wigs, scarves, or turbans can be used during and following chemotherapy until the hair grows back.

20. c. Rationale: Tissue that is actively proliferating, such as GI mucosa, esophageal and oropharyngeal mucosa, and bone marrow, exhibits early acute responses to radiation therapy. Cartilage, bone, kidney, and nervous tissue that proliferate slowly manifest subacute or late responses.

21. b. Rationale: Radiation ionization breaks chemical bonds in DNA, which renders cells incapable of surviving mitosis. This loss of proliferative capacity yields cellular death at the time of division for both normal cells and cancer cells, but cancer cells are more likely to be dividing because of the loss of control of cellular division. Cells are most radiosensitive in the M and G_2 phases, but damage

in cells that are not in the M phase will be expressed when division occurs. Normal tissues are usually able to recover from radiation damage but not always, and permanent damage may occur.

22. b. Rationale: Brachytherapy is the implantation or insertion of radioactive materials directly into the tumor or in proximity of the tumor and may be curative. The patient is a source of radiation, and in addition to implementing the principles of time, distance, and shielding, film badges should be worn by caregivers to monitor the amount of radiation exposure. Computerized dosimetry and simulation are used in external radiation therapy.

23. a. Rationale: Walking programs are a way for patients to keep active without overtaxing themselves and help combat the depression caused by inactivity. Ignoring the fatigue or overstressing the body can make symptoms worse, and the patient should rest only as necessary.

24. d. Rationale: Alkylating chemotherapeutic agents and high-dose radiation are most likely to cause secondary resistant malignancies as a late effect of treatment. The other conditions are not known to be later effects of radiation or chemotherapy.

25. b. Rationale: Biologic therapies are normal components of the immune system that have been identified and isolated and are used therapeutically to restore, augment, or modulate host immune system mechanisms to assist in immune activity against cancer cells.

26. a. Rationale: Virtually all biologic therapies may cause a flulike syndrome that includes headache, fever, chills, myalgias, fatigue, and anorexia. The other side effects may be caused by specific agents, but not by all biologic therapies.

27. c. Rationale: The nadir is the point of the lowest blood counts after chemotherapy is started, and it is the time when the patient is most at risk for infection. Because infection is the most common cause of morbidity and death in cancer patients, identification of risk and interventions to protect the patient are of the highest priority.

28. b. Rationale: An allogenic hematopoietic stem cell (bone marrow) transplant is one in which bone marrow from an HLA-matched donor is infused into a patient who has received high doses of chemotherapy, with or without radiation, to eradicate cancerous cells. In an autologous bone marrow transplant, the patient's own bone marrow is removed before therapy to destroy the bone marrow. The marrow is treated to remove cancer cells and may be infused right away or frozen and stored for later use. In either case, the new bone marrow will take several weeks to produce new blood cells, and protective isolation is necessary during this time.

29. b. Rationale: Hyperkalemia and hyperuricemia are characteristic of tumor lysis syndrome, which is the result of rapid destruction of large numbers of tumor cells. Signs include hyperuricemia that causes acute renal failure, hyperkalemia, hyperphosphatemia, and hypocalcemia. To prevent renal failure and other problems, the primary treatment includes increasing urine production using hydration therapy and decreasing uric acid concentrations using allopurinol (Zyloprim).

30. a. ability to cope with stressful events in the past
b. presence of effective support system
c. ability to express feelings and concerns
d. older age—usually have greater sense of mortality
e. feeling of control
f. possibility of cure or control
g. pain relief

Case Study

1. Chemotherapy-induced bone marrow suppression is probably the most relevant factor in the patient's decreased WBC and neutrophil count. Inadequate protein intake would also contribute to impaired recovery of normal blood cells.

2. A temperature of 99.4° F (37.4° C) in an immunosuppressed patient is a significant finding for infection. He also has warm skin, with some degree of dehydration. His risk of infection is high, with a WBC count of 3200/µL and neutrophils of 500/µL. The risk for infection increases when neutrophils are <1000/µL.

3. Assess for sore throat, chest pain, persistent cough, urinary symptoms, skin lesions, rectal pain, or confusion. Also note catheter site for chemotherapy as a possible source of infection.

4. His nausea, vomiting, and anorexia, as well as any other side effects of chemotherapy; negative attitude also promoted by lack of social support, an inability to cope with stress, and lack of information about expected results of treatment

5. *Nursing measures:*
   • Use antiemetic protocols to control treatment-related nausea and vomiting.
   • Offer small, frequent feedings of bland, high-calorie, high-protein foods in a pleasant environment.
   • Use relaxation techniques and distraction when the patient is nauseated.
   • Offer any fluids or foods the patient can tolerate and that may be appealing to him.
   • Avoid nagging or being judgmental about food intake.

6. *Teaching measures:*
   • Hand washing for staff, patient, and visitors
   • Careful sterile technique in caring for IV catheter site
   • Avoidance of visitors with infection

7. *Nursing diagnoses:*
   • Hopelessness related to uncertainty about outcomes and insufficient knowledge about cancer and treatment
   • Imbalanced nutrition: Less than body requirements related to decreased oral intake, increased metabolic demands of cancer

- Deficient fluid volume related to decreased oral fluid intake
- Risk for infection related to immunosuppression
Collaborative problems:
Potential complications: septicemia; negative nitrogen balance; myelosuppression

CHAPTER 17

1. a. F, 1000; b. F, 54 (90 kg × 60%); c. F, hyperkalemia; d. T; e. T; f. F, swell and burst, into; g. F, spaces that normally have little or no fluid; h. T
2. a. 4; b. 5; c. 6; d. 7; e. 2; f. 1; g. 3
3. 301 (2 × 147 + 126/18); increased
4. a. 1, 4; b. 2, 3; c. 1, 4; d. 2, 3
5. a. 1, oncotic pressure; b. 2, osmosis; c. 3, 4, osmosis; d. 4, interstitial hydrostatic pressure; e. 1, plasma hydrostatic pressure; f. 1, tissue oncotic pressure; g. 4, interstitial hydrostatic pressure
6. a. Serum osmolality increases as a large amount of sodium is absorbed.
   b. Stimulates antidiuretic hormone (ADH) release from the posterior pituitary, which increases water reabsorption from the kidney, lowering the sodium concentration but increasing vascular volume and hydrostatic pressure, perhaps causing fluid shift into interstitial spaces.
7. c. Rationale: Aldosterone is secreted by the adrenal cortex in response to a decrease in plasma volume (loss of water), serum sodium, or renal perfusion. It is also secreted in response to an increase in serum potassium.
8. b. Rationale: A decrease in renin and aldosterone and an increase in ADH and atrial natriuretic peptide (ANP) lead to decreased sodium reabsorption and increased water retention by the kidney, both of which lead to hyponatremia. Skin changes lead to increased insensible water loss, and plasma oncotic pressure is more often decreased because of lack of protein intake.
9. d. Rationale: A high sodium intake stimulates thirst and increased water intake. A total fluid excess occurs when water is ingested to balance sodium. The other symptoms are typical of fluid-volume deficit or other problems.
10. d. Rationale: A major cause of hypernatremia is a water deficit, which can occur in those with a decreased sensitivity to thirst, the major protection against hyperosmolality. All other conditions lead to hyponatremia.
11. d. Rationale: As water shifts into and out of cells in response to the osmolality of the blood, the cells that are most sensitive to shrinking or swelling are those of the brain, resulting in neurologic symptoms.
12. a. 8; b. 4; c. 6; d. 1; e. 7; f. 2; g. 9; h. 3; i. 6, 10; j. 6; k. 1; l. 5
13. a. hypernatremia, hypokalemia, hypomagnesemia

   b. Any three of these: hyperkalemia, hypocalcemia, hyperphosphatemia, hypermagnesemia
   c. hypokalemia, hyponatremia, hypocalcemia
14. d. Rationale: Because of the osmotic pressure of sodium, water will be excreted with the sodium lost with the diuretic. A change in the relative concentration of sodium will not be seen, but an isotonic fluid loss will occur.
15. c. Rationale: Potassium maintains normal cardiac rhythm, transmission and conduction of nerve impulses, and contraction of muscles. Cardiac cells demonstrate the most clinically significant changes with potassium imbalances because of changes in cardiac conduction. Although paralysis may occur with severe potassium imbalances, cardiac changes are seen earlier and much more commonly.
16. b. Rationale: In a metabolic acidosis, hydrogen ions in the blood are taken into the cell in exchange for potassium ions as a means of buffering excess acids. This results in an increase in serum potassium until the kidneys have time to excrete the excess potassium.
17. d. Rationale: Chvostek's sign is a contraction of facial muscles in response to a tap over the facial nerve. This indicates the neuromuscular irritability of low calcium levels, and IV calcium is the treatment used to prevent laryngeal spasms and respiratory arrest. Calcitonin is indicated for treatment of high calcium levels, and loop diuretics may be used to decrease calcium levels. Oral vitamin D supplements are part of the treatment for hypocalcemia but not for impending tetany.
18. c. Rationale: Kidneys are the major route of phosphate excretion, a function that is impaired in renal failure. A reciprocal relationship exists between phosphorus and calcium, and high serum phosphate levels of kidney failure cause low calcium concentration in the serum.
19. 7.35 to 7.45; 20 to 1
20. hydrogen ion concentration
21. a. 2; b. 4; c. 3; d. 2; e. 1; f. 4; g. 1; h. 2; i. 5; j. 1
22. c. Rationale: The amount of carbon dioxide in the blood directly relates to carbonic acid concentration and subsequently hydrogen ion concentration. The carbon dioxide combines with water in the blood to form carbonic acid, and in cases in which carbon dioxide is retained in the blood, acidosis occurs.
23. a. secretion of small amounts of hydrogen ions into renal tubule
    b. combining hydrogen ions with ammonia (NH_3) to form ammonium (NH_4)
    c. excreting weak acids
24. a. 4; b. 2; c. 1; d. 3
    Respiratory acid-base imbalances are associated with excesses or deficits of carbonic acid. Metabolic acid-base imbalances are associated with excesses or deficits of bicarbonate.

25. a. kidney conservation of bicarbonate and excretion of hydrogen ions
    b. deep, rapid respirations (Kussmaul breathing) to increase CO_2 excretion
    c. decreased respiratory rate and depth to retain carbon dioxide and kidney excretion of bicarbonate
26. a. 4; b. 3; c. 2; d. 1; e. 4; f. 3; g. 3; h. 2; i. 1
27. b. Rationale: Calculation of the anion gap by subtracting the serum chloride and bicarbonate levels from the serum sodium level should normally be 10 to 14 mmol/L. The anion gap is increased in metabolic acidosis associated with acid gain (e.g., diabetic acidosis) but remains normal in metabolic acidosis caused by bicarbonate loss (e.g., diarrhea).
28. a.
    1. pH >7.45 indicates alkalosis
    2. $PaCO_2$ is low, indicating respiratory alkalosis
    3. HCO_3^- is normal
    4. Respiratory alkalosis matches the pH
    5. Although uncommon, if the HCO_3^- were decreased, compensation would be present.
    Interpretation: respiratory alkalosis
    b.
    1. pH <7.35 indicates acidosis
    2. $PaCO_2$ is low, indicating a respiratory alkalosis
    3. HCO_3^- is low, indicating a metabolic acidosis
    4. Metabolic acidosis matches the pH
    5. The $PaCO_2$ does not match but is moving in the opposite direction, which indicates the lungs are attempting to compensate for the metabolic acidosis.
    Interpretation: Metabolic acidosis; partially compensated
    c.
    1. pH <7.35 indicates acidosis
    2. $PaCO_2$ is high, indicating a respiratory acidosis
    3. HCO_3^- is normal
    4. Respiratory acidosis matches the pH
    5. Normal HCO_3^- is found until the kidneys have time to retain bicarbonate.
    Interpretation: respiratory acidosis
    d.
    1. pH >7.45 indicates alkalosis
    2. $PaCO_2$ is high, indicating a respiratory acidosis
    3. HCO_3^- is high, indicating a metabolic alkalosis
    4. Metabolic alkalosis matches the pH
    5. The $PaCO_2$ does not match but is moving in the opposite direction, indicating that the lungs are attempting to compensate for the alkalosis.
    Interpretation: Metabolic alkalosis; partially compensated
    e.
    1. pH is within normal range but toward alkalosis
    2. $PaCO_2$ is high, indicating a respiratory acidosis
    3. HCO_3^- is high, indicating a metabolic alkalosis

4. Because the body will not overcompensate, the metabolic alkalosis is a closer match with the pH.
5. The high $PaCO_2$ indicates the ability of the lungs to compensate for the metabolic alkalosis.
Interpretation: Compensated or chronic metabolic alkalosis indicated by the high $PaCO_2$ and a pH within normal range
f.
1. pH is within normal range but toward acidosis
2. $PaCO_2$ is high, indicating a respiratory acidosis
3. HCO_3^- is high, indicating a metabolic alkalosis
4. Because the body will not overcompensate, the respiratory acidosis is a closer match with the pH.
5. The high HCO_3^- indicates the ability of the kidneys to compensate for the respiratory acidosis.
Interpretation: compensated respiratory acidosis as reflected by high HCO_3^- and pH in normal range
29. b. Rationale: Fluids such as 5% dextrose in water (D_5W) allow water to move from the extracellular fluid to the intracellular fluid. Although D_5W is physiologically isotonic, the dextrose is rapidly metabolized, leaving free water to shift into cells.
30. d. Rationale: An isotonic solution does not change the osmolality of the blood and does not cause fluid shifts between the extracellular fluid and intracellular fluid. In the case of extracellular fluid loss, an isotonic solution, such as lactated Ringer's solution, is ideal because it stays in the extracellular compartment. A hypertonic solution would pull fluid from the cells into the extracellular compartment, resulting in cellular fluid loss and possible vascular overload.
31. d. Rationale: Greatest risk with CVAD is systemic infection. Dressings that are loose should be changed immediately to reduce this risk.
32. a. F, back and forth; b. T; c. T; d. F, the invasiveness of the procedure.
33. a. Rationale: Catheters tunneled to the distal end of the superior vena cava or the right atrium are vascular access devices inserted into central veins, which decrease the incidence of extravasation, provide for rapid dilution of chemotherapy, and reduce the need for venipunctures. Most right atrial catheters, except for a Groshong, need to be flushed with heparin to prevent clotting in the tubing. Regional chemotherapy administration delivers the drug directly to the tumor and is the only administration route that can decrease the systemic effects of the drugs.
34. a. Rationale: With a low potassium there is an increased risk for dysrhythmias and severe muscle weakness. The sodium and magnesium levels are also not within normal limits. However, the implications are not as life-threatening. The calcium level is normal.

Case Study

1. Status: fluid-volume deficit
   Physical assessment: Decreased skin turgor; dry mucous membranes; weak pulses, low blood pressure; confusion
   Laboratory findings: Elevated blood urea nitrogen (BUN); elevated hematocrit
   Status: Hypokalemia
   Physical assessment: Weakness, confusion; irregular heart rhythm, tachycardia
   Laboratory findings: potassium 2.5 mEq/L
   Etiology: Diuretic therapy
2. Electrocardiographic (ECG) changes are associated with hypokalemia and metabolic alkalosis.
3. Metabolic alkalosis: pH 7.52 with base bicarbonate excess (43 mEq/L)
   Etiology: Diuretic-induced hypokalemia is the primary factor.
   Compensation: Not complete because the pH is out of normal range, but increased $PaCO_2$ and slow and shallow respirations indicate the attempt by the lungs to increase carbon dioxide to compensate for excess bicarbonate.
4. Less fluid reserve because older adults have less total body fluid; older adults also have decreased thirst sensation.
5. Aldosterone would be secreted in response to a hyperkalemia, and in her case its release would be inhibited by the hypokalemia. However, her low blood pressure and extracellular fluid deficit would stimulate secretion of aldosterone to increase sodium and water retention but cause even more potassium loss.
6. General care: Encourage and assist with oral fluid intake
   Provide skin care with assessment, changes in position, no soap
   Assessments:
   • Vital signs q4hr
   • I&O; daily weights
   • Cardiac monitoring until electrolytes and acid-base normal
   • Type and rate of IV fluid and electrolyte replacement
   • Lung sounds for signs of fluid overload in cardiac-compromised patient
   • Daily serum electrolyte and blood gas levels
7. *Nursing diagnoses:*
   • Deficient fluid volume related to excessive extracellular fluid (ECF) loss or decreased fluid intake
   • Ineffective health maintenance related to lack of knowledge of drugs and preventive measures
   • Risk for injury related to confusion, muscle weakness
   • Risk for impaired skin integrity related to dehydration

Collaborative problems:
Potential complications: dysrhythmias; hypovolemic shock; hypoxemia

CHAPTER 18

1. a. diagnosis; b. cosmetic; c. palliative; d. curative; e. curative
2. a. Rationale: Ambulatory surgery is usually less expensive and more convenient, generally involving fewer laboratory tests, fewer preoperative and postoperative medications, less psychologic stress, and less susceptibility to hospital-acquired infections. However, the nurse is still responsible for assessing, supporting, and teaching the patient undergoing surgery, regardless of where the surgery is performed.
3. a. Rationale: Excessive anxiety and stress can affect surgical recovery, and the nurse's role in psychologically preparing the patient for surgery is to assess for potential stressors that could negatively affect surgery. Specific fears should be identified and addressed by the nurse by listening and by explaining planned postoperative care. Falsely reassuring the patient, ignoring her behavior, and telling her not to be anxious are not therapeutic.
4. a. ginger; b. feverfew; c. garlic; d. ginkgo biloba; e. ginseng
5. c. Rationale: Risk factors for latex allergies include a history of hay fever and allergies to foods such as avocados, kiwi, bananas, potatoes, peaches, and apricots. When a patient identifies such allergies, the patient should be further questioned about exposure to latex and specific reactions to allergens. A history of any allergic responsiveness increases the risk for hypersensitivity reactions to drugs used during anesthesia, but the hay fever and fruit allergies are specifically related to latex allergy.
6. Findings are followed by risks/nursing needs in the bulleted lists.
   a. Personal or family history of:
   Problems with anesthesia
   • Possible malignant hyperthermia
   History of allergies
   • Possible drug reactions
   Smoking
   • Perioperative respiratory complications
   Medication/alcohol/drug use
   • Interaction with anesthetics
   • Lab tests that should be evaluated
   • Impaired liver function
   b. Obesity
   • Predisposed to dehiscence, infection, herniation
   • Need for increased anesthesia
   Nutritional deficiencies
   • Impaired healing
   c. Urinary retention
   • Surgical drugs may increase retention postoperatively.

Constipation
- Surgical drugs and analgesics may slow bowel motility.

d. Respiratory disease
- Upper respiratory infection may lead to cancellation of surgery.
- Increased laryngeal bronchospasm
- Increased secretions

Musculoskeletal problems
- Mobility restrictions affecting neck will alter intubation and airway management.
- Surgical positioning and postoperative ambulation may be altered.

e. Use of sleeping medication
- Interaction with anesthetics
- Need for preoperative sedation

f. Pain tolerance
- Postoperative pain management plan

Sensory devices
- Care of glasses, contacts, hearing aids

g. Body image
- Alterations in self-perception and body image from surgery

h. Fear and anxiety related to surgery; poor coping skills
- Stress management

7. d. Rationale: BUN, serum creatinine, and electrolytes are commonly abnormal in renal disease and should be evaluated before surgery. Other tests are often evaluated in the presence of diabetes, bleeding tendencies, and respiratory or heart disease.

8. a. Rationale: Obesity, as well as spinal, chest, and airway deformities, may compromise respiratory function during and after surgery. Dehydration may require preoperative fluid therapy, and an enlarged liver may indicate hepatic dysfunction that will increase perioperative risk related to glucose control, coagulation, and drug interactions. Weak peripheral pulses may reflect circulatory problems that could affect healing.

9. a, b, e. Rationale: Procedural information includes what will or should be done for surgical preparation, including what to bring and what to wear to the surgery center, food and fluid restrictions for how long, physical preparation required, pain control, need for coughing and deep breathing (if appropriate), and procedures done before and during surgery (such as vital signs, IV lines, and how anesthesia administered). Other options include sensory and process information.

10. a. Rationale: The nurse may be responsible for obtaining and witnessing the patient's signature on the consent form, but the health care provider is ultimately responsible for obtaining informed consent. The nurse may be a patient advocate during the signature of the consent form, verifying that consent is voluntary and that the patient understands the implications of consent, but the primary legal action by the nurse is witnessing the patient's signature.

11. a. Notify the health care provider because the patient needs further explanation of the planned surgery.
b. Sufficient comprehension

12. a. The preoperative fasting recommendations of the American Society of Anesthesiology indicate that clear liquids may be taken up to 2 hours before surgery for healthy patients undergoing elective procedures. There is evidence that longer fasting is not necessary.

13. b. Rationale: Preoperative checklists are a tool to ensure that the many preparations and precautions performed before surgery have been completed and documented. Patient identification, instructions to the family, and administration of preoperative medications are often documented on the checklist that ensures that no details are omitted.

14. c. Rationale: One of the major reasons the elderly need increased time preoperatively is the presence of impaired vision and hearing that slows understanding of preoperative instructions and preparation for surgery. Thought processes and cognitive abilities may also be impaired in some older adults. The older adult's decreased adaptation to stress because of physiologic changes may increase surgical risks, and overwhelming surgery-related losses may result in ineffective coping that is not directly related to time needed for preoperative preparation. The involvement of caregivers in preoperative activities may be appropriate for patients of all ages.

15. d. Rationale: This finding may indicate an infection. The surgeon will probably postpone the surgery until the cause of the elevated WBC has been found.

16. a, b, c, d, e. Rationale: All are actions that are needed to ensure the patient is ready for surgery. In addition, the nurse should verify that the ID band and allergy band (if applicable) are on, that the patient is not wearing any cosmetics, that nail polish has been removed, that valuables have been removed and secured, and that prosthetics, such as glasses, have been removed and secured.

Case Study

1. Family—children with cystic fibrosis who require extra care and expense, and concern that the wife will not be able to manage without him; fear of cancer and the unknown; anemia—contributes to fatigue and ability to cope

2. Three criteria:
- Adequate disclosure of the diagnosis; the nature and purpose of the proposed treatment; risks and consequences of the proposed treatment; the probability of a successful outcome; the availability, benefits, and risks of alternative

treatments; and the prognosis if treatment is not instituted.
- Sufficient comprehension of the information is provided.
- Voluntary consent is given without persuasion or coercion.

3. General preoperative instruction: Information related to preoperative routines and preparation, such as food and fluid restrictions; approximate length of surgery; and postoperative recovery
Outpatient instruction: When to arrive and the time of the surgery; how and where to register; what to wear and bring; and the need for a responsible adult for transportation home after the procedure

4. Smoking history increases the risk for postoperative respiratory complications—the longer the patient can stop smoking before surgery, the less the risk.
Mild obesity may contribute to problems with clearance of respiratory secretions and complete expansion of the lungs—should have preoperative instruction about deep-breathing and coughing techniques.
Fear of the diagnosis of cancer can alter adaptation and recovery—the nurse can help minimize risk with specific information about the experience and with supportive listening.

5. *Nursing diagnoses:*
- Fear related to possible diagnosis of cancer
- Interrupted family processes related to shift in family roles
- Ineffective health maintenance related to tobacco use
Collaborative problems:
Potential complications: hemorrhage; laryngospasm/bronchospasm; pneumonia; pneumothorax

CHAPTER 19

1. b. Rationale: Although all the factors are important to the safety and well-being of the patient, the first consideration in the physical environment of the surgical suite is prevention of transmission of infection to the patient.

2. b. Rationale: Persons in street clothes or attire other than surgical scrub clothing can interact with personnel of the surgical suite in unrestricted areas, such as the holding area, nursing station, control desk, or locker rooms. Only authorized personnel wearing surgical attire and hair covering are allowed in semirestricted areas, such as corridors, and masks must be worn in restricted areas, such as operating rooms, clean core, and scrub-sink areas.

3. a. 2; b. 1; c. 4; d. 1; e. 2; f. 5; g. 1; h. 6; i. 3; j. 2; k. 5

4. a. Allergy to skin preparation agents, adhesive tapes, or latex; b. musculoskeletal impairments requiring adaptations in positioning; c. pain requiring adaptation in moving or procedures; d. decreased level of consciousness requiring increased safety and protection

techniques; e. vision or hearing impairments requiring adaptations in communication; f. piercings that require removal of jewelry during electrosurgery.
Also: Skin conditions requiring special skin preparation and precautions against infection.

5. a. Rationale: The protection of the patient from injury in the operating room environment is maintained by the circulating nurse by ensuring functioning equipment, preventing falls and injury during transport and transfer, monitoring asepsis, and being with the patient during anesthesia induction.

6. c. Rationale: The Universal Protocol supported by the The Joint Commission (TJC) is used to prevent wrong site, wrong procedure, and wrong surgery in view of a high rate of these problems nationally. It involves pausing just before the procedure starts to verify identity, site, and procedure.

7. a. Rationale: The mask covering the face is not considered sterile, and if in contact with sterile gloved hands, contaminates the gloves. The gown at chest level and to 2 inches above the elbows is considered sterile, as is the drape placed at the surgical area.

8. c. Rationale: Musculoskeletal deformities can be a risk factor for positioning injuries and require special padding and support on the operating table. Skin lesions and break in sterile technique are risk factors for infection, and electrical or mechanical equipment failure may lead to other types of injury.

9. d. Rationale: The Perioperative Nursing Data Set includes outcome statements that reflect standards and recommended practices of perioperative nursing. Outcomes related to physiologic responses include those of physiologic function, such as respiratory function; perioperative safety includes the patient's freedom from any type of injury; and behavioral responses include knowledge and actions of the patient and family, including the consistency of the patient's care with the perioperative plan and the patient's right to privacy.

10. thiopental sodium (Pentothal) and sodium methohexital (Brevital)

11. b. Rationale: The volatile liquid inhalation agents have very little residual analgesia, and patients experience early onset of pain when the agents are discontinued. They are associated with a low incidence of nausea and vomiting. Prolonged respiratory depression is not common because of their rapid elimination. Hypothermia is not related to use of these agents, but they may precipitate malignant hyperthermia in conjunction with neuromuscular blocking agents.

12. a. Rationale: Midazolam (Versed) is a rapid, short-acting, sedative-hypnotic benzodiazepine that is used to prevent recall of events under anesthesia because of its amnestic properties.

13. a. Maintenance anesthesia—monitor for
    cardiopulmonary depression, early pain, and
    nausea and vomiting
    b. Dissociative anesthesia with analgesia and
    amnesia—monitor for agitation, hallucinations,
    nightmares
    c. Induction and maintenance of anesthesia; promote
    early analgesia—assess for nausea and vomiting,
    monitor respiratory status
    d. Produce deep muscle relaxation—monitor
    respiratory muscle movement, airway patency, and
    temperature
14. b. Rationale: MAC refers to sedation that allows the
    patient to manage his or her own airway and respond
    to commands, and yet the patient can emotionally
    and physically accept painful procedures. Drugs are
    used to provide analgesia, relieve anxiety, and/or
    provide amnesia. It can be administered by personnel
    other than anesthesiologists, but nurses should
    be specially trained in the techniques of MAC to
    carry out this procedure because of the high risk of
    complications resulting in clinical emergencies.
15. a. 5; b. 4; c. 1; d. 3; e. 2
16. b. Rationale: During epidural and spinal anesthesia,
    a sympathetic nervous system blockade may
    occur that results in hypotension, bradycardia,
    and nausea and vomiting. A spinal headache may
    occur after, not during, spinal anesthesia, and
    unconsciousness and seizures are indicative of IV
    absorption overdose. Upward extension of the effect
    of the anesthesia results in inadequate respiratory
    excursion and apnea.
17. b. Rationale: Although malignant hyperthermia can
    result in cardiac arrest and death, if the patient is
    known or suspected to be at risk for the disorder,
    appropriate precautions taken by the ACP can
    provide for safe anesthesia for the patient. Because
    preventive measures are possible if the risk is known,
    it is critical that preoperative assessment include a
    careful family history of surgical events.

Case Study

1. Ensure enough help is available to transfer the
   patient from the stretcher to the OR table. Position
   the patient carefully to prevent injury. Apply safety
   straps. Place ECG leads, BP cuff, and pulse oximetry.
   Check the IV to verify insertion and patency. Ensure
   the grounding pad is placed correctly. Complete the
   patient safety checklist. Implement the Universal
   Protocol—take a surgical time-out with the surgical
   team members to verify patient name, birthdate,
   operative procedure and location and compare the
   hospital ID number with the patient ID band and the
   chart.
2. Place in correct musculoskeletal alignment. Be sure
   no undue pressure is occurring to bony prominences,
   nerves, earlobes, and eyes. Be sure there can be

adequate thoracic wall movement. Prevent any
pressure/occlusion of veins/arteries. Secure the
patient's extremities and provide adequate padding.
Respect the patient's specific aches and pains.
3. Hypotension, bradycardia, nausea and vomiting,
   respiratory difficulties, apnea
4. Monitor the effect of anesthetic agents and adjuncts
   closely; ensure clear communication and verify
   patient understanding; closely monitor the patient's
   skin especially where tape, electrodes, and pads
   have been applied; position the older patient
   carefully with close attention to patient alignment
   and joint support.
5. *Nursing diagnoses:*
   • Risk for infection
   • Risk for impaired skin integrity related to
     positioning, immobility, and pressure
   • Risk for injury related to the surgical environment
     and equipment
   • Risk for hypothermia

CHAPTER 20

1. a. Rationale: Although some surgical procedures
   and drug administration require more intensive
   postanesthesia care, how fast and through which
   levels of care patients are moved depend on the
   condition of the patient. A physiologically unstable
   outpatient may stay an extended time in Phase I,
   whereas a patient requiring hospitalization but who
   is stable and recovering well may be transferred
   quickly to an inpatient unit.
2. c. Rationale: Physiologic status of the patient is
   always prioritized with regard to airway, breathing,
   and circulation, and respiratory adequacy is the
   first assessment priority of the patient on admission
   to the PACU from the operating room. Following
   assessment of respiratory function, cardiovascular,
   neurologic, and renal function should be assessed as
   well as the surgical site.
3. c. Rationale: The admission of the patient to the
   PACU is a joint effort between the ACP, who is
   responsible for supervising the postanesthesia
   recovery of the patient, and the PACU nurse, who
   provides care during anesthesia recovery. From
   the ACP it involves a verbal report that presents
   the details of the surgical and anesthetic course,
   preoperative conditions influencing the surgical and
   anesthetic outcome, and PACU treatment plans to
   ensure patient safety and continuity of care.
4. b. Rationale: Even before patients awaken from
   anesthesia, their sense of hearing returns, and all
   activities should be explained by the nurse from
   the time of admission to the PACU to assist in
   orientation and decrease confusion.
5. a. Rationale: ECG monitoring is performed on
   patients to assess initial cardiovascular problems
   during anesthesia recovery. Fluid and electrolyte

status is an indication of renal function, and determinations of arterial blood gases (ABGs) and direct arterial blood pressure monitoring are used only in special cardiovascular or respiratory problems.

6. a. 3; b. 1; c. 3; d. 1; e. 2; f. 2; g. 1; h. 3

7. d. Rationale: An unconscious or semiconscious patient should be placed in a lateral position to protect the airway from obstruction by the tongue. Deep breathing and elevation of the head of the bed are implemented to facilitate gas exchange when the patient is responsive. Oxygen administration is often used, but the patient must first have a patent airway.

8. c. Rationale: Incisional pain is often the greatest deterrent to patient participation in effective ventilation and ambulation, and adequate and regular analgesic medications should be provided to encourage these activities. Controlled breathing may help the patient to manage pain but does not promote coughing and deep breathing. Explanations of rationale and use of an incentive spirometer help to gain patient participation but are more effective if pain is controlled.

9. c. Rationale: Hypotension with normal pulse and skin assessment is typical of residual vasodilating effects of anesthesia and requires continued observation. An oxygen saturation of 88% indicates hypoxemia, whereas a narrowing pulse pressure accompanies hypoperfusion. A urinary output >30 mL/hr is desirable and indicates normal renal function.

10. a. Rationale: The most common cause of emergence delirium is hypoxemia, and initial assessment should evaluate respiratory function. When hypoxemia is ruled out, other causes, such as a distended bladder, pain, and fluid and electrolyte disturbances, should be considered. Delayed awakening may result from neurologic injury, and cardiac dysrhythmias most often result from specific respiratory, electrolyte, or cardiac problems.

11. a. Rationale: During hypothermia, oxygen demand is increased, and metabolic processes slow down. Oxygen therapy is used to treat the increased demand for oxygen. Antidysrhythmics and vasodilating drugs would be used only if the hypothermia caused symptomatic cardiac dysrhythmias and vasoconstriction. Sedatives and analgesics are not indicated for hypothermia.

12. a. patient awake; b. vital signs stable; c. no excess bleeding or drainage; d. no respiratory depression; e. oxygen saturation >90%

13. *Nursing diagnoses:*
- Ineffective airway clearance related to decreased respiratory excursion
- Impaired physical mobility related to decreased muscle strength
- Constipation related to decreased physical activity and impaired GI motility
- Risk for infection related to surgical incision, immobility, and decreased circulation

Collaborative problems:
Potential complications: Venous thromboembolism, paralytic ileus, urinary retention, atelectasis, pneumonia

14. c. Rationale: Secretion and release of aldosterone and cortisol from the adrenal gland and antidiuretic hormone (ADH) from the posterior pituitary as a result of the stress response cause fluid retention during the first 2 to 5 days postoperatively, and fluid overload is possible during this time. Aldosterone causes renal potassium loss with possible hypokalemia, and blood coagulation is enhanced by cortisol.

15. a. 1. slow progression to ambulation—elevate the head of the bed 1 to 2 minutes; dangle legs, stand by bed
     2. sit if feeling faint; if fainting occurs, lower to the floor
   b. 1. promote normal position for voiding or use bedside commode or ambulate to bathroom
     2. run water from a faucet; pour warm water over perineum
   c. 1. encourage to expel flatus
     2. reposition in bed frequently (at least every 2 hours); position on right side
   d. 1. use sterile technique for wound care; use proper drain management
     2. assessment of wound every 2-4 hours

16. a. 2; b. 4; c. 1; d. 3; e. 4

17. c. Rationale: Dressings over surgical sites are initially removed by the surgeon unless otherwise specified and should not be changed. Some drainage is expected for most surgical wounds, and the drainage should be evaluated and recorded to establish a baseline for continuing assessment.

18. d. Rationale: During the first 24 to 48 postoperative hours, temperature elevations to 100.4° F (38° C) are a result of the inflammatory response to surgical stress. Dehydration and lung congestion or atelectasis in the first 2 days will cause a temperature elevation above 100.4° F (38° C). Wound infections usually do not become evident until 3 to 5 days postoperatively and manifest with temperatures above 100° F (37.8° C).

19. d. Rationale: Before administering all analgesic medications, the nurse should first assess the nature and intensity of the patient's pain to determine whether the pain is expected, prior doses of the medication have been effective, and any undesirable side effects are occurring. The administration of PRN analgesic medication is based on the nursing assessment. If possible, pain medication should be in effect during painful activities, but activities may be scheduled around medication administration.

20. c. Rationale: All postoperative patients need discharge instruction regarding what to expect and what self-care can be assumed during recovery. Diet, activities, follow-up care, symptoms to report, and instructions about medications are individualized to the patient.

Case Study

1. Orienting as the patient recovers from the sedating medication, promoting voiding, providing oral fluids and intake
2. Syncope is possible because of the effects of the drug and instrumentation of the bladder. The patient should be slowly progressed to ambulation by elevating the head of the bed, then dangling the legs, and then standing at the side of the bed before attempting ambulation.
3. Inability to void is the most likely problem. The patient could also have respiratory depression or unstable vital signs because of the effects of the drugs or have complications such as bladder bleeding.
4. By standard discharge criteria for PACUs: stable vital signs, oxygen saturation >90%, awake and oriented, no excessive bleeding or drainage, and no respiratory depression, in addition to the specific criteria ordered for this patient.

5. In an outpatient setting, also needs to be alert and ambulatory with the ability to provide self-care near the level of preoperative functioning. Postoperative pain, nausea, and vomiting must be controlled, and the patient must be accompanied by an adult to drive her home. No opioids should have been given 30 minutes before discharge.
6. *Nursing diagnoses:*
   - Impaired urinary elimination related to bladder irritation
   - Acute pain related to bladder irritation
   - Risk for infection related to incomplete bladder emptying
   - Risk for injury related to sedation
   Collaborative problems:
   Potential complications: hemorrhage, infection.

CHAPTER 21

1. a. lens; b. pupil; c. cornea; d. anterior chamber; e. iris; f. posterior chamber; g. ciliary body; h. retina; i. choroid; j. sclera; k. vitreous cavity; l. optic nerve; m. optic disc
2. Word Search. a. zonules; b. aqueous humor; c. vitreous humor; d. cornea; e. ciliary body; f. rods; g. lens; h. cones; i. sclera; j. limbus; k. conjunctiva; l. puncta; m. optic disc; n. choroid; o. canal of Schlemm; p. iris; q. pupil

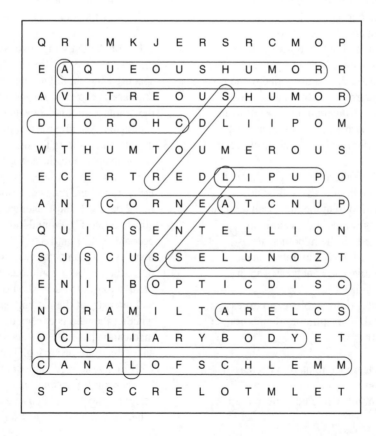

3. a. CN VII (facial)
   b. CN III (oculomotor)
   c. CN V (trigeminal)
   d. CN II (optic)
4. a. loss of orbital fat; b. chronic exposure to ultraviolet (UV) light or other environmental irritants;
   c. cholesterol deposits in the peripheral cornea;
   d. liquefaction and detachment of vitreous;
   e. decreased cones; f. increased rigidity of iris;
   g. deposition of lipids; h. decreased tear secretion
5. a. Rationale: The use of corticosteroids has been associated with the development of cataracts and glaucoma. Use of oral hypoglycemic agents alerts the nurse to the presence of diabetes and risk for diabetic retinopathy. Antihistamine and decongestant drugs may cause eye dryness; β-adrenergic blocking agents may cause additive effects in patients with glaucoma for whom these medications may be prescribed.
6. a. UV light exposure; age-related eye problems; improper contact lens care; family history of ocular problems; diseases affecting the eye
   b. Deficiencies of zinc or vitamins C and E
   c. Constipation and straining to defecate increases intraocular pressure
   d. Work and leisure activities that increase eye strain; lack of protective eyewear during sports; visual difficulties with activities
   e. Lack of sleep
   f. Presence of eye pain; unable to read
   g. Decreased self-concept and self-image; loss of independence
   h. Loss of roles and responsibilities; occupational eye injuries
   i. Eye medications that may cause fetal abnormalities; change in sexual activity related to self-image
   j. Grief related to loss of vision; emotional stress
   k. Values and beliefs that limit treatment decisions
7. With the right eye, the patient standing at 20 feet from a Snellen chart can read to the 40-foot line on the chart with two or fewer errors, and with the left eye, the patient can read only to the 50-foot line on the chart. This patient can read at 20 feet what a person with normal vision can read at 40 and 50 feet.
8. d. Rationale: PERRLA means pupils equal (in size), round, and react to light (pupil constricts when light shines into same eye and also constricts in the opposite eye) and accommodation (pupils constrict with focus on near object). Nystagmus on far lateral gaze is normal but is not part of the assessment of pupil function.
9. a. confrontation test; b. cardinal field of gaze; c. Jaeger chart; d. Snellen chart; e. Tono-pen tonometry
10. b. Rationale: A normal yellowish hue to the normally white sclera is found in dark-pigmented persons and in older adults. Infants and some older adults may exhibit a normal blue cast to the sclera because of

thin sclera. Iris color does not affect the color of the sclera, and infections of the eye may cause dilation of small blood vessels in the normally clear bulbar conjunctiva, reddening the sclera and conjunctiva.
11. b. Rationale: Fluorescein is a dye that is used topically to identify corneal irregularities; irregularities stain a bright green on application of the dye. A tonometer is used to measure intraocular pressure. Light from either a pen light or an ophthalmoscope often is not able to illuminate corneal injuries.
12. a. 3; b. 6; c. 5; d. 1; e. 7; f. 4; g. 2
13. c. Rationale: A break in the retina anywhere in the eye is abnormal and indicates a potential loss of vision. Depression of the center of the optic disc and blurring of the optic disc at the nasal border are normal findings. Pieces of liquified vitreous are "floaters" and are a normal finding in older adults and others.
14. b. Rationale: Although fluorescein dye can be used topically to identify corneal lesions, in angiography the dye is injected intravenously and outlines the vasculature of the retina, locating areas of retinopathy. Intraocular pressure is measured indirectly with a tonometer, and a keratometry is measurement of the corneal curvature.
15. a. 5; b. 1; c. 4; d. 7; e. 9; f. 6; g. 3; h. 8; i. 2
16. a. increased production and dryness of cerumen, increased hair; b. atrophy of the eardrum;
    c. decreased cochlear efficiency resulting from decreased blood supply, decreased hair cells, decreased neurons, and less effective vestibular apparatus in semicircular canals
17. d. Rationale: Presbycusis is a sensorineural hearing loss that occurs with aging and is associated with decreased ability to hear high-pitched sounds. Tinnitus is present in some, but not all, presbycusis. A sensation of fullness in the ears is related to a blocked eustachian tube, and difficulty in understanding the meaning of words is associated with a central hearing loss occurring with problems arising from the cochlea to the cerebral cortex.
18. a. Childhood middle ear infections with perforations and scarring of the eardrum lead to conductive hearing impairments in adulthood.
    b. Many medications are ototoxic, causing damage to the auditory nerve. OTC agents such as aspirin and NSAIDs are potentially ototoxic, as are prescription diuretics, antibiotics, and chemotherapeutic drugs.
    c. A head injury can damage areas of the brain to which auditory and vestibular stimuli are transmitted, with a resultant loss of hearing or balance.
    d. Some congenital hearing disorders are hereditary, and the age of onset of presbycusis also follows a familial pattern.

e. It is well documented that exposure to loud noises causes damage to the auditory organs and hearing loss. Noise exposure earlier in life also can result in increased hearing loss with age.

f. Persons with hearing loss may withdraw from social relationships because of difficulty with communication. A hearing loss often leaves the patient feeling isolated and cut off from valued relationships.

19. a. T; b. F, upward and backward; c. T; d. T; e. F, left; f. T; g. F, acute otitis media

20. a. SHL; b. CHL; c. CHL; d. SHL; e. CHL; f. SHL

21. b. Rationale: Hearing is most sensitive between 500 and 4000 Hz, and a 10-dB loss is not significant at 8000 Hz. A 40- to 45-dB loss in the frequency between 4000 and 8000 Hz will cause difficulty in distinguishing high-pitched consonants. A hearing aid is rarely recommended for a hearing loss of less than 26 dB, and problems in everyday communication situations occur only when the thresholds are 25 dB or higher.

22. b. Rationale: Irrigation of the external ear with water causes a disturbance in the endolymph that normally results in nystagmus directed opposite the side of instillation. The absence of nystagmus indicates that peripheral or central vestibular functions are impaired. An improvement in hearing would occur only if an obstruction of the ear canal was present, which would not be an indication for caloric testing. Severe pain upon irrigation would not be related to vestibular function.

CHAPTER 22

1. a. 4; b. 5; c. 2; d. 2; e. 1; f. 1; g. 1; h. 4; i. 3; j. 2; k. 2; l. 1

2. a. Rationale: A light shined at an angle over the cornea will illuminate a contact lens, and fluorescein should not have to be used. Cotton balls should not be placed on the cornea, and simply tensing the outer canthus will not dislodge the lens.

3. a, b, c, d, e. Rationale: Refractive errors are the most common visual problem and treatment may be nonsurgical corrections (corrective glasses, contect lenses, corneal molding), surgical therapy (LASIK, PRK), implants (ICRs) and thermal procedures (LTK, CK).

4. d. Rationale: A person who is legally blind has some usable vision that will benefit from vision-enhancement techniques. A person with total blindness has no light perception and no usable vision, and one with functional blindness has the loss of usable vision but some light perception. Dependency on others from visual impairment is individual and cannot be assumed.

5. a. Address patient, not others with the patient, in normal conversational tones.
   b. Face the patient and make eye contact.
   c. Introduce self when approaching the patient and let the patient know when you are leaving.
   d. Orient to sounds, activities, and physical surroundings.
   e. Use sighted-guide technique to ambulate and orient patient.
   (Other options: Do not move objects positioned by the patient without knowledge and consent of the patient; ask the patient what help is needed and how to provide it.)

6. c. Rationale: Emergency management of foreign bodies in the eye includes covering and shielding the eye, with no attempt to treat the injury, until an ophthalmologist can evaluate the injury. Irrigations are performed as emergency management in chemical exposure. Pressure should never be applied because it might further injure the eye.

7. Word Search. a. Chalazion; b. Hordeolum; c. Trachoma; d. Acute bacterial conjunctivitis; e. Corneal ulcer; f. Epidemic keratoconjunctivitis; g. Keratitis; h. Blepharitis; i. Conjunctivitis

```
I Q V S T P S E H J K J L B W Z O A E D
R P W T J F C D F Y E K C X O Y P C P N
C A J K Q F C F L J R F N U R L U U I S
E O M L J H O A P Y A U F X R U V T D I
V S R O J B V D U R T N T A B L B E E H
H B K N H N Y B O X I P Z J V E P B M B
P O N S E C I H H C T C B U L V T A I H
L T R T O A G N X I S I H B A E C C C Q
O I V D Z A L R R Z S J N S Y G Q T K C
N Q N N E C M U T I I I K E O H E E E R
G B A D H O A F L S H B G K E Z B R R M
U S F E I L L L N C O D D H Z G I I A L
J O W R N P P U I L E V G F D Q H A T H
W Z W X D W K Y M J Q R E P O S F L O Y
B L P J K P Y V M C G R C H S R C C K
F L V W O U D G S R T P M K R X K O O A
X J E A N U W J E T F X J E J J I N N L
F C P P L D Q F E I H S O Z J U R J J V
I R E D H G O U R S G K Y V F Z B U U H
R D F E D A R B N B O U I U Z X A N N V
U N Y T G C R Q F K E D U V R P R C C N
X O E K J O W I R V O Z I X D S R T T K
L I X F X I X T T H N I Z V A T I I I O
P Z Q H T C Y H L I G G K C K M V V V U
W A V U H N V J Z N S V L R T K B I I W
Z L S I T I V I T C N U J N O C H T T X
G A P K X H L G O G B I Z K X E J I I L
F H I B F R R E T S Z E G W U G U S S L
M C B U Z P W E J J Q Q H S T N G Z O I
M S O D Z V P Y Z T J F O G H J O Z I A
```

8. d. Rationale: All infections of the conjunctiva or cornea are transmittable, and frequent, thorough hand washing is essential to prevent spread from one eye to the other or to other persons. Artificial tears are not normally used in external eye infection. Photophobia is not experienced by all patients with eye infections, and cold compresses are indicated for some infections.

9. d. Rationale: Although cataracts do become worse with time, surgical extraction is considered an elective procedure and is usually performed when the patient decides that he or she wants or needs to see better for his or her lifestyle. There are no known measures to prevent cataract development or progression. Surgical extraction is safe, but the patient will still need glasses for near vision and for any residual refractive error of the implanted lens.

10. c. Rationale: The lens opacity of cataracts causes a decrease in vision, abnormal color perception, and glare. Blurred vision, halos around lights, and eye pain are characteristic of glaucoma; light flashes, floaters, and "cobwebs" or "hairnets" in the field of vision followed by a painless, sudden loss of vision are characteristic of detached retina.

11. a. Rationale: Assessment of the visual acuity in the patient's unoperated eye enables the nurse to determine how visually compromised the patient may be while the operative eye is patched and healing and to plan for assistance until vision improves. The patch on the operative eye is usually removed within 24 hours, and, although vision in the eye may be good, it is not unusual for visual acuity to be reduced immediately after surgery. Activities that are thought to increase intraocular pressure, such as bending, coughing, and Valsalva's maneuver, are restricted postoperatively.

12. a. vitreous shrinking during aging that pulls and tears the retina; b. rhegmatogenous; c. laser photocoagulation, cryopexy; d. scleral buckling

13. a. Rationale: Postoperatively the patient must position the head so that the bubble is in contact with the retinal break and may have to maintain this position for up to 16 hours a day for 5 days. The patient may go home within a few hours of surgery or may remain in the hospital for several days. No matter the type of repair, reattachment is successful in 90% of retinal detachments. Postoperative pain is expected and is treated with analgesics.

14. b. Rationale: The patient with age-related macular degeneration (AMD) can benefit from low-vision aids despite increasing loss of vision, and it is important to promote a positive outlook by not giving patients the impression that "nothing can be done" for them. Laser treatment may help a few patients with choroidal neovascularization, and photodynamic therapy is indicated for a small percentage of patients with wet AMD, but there is no treatment for the increasing deposit of extracellular debris in the retina.

15. c. Rationale: Verteporfin, the dye used with photodynamic therapy to destroy abnormal blood vessels, is a photosensitizing drug that can be activated by exposure to sunlight or other high-intensity light. Patients must cover all their skin to avoid thermal burns when exposed to sunlight. Blind spots occur with laser photocoagulation used for dry AMD. Head movements and position are not of concern following this procedure.

16. a. Rationale: In glaucoma, increased intraocular pressure ultimately damages the optic nerve and retina. Deposition of drusen and degeneration of the macula are characteristic of age-related macular degeneration, and aqueous humor clouding and ciliary body paralysis are not specifically related to eye disorders.

17. c. Rationale: Because glaucoma develops slowly and without symptoms, it is important that intraocular pressure be evaluated every 2 to 4 years in persons between the ages of 40 and 64 and every 1 to 2 years in those over 65 years old. More frequent measurement of intraocular pressure should be done in a patient with a family history of glaucoma, the African American patient, and the patient with diabetes or cardiovascular disease. The disease is chronic, but vision impairment is preventable in most cases with treatment.

18. a. POAG; b. PACG; c. PACG; d. PACG; e. POAG; f. PACG; g. POAG; h. POAG; i. POAG; j. PACG

19. a. β-Adrenergic blocking agent that decreases aqueous humor production
    b. an adrenergic agonist that decreases the production of aqueous humor
    c. a cholinergic agent that stimulates iris sphincter contraction, leading to miosis and opening of the trabecular network, increasing aqueous outflow
    d. carbonic anhydrase inhibitor that decreases aqueous humor production

20. b. Rationale: Patients receiving ototoxic drugs should be monitored for tinnitus, hearing loss, and vertigo to prevent further damage caused by the drugs. Ears should not be cleaned with anything but a washcloth and finger, and ear protection should be used in any environment with noise levels above 90 dB. Exposure to the rubella virus during the first 16 weeks of pregnancy may cause fetal deafness, and the vaccine should never be given during pregnancy.

21. a. 5; b. 2; c. 6; d. 1; e. 4; f. 3

22. Advanced age; use of three potentially ototoxic drugs (aspirin, quinidine, and furosemide)

23. d. Rationale: Antibiotic eardrops for external otitis should be applied without touching the auricle to avoid contaminating the dropper and the solution, and the patient should hold the ear upward for several minutes to allow the drops to run down the canal. An ear wick may be placed in the canal to help deliver the drops, but it remains in the ear throughout the course of treatment. The use of lubricating eardrops followed by irrigation is performed for impacted cerumen. "Swimmer's ear" is best prevented by avoiding swimming in contaminated waters; prophylactic antibiotics are not used.

24. a. F, antibiotics; b. F, a cholesteatoma; c. T; d. T; e. F, chronic; f. T; g. F, with the head of the bed elevated 30 degrees

25. a. Rationale: Otosclerosis is an autosomal-dominant hereditary disease that causes fixation of the footplate of the stapes, leading to conductive hearing loss. Tuning fork testing in conductive hearing loss would result in a negative Rinne test and lateralization to the poor ear or the ear with greater hearing loss upon Weber testing. During a stapedectomy, the patient often reports an immediate improvement in hearing, but the hearing level decreases temporarily postoperatively.

26. b. Rationale: Stimulation of the labyrinth intraoperatively may cause postoperative dizziness, increasing the risk for falls. Nystagmus on lateral gaze may result from perilymph disturbances but does not constitute a risk for injury. A tympanic graft is not performed in a stapedectomy, nor is postoperative tinnitus common.

27. a. vertigo; b. sensorineural hearing loss; c. tinnitus

28. b. Rationale: Nursing care should minimize vertigo by keeping the patient in a quiet, dark environment. Movement aggravates the whirling and roaring sensations, and the patient should be moved only for essential care. Fluorescent lights or television flickering may also increase vertigo and should be avoided. Side rails should be raised when the patient is in bed, but padding is not indicated.

29. c. Rationale: The benign acoustic neuroma can compress the facial nerve and arteries in the internal auditory canal and may expand into the cranium, but if removed when small, hearing and vestibular function can be preserved. During surgery for a tumor that has expanded into the cranium, preservation of hearing and the facial nerve is reduced.

30. a. C; b. C; c. C or S; d. C; e. S; f. C; g. S; h. S; i. S; j. C

31. c. Rationale: Initial adjustment to a hearing aid should include voices and household sounds and experimenting with volume in a quiet environment. The next recommended exposure is small parties; the outdoors; and, finally, uncontrolled areas, such as shopping areas.

Case Study

1. Her race, her family history of glaucoma, and her increasing age place her at a high risk for glaucoma. Glaucoma is the leading cause of blindness among African Americans, and in older persons, 1 in 10 African Americans has glaucoma. African Americans in every age category should have examinations more often than persons without risk factors because of the increased incidence and more aggressive course of glaucoma in these individuals.
2. To prevent systemic absorption of the drug; A.G. already uses one β-adrenergic blocker (metoprolol) for her hypertension, and systemic absorption of the betaxolol could cause additive effects.
3. The antihistamine comes into question because of its anticholinergic effects. It is allowed because A.G. has open-angle glaucoma (OAG) with no abnormal angle on gonioscopy. In angle-closure glaucoma, the drug is contraindicated because anticholinergic effects of the antihistamine would dilate the pupil, obstructing an already narrowed angle.
4. No, because glaucoma is a chronic disease with no cure. It can be controlled with medication and some surgical interventions, but it cannot be cured.
5. Alternatives to topical therapy for primary open-angle glaucoma (POAG) include a trabeculoplasty that opens outflow channels in the trabecular meshwork; a trabeculectomy, in which part of the iris and trabecular meshwork are removed; or cyclocryotherapy, in which parts of the ciliary body are destroyed, decreasing production of aqueous humor.
6. Optic disc cupping with the disc becoming wider, deeper, and paler occurs with progression of glaucoma. Visual complaints with increasing damage include increasing peripheral visual-field loss with eventual tunnel vision and loss of sight.
7. *Nursing diagnoses:*
   • Anxiety related to potential permanent visual impairment
   • Ineffective health maintenance related to lack of routine assessments for glaucoma
   • Ineffective self health management related to lack of knowledge about disease, treatment, administration of eyedrops, follow-up recommendations
   Collaborative problems:
   Potential complications: increased intraocular pressure, blindness

CHAPTER 23

1. a. hair shaft; b. stratum corneum; c. stratum germinativum; d. melanocyte; e. sebaceous gland; f. eccrine sweat gland; g. apocrine sweat gland; h. blood vessels; i. nerves; j. adipose tissue; k. hair follicle; l. arrector pili muscle; m. connective tissue; n. subcutaneous tissue; o. dermis; p. epidermis
2. a. 5; b. 3; c. 1; d. 6; e. 2; f. 8; g. 4; h. 4; i. 7; j. 2; k. 2
3. a. Decreased subcutaneous fat; decreased elasticity; collagen stiffening; UV exposure; gravity. b. Decreased extracellular fluid; decreased sweat and sebaceous gland activity. c. Increased capillary fragility and permeability. d. Decreased blood supply; increased keratin.
4. d. Rationale: A careful medication history is important because many medications cause dermatologic side effects, and patients also use many OTC preparations to treat skin problems. Freckles are common in childhood and are not related to skin disease. Communicable childhood illnesses are not directly related to skin problems, although varicella viruses may affect the skin in adulthood. Patterns of weight gain and loss are not significant, but the presence of obesity may cause skin problems in overlapping skin areas.
5. a. Poor skin hygiene; excessive or unprotected sun exposure; family history of alopecia, ichthyosis, psoriasis; history of skin cancer
   b. Decreased intake of vitamins A, D, E, or C; malnutrition; food allergies; obesity
   c. Incontinence; fluid imbalances
   d. Exposure to carcinogens or chemical irritants
   e. Itching that interferes with sleep
   f. Pain; decreased perception of heat, cold, and touch
   g. Feelings of rejection, prejudice, loss of self-esteem, and decreased body image
   h. Exposure to irritants and allergens; altered relationships with others
   i. Changes in sexual intimacy because of appearance, pain
   j. Skin problems exacerbated by stress
   k. High social value placed on appearance and skin condition with tanning, use of cosmetics
6. d. Rationale: It is necessary for the patient to be completely undressed for an examination of the skin. Gowns should be provided and exposure minimized as the skin is inspected generally first, followed by a lesion-specific examination. Skin temperature is best assessed with the back of the hand, and turgor is best assessed with the skin over the sternum.
7. b. Rationale: Discolored lesions that are caused by intradermal or subcutaneous bleeding do not blanch with pressure, whereas those caused by inflammation and dilated blood vessels will blanch and refill after palpation. Varicosities are engorged, dilated veins that may empty with pressure applied along the vein.

8. a. Vesicles. b. Discrete, localized to the chest and abdomen. c. Color, size, and configuration

9. d. Rationale: An excoriation is a focal loss of epidermis; it does not involve the dermis and, as such, does not scar with healing. Ulcers do penetrate into and through the dermis, and scarring does occur with these deeper lesions. Epidermal and dermal thinning is atrophy of the skin but does not involve a break in skin integrity. Both excoriations and ulcers have a break in skin integrity and may develop crusts or scabs over the lesions.

10. b. Rationale: During assessment of the skin in dark-skinned persons, inspection of skin color should be done where the epidermis is thin or in areas of least pigmentation. The mucosa of the eyes or mouth or the nail beds are acceptable sites. In African American individuals, the sclera is normally yellow-tinged and is not a good site for evaluating color changes. The palms of the hands and soles of the feet are secondary choices to the mucosa.

11. b. Rationale: A shave biopsy is done for superficial lesions that can be scraped with a razor blade, removing the full thickness of the stratum corneum. An excisional biopsy is done when the entire removal of a lesion is desired. Punch biopsies are done with larger nodules to examine for pathology, as are incisional biopsies.

12. a. Rationale: A culture can be performed to distinguish among fungal, bacterial, and viral infections. A Tzanck test is specific for herpes virus infections, potassium hydroxide slides are specific for fungal infections, and immunofluorescent studies are specific for infections that cause abnormal antibody proteins.

13. Word Search. a. Wheal; b. Vesicle; c. Petechiae; d. Macule; e. Fissure; f. Pustule; g. Papule; h. Scales; i. Angioma; j. Plaque; k. Ulcer; l. Excoriation; m. Telangiectasia; n. Vitiligo; o. Keloid; p. Hirsutism; q. Lichenification; r. Nevus; s. Hematoma; t. Intertrigo; u. Comedo; v. Alopecia

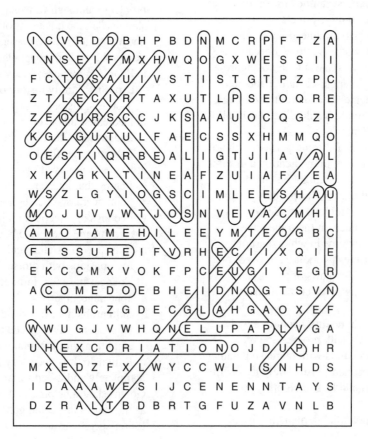

CHAPTER 24

1. a. F, UVB; b. T; c. T; d. F, sunscreen; e. F, vitamin A; f. T.

2. a. 5; b. 3; c. 5; d. 1; e. 1, 4; f. 1; g. 3; h. 4; i. 2, 5; j. 2; k. 3

3. A: Asymmetry—one half unlike the other half. B: Border—irregular and poorly circumscribed. C: Color—varied within lesion. D: Diameter—larger than 6 mm, E: Evolving—look appearance is changing.

4. b. Rationale: Thirty years ago, when the patient was a teenager, radiation therapy was used to treat cystic acne with the result that many of these patients now have developed basal cell carcinoma. For a person with dark skin, radiation therapy is a higher risk factor for skin cancer than exposure to the sun or other irritants.

5. a, b. Rationale: In the early stages, surgical excision with a margin of normal skin is the initial treatment for malignant melanoma. Mohs' surgery can also be used to treat malignant melanoma. Radiation may be used after excision for malignant melanoma, depending on staging of the disease. Topical nitrogen mustard may be used for treatment of cutaneous T-cell lymphoma.

6. a. Chronic disease. b. Obesity. c. Recent antibiotic therapy. d. Recent corticosteroid therapy.

7. Crossword Puzzle
   Across: 1. Warts; 7. Seborrheic keratosis; 11. Tinea; 13. Cellulitis; 14. Lentigo; 15. Pediculosis; 16. Scabies
   Down: 2. Acne; 3. Furuncle; 4. Herpes zoster; 5. Erysipelas; 6. Folliculitis; 8. Herpes simplex 1; 9. Candidiasis; 10. Impetigo; 12. Psoriasis

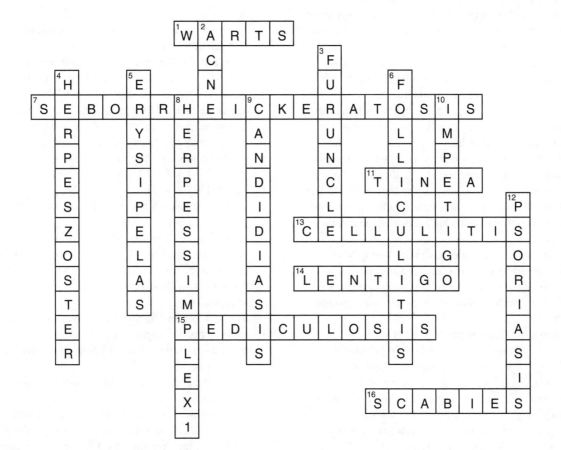

8. Kaposi's sarcoma, candidiasis, herpes zoster

9. b. Rationale: Urticaria is inflammation and edema in the upper dermis, most commonly caused by histamine released during an antibody-allergen reaction. The best treatment for all types of allergic dermatitis is avoidance of the allergen. Sunlight and warmth would increase the edema and inflammation. Antihistamines may be used for an acute outbreak, but not to prevent the dermatitis. Topical γ-benzene hexachloride is used to treat pediculosis.

10. a. Rationale: Pediculosis (head lice and body lice) causes very small, red, noninflammatory lesions that progress to papular wheal-like lesions and cause severe itching. Lice live on the body as nits (tiny white eggs) that are firmly attached to the hair shaft in head and body. Burrows, especially in interdigital webs, are found with scabies.

11. c. Rationale: A lotion is a suspension of insoluble powders in water, which has cooling and drying properties, useful when itching is present. Creams and ointments have an oil and water base that lubricates and protects skin, whereas a paste is a mixture of powder and ointment.

12. d. Rationale: Psoralen is absorbed by the lens of the eye, and eyewear that blocks 100% of UV light must be used for 24 hours after taking the medication. Because UVA penetrates glass, the eyewear must also be worn indoors when near a bright window. Psoralen does not affect the accommodative ability of the eye.

13. a. Clean skin; no occlusive dressings
    b. Diagnosis of the lesion first; thin layers; massaged in at prescribed frequency
    c. Advise of side effects and risks associated with driving or operating heavy machinery
    d. Avoid sunlight; causes photosensitivity; warn patient that it will cause painful, eroded dermatitis before healing

14. a. 4; b. 1, 2, 3, 5; c. 1, 3; d. 2, 3, 6; e. 2, 6
15. a. Rationale: Dressings used to treat pruritic lesions should be cool to cause vasoconstriction and to have an antiinflammatory effect. Water is most commonly used, and it does not need to be sterile. Acetic acid solutions are bacteriocidal and are used to treat skin infections.
16. b. Rationale: Tepid or warm solutions should be used when the purpose is debridement, and saline is a common debridement solution. Baths are appropriate for debridement, but sodium bicarbonate and oatmeal are used for pruritus.
17. a. vasoconstriction; b. decreased inflammation and blood flow, numbing of itch receptor; c. vasoconstriction and stopping itch sensation
18. b. Rationale: Defining characteristics for body-image problems include verbalization of self-disgust and reluctance to look at lesions as evidenced in this patient. Social isolation is indicated only if there is evidence of decreased social activities and of anxiety by verbalization of anxiety or frustration. Ineffective self health management is indicated by evidence of a lack of self-care or understanding of the disease process.
19. a. Rationale: Lichenification is thickening of the skin caused by chronic scratching or rubbing and can be prevented by controlling itching. It is not an infection, nor is it contagious, as the other options indicate.
20. a. Rationale: Improvement of body image is the most common reason for undergoing cosmetic surgery; appearance is an important part of confidence and self-assurance. Acne scars, pigmentation problems, and wrinkling can also be treated with cosmetic surgery, but the surgery does not prevent the skin changes associated with aging.
21. a. facelift; b. liposuction; c. laser
22. a. Rationale: Skin flaps as grafts include moving skin and subcutaneous tissue to another part of the body and are used to cover wounds with poor vascular beds, add padding, and cover wounds over cartilage and bone. Both types of free grafts include just skin, and soft tissue extension involves placement of an expander under the skin, which stretches the skin over time to provide extra skin for covering the desired area.

Case Study

1. W.B. should have cleansed the wound with soap and water and sought medical care for cleaning and suturing. A sterile dressing should have been applied and the arm elevated to reduce edema.
2. *Staphylococcus aureus* and streptococcus
3. That systemic antibiotics will be necessary and that warm, moist packs or dressings should be used to help localize the infection; hospitalization will be necessary if it becomes severe.

4. Gangrene of the extremity; possible septicemia
5. *Nursing diagnoses*:
   • Impaired skin integrity related to trauma
   • Acute pain related to inflammatory process
   • Hyperthermia related to inflammatory process
   Collaborative problems:
   Potential complications: gangrene, septicemia

CHAPTER 25

1. a. 4; b. 1; c. 2; d. 4; e. 1, 3; f. 3; g. 3
2. a. T; b. F, alkaline substances; c. F, chemical; d. T; e. F, electrical burn
3. a. Rationale: Dry, waxy white, leathery, or hard skin is characteristic of full-thickness burns in the emergent phase, and they may turn brown and dry in the acute phase. Deep partial-thickness burns in the emergent phase are red and shiny and have blisters. Edema may not be as extensive in full-thickness burns because of thrombosed vessels.
4. a. 3 1/2 + 1 + 7 1/2 + 2 + 3 1/2 = 17 1/2
   b. 4 1/2 + 9 + 4 1/2 = 18
   c. No, because edema and inflammation obscure the demarcation of zones of injury.
5. d. Rationale: The first intervention is to remove the source and stop the burning process. Airway maintenance would be second, then establishing IV access, followed by assessing for other injuries.
6. a. Fluid loss and formation of edema—usually 24 to 48 hours but might be up to 5 days.
   b. Mobilization of fluid and diuresis—weeks to months.
   c. Burned area covered and wounds healed—weeks to months
7. a. Rationale: With increased capillary permeability, water, sodium, and plasma proteins leave the plasma and move into the interstitial spaces, decreasing serum sodium and albumin. Serum potassium is elevated because injured cells and hemolyzed red blood cells (RBCs) release potassium from cells. An elevated hematocrit is caused by water loss into the interstitium, creating a hemoconcentration.
8. a. Rationale: Although all the selections add to the hypovolemia that occurs in the emergent burn phase, the initial and most pronounced effect is caused by fluid shifts out of the blood vessels as a result of increased capillary permeability.
9. b. Rationale: Burn injury causes widespread impairment of the immune system, with impaired WBC functioning, decrease in circulating immunoglobulins, and bone marrow depression.
10. b. Rationale: Shivering often occurs in a patient with a burn as a result of chilling that is caused by heat loss, anxiety, or pain. Severe pain is not common in full-thickness burns, nor is unconsciousness unless there are other factors present. Fever is a sign of infection in later burn phases.

11. d. Rationale: In circumferential burns, circulation to the extremities can be severely impaired, and pulses should be monitored closely for signs of obstruction by edema. Swelling of the arms would be expected, but it becomes dangerous when it occludes vessels. Pain and eschar are also expected.

12. b. Rationale: Patients with major injuries involving burns to the face and neck require intubation within 1 to 2 hours after burn injury to prevent the necessity for emergency tracheostomy, which is done if symptoms of upper respiratory obstruction occur. Carbon monoxide poisoning is treated with 100% oxygen, and eschar constriction of the chest is treated with an escharotomy.

13. To calculate fluid replacement, the patient's weight in pounds must be converted to kilograms: 132 lb = 60 kg.
    a. lactated Ringer's; 9600 mL (4 mL × 60 × 40)
    b. 4800 mL between 10:15 PM and 5:30 AM; 2400 mL between 5:30 AM and 1:30 PM; 2400 mL between 1:30 PM and 9:30 PM
    c. 720–1200 mL (0.3–0.5 mL/kg/%/TBSA or 0.3 or 0.5 mL × 60 × 40)
    d. urine output (30–50 mL/hr) and VS (BP 90 mm Hg, P 100, R 16–20).

14. b. Rationale: When the patient's wounds are exposed with the open method, the staff must wear caps, masks, gowns, and gloves. Sterile water is not necessary in the debridement tank, and topical antiinfective agents should be applied with sterile gloves. If some dressings are used with the open method, they are removed and wounds washed with clean gloves.

15. a. Rationale: Morphine is the drug of choice for pain control, and during the emergent phase, it should be administered IV because GI function is impaired and IM injections will not be absorbed adequately.

16. b. Rationale: The patient with large burns often develops paralytic ileus within a few hours, and a nasogastric tube is inserted and connected to low, intermittent suction. After GI function returns, feeding tubes may be used for nutritional supplementation and H_2R blockers may be used to prevent Curling's ulcers. Free water is not given to drink because of the potential for water intoxication.

17. c. Rationale: Patients with ear burns are not allowed to use pillows because of the danger of the burned ear sticking to the pillowcase, and patients with neck burns are not allowed to use pillows because contractures of the neck can occur.

18. a. hypermetabolic state resulting from increased plasma catecholamines and substrate mobilization
    b. massive catabolism resulting from protein breakdown and increased gluconeogenesis
    c. calories and protein used for tissue repair

19. c. Rationale: At the end of the emergent phase, fluid mobilization moves potassium back into the cells and sodium returns to the vascular space, causing hypokalemia and hypernatremia. As diuresis in the acute phase continues, sodium will be lost in the urine and potassium will continue to be low unless it is replaced. Excessive fluid replacement with 5% dextrose in water without potassium supplementation can cause hyponatremia with hypokalemia. Prolonged hydrotherapy and free oral water intake can cause a decrease in both sodium and potassium.

20. c. Rationale: The limited range of motion in this situation is related to the patient's inability or reluctance to exercise the joints because of pain, and the appropriate intervention is to help control the pain so that exercises can be performed. The patient is probably never without some pain, and although exercises and enlisting the help of the physical therapist are important, neither of these interventions addresses the cause.

21. a. Rationale: Early signs of sepsis include an elevated temperature and increased pulse and respiratory rate accompanied by decreased BP and, later, decreased urine output and perhaps paralytic ileus. A burn wound may become locally infected without causing sepsis.

22. a. confusion/delirium. b. Curling's ulcer.
    c. hyperglycemia

23. a. cultured epithelial autograft. b. eschar (or necrotic tissue), split-thickness grafts. c. aspirating the fluid with a TB syringe by individuals instructed on the skill.

24. a. Rationale: Midazolam is useful when patients' anticipation of the pain experience increases their pain because it causes a short-term memory loss; and, if given before a dressing change, the patient will not recall the event. A dosage range of morphine is useful, as is patient-controlled analgesia, but seldom will these doses effectively relieve the discomfort of dressing changes. Buprenorphine is an opioid agonist/antagonist and cannot be used with other opioids.

25. a. Rationale: Pressure garments help keep scars flat and prevent elevation and enlargement above the original burn injury area. Lotions and splinting are used to prevent contractures. Avoidance of sun is necessary for 1 year to prevent hyperpigmentation and sunburn injury to healed burn areas.

26. a. 3; b. 2; c. 1; d. 4: Rationale: Face and neck burns are frequently associated with airway inhalation. Therefore this patient requires airway assessment (priority = ABCs). Severe pain would be the next priority (high physiologic need). The patient returning from the OR will need to be seen soon to assess VS, LOC, IV fluids, and wounds. However, at the current time the transport personnel should be with her. The 18-year-old is not at risk related to the ABCs and it will probably take a few minutes to talk with him about why he doesn't want to go for the dressing change.

Case Study

1. Discharge planning should be initiated soon after admission, when the patient is stabilized. Resuming a functional role in society and accomplishing functional and cosmetic reconstruction are the end goals toward which all care is directed. The nurse should coordinate the discharge process with the whole health care team involved with D.K.'s care—the health care provider, physical and occupational therapists, dietitian, home care nurses, and counselors.

2. D.K. will continue to need a high-calorie, high-protein diet, but not to the same extent as during the acute phase. She should be taught about her diet as well as to monitor for unwanted weight gain and reduce calories as indicated. She may also have a functional disability in feeding herself and may need padded utensils or special assistive devices.

3. D.K. will need to continue the splinting and exercise routines diligently until healing is complete—probably for at least a year.

4. Stress that exercise and performance of activities of daily living will decrease the tightness and limitation of movement. Set achievable short-term goals with the patient that can be measured, or have her identify a few activities she wants most to do that are realistic and work toward success with those. She is receiving a secondary gain from her husband in her dependence and regression, and the nurse should help her husband see the importance of her reestablishing independence and enlist his help in coaching the patient with exercises.

5. Provide information and expected outcomes related to the healing of her injuries to both the patient and husband. Encourage both the patient and her husband to participate in the patient's care, and have them identify how care can be managed at home. Let them know that it is possible to maintain contact with hospital personnel after discharge to answer questions and give them support.

6. D.K. and her family may experience a wide range of emotional responses—fear, anxiety, anger, guilt, or depression—and D.K. may be very concerned about her children's reactions to the appearance of her injuries. The nurse should encourage the patient's expression of negative feelings and fears while still hospitalized. Arranging for short visits from her children while she is still hospitalized and while the visits can be controlled would be helpful. Preparation of the family can also be enhanced by helping all family members become aware of routines and activities that will need to be continued during rehabilitation.

7. The procedures for dressing changes and graft care should be formally demonstrated to the patient and her husband with time for them to practice and return the demonstrations. It is most likely the husband will need be involved because D.K. will be unable to manage applying dressings to her hands. Referral to home care nurses is essential for follow-up and evaluation when the patient is discharged to ensure that rehabilitation is continuing.

8. *Nursing diagnoses:*
   - Grieving related to impact of injury on appearance, relationships, and lifestyle
   - Anxiety related to appearance
   - Interrupted family processes related to altered health status of family member
   - Self-care deficit related to inability or unwillingness to participate in self-care
   - Ineffective self-health management related to insufficient knowledge of wound care and follow-up care
   - Situational low self-esteem related to effects of burn on appearance, increased dependence on others, and disruption of lifestyle and role responsibilities
   - Risk for disuse syndrome related to effects of immobility

   Collaborative problems:
   Potential complications: Graft rejection/infection; contractures

CHAPTER 26

1. a. nasal cavity; b. right main-stem bronchi; c. segmental bronchi; d. terminal bronchiole; e. alveolar duct; f. alveoli; g. septa; h. pores of Kohn; i. respiratory bronchiole; j. cilia; k. goblet cell; l. mucus; m. dust particle; n. left main-stem bronchi; o. carina; p. trachea; q. larynx; r. epiglottis; s. pharynx

2. a. right midclavicular line; b. right anterior axillary line; c. right upper lobe; d. right middle lobe; e. right lower lobe; f. left lower lobe; g. left upper lobe; h. angle of Louis; i. first rib; j. suprasternal notch; k. trachea; l. larynx; m. thyroid cartilage; n. midsternal line; o. vertebral line; p. spinal processes; q. left upper lobe; r. left lower lobe; s. right lower lobe; t. right upper lobe; u. scapular line

3. Word Search. a. thoracic cage; b. epiglottis; c. trachea; d. carina; e. dead space; f. surfactant; g. alveolar sacs; h. compliance; i. larynx; j. turbinates; k. angle of Louis; l. parietal pleura; m. phrenic nerve; n. cilia; o. visceral; p. empyema

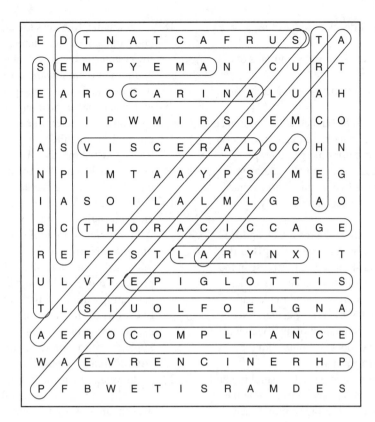

```
E  D (T  N  A  T  C  A  F  R  U  S) (T) (A)
(S)(E  M  P  Y  E  M  A) N  I  C  U  R  T
 E  A  R  O (C  A  R  I  N  A) L  U  A  H
 T  D  I  P  W  M  I  R  S  D  E  M  C  O
 A (S  V  I  S  C  E  R  A  L  O  C  H  N
 N  P  I  M  T  A  A  Y  P  S  I  M  E  G
 I  A  S  O  I  L  A  L  M  L  G  B  A  O
 B  C (T  H  O  R  A  C  I  C  C  A  G  E)
 R  E  F  E  S  T (L  A  R  Y  N  X) I  T
 U  L  V (E  P  I  G  L  O  T  T  I  S)
 T  L (S  I  U  O  L  F  O  E  L  G  N  A)
(A  E  R  O (C  O  M  P  L  I  A  N  C  E)
 W  A (E  V  R  E  N  C  I  N  E  R  H  P)
(P) F  B  W  E  T  I  S  R  A  M  D  E  S
```

4. a. F, arterial oxygen saturation (SaO_2), as a percentage; b. F, partial pressure of oxygen (PaO_2), in mm Hg; c. T; d. T; e. F, 65 mm Hg

5. a. Rationale: When the oxygen-hemoglobin curve shifts to the right, blood picks up less oxygen from the lungs but delivers oxygen more readily to the tissues; thus, low concentrations of oxygen may be given to prevent oxygen toxicity. Shifts to the right occur with acidosis, hyperthermia, and increased $PaCO_2$. Alkalosis, hypothermia, and decreases in $PaCO_2$ cause a leftward shift of the oxygen-hemoglobin curve, which may be treated with higher concentrations of oxygen to compensate for decreased oxygen unloading in the tissues.

6. c. Rationale: Normally, an SaO_2 of 85% correlates with a PaO_2 of about 60 mm Hg. In a leftward shift of the oxygen-hemoglobin curve, oxygen is less readily delivered to the tissues and a lower PaO_2 is present. In a rightward shift of the curve, an SaO_2 of 85% would reflect a higher PaO_2 than normal, about 65 mm Hg. Leftward shifts are commonly caused by alkalosis, hypothermia, and decreases in $PaCO_2$.

7. a. Rationale: Normal findings in arterial blood gases (ABGs) in the older adult include a decreased PaO_2 and SaO_2 but normal pH and $PaCO_2$. No interventions are necessary for these findings. Usual PaO_2 levels are expected in patients ≤60 years of age or younger.

8. d. Rationale: Normal venous blood gas values reflect the normal uptake of oxygen from arterial blood and the release of carbon dioxide from cells into the blood, resulting in a much lower PaO_2 and an increased $PaCO_2$. The pH is also decreased in mixed venous blood gases because of the higher $PvCO_2$. Normal mixed venous blood gases also have much lower PvO_2 and SvO_2 than arterial blood gases. Mixed venous blood gases are used when patients are hemodynamically unstable to evaluate the amount of oxygen delivered to the tissue and the amount of oxygen consumed by the tissues.

9. c. Rationale: Pulse oximetry is inaccurate if the probe is loose, if there is low perfusion, or when skin color is dark; before other measures are taken, the nurse should check the probe site. If the probe is intact at the site and perfusion is adequate, an ABG analysis should be done to verify accuracy, and oxygen may be administered, depending on the patient's condition and the assessment of respiratory and cardiac status.

10. c. Rationale: Poor peripheral perfusion that occurs with hypovolemia or other types of conditions that cause peripheral vasoconstriction will cause inaccurate pulse oximetry, and ABGs may need to be used to monitor oxygenation status and ventilation status in these patients. It would not be affected by fever or anesthesia and is a method of monitoring arterial oxygen saturation in patients receiving oxygen therapy.

11. a. How the patient's SpO_2 compares with the expected normal values

b. The trend and rate of development of the hypoxemia

c. The presence of other signs and symptoms of inadequate oxygenation

d. What the oxygenation status is with activity or exercise

12. c. Rationale: An SpO_2 of 88% and a PaO_2 of 55 mm Hg indicate inadequate oxygenation and are the criteria for prescription of continuous oxygen therapy (see Table 26-3). These values may be adequate for patients with chronic hypoxemia if no cardiac problems occur but will affect their activity tolerance.

13. c. Rationale: A combination of excess CO_2 and H_2O results in carbonic acid, which lowers the pH of the cerebrospinal fluid and stimulates an increase in the respiratory rate. Peripheral chemoreceptors in the carotid and aortic bodies also respond to increases in $PaCO_2$ to stimulate the respiratory center. Excess CO_2 does not increase the amount of hydrogen ions available in the body but does combine with the hydrogen of water to form an acid.

14. c. Rationale: Ciliary action impaired by smoking and increased mucus production may be caused by the irritants in tobacco smoke, leading to impairment of the mucociliary clearance system. Smoking does not directly affect filtration, the cough reflex, or reflex bronchoconstriction, but it does impair the respiratory defense mechanism provided by alveolar macrophages.

15. a. Decreased functional alveoli; small airway closure earlier in expiration

b. Decreased elastic recoil; decreased chest wall compliance

c. Decreased functional cilia; decreased force of cough

d. Decreased alveolar macrophage activity; decreased immunoglobulin A (IgA)

16. a. Smoking history; gradual change in health status; family history of lung disease

b. Decreased fluid intake; anorexia and rapid weight loss, obesity

c. Constipation; incontinence

d. Decreased exercise tolerance; dyspnea on rest or exertion; sedentary habits

e. Sleep apnea; awakening with dyspnea, wheezing, or cough; night sweats

f. Decreased cognitive function with restlessness, irritability; chest pain or pain with breathing

g. Inability to maintain lifestyle; altered self-esteem

h. Loss of roles at work or home; exposure to respiratory toxins at work

i. Sexual activity altered by respiratory symptoms

j. Dyspnea-anxiety-dyspnea cycle; poor coping with stress of chronic respiratory problems

k. Noncompliance with treatment plan; conflict with values

17. a. 3; b. 2; c. 3; d. 2; e. 1; f. 2; g. 4; h. 4; i. 1; j. 1; k. 4.

18. a. Rationale: To assess the extent and symmetry of chest movement, the nurse places the hands over the lower anterior chest wall along the costal margin and moves them inward until the thumbs meet at midline and then asks the patient to breathe deeply and observes the movement of the thumbs away from each other. To determine the tracheal position, the nurse places the index fingers on either side of the trachea just above the suprasternal notch and gently presses backward. The palms are placed against the chest wall to assess tactile fremitus.

19. b. Rationale: An increased AP diameter is characteristic of a barrel chest, in which the AP diameter is about equal to the side-to-side diameter. Normally the AP diameter should be one third to one half the side-to-side diameter. A prominent protrusion of the sternum is the pectus carinatum, and diminished movement of the two sides of the chest indicates decreased chest excursion. Lack of lung expansion caused by kyphosis of the spine results in shallow breathing with decreased chest expansion.

20. d. Rationale: Bronchovesicular breath sounds are normal breath sounds when they are heard anteriorly over the main-stem bronchi on either side of the sternum and posteriorly between the scapulae. If they are heard in the peripheral lung fields, they are considered abnormal breath sounds. Adventitious lung sounds are extra abnormal sounds that include crackles, rhonchi, wheezes, and pleural friction rubs.

21. a. 7; b. 6; c. 5; d. 8; e. 1; f. 2; g. 4; h. 3

22. d. Rationale: Because antibody production in response to infection with the TB bacillus may not be sufficient to produce a reaction to TB skin testing immediately after infection, two-step testing is recommended for individuals likely to be tested often, such as health care providers. An initial negative skin test should be repeated in 1 to 3 weeks, and if the second test is negative, the individual can be considered uninfected. All other answers indicate a negative response to skin testing but, as single testing, do not allow for delay in antibody production.

23. c. Rationale: Samples for ABGs must be iced to keep the gases dissolved in the blood (unless the specimen is to be analyzed in <1 minute) and taken directly to the lab. The syringe used to obtain the specimen is rinsed with heparin before the specimen is taken, and pressure is applied to the arterial puncture site for 5 minutes after obtaining the specimen. Changes in oxygen therapy or interventions should be avoided for 20 minutes before the specimen is drawn because these changes might alter blood gas values.

24. a. Rationale: A pulmonary angiogram involves the injection of an iodine-based radiopaque dye into the pulmonary artery or the right side of the heart,

and iodine or shellfish allergies should be assessed before injection. A bronchoscopy requires NPO status for 6 to 12 hours before the test, and invasive tests—such as bronchoscopy, mediastinoscopy, or biopsies—require informed consent. Nuclear scans use radioactive materials for diagnosis, but the amounts are very small, and no radiation precautions are indicated for the patient.

25. c. Rationale: To prevent damage to the lung tissue and to facilitate entry into the pleural cavity, the patient undergoing a thoracentesis is seated upright with the elbows or arms on an over-the-bed table.

26. c. Rationale: The greatest chance for a pneumothorax occurs with a thoracentesis because of the possibility of lung-tissue injury during this procedure. A ventilation-perfusion scan and positron emission tomography (PET) involve injections, but no manipulation of the respiratory tract is involved. Pulmonary function tests are noninvasive.

27. d. Rationale: A pulmonary angiogram outlines the pulmonary vasculature and is useful to diagnose obstructions or pathologic conditions of the pulmonary vessels, such as a pulmonary embolus. The tissue changes of TB and cancer of the lung may be diagnosed by chest x-ray, CT, MRI, or PET. Airway obstruction is most often diagnosed with pulmonary function testing.

28. a. 3; b. 7; c. 2; d. 4; e. 5; f. 6; g. 1; h. 8

CHAPTER 27

1. a. F, nasal septoplasty; b. T; c. T; d. F, persistent; e. T

2. a. Rationale: Direct pressure on the entire soft lower portion of the nose for 10 to 15 minutes is indicated for epistaxis, in addition to sitting the patient upright, leaning forward, to prevent swallowing of blood. Ice compresses to the nose may be used in addition to having the patient suck ice to constrict the nasal vessels.

3. d. Rationale: All the assessments are appropriate, but the most important is the patient's oxygen status. After the posterior nasopharynx is packed, some patients experience a decrease in PaO_2 and an increase in $PaCO_2$ because of impaired respiration, and the nurse should monitor the patient's respiratory rate and rhythm and SpO_2.

4. b. Rationale: The most important factor in managing allergic rhinitis is identification and avoidance of triggers of the allergic reactions. Immunotherapy may be indicated if specific allergens are identified and cannot be avoided. Drug therapy is an alternative to avoidance of the allergens, but long-term use of decongestants can cause rebound nasal congestion.

5. c. Rationale: Dyspnea and purulent sputum in a patient who has a viral upper respiratory infection (URI) indicate lower respiratory involvement and a possible secondary bacterial infection. Bacterial

infections are indications for antibiotic therapy, but unless symptoms of complications are present, injudicious administration of antibiotics may produce resistant organisms. Elevated temperature, purulent nasal drainage, cough, sore throat, and myalgia are common symptoms of viral rhinitis and influenza.

6. a. Rationale: The injected, inactivated influenza vaccine is recommended for individuals at increased risk for influenza-related complications, such as people aged 50 years and older, residents of long-term care facilities, adults with chronic diseases, health care workers, and providers of care to at-risk persons. The attenuated influenza vaccine is given intranasally and is recommended for all healthy people between the ages of 5 and 49. Antiviral agents will help reduce the duration and severity of influenza in those at high risk, but immunization is the best control.

7. c. Rationale: Classic antihistamines available without a prescription increase mucus viscosity and promote continued symptoms of sinusitis, and they should be avoided. Antibiotics should be taken for at least 1 week after symptoms are relieved, and aspirin products may be used to relieve sinus pain or fever. Nasal irrigations with a saline solution may also be used.

8. c. Rationale: Although inadequately treated β-hemolytic streptococcal infections may lead to rheumatic heart disease or glomerulonephritis, antibiotic treatment is not recommended until strep infections are definitely diagnosed with culture or antigen tests. The manifestations of viral and bacterial infections are similar, and appearance is not diagnostic except when candidiasis is present.

9. a. stridor; b. use of accessory muscles; c. suprasternal and intercostal retractions; d. wheezing.
Others: restlessness, tachycardia, cyanosis

10. b. Rationale: With a tracheostomy (versus an endotracheal [ET] tube), patient comfort is increased because there is no tube in the mouth; because the tube is more secure, mobility is improved. It is preferable to perform a tracheotomy in the operating room because it requires careful dissection, but it can be performed with local anesthetic in the ICU or in an emergency. With a cuff, tracheal pressure necrosis is as much a risk with a tracheostomy tube as with an ET tube, and infection is also as likely to occur because the defenses of the upper airway are bypassed.

11. a. 2; b. 1; c. 4; d. 2; e. 3; f. 4; g. 3; h. 1; i. 4

12. b. Rationale: An inner cannula is a second tubing that fits inside the outer tracheostomy tube and can be removed and cleaned of mucus that has accumulated on the inside of the tube. Many tracheostomy tubes today do not have inner cannulas because if humidification is adequate, accumulation of mucus should not occur.

13. a. Keep a replacement tube of equal or smaller size at the bedside for emergency reinsertion.
    b. Tracheostomy tapes should not be changed the first 24 hours after insertion.
    c. The first tube change is performed by the health care provider no sooner than 7 days after tracheostomy.

14. a, b, e. Rationale: LPNs may assess the need for suctioning, suction the tracheostomy, and evaluate whether the patient has improved after the suctioning when caring for stable patients. They may also perform tracheostomy care using sterile technique.

15. b. Rationale: Cuff pressure should be monitored every 8 hours to ensure that an air leak around the cuff does not occur and that the pressure is not too high to allow adequate tracheal capillary perfusion. Tracheostomy tubes are not usually changed sooner than 7 days after a tracheotomy. Mouth care should be performed a minimum of every 8 hours and more often as needed to remove dried secretions. ABGs are not routinely assessed with tracheostomy tube placement unless symptoms of respiratory distress continue.

16. a. Rationale: If a tracheostomy tube is dislodged, the nurse should immediately attempt to replace the tube by grasping the retention sutures (if available) and spreading the opening. The obturator is inserted in the replacement tube, water-soluble lubricant is applied to the tip, and the tube is inserted in the stoma at a 45-degree angle to the neck. The obturator is immediately removed to provide an airway. If the tube cannot be reinserted, the health care provider should be notified, and the patient should be assessed for the level of respiratory distress, positioned in semi-Fowler's position, and ventilated with a manual resuscitation bag (MRB) only if necessary until assistance arrives.

17. d. Rationale: If colored secretions are coughed or suctioned from the trachea after the patient has attempted to swallow colored water, swallowing is probably not functional and aspiration has occurred. Uncolored water is not discernable as aspirate, and aspiration of small amounts may not cause any respiratory symptoms. The presence of a gag reflex does not ensure that a patient can adequately swallow with a tracheostomy tube in place, and no fluids except clear liquids should be used to assess aspiration risk.

18. b. Rationale: The primary risk factors associated with head and neck cancers are heavy tobacco and alcohol use and family history. Chronic infections are not known to be risk factors, and although oral cancer may cause a change in the fit of dentures, denture use is not a risk factor for oral cancer.

19. a. Rationale: If laryngeal tumors are small, radiation is the treatment of choice because it can be curative and can preserve voice quality. Surgical procedures are used if radiation treatment is not successful or if larger or advanced lesions are present.

20. a. Rationale: With removal of the larynx, the patient will not be able to communicate verbally, and it is important to arrange with the patient a method of communication before surgery so that postoperative communication can take place. Dry mouth and stomatitis result from radiation therapy. Vigorous coughing is not encouraged immediately postoperatively, and information related to community resources is usually introduced during the postoperative period.

21. a. Rationale: Following a radical neck dissection, drainage tubes are often used to prevent fluid accumulation in the wound as well as possible pressure on the trachea. A tracheostomy tube is in place, but mechanical ventilation is usually not indicated. The patient has placement of a nasogastric tube to suction immediately after surgery, which will later be used to administer tube feedings until swallowing can be accomplished.

22. c. Rationale: A supraglottic laryngectomy involves removal of the epiglottis and false vocal cords, and the removal of the epiglottis allows food to enter the trachea. Supraglottic swallowing requires performance of the Valsalva maneuver before placing food in the mouth and swallowing. The patient then coughs to remove food from the top of the vocal cords, swallows again, and then breathes after the food has been removed from the vocal cords.

23. b. Rationale: Suctioning of the tracheostomy with the use of a mirror is a self-care activity taught to the patient before discharge. Voice rehabilitation is usually managed by a speech therapist or speech pathologist, but the nurse should discuss the various types and the advantages and disadvantages of each option. The laryngectomy stoma should be covered with a shield during showering and covered with light scarves or fabric when aspiration of foreign materials is likely.

24. a. Rationale: The voice prosthesis provides the most normal voice reproduction but requires surgical insertion of the device into a fistula made between the esophagus and the trachea. Esophageal speech involves trapping air in the esophagus and releasing it to form sound, but only 10% of patients can develop fluent speech with this method. The electrolarynx, whether mouth-placed or held to the neck, allows speech with a metallic or robotic sound.

Case Study

1. Clear drainage in the nose after facial trauma may be cerebrospinal fluid (CSF) that is leaking from the central nervous system following fractures of the face. Testing at the bedside or in the laboratory with strips that indicate glucose can differentiate CSF from mucus.

2. The vascularity of the face may cause excessive edema following facial trauma, and surgery to repair fractures may need to be delayed until the edema subsides.

3. Airway can be maintained best by keeping the patient in an upright position and controlling edema of the upper airway. After surgery, the head of the bed should continue to be elevated to decrease edema and reduce dyspnea. Application of 4 × 4 dressings dipped in ice water can be placed over the incision for the first 24 hours; the patient may have PO fluids when awake, and cold fluids will help decrease the swelling.

4. Respiratory status—rate, depth, and rhythm—should be assessed frequently to note respiratory distress; vital signs; observation of the surgical site for hemorrhage and edema should also be done often.

5. The patient needs to be taught how to clean the nose and nares with cotton swabs and water or hydrogen peroxide and to apply water-soluble jelly to the nares; to report any continued drainage of serosanguineous fluid from nose after 24 hours or any fresh bleeding; and not to use aspirin or aspirin-containing products for pain relief.

6. *Nursing diagnoses:*
   - Disturbed body image related to postoperative edema and changed facial appearance
   - Acute pain related to incisional edema
   - Risk for ineffective breathing pattern related to presence of packing and nasal edema
   Collaborative problems:
   Potential complications: nasal hemorrhage, nasal hematoma

CHAPTER 28

1. a. aspiration from the nasopharynx or oropharynx; b. inhalation of microbes in the air; c. hematogenous spread from infections elsewhere in the body

2. c. Rationale: Pneumonia that has its onset in the community is usually caused by different microorganisms than pneumonia that develops during hospitalization, and treatment can be empiric—based on observations and experience without knowing the exact cause. In at least half the cases of pneumonia, a causative organism cannot be identified from cultures, and treatment is based on experience.

3. a. 3; b. 2; c. 2; d. 1; e. 1, 2; f. 1, 2; g. 2; h. 2; i. 1; j. 3; k. 1

4. a. red hepatization; b. resolution; c. congestion; d. gray hepatization

5. c. Rationale: Community-acquired pneumonia (CAP) is most commonly caused by *Staphylococcus pneumoniae* and is associated with an acute onset with fever, chills, productive cough with purulent or bloody sputum, and pleuritic chest pain. Other causes of pneumonia have a more gradual onset with dry, hacking cough; headache; and sore throat. A recent loss of consciousness or altered consciousness is common in those pneumonias associated with aspiration, such as anaerobic bacterial pneumonias.

6. d. Rationale: Prompt treatment of pneumonia with appropriate antibiotics is important in treating bacterial and mycoplasma pneumonia, and antibiotics are often administered on the basis of the history, physical examination, and a chest x-ray showing a typical pattern characteristic of a particular organism without further testing. Sputum and blood cultures take 24 to 72 hours for results, and microorganisms often cannot be identified with either Gram stains or cultures. Whether the pneumonia is community acquired or hospital acquired is more significant than the severity of symptoms.

7. c. Rationale: A sputum specimen for Gram stain and culture should be done before initiating antibiotic therapy in a hospitalized patient with suspected pneumonia, and then antibiotics should be started without delay. Chest x-rays and blood cell tests will not be altered significantly by delaying the tests until after the first dose of antibiotics.

8. a. Patient with altered consciousness: Position to side, protect airway
   b. Patient with a feeding tube: Check placement of the tube before feeding, residual feeding; keep head of bed up after feedings or continuously with continuous feedings.
   c. Patient with local anesthetic to throat: Check gag reflex before feeding or offering fluids
   d. Patient with difficulty swallowing: Cut food in small bites, encourage thorough chewing, and provide soft foods that are easier to swallow than liquids

9. a. Rationale: Oxygen saturation obtained by pulse oximetry should be between 90% and 100%. An SpO_2 lower than 90% indicates a hypoxemia and impaired gas exchange. Crackles, purulent sputum, and fever are all symptoms but do not necessarily relate to impaired gas exchange.

10. a. Rationale: The patient with pneumococcal pneumonia is acutely ill with fever and the systemic manifestations of fever, such as chills, thirst, headache, and malaise. Interventions that monitor temperature and aid in lowering body temperature are appropriate. Ineffective airway clearance would be manifested by adventitious breath sounds and difficulty producing secretions. Disorientation and confusion are not noted in this patient and are not typical unless the patient is very hypoxemic. Pleuritic pain is an acute pain that is due to inflammation of the pleura.

11. a. Rationale: Secretions are liquefied and more easily removed by coughing when fluid intake is at least 3 L/day. Positioning and oxygen administration may help ineffective breathing patterns and impaired oxygen exchange but are not indicated for retained secretions. Deep breaths are necessary to move mucus from distal airways.

12. b. Rationale: A second dose of the pneumococcal vaccine should be provided to all persons 65 years of age or older who have not received vaccine within 5 years and were younger than 65 years of age at the time of vaccination. Influenza vaccine should be taken each year by those older than 65 years of age. Antibiotic therapy is not appropriate for all upper respiratory infections unless secondary bacterial infections develop.

13. b. Rationale: Drug-resistant strains of TB have developed because TB patients' compliance to drug therapy has been poor and there has been general decreased vigilance in monitoring and follow-up of TB treatment. Antitubercular drugs are almost exclusively used for TB infections. TB can be effectively diagnosed with sputum cultures. The incidence of TB is at epidemic proportions in patients with HIV, but this does not account for drug-resistant strains of TB.

14. b. Rationale: A patient with class 3 TB has clinically active disease, and airborne infection isolation is required for active disease until the patient has been on drug therapy for at least 2 weeks or until smears are negative on different days. Cardiac monitoring and observation will need to be done with the patient in isolation. The nurse will administer the antitubercular drugs after the patient is in isolation. There should be no need for suction or extra linens after the TB patient is receiving drug therapy.

15. b. Rationale: TB usually develops insidiously with fatigue, malaise, low-grade fevers, and night sweats. Chest pain and a productive cough may also occur, but hemoptysis is a late symptom.

16. For the first 2 months, a four-drug regimen consists of isoniazid (INH), rifampin (Rifadin), pyrazinamide (PZA), and ethambutol (Myambutol).

17. d. Rationale: The nurse should notify the public health department if drug compliance is questionable so that follow-up of patients can be made by directly observed treatment (DOT) by a public health nurse or a responsible family member. A patient who cannot remember to take the medication usually will not remember to come to the clinic daily or will find it too inconvenient. Additional teaching, or support from others, is not usually effective for this type of patient.

18. a, c, d. Rationale: Amphotericin B is a toxic drug with many side effects, including hypersensitivity reactions, fever, chills, malaise, nausea and vomiting, and abnormal renal function, but it does not commonly cause immunosuppression. The side effect that would most commonly intensify when a patient also receives chemotherapeutic agents would be nausea and vomiting.

19. b. Rationale: Although all of the precautions identified in this question are appropriate in decreasing the risk of occupational lung diseases, using masks and effective ventilation systems to reduce exposure is the most efficient and affects the greatest number of employees.

20. a, b, d, e. Rationale: Smoking by women is taking a great toll, as reflected by the incidence of lung cancer in women. Lung cancer incidence and deaths are decreasing in men, whereas almost all other statistics indicate increased risk in women. The incidence of small cell carcinoma is higher in women than in men. Men still have a worse prognosis than women from lung cancer.

21. d. Rationale: The use of radiography, CT, and sputum cytology has been shown to detect lung cancer at earlier stages but has not decreased lung cancer mortality. There is no recommended screening for lung cancer; if screening is done, the patient should be informed of the advantages and disadvantages of each method. A patient who has a smoking history always has an increased risk for lung cancer compared with an individual who has never smoked, but the risk decreases the longer the period of nonsmoking.

22. d. Rationale: Although chest radiographs, lung tomograms, CT scans, MRI, and PET can identify tumors and masses, exact diagnosis of a lung malignancy requires identification of malignant cells either in sputum specimens or biopsies.

23. a. 3; b. 6; c. 8; d. 7; e. 1; f. 9; g. 5; h. 2; i. 4

24. b. Rationale: Before making any judgments about the patient's statement, it is important to explore what meaning he finds in the pain. It may be that he feels it is deserved punishment for smoking, but further information needs to be obtained from the patient. Immediate referral to a counselor negates the nurse's responsibility in helping the patient, and there is no indication that he is not dealing effectively with his feelings.

25. a. open pneumothorax; b. hemothorax; c. closed pneumothorax; d. tension pneumothorax; e. chylothorax; f. chest tube, water-seal drainage

26. b. Rationale: A tension pneumothorax causes many of the same symptoms as a pneumothorax, but severe respiratory distress from collapse of the entire lung with movement of the mediastinal structures and trachea to the unaffected side are present in a tension pneumothorax. Percussion dullness on the injured site indicates the presence of blood or fluid, and decreased movement and diminished breath sounds are characteristic of a pneumothorax. Muffled and distant heart sounds indicate a cardiac tamponade.

27. d. Rationale: Flail chest may occur when two or more ribs are fractured, causing an unstable segment. The chest wall cannot provide the support for ventilation and the injured segment will move paradoxically to the stable portion of the chest (in on expiration; out on inspiration). Absent breath sounds occur following pneumothorax or hemothorax; hypotension occurs with a number of conditions that

impair cardiac function; chest pain occurs with a single fractured rib and will be of high priority with flail chest.

28. A. suction control chamber; B. water-seal chamber; C. collection chamber.

29. The *collection chamber* receives the fluid and air from the pleural or mediastinal space. Nursing keeps track of the amount of drainage and can mark the container for easy measuring. The *water-seal chamber* contains 2 cm of water, which will act as a one-way valve. Incoming air will enter from the collection chamber and bubble up through the water. The water will prevent backflow of the air into the patient from the system. The *suction control chamber* applies suction to the chest drainage. The water suction type system contains a column of water with the top end vented to the atmosphere to control the amount of suction. The amount of suction applied is controlled by the amount of water in the chamber (usually −20 cm), not the wall suction applied to it. The dry suction device contains no water and uses a regulator to dial the desired negative pressure.

30. b. Rationale: The water-seal chamber should bubble intermittently as air leaves the lung with exhalation in a spontaneously breathing patient, and continuous bubbling indicates a leak. The water in the suction control chamber will bubble continuously, and the fluid in the tubing in the water-seal chamber fluctuates with the patient's breathing. Water in the suction control chamber, and perhaps in the water-seal chamber, evaporates and may need to be replaced periodically.

31. c. Rationale: If chest tubes are to be milked or stripped, this procedure should be done only by the professional nurse. This procedure is somewhat controversial because it may dangerously increase pleural pressure, but there is no indication to milk the tubes when there is no bloody drainage, as in a pneumothorax. The nursing assistant can loop the chest tubing on the bed to promote drainage, and patients should be reminded to cough and deep-breathe at least every 2 hours to aid in lung reexpansion. Securing the drainage container in an upright position is also a necessary activity that can be completed by a nursing assistant.

32. a. 3; b. 5; c. 1; d. 6; e. 7; f. 4; g. 2

33. d. Rationale: A thoracotomy incision is large and involves cutting into bone, muscle, and cartilage, resulting in significant postoperative pain. The patient has difficulty deep-breathing and coughing because of the pain, and analgesics should be provided before attempting these activities. Water intake is important to liquefy secretions but is not indicated in this case, nor should a patient with chest trauma or surgery be placed in Trendelenburg position because it increases intrathoracic pressure.

34. a. 2; b. 6; c. 5; d. 7; e. 9; f. 8; g. 1; h. 3; i. 4

35. a. Rationale: All of the activities are correct, but the first thing to do is to raise the head of the bed to promote respiration in the patient who is dyspneic. The health care provider would not be called until the nurse had assessment data relating to vital signs, pulse oximetry, and any other patient complaints.

36. b. Rationale: A spiral (helical) CT is the most frequently used test to diagnose pulmonary emboli because it allows illumination of all anatomic structures and produces a 3-D picture. If a patient cannot have contrast media, a ventilation-perfusion (V/Q) scan is done. Pulmonary angiography is invasive and carries more risk for complications. Chest radiographs do not detect pulmonary emboli until necrosis or abscesses occur.

37. a. 3; b. 1; c. 2

38. b. Rationale: High pressure in the pulmonary arteries increases the workload of the right ventricle and eventually causes right ventricular hypertrophy and dilation, known as cor pulmonale. Eventually, decreased left ventricular output may occur because of decreased return to the left atrium, but it is not the primary effect of pulmonary hypertension. Alveolar interstitial edema is pulmonary edema associated with left ventricular failure. Pulmonary hypertension does not cause systemic hypertension.

39. d. Rationale: If possible, the primary management of cor pulmonale is treatment of the underlying pulmonary problem that caused the heart problem. Low-flow oxygen therapy will help prevent hypoxemia and hypercapnia, which cause pulmonary vasoconstriction.

40. c. Rationale: Acute rejection may occur as early as 5 to 7 days after surgery and is manifested by low-grade fever, fatigue, and oxygen desaturation with exertion. Complete remission of symptoms can be accomplished with bolus corticosteroids. Cytomegalovirus (CMV) and other infections can be fatal but usually occur weeks after surgery and manifest with symptoms of pneumonia. Obliterative bronchiolitis is a late complication of lung transplantation, reflecting chronic rejection.

Case Study

1. Low-flow oxygen; calcium-channel blocking agents (nifedipine [Adalat], diltiazem [Cardizem]), prostacyclins (epoprostenol [Flolan], bosentan [Tracleer]), diuretics

2. Yes, because her medical treatment has failed, and she can be potentially treated with either a lung or heart-lung transplant. She meets additional criteria of being less than 60 years old and a nonsmoker.

3. A heart-lung transplant is indicated for the patient because she has heart damage from the pulmonary hypertension, although there is evidence that even a single-lung transplant can markedly correct pulmonary hypertension and the resultant cor pulmonale.

4. Ability to cope with the postoperative regimen that includes the following:
   - Strict adherence to immunosuppressive drugs
   - Continuous monitoring and reporting of manifestations of infection
   - Financial resources for the procedure, drugs, and follow-up care
   - Social and emotional support system because she is a single mother
5. *Nursing diagnoses:*
   - Activity intolerance related to fatigue as a result of hypoxemia
   - Excess fluid volume related to pump failure
   - Impaired gas exchange related to mechanical failure
   - Ineffective role performance related to inability to perform role responsibilities
   - Anxiety related to breathlessness
   - Risk for impaired skin integrity related to edema
   Collaborative problems:
   Potential complications: dysrhythmias; hypoxemia

CHAPTER 29

1. d. Rationale: Respiratory infections are one of the most common precipitating factors of an acute asthma attack. Sensitivity to food and drugs may also precipitate attacks, and exercise-induced asthma probably occurs to some extent in all patients with asthma. Psychologic factors can interact with the asthmatic response to worsen the disease, but it is not a psychosomatic disease.
2. b. Rationale: Diminished or absent breath sounds may indicate a significant decrease in air movement resulting from exhaustion and an inability to generate enough muscle force to ventilate and is an ominous sign. The other symptoms are expected in an asthma attack.
3. c. Rationale: Early in an asthma attack, an increased respiratory rate and hyperventilation create a respiratory alkalosis with increased pH and decreased $PaCO_2$, accompanied by a hypoxemia. As the attack progresses, pH shifts to normal, then decreases, with ABGs that reflect respiratory acidosis with hypoxemia. During the attack, high-flow oxygen should be provided; breathing in a paper bag, although used to treat some types of hyperventilation, would increase the hypoxemia.
4. a. Salicylates are associated with the asthma triad—people with nasal polyps, asthma, and sensitivity to salicylates and nonsteroidal antiinflammatory drugs (NSAIDs). b. β-adrenergic blocking agents are contraindicated for patients with asthma because they prevent bronchodilation. c. Beer, wine, and other foods contain sulfites that are common triggers of asthma.
5. b. Rationale: Peak expiratory flow rates (PEFRs) are normally up to 600 L/min and in status asthmaticus may be as low as 100 to 150 L/min. An SaO_2 of 85% and FEV_1 of 85% of predicted are typical of mild to moderate asthma, and a flattened diaphragm may be present in the patient with long-standing asthma but does not reflect current bronchoconstriction.
6. a. 2, 3; b. 1, 6; c. 1, 6; d. 2, 8; e. 1, 7; f. 1, 4; g. 1, 6; h. 1, 5; i. 1, 9; j. 1, 5; k. 1, 6; l. 1, 4; m. 1, 3
7. Correct instructions are a, b, d, e, g, h, i
8. b. Rationale: The patient in an acute asthma attack is very anxious and fearful. It is important to stay with the patient and interact in a calm, unhurried manner. Helping the patient breathe with pursed lips will facilitate expiration of trapped air and help the patient gain control of breathing.
9. d. Rationale: Initial drug therapy for acute respiratory distress involves the use of aerosolized albuterol or other β-adrenergic agonists by nebulization every 20 minutes to 4 hours as necessary. The other medications may be added if the patient does not respond to inhaled β-adrenergic agonists.
10. b. Rationale: A yellow zone indicated on the peak flow meter indicates that the patient's asthma is getting worse, and quick-relief medications should be used. The meter is routinely used only each morning before taking medications and does not have to be on hand at all times. The meter measures the ability to empty the lungs and involves blowing through the meter.
11. b. Rationale: Nonprescription drugs should not be used by patients with asthma because of dangers associated with rebound bronchospasm, interactions with prescribed drugs, and undesirable side effects. All the other responses are appropriate for the patient with asthma.
12. a. F, lower; b. T; c. T; d. T; e. F, African Americans
13. See table below.

	Acute Effect	Long-Term Effect
a. Alveolar macrophages	Decreased function	Increased risk of infection
b. Tongue	Decreased taste	Cancer
c. Cilia	Paralysis, sputum accumulation, cough	Chronic bronchitis, cancer
d. Vocal cords	Hoarseness	Chronic cough, cancer
e. Mucous glands	Increased secretions and cough	Hyperplasia of glands, chronic bronchitis
f. Nasopharyngeal	Decreased smell	Cancer
g. Bronchioles	Bronchospasm, cough	Chronic bronchitis, asthma, cancer

14. a. C; b. B; c. C; d. C; e. B; f. C; g. C; h. A; i. A; j. B; k. C

15. b. Rationale: Constriction of the pulmonary vessels, leading to pulmonary hypertension, is caused by alveolar hypoxia and the acidosis that results from hypercapnia. Polycythemia is a contributing factor in cor pulmonale because it increases the viscosity of blood and the pressure needed to circulate the blood. Long-term low-flow oxygen therapy dilates pulmonary vessels and is used to treat cor pulmonale; high oxygen administration is not related to cor pulmonale.

16. d. Rationale: Smoking cessation is one of the most important factors in preventing further damage to the lungs in COPD, but prevention of infections that further increase lung damage is also important. The patient is very susceptible to infections, and infections make the disease worse, creating a vicious cycle. Bronchodilators, inhaled steroids, and lung-volume–reduction surgery help to control symptoms, but these are symptomatic measures.

17. a. 4; b. 6; c. 5; d. 1; e. 3; f. 2

18. a. Rationale: Liquid oxygen reservoirs will last approximately 7 to 10 days when used at 2 L/min, and the portable units will hold about 6 to 8 hours of oxygen. Compressed oxygen comes in various tank sizes, but generally it requires weekly deliveries of four to five large tanks to meet a 7- to 10-day supply. Oxygen concentrators or extractors are more expensive; they continuously supply oxygen, but they must be kept out of the bedroom because they are noisy and interfere with sleep.

19. c. Rationale: Pursed-lip breathing prolongs exhalation and prevents bronchiolar collapse and air trapping. Diaphragmatic breathing emphasizes the use of the diaphragm to increase maximum inhalation, but it has not been shown to be helpful for patients with COPD. Thoracic breathing is not as effective as diaphragmatic breathing and is the method most naturally used by patients with COPD. Huff coughing is a technique used to increase coughing patterns to remove secretions.

20. c. Rationale: Many postural drainage positions require placement in Trendelenburg position, but patients with heart disease, hemoptysis, chest trauma, or severe dyspnea should not be placed in these positions. Postural drainage should be done 1 hour before and 3 hours after meals if possible. Coughing, percussion, and vibration are all performed after the patient has been positioned.

21. b. Rationale: Eating is an effort for patients with COPD, and frequently these patients do not eat because of fatigue, dyspnea, and difficulty holding their breath while swallowing. Foods that require much chewing cause more exhaustion and should be avoided. A low-carbohydrate diet is indicated if the patient has hypercapnia because carbohydrates are metabolized into carbon dioxide. Fluids should be avoided at meals to prevent a full stomach, and cold foods seem to give less of a sense of fullness than hot foods.

22. a. Rationale: Positioning and activities of daily living (ADL) assistance are within the educational preparation of NAPs. Teaching, assessing, and planning are all more appropriate for the RN's practice.

23. c. Rationale: Venturi masks deliver the most precise oxygen concentration and can be set to give 24%, 28%, 31%, 35%, 40%, or 50%. In COPD patients, the Venturi mask can be set to deliver low, constant oxygen. The other delivery systems deliver a range of oxygen concentration, but delivery is variable.

24. d. Rationale: The tripod position with an elevated backrest and supported upper extremities to fix the shoulder girdle maximizes respiratory excursion and an effective breathing pattern. Staying with the patient and encouraging pursed-lip breathing also helps. Bronchodilators may help but can also increase nervousness and anxiety. Postural drainage is not tolerated by a patient in acute respiratory distress, and oxygen is titrated to an effective rate based on ABGs because of the possibility of carbon dioxide narcosis.

25. d. Rationale: Specific guidelines for sexual activity help to preserve energy and prevent dyspnea, and maintenance of sexual activity is important to the healthy psychologic well-being of the patient. Open communication between partners is needed so that the modifications can be made with consideration of both partners.

26. c. Rationale: Shortness of breath usually increases during exercise, but the activity is not being overdone if breathing returns to baseline within 5 minutes after stopping. Bronchodilators can be administered 10 minutes before exercise but should not be administered for at least 5 minutes after activity to allow recovery. Patients are encouraged to walk 15 to 20 minutes a day with gradual increases, but actual patterns will depend on patient tolerance. Dyspnea most frequently limits exercise and is a better indication of exercise tolerance than is heart rate in the patient with COPD.

27. c. Rationale: Cystic fibrosis (CF) is an autosomal-recessive, multisystem disease involving altered function of the exocrine glands of the lungs, pancreas, and sweat glands. Abnormally thick, abundant secretions from mucous glands lead to a chronic, diffuse, obstructive pulmonary disorder in almost all patients, whereas exocrine pancreatic insufficiency occurs in about 85% to 90% of patients with CF.

28. d. Rationale: The major objective of therapy in CF is to promote removal of the secretions, and performance of postural drainage, vibration, and percussion has been the mainstay of treatment. Aerobic exercise also seems to be effective in clearing the airways and is an important part of treatment. Antibiotics are used for early signs of

infection, and long courses are necessary, but they are not used prophylactically. Bronchodilators have no long-term benefit. Although CF has become a leading indication for heart-lung transplant, such a remedy is not available for most patients.

29. a. Rationale: The presence of a chronic disease that is present at birth and significantly lowers life span affects all relationships and development of those patients who live to young adulthood. Children of a parent with CF will either be carriers of CF or have the disease; many men with CF are sterile, and women have difficulty becoming pregnant. Educational and vocational goals may be met in those who maintain treatment programs and health.

30. d. Rationale: Almost all forms of bronchiectasis are associated with bacterial infections that damage the bronchial walls. The incidence of bronchiectasis has decreased with use of measles and pertussis vaccines and better treatment of lower respiratory tract infections.

31. d. Rationale: Mucus production is increased in bronchiectasis and collects in the dilated, pouched bronchi. A major goal of treatment is to promote drainage and removal of the mucus, primarily through deep breathing, coughing, and postural drainage.

Case Study

1. Oxygen therapy needs to be started on E.S. immediately. The goal is to get her oxygen saturation above 90% and to maintain it at or above that level. Although oxygen could be administered using nasal cannula or face mask, it is important to ensure that the patient is receiving the oxygen supplement. Monitor the patient's SpO_2 or PaO_2 closely. Also assess whether the patient with a nasal cannula or face mask device keeps it on (some patients complain that the face mask is suffocating them).

2. E.S. is using accessory muscles, has audible wheezing, a respiratory rate >30, and a pulse >120. Her responses to questions are very short (one- to three-word sentences). She is sitting upright and is extremely anxious and restless. Her breath sounds are not audible in the bases of her lungs and her oxygen saturation is <90%. These are all manifestations of a severe asthma attack. Other observations that might be evident during severe attacks are agitation, PEFR <150 mL, neck vein distention, and a pulsus paradoxus of ≥40 mmHg. Patients with life-threatening asthma are usually too dyspneic to speak and are perspiring profusely. They may be drowsy and the ABGs will reveal further deterioration (lower PaO_2, lower O_2 saturation, rising $PaCO_2$ and pH that is acidotic). Breath sounds may be very difficult to hear and wheezing may no longer be present (very little airflow). These patients become bradycardic and may require airway intubation, mechanical ventilation, and admission to the ICU.

3. Short acting β_2-adrenergic agonists (SABA) stimulate the β-adrenergic receptors in the bronchioles producing bronchodilation (relieve bronchospasm) as well as increase mucociliary clearance. The SABA medications will be given by nebulizer repetitively. Often a SABA plus ipratropium (Atrovent) is given in severe asthma attacks and provides partial relief. Systemic corticosteroids are the second classification of medications given in severe attacks. They can be administered orally or intravenously. Corticosteroids are antiinflammatory agents that reduce bronchial hyperresponsiveness, block the late phase reaction, and inhibit migration of inflammatory cells.

4. Patients experiencing a severe asthma attack are extremely anxious and may not be able to follow the direction of health care providers. Nurses can decrease the patient's sense of panic by providing a calm, quiet, reassuring attitude. Position the patient for comfort (usually sitting upright), stay with the patient, and be available to provide comfort. Gain eye contact with the patient, and in a firm and calm voice coach the patient to use pursed-lip breathing and abdominal breathing (technique called "talking down"). This helps the patient remain calm and improves ventilation (maintains a positive airway pressure, slows down the respiratory rate, and encourages deeper breaths).

5. PEFR is peak expiratory flow rate measured by the peak flow meter, which correlates with forced expiratory volume in 1 second (FEV_1) and is helpful to diagnose and manage asthma. Since there are no standardized PEFR reference values, spirometry is preferred. PEFR can be useful to monitor the asthma patient's response to treatments.

6. *Nursing Diagnoses:*
   - Ineffective airway clearance related to bronchospasm and fatigue
   - Anxiety related to difficulty breathing and fear
   - Deficient knowledge related to lack of information and education about asthma
   - Ineffective health maintenance related to lack of primary health care provider
   Collaborative problems:
   Potential complications: Severe acute asthma, life-threatening asthma

CHAPTER 30

1. a. 7; b. 8; c. 6; d. 7; e. 1; f. 4; g. 3; h. 5; i. 3; j. 6; k. 4; l. 8; m. 3; n. 2; o. 5; p. 3
2. a. neutrophils, basophils, eosinophils; b. erythropoietin; c. iron, vitamin B_{12}, folic acid; d. lymphedema; e. liver, spleen, lymph nodes; f. ferritin, hemosiderin
3. a. 3; b. 2; c. 2; d. 4; e. 2; f. 4; g. 4; h. 1; i. 3; j. 1; k. 3; l. 2
4. b. Rationale: During fibrinolysis by plasmin, the fibrin clot is split into smaller molecules known as fibrin split products (FSPs) or fibrin degradation

products (FDPs). Increased FSPs impair platelet aggregation, reduce prothrombin, and prevent fibrin stabilization and lead to bleeding.

5. c. Rationale: In aging, the partial thromboplastin time (PTT) is normally decreased, so an abnormally high PTT of 60 seconds is an indication that bleeding could readily occur. Platelets are unaffected by aging, and 150,000/μL is a normal count. Serum iron levels are decreased and the erythrocyte sedimentation rate (ESR) is significantly increased with aging, as are reflected in these values.

6. a, c, d. Rationale: The myeloblast is a committed hematopoietic cell found in the bone marrow from which granulocytes develop. A disorder in which myeloblasts are overproduced would result in increased basophils, eosinophils, and neutrophils.

7. a. Rationale: The parietal cells of the stomach secrete intrinsic factor, a substance necessary for the absorption of cobalamin (vitamin B_{12}), and if all or part of the stomach is removed, the lack of intrinsic factor can lead to impaired RBC production and pernicious anemia. Recurring infections indicate decreased WBCs and immune response, and corticosteroid therapy may cause a neutrophilia and lymphopenia. Oral contraceptive use is strongly associated with changes in blood coagulation.

8. a. family history of hematologic disorders; alcohol and cigarette use
 b. deficiencies of iron, vitamin B_{12}, and folic acid; GI bleeding; petechiae or bruising of the skin; fever; lymph node swelling
 c. frankly bloody or dark, tarry stools; dark or bloody urine
 d. fatigue and weakness; change in ability to perform normal activities of daily living
 e. fatigue unrelieved by sleep
 f. pain, especially in joints, bones; paresthesias, numbness, tingling; changes in hearing, vision, taste, mental status
 g. altered self-perception because of lymph node enlargement, skin changes
 h. home or work exposure to radiation or chemicals; military history
 i. menstrual history and characteristics of bleeding; intrapartum or postpartum bleeding problems; impotence
 j. lack of support to meet daily needs; methods of coping with stress
 k. values conflict with treatment, especially blood product or bone marrow transplants

9. a. Rationale: Superficial lymph nodes are evaluated by light palpation, but they are not normally palpable. It may be normal to find small (≤1.0 cm), mobile, firm, nontender nodes. Deep lymph nodes are detected radiographically.

10. b. Rationale: Petechiae are small, flat, red or reddish-brown pinpoint microhemorrhages that occur on the skin when platelet levels are low; when they are numerous, they group, causing reddish bruises known as purpura. Jaundice occurs when anemias are of a hemolytic origin, resulting in accumulation of bile pigments from red blood cells (RBCs). Enlarged, tender lymph nodes are associated with infection, and sternal tenderness is associated with leukemias.

11. b. Rationale: Any smooth, shiny, reddened tongue is an indication of iron-deficiency anemia or pernicious anemia that would be reflected by a decreased hemoglobin level. The increased WBC count could be indicative of an infection; the decreased neutrophils, of neutropenia; and the increased RBCs, of polycythemia.

12. d. Rationale: Any platelet count < 150,000/μL is considered thrombocytopenia and could place the patient at risk for bleeding, necessitating consideration in nursing care. Chemotherapy may cause bone marrow suppression and a depletion of all blood cells. The other factors are all within normal range.

13. a. iron-deficiency anemia; b. inflammatory conditions of any kind; c. infection; d. heparin therapy; e. hemolysis of RBCs; f. multiple myeloma

14. c. Rationale: A patient with O Rh⁺ blood has no A or B antigens on the RBC but does have anti-A and anti-B antibodies in the blood and has an Rh antigen. AB Rh⁻ blood has both A and B antigens on the RBC but no Rh antigen and no anti-A or anti-B antibodies. If the AB Rh⁻ blood is given to the patient with O Rh⁺ blood, the antibodies in the patient's blood will react with the antigens in the donor blood, causing hemolysis of the donor cells. There will be no Rh reaction because the donor blood has no Rh antigen.

15. a. Rationale: A contrast CT involves the use of an iodine-based dye that could cause a reaction if the patient is sensitive to iodine. Metal implants or internal appliances and claustrophobia should be determined before magnetic resonance imaging (MRI). Prior blood transfusions are not a factor in this diagnostic test.

16. c. Rationale: The aspiration of bone marrow contents is done with local anesthesia at the site of the puncture, but the aspiration causes a suction pain that is quite painful, but very brief. There generally is no residual pain following the test.

17. d. Rationale: Lymph node biopsy is usually done to determine whether malignant cells are present in lymph nodes and can be used to diagnose lymphomas as well as metastatic spread from any malignant tumor in the body. Leukemias may infiltrate lymph nodes, but biopsy of the nodes is more commonly used to detect any type of neoplastic cells.

18. Word Search. a. Ecchymosis; b. Erythropoiesis; c. Fibrinolysis; d. Hematopoiesis; e. Hemolysis; f. Leukopenia; g. Neutropenia; h. Pancytopenia; i. Petechiae; j. Reticulocyte; k. Thrombocytopenia; l. Thrombocytosis; m. Phagocytosis; n. Lymphadenopathy; o. Splenomegaly

```
A S R S Q K R U I Y I H B B E T H B E A
S I E E M O C C K E E I L R H N S C P
P I N S T C J N N X N M L O Y R K I C I
I E S E I O P D W F O F E T O Q S H O N
J E T Y P I C I I R T L L Y H M I O Y N U
Z D R E L O O U Y O U Y S F R B W T M U H
G H B L C O T P L Z H S R W O O Z Y O H
S Y N A Z H N Y O O T I C Q P C P C S N
D M A F X Y I I C T C S S C O Y A O I O
D X L A P Z W A R O A Y U G I T N G S J
D J Y K Q W L B E B B M T R E O C A F L
A I N E P O K U E L I M E E S S Y H D L
D D G W Q Q A B U B F F O H I I T P O S
O S P L E N O M E G A L Y R S S O I L N
U P Y F L Y F W G B B B H S H F P K D U
L Y M P H A D E N O P A T H Y T E G T E
W S K E D K E Q O R B K K B J F N X G E
W C F Q N H O C A H D Z Y E Y F I H H L
S B I Q J N Y A Y D I E M N H F A Y S H
A I N E P O R T U E N X Y P B N X X D N
```

CHAPTER 31

1. a. 2, 4; b. 3, 4; c. 2, 4; d. 1, 4; e. 1, 4; f. 3, 4; g. 1, 6; h. 1, 6; i. 1, 5; j. 3, 4; k. 1, 4; l. 3, 4

2. b. Rationale: The patient's hemoglobin (Hb) level indicates a moderate anemia, and at this severity, additional findings usually include dyspnea and fatigue. Pallor, smooth tongue, and sensitivity to cold usually manifest in severe anemia when the Hb level is below 6 g/dL (60 g/L).

3. c. Rationale: In the older adult, confusion, ataxia, and fatigue are common manifestations of anemia and place the patient at risk for injury. Nursing interventions should include safety precautions to prevent falls and injury when these symptoms are present. The nurse is responsible for the patient, not the patient's family, and, although a quiet room may promote rest, it is not as important as protection of the patient.

4. d. Rationale: Dyspnea at rest indicates that the patient is making an effort to provide adequate amounts of oxygen to the tissues. If oxygen needs are not met, angina, myocardial infarction, heart failure, and pulmonary and systemic congestion can occur. The other manifestations are present in severe anemia, but they do not reflect hypoxemia, a priority problem.

5. d. Rationale: Patients with any type of anemia have decreased Hb and symptoms of hypoxemia, leading to activity intolerance. Impaired skin integrity and body image disturbance may be appropriate for patients with jaundice from hemolytic anemias, and altered nutrition is indicated when iron, folic acid, or vitamin B intake is deficient.

6. a. 2; b. 7; c. 5; d. 1; e. 4; f. 3; g. 1; h. 3; i. 2; j. 3; k. 7; l. 6; m. 5; n. 1; o. 2; p. 4

7. a. The hypoxia resulting from loss of RBCs in chronic blood loss stimulates the kidney to release erythropoietin, stimulating production of RBCs and reticulocytes, but in pernicious anemia, normal reticulocytes are not produced because of the lack of cobalamin.

   b. Sickle cell anemia is a hemolytic anemia involving an accelerated RBC breakdown, leading to increased serum bilirubin levels, whereas acute blood loss results in loss of the RBC and the bile pigments from the body.

   c. The mean corpuscular volume (MCV) is a determination of the relative size of an RBC, and macrocytic anemias, such as folic acid deficiency and cobalamin deficiency, are characterized by the production of large, immature RBCs that would reflect an increased MCV. In iron-deficiency anemia, the MCV is low because of the lack of Hb in the cells.

8. b. Rationale: Constipation is a common side effect of oral iron supplementation, and increased fluids and fiber should be consumed to prevent this effect. Because iron can be bound in the GI tract by food, it should be taken before meals unless gastric side effects of the supplements necessitate its ingestion with food. Black stools are an expected result of oral iron preparations. Taking iron with ascorbic acid or orange juice enhances absorption of the iron, but enteric-coated iron often is ineffective because of unpredictable release of the iron in areas of the GI tract where it can be absorbed.

9. b. Rationale: Pernicious anemia is a type of cobalamin (vitamin B_{12}) deficiency that results when parietal cells in the stomach fail to secrete enough intrinsic factor to absorb ingested cobalamin. Extrinsic factor is cobalamin and may be a factor in some cobalamin deficiencies, but not in pernicious anemia.

10. c. Rationale: Neurologic manifestations of weakness, paresthesias of the feet and hands, and impaired thought processes are characteristic of cobalamin deficiency and pernicious anemia. Hepatomegaly and jaundice often occur with hemolytic anemia and the patient with cobalamin deficiency often has achlorhydria or decreased stomach acidity and would not experience effects of gastric hyperacidity.

11. a. Rationale: Without cobalamin replacement, individuals with pernicious anemia will die in 1 to 3 years, but the disease can be controlled with cobalamin supplements for life. Hematologic manifestations can be completely reversed with therapy, but long-standing neuromuscular complications might not be reversed. Because pernicious anemia results from an inability to absorb cobalamin, dietary intake of the vitamin is not a treatment option, nor is a bone marrow transplant.

12. d. Rationale: Because red meats are the primary dietary source of cobalamin, a strict vegetarian is most at risk for cobalamin-deficiency anemia. Meats are also an important source of iron and folic acid, but whole grains, legumes, and green leafy vegetables also supply these nutrients. Thalassemia is not related to dietary deficiencies.

13. a, b, c. Rationale: The anemia of aplastic anemia may cause an inflamed, painful tongue; the thrombocytopenia may contribute to blood-filled bullae in the mouth and gingival bleeding; and the leukopenia may lead to stomatitis and oral ulcers and infections. Coagulation factors are not affected in aplastic anemia.

14. b. Rationale: Hemorrhage from thrombocytopenia and infection from neutropenia are the greatest risks for the patient with aplastic anemia. The patient will experience fatigue from anemia, but bleeding and infection are the major causes of death in aplastic anemia.

15. a. *F*, clinical symptoms; b. *T*; c. *F*, blood transfusions or iron supplements; d. *T*; e. *F*, kidney.

16. b. Rationale: Because RBCs are abnormal in sickle cell anemia, the mean RBC survival time is 10 to 15 days (rather than the normal 120 days) because of accelerated RBC breakdown by the liver and spleen. Antibody reactions with RBCs may be seen in other types of hemolytic anemias but are not present in sickle cell anemia.

17. b. Rationale: During a sickle cell crisis, the sickling cells clog small capillaries, and the resulting hemostasis promotes a self-perpetuating cycle of local hypoxia, deoxygenation of more erythrocytes, and more sickling. Administration of oxygen may help control further sickling, but additional oxygen does not reach areas of local hypoxia caused by occluded vessels.

18. d. Rationale: Because pain usually accompanies a sickle cell crisis and may last for 4 to 6 days, pain control is an important part of treatment. Rest is indicated to reduce metabolic needs, and fluids and electrolytes are administered to reduce blood viscosity and maintain renal function. Although thrombosis does occur in capillaries, elastic stockings that primarily affect venous circulation are not indicated.

19. d. Rationale: The patient with sickle cell disease is particularly prone to infection, and infection can precipitate a sickle cell crisis. Patients should seek medical attention quickly to counteract upper respiratory infections because pneumonia is the most common infection of the patient with sickle cell disease. Fluids should be increased to decrease blood viscosity, which may precipitate a crisis, and moderate activity is permitted.

20. a. *T*; b. *T*; c. *F*, Immune thrombocytopenia purpura (ITP); d. *F*, increased agglutination function of platelets; e. *F*, petechiae; f. *T*; g. *T*; h. *F*, increased

21. b. Rationale: Thrombus and embolization are the major complications of polycythemia vera because of increased hypervolemia and hyperviscosity. Active or passive leg exercises and ambulation should be implemented to prevent thrombus formation. Hydration therapy is important to decrease blood viscosity, but because the patient already has hypervolemia, a careful balance of intake and output must be maintained and fluids are not injudiciously increased.

22. b. Rationale: Corticosteroids are used in initial treatment of idiopathic thrombocytopenic purpura (ITP) because they suppress the phagocytic response of splenic macrophages, decreasing platelet destruction. They also depress autoimmune antibody formation and reduce capillary fragility and bleeding time. All of the other therapies may be used but only in patients who are unresponsive to corticosteroid therapy.

23. c. Rationale: The major complication of thrombocytopenia is hemorrhage, and it may occur in any area of the body. Cerebral hemorrhage may be fatal, and evaluation of mental status for central nervous system (CNS) alterations to identify CNS bleeding is very important. Fever is not a common finding in thrombocytopenia. Protection from injury to prevent bleeding is an important nursing intervention, but strict bed rest is not indicated. Oral care is performed very gently with minimum friction and soft swabs.

24. Any five of these are appropriate: Monitor for signs and symptoms of bleeding (check IV sites, wounds, any secretions); Monitor ordered coagulation studies; Avoid injections; Use an electric razor; Protect the patient from trauma; Administer ordered blood products; Instruct the patient/caregiver to avoid aspirin and other anticoagulants; Instruct the patient to avoid high-contact activities (many sports).

25. d. Rationale: A prolonged PTT occurs when there is a deficiency of clotting factors, such as factor VIII associated with hemophilia A. Factor IX is deficient in hemophilia B, and prolonged bleeding time and decreased platelet counts are associated with platelet deficiencies.

26. c. Rationale: Although whole blood and fresh frozen plasma contain the clotting factors that are deficient in hemophilia, specific factor concentrates have been developed that are more pure and safer in preventing infection transmission. Thromboplastin is factor III and is not deficient in patients with hemophilia.

27. b. Rationale: During an acute bleeding episode in a joint, it is important to totally rest the involved joint and slow bleeding with application of ice. Drugs that decrease platelet aggregation, such as aspirin or NSAIDs, should not be used for pain. As soon as bleeding stops, mobilization of the affected area is encouraged with ROM exercises and physical therapy.

28. a. 5; b. 8; c. 3; d. 6; e. 2; f. 7; g. 1; h. 4

29. a. yes—WBC below 4000/μL; b. 920/μL (2300 × 40%); c. yes—neutrophils less than 1000/μL; d. moderate—neutropenia of 500 to 1000/μL

30. a. Rationale: An elevated temperature is of most significance in recognizing the presence of an infection in the neutropenic patient because there is no leukocytic response; when the WBC count is depressed, the normal phagocytic mechanisms of infection are impaired, and the classic signs of inflammation may not occur. Cultures are indicated if the temperature is elevated but are not used to monitor for infection.

31. d. Rationale: Despite its seeming simplicity, hand washing before, during, and after care of the patient with neutropenia is the major method to prevent transmission of harmful pathogens to the patient. HEPA filtration and laminar airflow (LAF) rooms may reduce the number of aerosolized pathogens, but they are expensive and LAF use is controversial. Antibiotics are administered when febrile episodes occur but are not used prophylactically to prevent development of resistance.

32. a. Rationale: Although myelodysplastic syndromes, like leukemia, are a group of disorders in which hematopoietic stem cells of the bone marrow undergo clonal change and may cause eventual bone marrow failure, the primary difference from leukemias is that myelodysplastic cells have some degree of maturation, and the disease progression is slower than in acute leukemias.

33. a. 4; b. 4; c. 1; d. 2; e. 3; f. 2; g. 3; h. 1; i. 3; j. 2; k. 4

34. c. Rationale: Almost all leukemias cause some degree of hepatosplenomegaly because of infiltration of these organs as well as the bone marrow, lymph nodes, bones, and central nervous system by excessive WBCs in the blood.

35. d. Rationale: Whether the donor bone marrow is from a matched donor or taken from the patient during a remission for later use, hematopoietic stem cell transplant always involves the use of combinations of chemotherapy and total-body radiation to eliminate leukemic cells and the patient's bone marrow stem cells totally before IV infusion of the donor cells. A severe pancytopenic period follows the transplant, during which the patient must be in protective isolation and during which RBC and platelet transfusions may be given.

36. b. Rationale: A patient newly diagnosed with leukemia is most likely to respond with anxiety about the effects and outcome of the disease, and the risk of infection from altered WBCs is always present, even if other blood cells are not yet affected by the disease.

37. a. NHL; b. HL; c. B; d. NHL; e. HL; f. NHL; g. HL; h. B; i. HL; j. HL

38. a. *F*, determine treatment; b. *T*; c. *F*, B cells, bone; d. *T*

39. c. Rationale: Splenectomy may be indicated for treatment for ITP, and when the spleen is removed, platelet counts increase significantly in most patients. In any of the disorders in which the spleen removes excessive blood cells, splenectomy will most often increase peripheral RBC, WBC, and platelet counts.

40. b. Rationale: Chills and fever are symptoms of an acute hemolytic or febrile transfusion reaction, and if these develop, the transfusion should be stopped, saline infused through the IV line, the health care provider and blood bank notified immediately, the ID tags rechecked, and vital signs and urine output monitored. The addition of a leukocyte reduction filter may prevent a febrile reaction but is not helpful once the reaction has occurred. Mild and transient allergic reactions indicated by itching and hives might permit restarting of the transfusion after treatment with antihistamines.

41. b. Rationale: Because platelets adhere to the plastic bags, the bag should be gently agitated throughout the transfusion. Platelets do not have A, B, or Rh antibodies, and ABO compatibility is not a consideration. Baseline vital signs should be taken before the transfusion is started, and the nurse should stay with the patient during the first 15 minutes. Platelets are stored at room temperature and should not be refrigerated.

42. a. 3; b. 2; c. 1; d. 1; e. 5; f. 2; g. 1; h. 5; i. 3; j. 4
43. b, d. Rationale: All other actions are the responsibility of the RN. The LPN may be able to assist with the ID checks (depending on the state and the facility policy).
44. a. 1; b. 3; c. 6; d. 2; e. 4; f. 5; g. 10; h. 9; i. 8; j. 7.

Case Study

1. Traumatized placental and uterine tissues that release tissue factor into circulation, initiating the coagulation cascade
2. Venipuncture site bleeding; oozing of blood from other sites; respiratory problems, such as tachypnea, hemoptysis, and orthopnea; hematuria; hematemesis
3. Elevated fibrin split products; reduced factors V, VII, VIII, X; elevated D-dimers (cross-linked fibrin fragments); prolonged prothrombin and partial thromboplastin time (PTT); prolonged activated partial thromboplastin time; prolonged thrombin time; reduced fibrinogen, platelets
4. In the bleeding patient, therapy is administered on the basis of specific component deficiencies. Platelets are given to correct thrombocytopenia, cryoprecipitate replaces factor VIII and fibrinogen, and fresh frozen plasma replaces all clotting factors except platelets and provides a source of antithrombin. This patient is not manifesting symptoms of thrombosis, so anticoagulation is probably not indicated at this time. Treatment of the underlying condition may include a dilation and curettage or even a hysterectomy, if necessary, to remove the stimulus of DIC.
5. *Nursing diagnoses:*
   - Ineffective tissue perfusion: cardiopulmonary, cerebral, peripheral, and renal related to blood loss and thrombosis
   - Decreased cardiac output related to fluid volume deficit
   - Risk for impaired tissue integrity related to altered coagulation
   - Anxiety or fear related to disease process and therapy

   Collaborative problems:
   Potential complication: hemorrhage, thrombosis, hypovolemia/shock, renal failure

CHAPTER 32

1. a. tricuspid valve; b. interventricular septum; c. papillary muscle; d. chordae tendineae; e. mitral valve
2. a. aorta; b. superior vena cava; c. aortic semilunar valve; d. right atrium; e. right coronary artery; f. right marginal artery; g. posterior descending artery; h. right ventricle; i. left ventricle; j. left anterior descending artery; k. left marginal artery; l. circumflex artery; m. left atrium; n. left coronary artery; o. pulmonary trunk; p. aorta; q. superior vena cava; r. right atrium; s. small cardiac vein; t. middle cardiac vein; u. right ventricle; v. left ventricle; w. great cardiac vein; x. coronary sinus; y. posterior vein; z. left atrium; aa. pulmonary trunk
3. a. right coronary artery, left anterior descending artery, left circumflex artery; b. right coronary; c. diastolic
4. a. 4; b. 7; c. 2; d. 5; e. 8; f. 1; g. 3; h. 6
5. a. P; b. Q; c. R; d. S; e. T; f. PR interval; g. QRS interval; h. QT interval
6. a. 2; b. 4; c. 2; d. 4; e. 5; f. 3; g. 3; h. 1
7. See table below.

	Stroke Volume	Cardiac Output
a. Valsalva maneuver	preload ↓	↓
b. Venous dilation	preload ↓	↓
c. Hypertension	afterload ↑	↓
d. Administration of epinephrine	contractility ↑	↑
e. Obstruction of pulmonary artery	preload ↓	↓
f. Hemorrhage	preload ↓	↓

8. a. 2; b. 3; c. 1; d. 2; e. 2; f. 3
9. a. loss of vascular distensibility and elastic recoil during systole; b. increased collagen and decreased elastin; c. decrease in SA node cells and bundle of His fibers; d. decreased number and function of receptors; e. valvular lipid accumulation and calcification
10. d. Rationale: Recreational or abused drugs, especially stimulants such as cocaine and methamphetamine, are a growing cause of cardiac dysrhythmias and problems associated with tachycardia, and intravenous (IV) injection of abused drugs is a risk factor for inflammatory and infectious conditions of the heart. Streptococcal, but not viral, pharyngitis is a risk factor for rheumatic heart disease. Although calcium is involved in the contraction of muscles, calcium supplementation is not a significant factor in heart disease, nor is metastatic cancer.
11. a. hyperlipidemia, hypertension, smoking, obesity, sedentary or stressful lifestyle, history of hereditary or familial cardiovascular disease, diabetes mellitus
    b. underweight, obesity, high intake of sodium, fat, cholesterol, and triglycerides
    c. dependent edema, incontinence or constipation; use of diuretics with increased urinary output
    d. lack of aerobic exercise; decreased activity tolerance; symptoms during exercise
    e. attacks of shortness of breath interrupting sleep; use of several pillows to sleep

f. chest pain; pain in legs with walking; vertigo, cognitive changes

g. loss of self-esteem resulting from fatigue and decreased activity tolerance

h. stress or conflict in roles

i. change in sexual activity caused by shortness of breath or fatigue; impotence

j. depression, high stress, anxiety, denial/anger/ hostility as coping mechanisms

k. diagnosis or treatment conflict with value system

12. d. Rationale: A palpable vibration of a blood vessel is called a thrill and usually indicates turbulent blood flow through the vessel. A weak, thready pulse has little pressure and is difficult to palpate. A bruit is an abnormal buzzing or humming sound that may be auscultated over pathologic vessels, and a bounding pulse is an extra full, hard pulse that may occur with atherosclerosis or hypervolemia.

13. a. Angle of Louis; b. Second rib; c. Aortic area; d. Second ICS; e. Mitral area (apex) and PMI; f. Tricuspid area; g. Erb's point; h. Pulmonic area.

14. a. S_2; b. S_1; c. S_2; d. S_1; e. S_1; f. S_1; g. S_2; h. S_2; i. S_1

15. a. 7; b. 4; c. 9; d. 10; e. 8; f. 2; g. 1; h. 3; i. 6; j. 5

16. c. Rationale: In an exercise nuclear imaging scan, technetium-99 sestamibi is injected at the maximum heart rate on a bicycle or treadmill and used to evaluate blood flow in different parts of the heart. Simply monitoring ECG activity during exercise is an exercise stress test, and an echocardiogram uses transducers to bounce sound waves off the heart. Insertion of electrodes into the heart chambers via the venous system to record intracardiac electrical activity is an electrophysiology study.

17. d. Rationale: In order to perform a TEE, the throat must be numbed. Until sensation returns, as evidenced by the gag reflex, the patient is at risk of aspiration (priority related to airway—ABCs).

18. b. Rationale: Holter monitoring involves placing electrodes on the chest attached to a recorder that will record ECG rhythm for 24 to 48 hours while the patient engages in normal daily activities. The recording is later analyzed for cardiac dysrhythmias. Frequent, but not continuous, ECGs are serial ECGs. An electrophysiology study is an invasive test that records intracardiac electrical activity in different cardiac structures, and positron emission tomography (PET) uses radioisotopes to evaluate myocardial perfusion and metabolic function.

19. c. Rationale: An absence of pulses distal to the catheter insertion site indicates that clotting around the site is occluding blood flow to the extremity and is an emergency that requires immediate medical attention. Some swelling and pain at the site are expected, but the site is also monitored for bleeding, and a pressure dressing and perhaps a sandbag may be applied. Hives may occur as a result of iodine sensitivity and will require treatment, but the priority is the lack of pulses.

20. d. Rationale: A risk assessment for coronary artery disease (CAD) is determined by comparing the total cholesterol to HDL, and a ratio can be calculated by dividing the total cholesterol level by the HDL level. The ratio provides more information than either value alone, and an increased ratio indicates an increased risk. The female patient has a ratio of 3.56 compared with the male patient's ratio of 6.56.

21. b, c, e. Increased levels of C-reactive protein, troponin, and lipoprotein-associated phospholipase A_2 are indicators of risk for, or evidence of, MI. Increased BNP is a marker for heart failure and increased creatine kinase MM is most commonly associated with skeletal muscle injury.

CHAPTER 33

1. See table below.

	Increased CO	Increased SVR	Mechanisms Causing Increases
a. β_1-Adrenergic stimulation	X	X	Increased rate and contractility of the heart increases CO. Stimulation of renin production that activates the renin-angiotensin-aldosterone system (RAAS).
b. α_1-Adrenergic stimulation	X	X	Peripheral arteriole vasoconstriction and increased contractility of the heart
c. α_2-Adrenergic stimulation		X	Constriction of selected vascular beds
d. Endothelin release		X	Vasoconstriction
e. Angiotensin II		X	Arteriole vasoconstriction
f. Aldosterone release	X		Increased vascular volume
g. Antidiuretic hormone (ADH) release	X		Increased vascular volume

2. The vasoconstriction caused by the α_1-adrenergic agent raises the BP, stimulating the baroreceptors. The baroreceptors send impulses to the sympathetic vasomotor center in the brainstem, which inhibit the sympathetic nervous system, resulting in a decreased heart rate (HR), decreased force of contraction, and vasodilation.

3. Lower BP because of decreased stroke volume and decreased HR, both of which decrease CO

4. a. Age—hypertension progresses with increasing age. b. Gender—hypertension is more prevalent in men up to age 45 and above the age of 64 in women. c. Ethnicity—African Americans have a higher incidence of hypertension than do white Americans. d. Family history—children and siblings should be screened and taught about healthy lifestyles.

5. c. Rationale: Secondary hypertension has an underlying cause that can often be treated, in contrast to primary or essential hypertension, which has no single known cause. Isolated systolic hypertension occurs when the systolic blood pressure (SBP) is consistently elevated over 140 mm Hg, but the diastolic blood pressure (DBP) remains less than 90 mm Hg, which is more prevalent in older adults. The only type of hypertension that does not cause target organ damage is pseudohypertension.

6. a. Rationale: Hypertension is often asymptomatic, especially if it is mild or moderate, and has been called the "silent killer." The absence of symptoms often leads to noncompliance with medical treatment and a lack of concern about the disease in patients. With severe hypertension, symptoms usually occur and may include a morning occipital headache, fatigability, dizziness, palpitations, angina, and dyspnea.

7. b. Rationale: Elevated BP causes the entire inner lining of arterioles to become thickened from hyperplasia of connective tissues in the intima and affects coronary circulation, cerebral circulation, peripheral vessels, and renal and retinal blood vessels. The narrowed vessels lead to ischemia and, ultimately, to damage of these organs.

8. b. Rationale: The increased SVR of hypertension directly increases the workload of the heart, and heart failure occurs when the heart can no longer pump effectively against the increased resistance. The heart may be indirectly damaged by atherosclerotic changes in the blood vessels, as are the brain, retina, and kidney.

9. a. Elevated BUN and creatinine may indicate destruction of glomeruli and tubules of the kidney resulting from hypertension.
   b. Serum potassium levels are decreased when hypertension is associated with hyperaldosteronism.
   c. Fasting glucose levels are elevated when hypertension is associated with glucose intolerance and insulin resistance.

d. An increased uric acid level may be caused by diuretics used to treat hypertension.
   e. An elevated LDL level indicates an increased risk for atherosclerotic changes in the patient with hypertension.

10. a. Dietary modifications to restrict sodium; maintain intake of potassium, calcium, and magnesium; and promote weight reduction if overweight
    b. Moderation or cessation of alcohol intake
    c. Daily moderate-intensity physical activity for at least 30 minutes on most days of the week
    d. Cessation of smoking (if a smoker)
    Also: Psychosocial risk factors must be addressed.

11. a. 4; b. 5; c. 8; d. 6; e. 2; f. 7; g. 1; h. 3

12. d. Rationale: Hydrochlorothiazide is a thiazide diuretic that causes sodium and potassium loss through the kidneys. High-potassium foods should be included in the diet, or potassium supplements used, to prevent hypokalemia. Enalapril and spironolactone may cause hyperkalemia by inhibiting the action of aldosterone, and potassium supplements should not be used by patients taking these drugs. As a combined α/β-blocker, labetalol does not affect potassium levels.

13. b. Rationale: Prazosin is an α-adrenergic blocker that causes dilation of arterioles and veins and causes orthostatic hypotension. The patient may feel dizzy, weak, and faint when assuming an upright position after sitting or lying down and should be taught to change positions slowly, avoid standing for long periods, do leg exercises to increase venous return, and lie or sit down when dizziness occurs. Direct-acting vasodilators often cause fluid retention, dry mouth occurs with diuretic use, and centrally acting α- and β-blockers may cause bradycardia.

14. c. Rationale: Sexual dysfunction, which can occur with many of the antihypertensive drugs, including thiazide and potassium-sparing diuretics and β-blockers, can be a major reason that a male patient does not adhere to his treatment regimen. It is helpful for the nurse to raise the subject because sexual problems may be easier for the patient to discuss and handle once it has been explained that the drug might be the source of the problem.

15. a. Rationale: Centrally acting α-blockers may cause severe rebound hypertension if the drugs are abruptly discontinued, and patients should be taught about this effect because many are not consistently compliant with drug therapy. Diuretics should be taken early in the day to prevent nocturia, and the profound orthostatic hypotension that occurs with first-dose α-adrenergic blockers can be prevented by taking the initial dose at bedtime. Aspirin use may decrease the effectiveness of ACE inhibitors.

16. d. Rationale: Correct technique in measuring BP includes taking two or more readings at least 1 minute apart. Initially BP measurements should

be taken in both arms to detect any differences; if there is a difference, the arm with the higher reading should be used for all subsequent BP readings. The patient may be supine or sitting. The important point is that the arm being used is at the heart level and the cuff needs to fit snugly.

17. c. Rationale: Hypertensive emergency, a type of hypertensive crisis, is a situation that develops over hours or days in which a patient's BP is severely elevated with evidence of acute target-organ damage, especially to the central nervous system (CNS). The neurologic manifestations are often similar to the presentation of a stroke but do not show the focal or lateralizing symptoms of stroke. Hypertensive crises are defined by the degree of organ damage and how rapidly the BP must be lowered, not by specific BP measurements. A hypertensive urgency is a less severe crisis in which a patient's BP becomes severely elevated over days or weeks, but there is no evidence of target-organ damage.

18. d. Rationale: Hypertensive crises are treated with IV administration of antihypertensive drugs, including the vasodilators sodium nitroprusside, nitroglycerin, diazoxide, and hydralazine; adrenergic blockers such as phentolamine, labetalol, and methyldopa; and the ACE inhibitor IV enalaprilat. Sodium nitroprusside is the most effective parenteral drug for hypertensive emergencies. Drugs that are used specifically for hypertensive emergencies include sodium nitroprusside, nitroglycerin, and diazoxide.

19. b. Rationale: Initially the treatment goal in hypertensive emergencies is to reduce the MAP by no more than 25% in the first hour, with further gradual reduction over the next 24 hours. Lowering the BP too far or too fast can cause hypotension in a person whose body has adjusted to hypertension and could cause a stroke, myocardial infarction (MI), or visual changes. Only when the patient has an aortic dissection, angina, or signs of MI does the systolic BP need to be lowered to 100 mm Hg or less as quickly as possible.

20. d. Rationale: Hypertensive urgencies are often treated with oral drugs on an outpatient basis, but it is important for the patient to be seen by a health professional within 24 hours to evaluate the effectiveness of the treatment. Hourly urine measurements, ECG monitoring, and titration of IV drugs are indicated for hypertensive emergencies.

Case Study

1. Increasing age, which leads to loss of elasticity in large arteries from atherosclerosis; more prevalent in women (and African Americans)

2. High sodium intake from canned foods; sedentary lifestyle; weight gain

3. Sodium restriction to 2 g/day; decrease fat to no more than 30% of diet; cholesterol intake of less than 200 mg/day; increase high-potassium foods

4. Regular daily aerobic exercise; need for stress management indicated by weight gain in response to husband's death; teaching about pathology, complications, and management of hypertension

5. Because of her low potassium level, a potassium-saving diuretic, such as spironolactone, amiloride, or triamterine, could be used. If a stronger diuretic were needed, potassium supplementation would be indicated.

6. *Nursing diagnoses:*
   - Ineffective health maintenance related to increased caloric intake and deficiency of potassium sources
   - Ineffective coping related to use of food as coping mechanism
   - Deficient knowledge related to inadequate teaching related to hypertension and treatment
   Collaborative problems:
   Potential complications: cerebrovascular accident, MI, renal failure

CHAPTER 34

1. a. fatty streak, age 15; b. raised fibrous plaque, age 30; c. complicated lesion, over age 30

2. a. *T*; b. *T*; c. *F*, complicated lesion; d. *F*, older patient with chronic ischemia

3. c. Rationale: The white woman has one unmodifiable risk factor (age) and two major modifiable risk factors (hypertension and physical inactivity). Her gender risk is as high as a man's because of her age. The white man has one unmodifiable risk factor (gender), one major modifiable risk factor (smoking), and one minor modifiable risk factor (stressful lifestyle). The African American man has an unmodifiable risk factor related to age and one minor modifiable risk factor (obesity). The Asian woman has only one major modifiable risk factor (hyperlipidemia), and Asians in the United States have fewer myocardial infarctions (MIs) than do whites.

4. d. Rationale: CAD is the number-one killer of American women, and women have a much higher mortality rate within 1 year following MI than do men. Recent research indicates that estrogen replacement does not reduce the risk for CAD, even though estrogen lowers low-density lipoprotein (LDL) and raises high-density lipoprotein (HDL) cholesterol. Smoking carries specific problems for women because smoking has been linked to a decrease in estrogen levels and to early menopause, and it has been identified as the most powerful contributor to CAD in women under the age of 50. Men have a higher incidence of sudden cardiac death.

5. a. 3; b. 2; c. 1; d. 1; e. 3; f. 1; g. 2; h. 2

6. a. >200 mg/dL (5.2 mmol/L); b. >150 mg/dL (3.7 mmol/L); c. >160 mg/dL (4.14 mmol/L) d. < 37 mg/dL (0.97 mmol/L) for men and <40 mg/dL (1.05 mmol/L) for women

7. a. Rationale: Increased exercise without an increase in caloric intake will result in weight loss, reducing the risk associated with obesity, and exercise increases lipid metabolism and increases HDL, reducing CAD risk. Exercise may also indirectly reduce the risk of CAD by controlling hypertension, promoting glucose metabolism in diabetes, and reducing stress. Although research is needed to determine whether a decline in homocysteine can reduce the risk of heart disease, it appears that dietary modifications are indicated for risk reduction.

8. a, c, e. Rationale: Therapeutic Lifestyle Changes diet recommendations emphasize reduction in saturated fat and cholesterol intake. Red meats, whole-milk products, and eggs should be reduced or eliminated from diets. Alcohol and simple sugars should be reduced if triglyceride levels are high.

9. a. Rationale: Therapeutic Lifestyle Changes include recommendations for all people to decrease CAD, not just those with risk factors for CAD.

10. a. Rationale: Diet therapy is indicated for a patient without CAD who has two or more risk factors and an LDL level ≥130 mg/dL. When the patient's LDL levels are ≥160 mg/dL, drug therapy would be added to diet therapy. Exercise is indicated to reduce risk factors throughout treatment.

11. a. stable angina
    b. unstable angina, non-ST-segment-elevation MI, ST-segment-elevation MI
    c. infarct

12. a. increased oxygen demand, decreased oxygen supply; b. increased oxygen demand; c. decreased oxygen supply; d. decreased oxygen supply; e. decreased oxygen supply; f. increased oxygen demand; g. increased oxygen demand; h. increased oxygen demand

13. c. Rationale: When the coronary arteries are occluded, contractility ceases after several minutes, depriving the myocardial cells of glucose and oxygen for aerobic metabolism. Anaerobic metabolism begins and lactic acid accumulates, irritating myocardial nerve fibers that then transmit a pain message to the cardiac nerves and upper thoracic posterior roots. The other factors may occur during vessel occlusion but are not the source of pain.

14. a. 6; b. 3; c. 5; d. 1; e. 5; f. 3; g. 1; h. 2; i. 4; j. 2, 7

15. d. Rationale: An increased HR decreases the time the heart spends in diastole, which is the time of greatest coronary blood flow. Unlike other arteries, coronary arteries are perfused when the myocardium relaxes and blood backflows from the aorta into the sinuses of Valsalva, which have openings to the right and left coronary arteries. Thus the heart has a decreased oxygen supply at a time when there is an increased oxygen demand.

16. a. nitrates; b. nitrates, calcium-channel blocking agents; c. antiplatelet aggregation agents, including aspirin; d. calcium-channel blocking agents, β-adrenergic blocking agents; e. nitrates, β-adrenergic blocking agents; f. β-adrenergic blocking agents, calcium-channel blocking agents

17. a. Rationale: A common complication of nitrates is dizziness caused by orthostatic hypotension, so the patient should sit or lie down and place the tablet under the tongue. The tablet should be allowed to dissolve under the tongue; to prevent the tablet from being swallowed, water should not be taken with it. The recommended dose for the patient for whom nitroglycerin (NTG) has been prescribed is one tablet taken sublingually (SL) or one metered spray for symptoms of angina. If symptoms are unchanged or worse after 5 minutes, the patient should contact the emergency medical services (EMS) system before taking additional NTG. If symptoms are significantly improved by one dose of NTG, instruct the patient or caregiver to repeat NTG every 5 minutes for a maximum of three doses and contact EMS if symptoms have not resolved completely. Headache is also a common complication of nitrates but usually resolves with continued use of nitrates and may be controlled with mild analgesics.

18. a. Rationale: Orthostatic hypotension may cause dizziness and falls in older adults taking antianginal agents that decrease preload, and patients should be cautioned to change positions slowly. Exercise programs are indicated for older adults and may increase performance, endurance, and ability to tolerate stress. A change in lifestyle behaviors may increase the quality of life and reduce the risks of CAD, even in the older adult. Aspirin is commonly used in these patients and is not contraindicated.

19. c. Rationale: Unstable angina is associated with deterioration of a once-stable atherosclerotic plaque that ruptures, exposing the intima to blood and stimulating platelet aggregation and local vasoconstriction with thrombus formation. Patients with unstable angina require immediate hospitalization and monitoring because the lesion is at increased risk of complete thrombosis of the lumen with progression to MI. Any type of angina may be associated with severe pain, ECG changes, and dysrhythmias; and Prinzmetal's, or variant, angina is characterized by coronary artery spasm.

20. a. Rationale: One of the primary differences between the pain of angina and the pain of an MI is that angina pain is usually relieved by rest or nitroglycerin, which reduces the oxygen demand of

the heart, whereas MI pain is not. Both angina and MI pain can cause a pressure or squeezing sensation; may radiate to the neck, back, arms, fingers, and jaw; and may be precipitated by exertion.

21. b. Rationale: An exercise stress test will reveal ECG changes that indicate impaired coronary circulation when the oxygen demand of the heart is increased. A single ECG is not conclusive for CAD, and negative findings do not rule out CAD. Echocardiograms of various types may identify abnormalities of myocardial wall motion under stress but are indirect measures of CAD. Coronary angiography can detect narrowing of coronary arteries but is an invasive procedure.

22. d. Rationale: The pain of an MI is usually severe; is usually unrelieved by nitroglycerin, rest, or position change; and usually lasts more than the 15 or 20 minutes typical of angina pain. All the other symptoms may occur with angina as well as with an MI.

23. c. Rationale: At 10 to 14 days after MI, the myocardium is considered especially vulnerable to increased stress because of the unstable state of healing at this point, and this is the time that the patient is also increasing physical activity. At 2 to 3 days, removal of necrotic tissue is taking place by phagocytic cells; by 4 to 10 days, the tissue has been cleared and a collagen matrix for scar tissue has been deposited. Healing with scar-tissue replacement of the necrotic area is usually complete by 6 weeks.

24. c. Rationale: The most common complication of MI is cardiac dysrhythmias, especially ventricular dysrhythmia, which may be life-threatening. Continuous cardiac monitoring allows identification and treatment of dysrhythmias that may cause further deterioration of the cardiovascular status. Measurement of hourly urine output and vital signs is indicated to detect symptoms of the complication of cardiogenic shock; crackles, dyspnea, and tachycardia may indicate the onset of heart failure.

25. a. 4; b. 5; c. 2; d. 1; e. 3

26. c. Rationale: Creatine kinase–muscle and brain subunits band (CK-MB) is a tissue enzyme that is specific to cardiac muscle and is released into the blood when myocardial cells die. CK-MB levels begin to rise about 6 hours after an acute MI, peak in about 18 hours and return to normal within 24 to 36 hours. This increase can demonstrate the presence of cardiac damage and the approximate extent of the damage. Troponin, a myocardial muscle protein released with myocardial damage, rises as quickly as CK does and remains elevated for 2 weeks. ECG changes are often not apparent immediately after infarct and may be normal when the patient seeks

medical attention. An enlarged heart, determined by x-ray, indicates cardiac stress but is not diagnostic of acute MI.

27. c. Rationale: A differentiation is made between MIs that have ST-segment elevations on ECG and those that do not because chest pain accompanied by ST-segment elevations is associated with prolonged and complete coronary thrombosis and is treated with reperfusion therapy.

28. a. 4; b. 2; c. 1; d. 2; e. 3; f. 1

29. c. Rationale: NAP can check VS and report results to the RN. The other actions include assessment, teaching, and monitoring of IV fluids, which are all responsibilities of the RN.

30. c. Rationale: The most common method of coronary artery bypass involves leaving the internal mammary artery attached to its origin from the subclavian artery but dissecting it from the chest wall and anastomosing it distal to an obstruction in a coronary artery. Synthetic grafts are not commonly used as coronary bypass grafts, although research continues for this option. Saphenous veins are used for bypass grafts when additional conduits are needed.

31. c. Rationale: Because a NSTEMI is an acute coronary syndrome that indicates a transient thrombosis or incomplete coronary artery occlusion, treatment involves intensive drug therapy with antiplatelets, GPIIB inhibitors, antithrombotics, and heparin to prevent clot extension, in addition to nitroglycerin IV. Reperfusion therapy using fibrinolytics, coronary artery bypass graft (CABG), or PCI is used for treatment of STEMI.

32. c. Rationale: Decreasing level of consciousness (LOC) may reflect hypoxemia resulting from internal bleeding, which is always a risk with fibrinolytic therapy. Oozing of blood is expected, as are reperfusion dysrhythmias. BP is low but not considered abnormal because the pulse is within normal range.

33. a. Rationale: Indications that the occluded coronary artery is patent, and blood flow to the myocardium is reestablished following thrombolytic therapy, including relief of chest pain; return of ST segment to baseline on the ECG; the presence of reperfusion dysrhythmias; and marked, rapid rise of the CK enzyme within 3 hours of therapy. If chest pain is unchanged, it is an indication that reperfusion was not successful.

34. a. 4; b. 5; c. 6; d. 2; e. 1; f. 3

35. a. Rationale: This patient is indicating positive coping with a realization that recovery takes time and that lifestyle changes can be made as needed. The patient who is "just going to get on with life" is probably in denial about the seriousness of the condition and the changes that need to be made.

Nervous questioning about the expected duration and effect of the condition indicates the presence of anxiety, as does the statement regarding the health care professionals' role in treatment.

36. d, c, f, e, b, a. Rationale: A patient having chest pain needs to have the pain assessed and relieved as quickly as possible. The administration of oxygen may help relieve the pain; following an assessment of the pain, analgesia may be administered; and it is important to know if the pain is accompanied by a change in VS and if any other manifestations or ECG changes exist before the report is given to the physician.

37. a. dependence; b. anxiety/fear; c. depression; d. anger; e. denial

38. a. Rationale: Golfing is a moderate-energy activity that expends about 5 metabolic equivalents (METs) and is within the 3 to 5 METs activity level desired for a patient by the time of discharge from the hospital following an MI. Walking at 5 mph and mowing the lawn by hand are high-energy activities, and cycling at 13 mph is an extremely high-energy activity.

39. a. Rationale: Any activity or exercise that causes dyspnea and chest pain should be stopped in the patient with CAD. The training target for a healthy 58-year-old is 80% of maximum HR, or 132 beats/min; in a patient with cardiac disease undergoing cardiac conditioning, however, the HR should not exceed 20 beats/min over the resting pulse rate. HR, rather than respiratory rate (RR), determines the parameters for exercise.

40. b. Rationale: Resumption of sexual activity is often difficult for patients to approach, and it is reported that most cardiac patients do not resume sexual activity after MI. The nurse can give the patient permission to discuss concerns about sexual activity by introducing it as a physical activity when other physical activities are discussed. Health care providers may have preferences regarding the timing of resumption of sexual activity, and the nurse should discuss this with the health care provider and the patient, but addressing the patient's concerns is a nursing responsibility. Patients should be informed that impotence after MI is common but that it usually disappears after several attempts.

41. c. Rationale: It is not uncommon for a patient who experiences chest pain on exertion to have some angina during sexual stimulation or intercourse, and the patient should be instructed to use nitroglycerin prophylactically. Positions during intercourse are a matter of individual choice, and foreplay is desirable because it allows a gradual increase in HR. Sildenafil (Viagra) should be used cautiously in men with CAD and should not be used with nitrates.

42. a. Rationale: Most patients who experience sudden cardiac death as a result of CAD do not have an acute MI but have dysrhythmias that cause death, probably as a result of electrical instability of the myocardium. To identify and treat those specific dysrhythmias, continuous monitoring is important.

Case Study

1. Diabetes mellitus; smoking history; obesity; physical inactivity; stress response

2. H.C. appears little motivated to assume responsibility for her health and, in the absence of symptoms, has not had a desire to make lifestyle changes. First, assist H.C. to clarify her personal values. Then, by explaining the symptoms related to her risk factors and having her identify her personal vulnerability to various risks, you may help her recognize her susceptibility to CAD. Help her set realistic goals, and allow her to choose which risk factor to change first.

3. Anxiousness with fist clutching; radiation of the burning from epigastric area into the sternum; prior episodes of chest pain with activity, relieved by rest

4. Depressed ST segment; T wave inversion

5. Inform the patient that she will have continuous cardiac monitoring while she walks on a treadmill with increasing speed and elevation to evaluate the effects of exercise on the blood supply to her heart. Her pulse, respiration, BP, and heart rhythm will be measured while she walks and after the test until they return to normal, and the cardiac monitor will be used after the test until any changes return to normal.

6. *Nursing diagnoses:*
   - Acute pain related to ischemic myocardium
   - Anxiety related to possible diagnosis and uncertain future
   - Ineffective denial related to reluctance to receive medical care or change lifestyle
   - Ineffective coping related to lack of effective coping skills
   - Imbalanced nutrition: more than body requirements related to intake of calories in excess of calorie expenditure

   Collaborative problems:
   Potential complications: MI; cardiac dysrhythmias

CHAPTER 35

1. a. *F*, diastolic failure; b. *T*; c. *T*; d. *F*, dysrhythmia; e. *F*, reduced

2. a. ↑ CO: Increased force of contraction by stretching of cardiac muscle
   Detrimental effect: Overstrains the muscle fibers; mitral valve incompetence
   b. ↑ CO: Increased contractile force of muscle
   Detrimental effect: Increased myocardial oxygen need

c. ↑ CO: Increased heart rate (HR) and force of contraction; increased preload
Detrimental effect: Increased myocardial oxygen need; overwhelming preload; increased afterload

d. 1. ↑ CO: Increased fluid retention and vasoconstriction to maintain blood pressure (BP)

Detrimental effect: Increased preload and afterload

2. ↑ CO: Increased water retention
Detrimental effect: increased blood volume when already overloaded

3. See table below.

Substances	Trigger	Mechanism of Action
Atrial natriuretic peptide (ANP)	Increase in volume stimulates granules in the atria and ventricles.	Endothelin and aldosterone antagonist. Will increase glomerular filtration rate and decrease preload, inhibit development of cardiac hypertrophy, and have antiinflammatory effect.
Brain natriuretic peptide (BNP)	Increase in pressure on granules located in the ventricles, especially in the left ventricle.	Same as above
Nitrous oxide (NO)	Response to the compensatory mechanisms.	Relaxes smooth muscle, promotes vasodilation, decreases afterload.

4. F = Fatigue; A = Activity limitations; C = Congestion/cough; E = Edema; S = Shortness of breath

5. b. Rationale: In left-sided heart failure, blood backs up into the pulmonary veins and capillaries. This increased hydrostatic pressure in the vessels causes fluid to move out of the vessels and into the pulmonary interstitial space. When increased lymphatic flow cannot remove enough fluid from the interstitial space, fluid moves into the alveoli, resulting in pulmonary edema and impaired alveolar oxygen and carbon dioxide exchange. Initially the right side of the heart is not involved.

6. a. Rationale: Clinical manifestations of acute left-sided heart failure are those of pulmonary edema, with bubbling crackles and tachycardia; frothy, blood-tinged sputum; severe dyspnea; tachypnea; and orthopnea. Severe tachycardia and cool, clammy skin are present as a result of stimulation of the sympathetic nervous system from hypoxemia. Systemic edema reflected by jugular vein distention, peripheral edema, and hepatosplenomegaly are characteristic of right-sided heart failure.

7. d. Rationale: Paroxysmal nocturnal dyspnea (PND) is awakening from sleep with a feeling of suffocation and a need to sit up to be able to breathe, and patients learn that sleeping with the upper body elevated on several pillows helps prevent PND. Orthopnea is an inability to breathe effectively when lying down, and nocturia occurs with heart failure as fluid moves back into the vascular system during recumbency, increasing renal blood flow.

8. a. SpO_2 of 84% on 2 L/nasal cannula indicates impaired oxygen saturation. Patient is having trouble with gas exchange. Airway/breathing are a priority (follow ABCs).
b. Assess the patient immediately, recheck SpO_2, auscultate breath sounds, assess level of consciousness (LOC), and talk with the patient about her/his breathing.

9. b. Rationale: Thrombus formation occurs in the heart when the chambers do not contract normally and empty completely. Both atrial fibrillation and very low left ventricular output (LV ejection fraction <20%) lead to thrombus formation, which is treated with anticoagulants to prevent the release of emboli into the circulation.

10. c. Rationale: bNP is released from the ventricles in response to ventricular stretch and is a good marker for heart failure. If bNP is elevated, shortness of breath is due to heart failure; if the bNP is normal, dyspnea is due to pulmonary disease. bNP opposes the actions of the renin-angiotensin-aldosterone system, resulting in vasodilation and reduction in blood volume. Exercise stress testing and cardiac catheterization are more important tests to diagnose coronary artery disease, and although the BUN may be elevated in heart failure, it is a reflection of decreased renal perfusion.

11. Crossword Puzzle
Across: 4. valsartan; 6. carvedilol; 7. milrinone; 12. isosorbide nitrate and hydralazine; 13. furosemide
Down: 1. enalapril; 2. IV nitroglycerin; 3. digoxin; 5. IV nitroprusside; 8. IV morphine; 9. spironolactone; 10. dopamine; 11. nesiritide

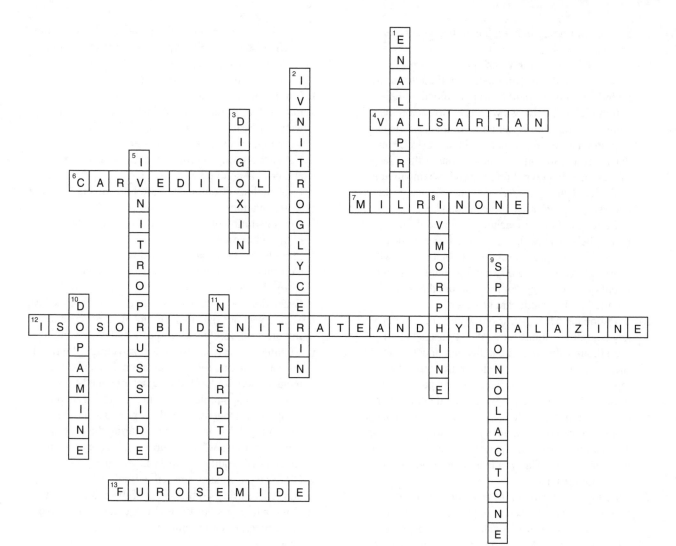

12. c. Rationale: Hypokalemia is one of the most common causes of digitalis toxicity because low serum potassium levels enhance ectopic pacemaker activity. When a patient is receiving potassium-losing diuretics, such as hydrochlorothiazide and furosemide, it is essential to monitor the patient's serum potassium levels to prevent digitalis toxicity.

13. a. Rationale: Spironolactone is a potassium-sparing diuretic, and when it is the only diuretic used in the treatment of heart failure, moderate to low levels of potassium should be maintained to prevent development of hyperkalemia. Sodium intake is usually reduced to at least 2400 mg/day in patients with heart failure, but salt substitutes cannot be freely used because most contain high concentrations of potassium.

14. d. Rationale: Although all these drugs may cause hypotension, nitroprusside is a potent dilator of both arteries and veins and may cause such marked hypotension that dobutamine administration may be necessary to maintain the BP during its administration. Milrinone has a positive inotropic effect, in addition to direct arterial dilation, and nitroglycerin primarily dilates veins. Furosemide may cause hypotension because of diuretic-induced depletion of intravascular fluid volume.

15. c. Rationale: All foods that are high in sodium should be eliminated in a 2400-mg sodium diet, in addition to the elimination of salt during cooking. Examples include obviously salted snack foods as well as pickles, processed prepared foods, and many sauces and condiments.

16. a. Hypertension: Use medications, diet, and exercise to control
    b. Valvular defects: Surgical replacement before heart failure occurs; prophylactic antibiotics
    c. Ischemic heart disease: percutaneous coronary intervention (PCI), coronary artery bypass surgery, fibrinolytic therapy for occlusions
    d. Dysrhythmias: Antidysrhythmic agents, pacemakers, or defibrillators to control

17. c. Rationale: Successful treatment of heart failure is indicated by an absence of symptoms of pulmonary edema and hypoxemia, such as clear lung sounds and a normal HR. Weight loss and diuresis, warm skin, less fatigue, and improved LOC may occur without resolution of pulmonary symptoms. Chest pain is not

a common finding in heart failure unless coronary artery perfusion is impaired.

18. d. Rationale: A high Fowler's position increases the thoracic capacity, improving ventilation; sitting with the legs dependent helps pool blood in the extremities and decrease venous return, or preload. Coughing and deep breathing will not clear the lungs of pulmonary edema. Intake and output (I&O) and daily weights should be done to monitor the effects of treatment but do not directly address impaired gas exchange. During periods of acute dyspnea, rest is necessary to decrease oxygen demand.

19. d. Rationale: Further teaching is needed if the patient believes a weight gain of 2 to 3 pounds in 2 days is an indication for dieting. In a patient with heart failure, this type of weight gain reflects fluid retention and is a sign of heart failure that should be reported to the health care provider.

20. d. Rationale: The 52-year-old woman does not have any contraindications for cardiac transplantation, even though she lacks the indication of adequate financial resources. The postoperative transplant regimen is complex and rigorous, and patients who have not been complian t with other treatments or who might not have the means to understand the care would not be good candidates. A history of drug or alcohol abuse is usually a contraindication to heart transplantation. (This would add rationale for why "a" is not the answer.)

21. a. Rationale: Because of the need for long-term immunosuppressant therapy to prevent rejection, the patient with a transplant is at high risk for infection, a leading cause of death in transplant patients. Acute rejection episodes may also cause death in patients with transplants, but many can be successfully treated with augmented immunosuppressive therapy. Malignancies occur in patients with organ transplants after taking immunosuppressants for a number of years.

Case Study

1. Right-sided failure: Jugular vein distention, peripheral edema, hepatomegaly
   Left-sided failure: dyspnea, $\downarrow$ SpO_2, PMI displacement, pulmonary crackles, frothy pink sputum, $\downarrow$ BP, S_3, S_4 heart sounds
   Present with both: fatigue, $\uparrow$ HR, dysrhythmias
2. Diagnostic procedures include the following:
   Chest radiography: Cardiomegaly, pulmonary venous hypertension, pleural effusion
   ECG: Tachycardia and dysrhythmias of conduction disturbances
   Echocardiogram: To determine the presence of a low LV ejection fraction
   Cardiac catheterization and coronary angiography: normal coronary arteries, ventricular pressures
   Nuclear imaging studies: cardiac contractility, myocardial perfusion, low ejection fraction

Blood analysis: Arterial blood gases (ABGs), serum chemistries, cardiac enzymes, BNP level, cardiac damage, oxygenation status, liver damage, confirm dyspnea of cardiac source

3. Continuous ECG monitoring; hemodynamic monitoring (intraarterial BP, SaO_2, pulmonary artery wedge pressure [PAWP], CO); BP, HR, RR, pulse oximetry, urine output every hour
4. Calm, reassuring approach because of his anxiety and critical condition
   Explanations of rationales for all diagnostic tests and medications
   Administration of oxygen, sit upright with legs out straight or dependent
   Provide emotional and physical rest
   Constant monitoring of cardiovascular and respiratory function
   Evaluation and documentation of the effects of medical interventions (i.e., to determine if HF is resolving)
   Initiate strict I&O measurements and daily weights
5. Nursing can be responsible for providing (1) written discharge instructions or educational material that includes activity level, diet, discharge medications, follow-up appointment, weight monitoring, and symptom management; and (2) provide smoking cessation advice or counseling during the hospital stay for patients who are current smokers or former smokers who quit in the past 12 months.
6. CRT is a pacemaker that will stimulate both the right and left ventricles (chambers) of the heart so they will contract in coordination (together) to improve the way your heart pumps blood with each heart beat.
7. *Nursing diagnoses:*
   • Death anxiety related to question: "Am I going to die?"
   • Impaired gas exchange related to alveolar-capillary membrane changes
   • Ineffective tissue perfusion related to pump failure
   • Decreased CO related to altered contractility
   • Activity intolerance related to imbalance between oxygen supply and demand
   • Risk for impaired skin integrity related to edema
   • Deficient knowledge related to lack of information about complications, medications, and disease management
   Collaborative problems:
   Potential complications: Cardiogenic shock, ventricular dysrhythmias, emboli, liver/renal failure, cardiac arrest

CHAPTER 36

1. a. *F*, depolarization; b. *F*, QRS complex; c. *F*, 80 beats/min; d. *T*; e. *T*, f. *F*, 40 to 60; g. *T*; h. *F*, ectopic foci
2. a. 6; b. 5; c. 1; d. 2; e. 3; f. 4
3. d. Rationale: The normal PR interval is 0.12 to 0.20 sec and reflects the time taken for the impulse

to spread through the atria, AV node and bundle of His, the bundle branches, and Purkinje fibers. A PR interval of six small boxes is 0.24 sec and indicates that the conduction of the impulse from the atria to the Purkinje fibers is delayed.

4. d. Rationale: Electrophysiologic testing involves electrical stimulation to various areas of the atrium and ventricle to determine the inducibility of dysrhythmias and frequently induces ventricular tachycardia or ventricular fibrillation. The patient may have "near-death" experiences and requires emotional support if this occurs.

5. Word Search. a. Asystole; b. Premature ventricular contraction (PVC); c. Paroxysmal supraventricular tachycardia (PSVT); d. Type II AV block; e. Ventricular fibrillation; f. Sinus bradycardia; g. Junctional escape rhythm; h. Premature atrial contractions; i. Third-degree AV block; j. Ventricular tachycardia; k. First-degree AV block; l. Atrial fibrillation; m. Sinus tachycardia; n. Pulseless electrical activity

```
Q K C I A O F Y R O P J V U K T N K I P N J L M D R D W S H
A B S H F L B U O G J V Q R J V P E T D Y A V B T J L M C Z
R B N L Z N D P N G I C X O E S R U V K F B W P R U B Y N A
S G O C X G E E N G W X V B P P E Q K F R W K Q N N T R Z C
F I I K C S V I G M E L J R W A M P M U M E S K A C L O A S
E C T R L M F E Q A Q I Q D D I A J B J Z T S I S T U K G E
U D C W Y Y O F N K L J U Z M D T E A N W Q I Y X I X Q K Q
K A A G G I H R P T Y U G C Z R U H A Z V M Q R K O T V G H
U C R P C B Q J X O R P K F P A R O K A G C V Y B N I Z E P
V L T X X N U T D A H I U R P C E E J K F B U F U A W M L U
X X N C N X R O V Y R L C V N Y V U E U C S N M E L A J Z D
M B O R E F E K Z C C B R U A H E K E S L D O C R E T L S J
T R C Y N H F W G T N D M N L C N U R B I B G O P S R D L C
S Q L O Z T X D O J J O A Y Q A T V W Z E H N C X C I G L I
P I A F B E I D A P L B I T J T R V D B V H K H J A A L T Z
C V I D S Q L Z K C P Z D T J R I F Q W X M T K Z P L M I I
G A R O Q T F M S K X M R U A C I I A T H B K D E F V P S
Y I T O G K C S C X T O A O J L U T E B X G E G J R L J T F
T D A J J P B M F P H X C V W U L W Y O R P N M D H U R C F
S R E R W V J S E W I R Y Y L C A I P P C I Z L G Y T I Y W
K A R W I Y U A K R R C H V U I R X R I E U L K Y T T C F H
G C U M E D P Y U W D D C J K R C I C B V I K L L H E K Z B
Q Y T U D O F C P O D I A O W T O T A Y I O I S A M R F D C
C H A Y K A G X S T E J T S T N N M Z X N F N A A T P D M U
D C M V C G E U K Z G Z R H K E T H W J T A L S V J I Z F
G A E L O B B Z D B R O A P J V R F M S Q Z Y A V B H O N V
Y T R X V R J A U D E J L L O A A G C V S P O I D L W N K
U S P A R R A G L F E D U Z G R C A D B T C O R J R Y O D W
F U H N M G X X D I A Q C V Z P T Y U O Y K N J H I T L C B
I N F U W E Z Y P V V O I S E U I Z L D J G R K Q K R A F K
V I D U I N J K M D B H R N W S O E E B V L H F A B Y A Q I
A S G T B B Z F S H L C T A J L N G I Y V Q J K R E O U G Y
D L C Y U V H T H X O S N Q J A P R O U C J G U E C L M T U
J W H I M L V Y G U C K E U D M V C U X C L K J A X N Q P E
T E N E T J O G C T K J V I Q S C F F L S U A O E O U L A P
D E V Q C K S I N U S B R A D Y C A R D I A B M G G W A Y J
Z I B C Z C Q Z R E C Q V P M X S D P D C J C J M X G S H L
F I R S T D E G R E E A V B L O C K L D H U I R H I J E L E
A E P Y T I V I T C A L A C I R T C E L E S S E L E S L U P
F N Y S E C O N D D E G R E E A V B L O C K T Y P E I E W V
G Q S D F O V C N G V D T X M P V Z L C J L A T M V D D L Z
```

(PEA); o. Atrial flutter; p. Second-degree AV block Type I

6. a. third-degree (total) heart block, a pacemaker; b. sinus tachycardia; c. paroxysmal supraventricular tachycardia; d. type I, second-degree heart block; e. ventricular tachycardia, ventricular fibrillation

7. d. Rationale: Although many factors can cause a sinus tachycardia, in the patient who has had an acute MI, a tachycardia increases myocardial oxygen need in a heart that already has impaired circulation and may lead to increasing angina and further ischemia and necrosis.

8. a. Rationale: A distorted P wave with normal conduction of the impulse through the ventricles is characteristic of a premature atrial contraction. In a normal heart, this dysrhythmia is frequently associated with emotional stress or the use of caffeine, tobacco, or alcohol. Aerobic conditioning and holding of breath during exertion (Valsalva's maneuver) often cause bradycardia. Sedatives rarely slow the HR.

9. a. Rationale: A rhythm pattern that is normal except for a prolonged PR interval is characteristic of a first-degree heart block. First-degree heart blocks are not treated but are observed for progression to higher degrees of heart block. Defibrillation is used only for ventricular fibrillation, atropine is administered for bradycardias, and pacemakers are used for higher-degree heart blocks.

10. b. Rationale: Symptoms of decreased cardiac output (CO) related to cardiac dysrhythmias include a sudden drop in BP and symptoms of hypoxemia, such as decreased mentation, chest pain, and dyspnea. Peripheral pulses are weak, and the HR may be increased or decreased, depending on the type of dysrhythmia present.

11. c. Rationale: Premature ventricular contractions (PVCs) in a patient with an MI indicate significant ventricular irritability that may lead to ventricular tachycardia or ventricular fibrillation. Antidysrhythmics, such as α-adrenergic blockers, procainamide, amiodarone, or lidocaine, may be used to control the dysrhythmias. Valsalva maneuver may be used to treat paroxysmal supraventricular tachycardia.

12. a. Rationale: The PVC is an ectopic beat that causes a wide, distorted QRS complex, > 0.12 sec, because the impulse is not conducted normally through the ventricles. Because it is premature, it precedes the P wave and the P wave may be hidden in the QRS complex, or the ventricular impulse may be conducted retrograde and the P wave may be seen following the PVC. Continuous wide QRS complexes with a rate between 110 and 250 are seen in ventricular tachycardia, whereas saw-toothed P waves are characteristic of atrial flutter.

13. c. Rationale: The intent of defibrillation is to apply an electrical current to the heart that will depolarize the cells of the myocardium so that subsequent repolarization of the cells will allow the SA node to resume the role of pacemaker. An artificial pacemaker provides an electrical impulse that stimulates normal myocardial contractions. Cardioversion involves delivery of a shock that is programmed to occur during the QRS complex of the ECG, but this cannot be done during ventricular fibrillation because there is no normal ventricular contraction or QRS complex.

14. a. Rationale: During asystole or pulseless electrical activity, cardiopulmonary resuscitation (CPR) must be initiated immediately to maintain minimal CO and oxygenation, followed by intubation and administration of epinephrine and atropine. Defibrillation is not effective because the myocardial cells are in a state of depolarization.

15. a. Rationale: In preparation for defibrillation, the nurse should apply conductive materials, such as saline pads, electrode gel, or defibrillator gel pads, to the patient's chest to decrease electrical impedance and prevent burns. For defibrillation, the initial shock is 200 joules, and the synchronizer switch used for cardioversion must be turned off. Sedatives may be used before cardioversion if the patient is conscious, but the patient in ventricular fibrillation is unconscious.

16. a, b. Rationale: If the cardioverter-defibrillator delivers a shock, the patient has experienced a lethal dysrhythmia and needs to lie down to allow recovery from the dysrhythmia. In the event that the patient loses consciousness or there is repetitive firing, a call should be placed to 911 by anyone who finds the patient.

17. b. Rationale: High-output electrical generators or large magnets, such as those used in magnetic resonance imaging (MRI), can reprogram pacemakers and should be avoided. Microwave ovens pose no problems to pacemaker function, but the arm should not be raised above the shoulder for 1 week after placement of the pacemaker. The pacing current of an implanted pacemaker is not felt by the patient, but an external pacemaker may cause uncomfortable chest muscle contractions.

18. d. Rationale: Until the defibrillator is available, the patient needs CPR. Defibrillation is needed as soon as possible, so someone should bring the crash cart to the room. Defibrillation would be with 360 joules for monophasic defibrillators and 120-200 joules with biphasic defibrillators. Amiodarone is an antidysrhythmic that is part of the ACLS protocol for ventricular fibrillation.

19. c. Rationale: Catheter ablation therapy uses radiofrequency energy to ablate or "burn" accessory pathways or ectopic sites in the atria, atrioventricular (AV) node, or ventricles that cause tachydysrhythmias.

20. c. Rationale: ST elevation indicates injury/infarction of an area of the heart. An inverted

T wave is most often associated with ischemia and resolves when blood flow is restored. Occasional PVCs may be normal or may be the result of electrolyte imbalance or hypoxia. They require continued observation. A PR interval of 0.18 sec indicates a first-degree block that requires only careful observation.

21. d. Rationale: One of the most common causes of syncope is neurocardiogenic syncope, or "vasovagal" syncope. In this type of syncope, there is accentuated adrenergic activity in the upright position, with intense activation of cardiopulmonary receptors resulting in marked bradycardia and hypotension. Normally testing with the upright tilt table causes activation of the renin-angiotensin system and compensation to increase CO and maintain BP when blood pools in the extremities. However, patients with neurocardiogenic syncope experience a marked decrease in BP and HR.

22. a. third-degree block; b. atrial flutter; c. premature ventricular contraction, bigeminal; d. sinus bradycardia; e. second-degree block, type I; f. premature atrial contraction; g. second-degree block, type II; h. sinus tachycardia; i. first-degree block; j. ventricular fibrillation; k. PVC, trigeminal; l. atrial fibrillation; m. premature atrial contraction; n. normal sinus rhythm; o. ventricular tachycardia

Case Study

1. The immediate goal of drug therapy is to decrease the rapid ventricular response to the atrial fibrillation because it leads to decreased CO.

2. Cardioversion may be used to convert the fibrillation to a normal sinus rhythm. Cardioversion is administered with an initial dose of 50 joules synchronized with the QRS complex of the ECG, and the patient may be sedated before the procedure.

3. Diltiazem is indicated for treatment of atrial fibrillation because it inhibits the influx of calcium ions during depolarization of cardiac cells and slows the AV nodal conduction time, decreasing the ventricular response. Since this patient is unstable, a bolus dose would be ordered followed by a continuous drip and then PO med would be started.
   Digoxin is used to treat atrial fibrillation because it decreases the ventricular response by increasing the refractory period of the AV node, and it also decreases atrial automaticity.
   Lovenox and Coumadin are used to prevent thrombus formation, or extension, in the atria, where blood pools because of ineffective atrial contraction. If thrombi form in the left atria, arterial embolization may occur.

4. During atrial fibrillation, there is total disorganization of atrial electrical activity and no effective atrial contraction. Fibrillatory waves or undulations occur at a rate of 300-600/min in the atria, and although not all electrical activity is conducted to the ventricles, the ventricular rate is usually 100-160 beats/min and irregular. "Atrial kick" is lost and result is a 15% to 20% decrease in CO; CO is also decreased due to tachycardia

5. Atrial rhythm is chaotic, and although no definite P wave can be observed, fibrillatory waves can be seen as a jagged, irregular baseline between QRS complexes. The PR interval cannot be measured. The ventricular rhythm is usually irregular, but QRS complexes are usually of normal contour.

6. *Nursing diagnoses:*
   Decreased cardiac output related to dysrhythmia
   Activity intolerance related to inadequate cardiac output
   Impaired gas exchange related to alveolar-capillary membrane changes
   Anxiety related to vulnerability and cardiac disease
   Collaborative problems:
   Potential complications: Embolism; heart failure; cardiogenic shock

CHAPTER 37

1. a, b, c, d, e. Rationale: recent dental, urologic, surgical, or gynecologic procedures and history of IV drug abuse, heart disease, cardiac catheterization or surgery, renal dialysis, and infections all increase the risk of IE.

2. a. Rationale: Although a complete blood cell count (CBC) will reveal a mild leukocytosis and erythrocyte sedimentation rates (ESRs) will be elevated in patients with infective endocarditis, these are nonspecific findings, and blood cultures are the primary diagnostic tool for infective endocarditis. Transesophageal echocardiograms can identify vegetations on valves but are used when blood cultures are negative, and cardiac catheterizations are used when surgical intervention is being considered.

3. a. 3; b. 5; c. 2; d. 1; e. 4

4. b. Rationale: Drug therapy for patients who develop endocarditis of prosthetic valves is often unsuccessful in eliminating the infection and preventing embolization, and early valve replacement followed by prolonged drug therapy is recommended for these patients.

5. d. Rationale: The dyspnea, crackles, and restlessness the patient is manifesting are symptoms of heart failure and decreased cardiac output (CO) that occurs in up to 80% of patients with aortic valve endocarditis as a result of aortic valve incompetence. Vegetative embolization from the aortic valve occurs throughout the arterial system and may affect any body organ. Pulmonary emboli occur in right-sided endocarditis.

6. d. Rationale: The patient with outpatient antibiotic therapy requires vigilant home nursing care, and it is most important to determine the adequacy of the home environment for successful management of the patient. The patient is at risk for life-threatening complications, such as embolization and pulmonary edema, and must be able to access a hospital if needed. Bed rest will not be necessary for the patient without heart damage. Avoiding infections and planning diversional activities are indicated for the patient but are not the most important step while he is on outpatient antibiotic therapy.

7. d. Rationale: Prophylactic antibiotic therapy should be initiated before invasive dental, medical, or surgical procedures to prevent recurrence of endocarditis. Continuous antibiotic therapy is indicated only in patients with implanted devices or ongoing invasive procedures. Symptoms of infection should be treated promptly, but antibiotics are not used for exposure to infection.

8. c. Rationale: The stethoscope diaphragm at the left sternal border is the best method to use to hear the high-pitched, grating sound of a pericardial friction rub. The sound does not radiate widely and occurs with the heartbeat.

9. b. Rationale: The patient is experiencing a cardiac tamponade that consists of excess fluid in the pericardial sac, which compresses the heart and the adjoining structures, preventing normal filling and cardiac output. Fibrin accumulation, a scarred and thickened pericardium, and adherent pericardial membranes occur in chronic constrictive pericarditis.

10. a. *F*, at expiration; heard throughout the respiratory cycle; b. *T*; c. *F*, presence of acute tamponade, purulent pericarditis, or suspicion of a neoplasm; d. *T*; e. *T*

11. d. Rationale: Relief from pericardial pain is often obtained by sitting up and leaning forward. Pain is increased by lying flat. The pain has a sharp, pleuritic quality that changes with respiration, and patients take shallow breaths. Antiinflammatory medications may also be used to help control pain, but opioids are not usually indicated.

12. c. Rationale: Viruses are the most common cause of myocarditis in the United States, and early manifestations of myocarditis are often those of systemic viral infections. Myocarditis may also be associated with systemic inflammatory and metabolic disorders as well as with other microorganisms, drugs, or toxins. The heart has increased sensitivity to digoxin in myocarditis, and it is used very cautiously, if at all, in treatment of the condition.

13. d. Rationale: Initial attacks of rheumatic fever and the development of rheumatic heart disease can be prevented by adequate treatment of group A streptococcal pharyngitis. Because streptococcal

infection accounts for only about 20% of acute pharyngitis, cultures should be done to identify the organism and direct antibiotic therapy. Viral infections should not be treated with antibiotics. Prophylactic therapy is indicated in those who have valvular heart disease or have had rheumatic heart disease.

14. a. Rationale: Major criteria for the diagnosis of rheumatic fever include evidence of carditis, polyarthritis, chorea (often very late), erythema marginatum, and subcutaneous nodules. Minor criteria include all laboratory findings as well as fever, arthralgia, and a history of previous rheumatic fever.

15. a. To eliminate any residual group A β-hemolytic streptococci; prevent spread of infection; prevent recurrent infection
    b. Antiinflammatory effect to control fever and arthritic and joint manifestations
    c. Antiinflammatory effect to control fever, inflammation of severe carditis
    d. Antiinflammatory effect to control fever and joint manifestations

16. b. Rationale: When carditis is present in the patient with rheumatic fever, ambulation is postponed until any symptoms of heart failure are controlled with treatment, and full activity cannot be resumed until antiinflammatory therapy has been discontinued. In the patient without cardiac involvement, ambulation may be permitted as soon as acute symptoms have subsided, and normal activity can be resumed when antiinflammatory therapy is discontinued.

17. a. *F*, decreased, hypertrophy; b. *F*, valvular stenosis; c. *F*, mitral; d. *F*, mitral valve prolapse

18. c. Monitoring vital signs before and after ambulation is the collection of data. Instructions should be provided to the LPN regarding what changes in these should be reported to the RN. Other actions listed are RN responsibilities.

19. a. 6; b. 8; c. 2; d. 1; e. 3; f. 4; g. 5; h. 7; i. 5; j. 1; k. 8; l. 2; m. 3

20. b. Rationale: Patients with mechanical valves have an increased risk for thrombus formation. Therefore prophylactic anticoagulation therapy is used to prevent thrombus formation and systemic or pulmonary embolization. Nitrates are contraindicated for the patient with aortic stenosis because an adequate preload is necessary to open the stiffened aortic valve. Antidysrhythmics are used only if dysrhythmias occur, and α- or β-adrenergic blocking agents may be used to control the HR as needed.

21. b. Rationale: Dysrhythmias frequently cause palpitations, lightheadedness, and dizziness, and the patient should be carefully attended to prevent falls. Hypervolemia and paroxysmal nocturnal dyspnea (PND) would be apparent in the patient with heart failure.

22. c. Rationale: This procedure has been used for repair of pulmonic, tricuspid, and mitral stenosis, but usually for those patients that are poor surgical risks.

23. c. Rationale: Repair of mitral or tricuspid valves has a lower operative mortality rate than does replacement and is becoming the surgical procedure of choice for these valvular diseases. Open repair is more precise than closed repair and requires cardiopulmonary bypass during surgery. All types of valve surgery are palliative, not curative, and patients require lifelong health care. Anticoagulation therapy is used for all valve surgery for at least some time postoperatively.

24. c. Rationale: Mechanical prosthetic valves require long-term anticoagulation, and this is a factor in making a decision about the type of valve to use for replacement. Patients who cannot take anticoagulant therapy, such as women of childbearing age, patients at risk for hemorrhage, or patients who may not be compliant with anticoagulation therapy, may be candidates for the less durable biologic valves.

25. d. Rationale: The greatest risk to a patient who has an artificial valve is the development of endocarditis with invasive medical or dental procedures; before any of these procedures, antibiotic prophylaxis is necessary to prevent infection. Health care providers must be informed of the presence of the valve and the anticoagulant therapy, but the most important factor is using antibiotic prophylaxis before invasive procedures.

26. a. H; b. D; c. R; d. D; e. H; f. D; g. D; h. H; i. D; j. H; k. R; l. H

27. a, b, c, d, e. Rationale: These are all points that can apply to any cardiomyopathy.

Case Study

1. His age—incidence is higher in older adults; the invasive endoscopic cholecystectomy
2. Mitral valve prolapse
   Degenerative valve lesions: calcification degeneration of a bicuspid aortic valve; senile calcification degeneration of a normal aortic valve
3. Stroke symptoms: Embolization of vegetations to cerebral circulation with cerebral infarction
   Petechiae: Occur as a result of fragmentation and embolization of vegetative lesions
   Systolic, crescendo-decrescendo murmur: Aortic valve involvement
   Fever: Infection; occurs in 90% of patients with infective endocarditis
4. It provided a route for introduction of bacteria into the bloodstream to trigger the infectious process.

5. Identification of the organism with blood cultures and appropriate IV antibiotic therapy; antipyretics to control fever; rest—with increase in activity after fever abates and if there are no symptoms of heart failure; valve replacement if there is no response to antibiotic therapy
6. Preoperative prophylactic antibiotic therapy
7. *Nursing diagnoses:*
   - Hyperthermia related to infection, elevated temperature
   - Decreased CO related to valvular insufficiency
   - Risk for impaired skin integrity related to immobility
   Collaborative problems:
   Potential complications: Emboli; heart failure

CHAPTER 38

1. d. Rationale: Regardless of the location, atherosclerosis is responsible for peripheral arterial disease (PAD) and is related to other cardiovascular disease and its risk factors, such as coronary artery disease and carotid artery disease. Venous thrombosis, venous stasis ulcers, and pulmonary embolism are diseases of the veins and are not related to atherosclerosis.
2. a. 2; b. 3; c. 1
3. c. Rationale: Although most abdominal aortic aneurysms (AAAs) are asymptomatic, on physical examination, a pulsatile mass in the periumbilical area slightly to the left of the midline may be detected, and bruits may be audible with a stethoscope placed over the aneurysm. Hoarseness and dysphagia may occur with aneurysms of the ascending aorta and the aortic arch. Severe back pain with flank ecchymosis is usually present on rupture of an AAA, and neurologic loss in the lower extremities may occur from pressure of a thoracic aneurysm.
4. d. Rationale: A computed tomography (CT) scan is the most accurate test to determine the diameter of the aneurysm and whether a thrombus is present. The other tests may also be used, but the CT yields the most descriptive results.
5. b. Rationale: Increased systolic blood pressure (SBP) continually puts pressure on the diseased area of the artery, promoting its expansion. Small aneurysms can be treated by decreasing blood pressure (BP), modifying atherosclerosis risk factors, and monitoring the size of the aneurysm. Anticoagulants are used during surgical treatment of aneurysms, but physical activity is not known to increase their size. Calcium intake is not related to calcification in arteries.
6. b. Rationale: Because atherosclerosis is a systemic disease, the patient with an AAA is likely to have cardiac, pulmonary, cerebral, or lower-extremity vascular problems that should be noted and monitored throughout the perioperative period. Postoperatively,

the BP is balanced: high enough to keep adequate flow through the artery to prevent thrombosis but low enough to prevent bleeding at the surgical site.

7. a. saccular; b. synthetic graft; c. all; d. iliac; e. endovascular graft; f. renal

8. b. Rationale: The BP and peripheral pulses are evaluated every hour in the acute postoperative period to ensure that BP is adequate and that extremities are being perfused. BP is kept within normal range. If it is too low, thrombosis of the graft may occur; if it is too high, it may cause leaking or rupture at the suture line. Hypothermia is induced during surgery, but the patient is rewarmed as soon as the surgery is completed. Fluid replacement to maintain urine output at 100 mL/hr would increase the BP too much.

9. a. Rationale: During repair of an AAA, the blood supply to the carotid arteries may be interrupted, leading to neurologic complications manifested by a decreased level of consciousness (LOC) and altered pupil responses to light as well as changes in facial symmetry, speech, and movement of upper extremities. The thorax is opened for ascending aortic surgery, and shallow breathing, poor cough, and decreasing chest drainage are expected. Often, lower limb pulses are normally decreased or absent for a short time following surgery.

10. a. decreased or absent pulses in conjunction with cool, painful extremities below the level of repair; b. cardiac dysrhythmias, chest pain; c. absent bowel sounds, abdominal distention, diarrhea, bloody stools; d. increased temperature and white blood cells; surgical site inflammation or drainage.

11. b. Rationale: The decreasing urine output is evidence that either the patient needs volume or there is reduced renal blood flow. The physician will want to be notified as soon as possible of this change in condition and may order labs.

12. d. Rationale: Patients are taught to palpate peripheral pulses to identify changes in their quality or strength, but the rate is not a significant factor in peripheral perfusion. The color and temperature of the extremities are also important for patients to observe. The remaining statements are all true.

13. d. Rationale: The onset of an aortic dissection involving the distal descending aorta is usually characterized by a sudden, severe, tearing pain in the back, and as it progresses down the aorta, the kidneys, abdominal organs, and lower extremities may begin to show evidence of ischemia. Aortic dissections of the ascending aorta and aortic arch may affect the heart and circulation to the head, with the development of murmurs, ventricular failure, and cerebral ischemia.

14. a. Rationale: Although most initial treatment for aortic dissection involves a period of lowering the BP and myocardial contractility to diminish the pulsatile forces in the aorta, immediate surgery is indicated when complications (such as occlusion of the carotid arteries) occur. Anticoagulants would prolong and intensify the bleeding, and blood is administered only if the dissection ruptures.

15. a. Rationale: Relief of pain is an indication that the dissection has stabilized, and it may be treated conservatively for an extended time with drugs that lower the BP and decrease myocardial contractility. Surgery is usually indicated for dissections of the ascending aorta or if complications occur.

16. a. A; b. V; c. V; d. A; e. A; f. V; g. A; h. V; i. A; j. V; k. V

17. a. intermittent claudication; b. nonhealing ischemic ulcers, gangrene; c. 0.77, mild; d. rest

18. c. Rationale: Oral anticoagulants (warfarin) are not recommended for treatment of peripheral artery disease, but all the other statements are correct in relation to treatment of peripheral artery disease.

19. a, b, e. Rationale: Warm legs and feet increase circulation. The lower extremities should be assessed at a regular interval for changes. Walking exercise increases oxygen extraction in the legs and improves skeletal muscle metabolism. The patient with PAD should walk at least 30 minutes a day, preferably twice a day. Exercise should be stopped when pain occurs and resumed when the pain subsides. Nicotine in all forms causes vasoconstriction and must be eliminated.

20. b. Rationale: Peripheral artery disease occurs as a result of atherosclerosis, and the risk factors are the same as for other diseases associated with atherosclerosis, such as CAD, cerebral vascular disease, and aneurysms. Major risk factors are hypertension, cigarette smoking, and hyperlipidemia. The risk for amputation is high in patients with severe occlusive disease, but it is not the best approach to encourage patients to make lifestyle modifications.

21. c. Rationale: Loss of palpable pulses and numbness and tingling of the extremity are indications of occlusion of the bypass graft and need immediate medical attention. Pain, redness, and serous drainage at the incision site are expected postoperatively, but decreasing ankle-brachial indices may indicate graft obstruction.

22. a. pain; b. pallor; c. pulselessness; d. paresthesia; e. paralysis; f. poikilothermia

23. a. R; b. B; c. R; d. B; e. R; f. R; g. B; h. R; i. B; j. R

24. a. damage of the endothelium; b. venous stasis; c. hypercoagulability; d. venous stasis; e. hypercoagulability; f. venous stasis

25. a. *F*, varicose veins; b. *F*, superficial vein thrombosis; c. *T*

26. d. Rationale: Prevention of emboli formation can be achieved by bed rest and limiting movement of the involved extremity until the clot is stable, inflammation has receded, and anticoagulation is achieved. Elevating the affected limb will promote venous return, but it does not prevent embolization, and dangling the legs promotes venous stasis and further clot formation.

27. a. 3, 5; b. 3; c. 4; d. 2; e. 2; f. 1; g. 1; h. 4; i. 4; j. 1, 3, 5.
28. b. Rationale: Anticoagulant therapy with heparin or warfarin (Coumadin) does not dissolve clots but prevents propagation of the clot, development of new thrombi, and embolization; lysis of the clot occurs through the action of the body's intrinsic fibrinolytic system or by the administration of fibrinolytic agents.
29. d. Rationale: Exercise programs for patients recovering from venous thromboembolism (VTE) should emphasize swimming, which is particularly beneficial because of the gentle, even pressure of the water. Coumadin will not blacken stools; if this occurs, it could be a sign of gastrointestinal bleeding. Dark green and leafy vegetables have high amounts of vitamin K and should not be increased during Coumadin therapy, but they do not need to be restricted. The legs must not be massaged because of the risk for dislodging any clots that may be present.
30. a. Rationale: During walking, the muscles of the legs continuously knead the veins, promoting movement of venous blood toward the heart, and walking is the best measure to prevent venous stasis. The other methods will help venous return, but they do not provide the benefit that ambulation does.
31. a. 4; b. 7; c. 1; d. 5; e. 8; f. 3; g. 9; h. 6; i. 2
32. b. Rationale: Although leg elevation, moist dressings, and topical antibiotics are useful in treatment of venous stasis ulcers, the most important factor appears to be extrinsic compression to minimize venous stasis, venous hypertension, and edema. Extrinsic compression methods include compression gradient stockings, elastic bandages, and Unna's boot.

Case Study

1. Smoking history; history of atherosclerosis with CAD; age; sex
2. The primary etiology of an AAA is atherosclerotic plaquing that causes degenerative changes in the media lining of the aorta. The changes lead to loss of elasticity, weakening, and eventual dilation of the aorta. Trauma and infections and a possible genetic component are responsible for a small number of AAAs.
3. The severe back pain
   The shock symptoms: BP 88/68 mm Hg; cool, clammy extremities
4. The first priority is to control the bleeding, which will require immediate surgical repair of the aneurysm. Fatal hemorrhage is likely if the bleeding is not controlled.
5. The patient will most likely be taken to surgery from the emergency department, and emergency departments are not the most private or supportive environments. It is important for the nurse to provide privacy as much as possible and allow the patient and family to be together and ask questions as necessary. The nurse should also provide explanations of the procedures and interventions that are being implemented and be supportive during this critical time.

6. The only effective treatment for AAA is surgery, and the only way to prevent rupture is to repair the aneurysm surgically before it ruptures. Patients with AAAs should have close medical observation to detect increases in aneurysm size because surgical repair is generally required when the aneurysm is ≥5.5 cm for men and ≥5 cm for women.
7. *Nursing diagnoses:*
   • Acute pain related to compression of internal structures with blood
   • Decreased cardiac output related to hypovolemia
   • Deficient knowledge related to lack of information about surgical aneurysm repair and postoperative care
   Collaborative problems:
   Potential complications: Organ ischemia; hypovolemic shock; myocardial infarction

CHAPTER 39

1. a. parotid gland; b. submandibular gland; c. pharynx; d. trachea; e. esophagus; f. diaphragm; g. liver; h. hepatic flexure; i. transverse colon; j. ascending colon; k. ileum; l. cecum; m. ileocecal valve; n. vermiform appendix; o. anal canal; p. rectum; q. sigmoid colon; r. descending colon; s. stomach; t. splenic flexure; u. spleen; v. larynx; w. sublingual gland; x. tongue
2. a. gallbladder; b. cystic duct; c. ampulla of Vater; d. pancreas (head); e. main pancreatic duct; f. duodenum; g. pancreas (tail); h. pancreas (body); i. common bile duct; j. common hepatic duct; k. left hepatic duct; l. right hepatic duct
3. c. Rationale: The parasympathetic nervous system stimulates activity of the gastrointestinal (GI) tract, increasing motility and secretions and relaxing sphincters to promote movement of contents. A drug that blocks this activity decreases secretions and peristalsis, slows gastric emptying, and contracts sphincters. The enteric nervous system of the GI tract is modulated by sympathetic and parasympathetic influence.
4. d. Rationale: Cholecystokinin is secreted by the duodenal mucosa when fats and amino acids enter the duodenum and stimulates the gallbladder to release bile to emulsify the fats for digestion. The bile is produced by the liver but stored in the gallbladder. Secretin is responsible for stimulating pancreatic bicarbonate secretion, and gastrin increases gastric motility and acid secretion.
5. c. Rationale: The stomach secretes intrinsic factor, necessary for cobalamin (vitamin B_{12}) absorption in the intestine. In removal of part or all of the stomach, cobalamin must be supplemented for life.
6. a. *F*, lower esophageal sphincter; b. *T*; c. *F*, parietal cells; d. *T*; e. *F*, conjugated (direct); f. *T*
7. a. 3; b. 5; c. 7; d. 8; e. 10; f. 9; g. 1; h. 4; i. 2; j. 6
8. a. Rationale: Bacteria in the colon (1) synthesize vitamin K, which is needed for the production of

prothrombin by the liver and (2) deaminate undigested or nonabsorbed proteins, producing ammonia, which is converted to urea by the liver. A reduction in normal flora bacteria by antibiotic therapy can lead to decreased vitamin K, resulting in decreased prothrombin and coagulation problems. Bowel bacteria do not influence protein absorption or the secretion of mucus.

9. c. Rationale: The ampulla of Vater is the site where the pancreatic duct and common bile duct enter the duodenum, and the opening and closing of the ampulla is controlled by the sphincter of Oddi. Because bile from the common bile duct is needed for emulsification of fat to promote digestion, and pancreatic enzymes from the pancreas are needed for digestion of all nutrients, a blockage at this point would affect the digestion of all nutrients. Gastric contents pass into the duodenum through the pylorus or pyloric valve.

10. The bilirubin from hemoglobin is insoluble (unconjugated) and attached to albumin in the blood, removed by the liver, combined with glucuronic acid to become soluble (conjugated), and excreted in bile into the intestine. Bowel bacteria convert some of the bilirubin to urobilinogen; urobilinogen is absorbed into the blood; and a small amount of urobilinogen is excreted by the kidneys in urine, with the rest being removed by the liver and re-excreted in the bile.

11. d. Rationale: There is decreased tone of the lower esophageal sphincter with aging, and regurgitation of gastric contents back into the esophagus occurs, causing heartburn and belching. There is a decrease in hydrochloric acid secretion in aging. Jaundice and intolerance to fatty foods are symptoms of liver or gallbladder disease and are not normal age-related findings.

12. a. Excessive alcohol intake, smoking, exposure to hepatotoxins, recent foreign travel
    b. Anorexia and weight loss, excessive weight gain, inadequate diet
    c. Change in bowel patterns, laxative/enema use, decreased fluid/fiber intake
    d. Weakness, fatigue, inability to procure and prepare food, inability to feed self

e. Interruption of sleep with GI symptoms
f. Changes in taste or smell, use of pain medications, sensory problems that interfere with food preparation or intake
g. Self-esteem and body image problems related to weight, symptoms affecting appearance
h. Loss of employment because of chronic illness, altered relationships with others
i. Anorexia, alcohol intake, decreased acceptance by sexual partner
j. GI problems or symptoms induced by stress, depression
k. Religious dietary restrictions, vegetarianism

13. c. Rationale: A thin, white coating of the dorsum (top) of the tongue is normal. A red, slick appearance is characteristic of cobalamin deficiency; and scattered red, smooth areas on the tongue are known as *geographic tongue*. The uvula should remain in the midline while the patient is saying "Ahh."

14. b. Rationale: The pulsation of the aorta in the epigastric area is a normal finding. Bruits indicate that blood flow is abnormal, the liver is percussed in the right midclavicular line, and a normal spleen cannot be palpated.

15. b. Rationale: The pancreas is located in the left upper quadrant, the liver is in the right upper quadrant, the appendix is in the right lower quadrant, and the gallbladder is in the right upper quadrant.

16. a. Rationale: Borborygmi are loud gurgles (stomach growling) that indicate hyperperistalsis. Normal bowel sounds are relatively high-pitched and are heard best with the diaphragm of the stethoscope. High-pitched, tinkling bowel sounds occur when the intestines are under tension, as in bowel obstructions. Absent bowel sounds may be reported only when no sounds are heard for 5 minutes in each quadrant.

17. d. Rationale: The abdomen should be assessed in the following sequence: inspection, auscultation, percussion, palpation. The patient should empty his or her bladder before assessment begins.

18. See table below.

	(1) NPO	(2) Bowel	(3) Consent	(4) Allergy
Upper GI series	X			
Barium enema	X	X		
Percutaneous transhepatic cholangiogram	X		X	X
Gallbladder ultrasound	X			
Hepatobiliary scintigraphy	X			
Upper GI endoscopy	X		X	
Colonoscopy	X	X	X	
Endoscopic retrograde cholangiopancreatography (ERCP)	X		X	

19. c. Rationale: The aspartate aminotransferase (AST) level is elevated in liver disease, but it is important to note that it is also elevated in damage to the heart and lungs and is not a specific test for liver function. Measurement of most of the transaminases are nonspecific tests unless isoenzyme fractions are determined. Hepatic encephalopathy is related to elevated ammonia levels.

20. a. 1; b. 5 (signs of peritonitis); c. 1; d. 2; e. 3; f. 4, 5; g. 3; h. 3; i. 4; j. 2

CHAPTER 40

1. a. protein: 120 g × 4 = 480 cal = 16% of 3000 cal; fat: 160 g × 9 = 1440 cal = 48% of 3000 cal; carbohydrate: 270 g × 4 = 1080 cal = 36% of 3000 cal
   b. protein: 64 g (0.8 g/kg body weight) = 256 cal; fat: 100 g (30% of 3000 cal) = 900 cal; carbohydrate: should be the balance—461 g carbohydrate = 1844 cal
   c. An average adult requires an estimated 20 to 35 calories/kg of body weight per day. In his case it would be between 1600 and 2800 calories per day (80 kg × 20 and 80 kg × 35).
   d. Increase breads, cereals, rice, and pasta as sources of complex carbohydrate. Decrease meat and egg group to three servings a day to lower protein and fat.
   Use 3 servings of milk group to lower fat intake.
   Use all fats, oils, and sweets sparingly.

2. a. *T*; b. *F*, cobalamin (vitamin B$_{12}$) and iron; c. *F*, fat; d. *F*, kwashiorkor

3. d. Rationale: In the United States, where protein intake is high and of good quality, protein-calorie malnutrition most commonly results from problems of the gastrointestinal (GI) system. In developing countries, adequate food sources might not exist, the inhabitants may not be well educated about nutritional needs, and economic conditions can prevent purchase of balanced diets.

4. a. Carbohydrates stored in the liver and muscles in the form of glycogen are used and may be quickly depleted.
   b. Protein, primarily the amino acids alanine and glutamine, is converted to glucose for energy, and a negative nitrogen balance occurs.
   c. Body fat is mobilized and used as the primary source of energy, conserving protein.
   d. Fat stores are usually depleted in 4 to 6 weeks, and body proteins are used because they are the only source of energy available.

5. c. Rationale: The sodium-potassium exchange pump uses 20% to 50% of all calories ingested. When energy sources are decreased, the pump fails to function, sodium is left in the cell, and potassium remains in extracellular fluids. Hyperkalemia, as well as hyponatremia, occurs.

6. a. *F*, 7% increase per Fahrenheit degree; b. *F*, peripheral nervous system; c. *T*

7. a, b, d, e. Rationale: In malnutrition, metabolic processes are slowed, leading to increased sensitivity to cold, slowed heart rate (HR) and cardiac output (CO), and decreased neurologic function. Because of slowed GI motility and absorption, the abdomen becomes distended and protruding, bowel sounds are decreased. Skin is rough, dry, and scaly whereas bone structures protrude because of muscle loss.

8. d. Rationale: Malnutrition that results from a decreased intake of food is most common in individuals with severe anorexia that decreases the desire to eat. Infections create a hypermetabolic state that increases nutritional demand, malabsorption causes loss of nutrients that are ingested, and draining decubitus ulcers are examples of disorders that cause both loss of protein and hypermetabolic states.

9. c. Rationale: Serum transferrin is a protein that is synthesized by the liver and used for iron transport and decreases when there is protein deficiency. An increase in the protein would indicate a more positive nitrogen balance with amino acids available for synthesis. Decreased lymphocytes and serum prealbumin are indicators of protein depletion, and an increased serum potassium shows continuing failure of the sodium-potassium pump.

10. d. Rationale: Anthropometric measurements, including mid-upper arm circumference and triceps skinfold measurements, are good indicators of lean body mass and skeletal protein reserves and are valuable in evaluating persons who may have or are being treated for acute protein malnutrition. The other measurements do not specifically address muscle mass.

11. a. Rationale: The breakfast with the eggs provides 24 g of protein, compared with 14 g for the protein-fortified cream of wheat and milkshake breakfast. Whole milk instead of skim helps meet the calorie requirements. The toast breakfast has 10 g of protein, and the pancakes have about 6 g. Bacon is considered a fat rather than a meat serving.

12. b. Rationale: Although calorie intake should be decreased in the older adult because of decreased activity and basal metabolic rate, the need for specific nutrients, such as proteins and vitamins, does not change.

13. a. Rationale: Socioeconomic conditions frequently have the greatest effect on the nutritional status of the healthy older adult. Limited income and social isolation can result in the "tea and toast" meals of the older adult.

14. a. Rationale: Standard nasogastric (NG) tubes are used for tube feedings for short-term feeding problems because prolonged therapy can result in irritation and erosion of the mucosa of the upper GI tract.

Gastric reflux and the potential for aspiration can occur with both tubes that deliver fluids into the stomach. Both NG and gastrostomy tubes can become displaced and deprive the patient of the sensations associated with eating.

15. a. Position the patient with the head of the bed elevated 30 to 45 degrees. Following intermittent feedings, keep the head of the bed elevated for 30 to 60 minutes. Measure residual feeding to detect retention of solution in the stomach so that the stomach does not become overdistended.
    b. Start tube feedings with small amounts and/ or decrease rate of infusion. Refrigerate opened solutions to prevent bacterial growth but warm them to room temperature before administration; discard outdated formula; use closed systems; use sterile water to flush.
    c. Flush the tube with 30 mL water before and after feedings and medication administration. In continuous feedings, flush the tube with water every 4 hours; flush after residual measurements.
    d. Confirm placement initially with chest x-ray; mark exit point of tube following x-ray confirmation and look for changes in the external length of the tube. If lengthened, check pH of aspirate (<5).
    e. Stop feeding and flush with 15 mL of water, dilute medications and use clean oral syringe to administer medication; flush again taking into account the patient's fluid status; separately dilute and administer medications; use liquid forms of medications, if available; use immediate release form, if liquid not available.

16. b. Rationale: <250 mL residual does not require further action.

17. a. RN; b. NAP; c. RN; d. RN; e. NAP; f. NAP; g. RN; h. NAP

18. a. PPN; b. CPN; c. CPN; d. PPN; e. CPN; f. PPN; g. CPN

19. c. Rationale: In malabsorption syndromes, foods that are ingested into the intestinal tract cannot be digested or absorbed, and tube feedings infused into the intestinal tract would also not be absorbed. All the other conditions can be treated with enteral or parenteral nutrition, depending on the patient's needs.

20. a. Refrigerate solutions until 30 minutes before use; change dressing to catheter site per institutional protocol; label date and time started; change filter and tubing every 24 hours if lipids are being administered or every 72 hours if amino acids and dextrose are being administered; do not infuse solution in one bottle more than 24 hours.
    b. Start infusions slowly, gradually increasing rate for 24 to 48 hours; check capillary blood glucose levels every 4 to 6 hours; provide sliding-scale doses of insulin as prescribed; do not speed up infusion rates or remove infusion from infusion controllers/pumps; visually check the amount infused every 30 to 60 minutes

21. a. Rationale: Bacterial growth occurs at room temperature in nutritional solutions; therefore, solutions must not be infused for longer than 24 hours. Remaining solution should be discarded. Speeding up the solution may cause hyperglycemia and should not be done.

22. a. AB; b. A; c. B; d. AB; e. AB; f. A

23. b. Rationale: The potential life-threatening cardiac complications related to the hypokalemia are the most important considerations in the patient's care. The other nursing diagnoses are important considerations in the patient's care but do not pose the immediate risk that the hypokalemia does.

Case Study

1. Her position on the weight for height and body frame chart; food intake history; assessment of each body system

2. The chemotherapy and radiation have greatly increased nutritional need, but food intake is decreased because of side effects of cancer treatment; weakness may lead to inability to procure and prepare food; she lives alone and has no socialization with meals, and she has feelings of hopelessness about treatment for cancer.

3. Edema and possible ascites indicated by hypoalbuminemia; paleness of skin, mucous membranes indicated by her hemoglobin and hematocrit levels

4. Liver damage with fatty infiltration; susceptibility to infection very high because of chemotherapy and radiation immunosuppression in addition to that of malnutrition

5. Easy-to-prepare foods
   How to add protein supplement or powdered milk to foods; decrease fluids with meals so that more calories are consumed; eat small multiple feedings that are of nutritional value; provide all written instructions in Spanish; refer to community resources for socialization and Meals on Wheels

6. *Nursing diagnoses:*
   • Imbalanced nutrition: Less than body requirements related to anorexia and decreased food intake
   • Activity intolerance related to fatigue and weakness
   • Hopelessness related to belief that cancer therapy is ineffective
   • Risk for infection related to decreased host defense mechanisms
   Collaborative problems:
   Potential complications: Liver failure; electrolyte imbalance

CHAPTER 41

1. a. *F*, 40-59; b. T; c. *F*, second; d. *T*
2. a. 33.6 kg/m², obesity; b. 0.88; c. an increased risk for health complications

3. b. Rationale: The 56-year-old has a body mass index (BMI) of 38 (obese) with waist-to-hip ratio of 1.1 with central obesity and is more at risk than the others. The 30-year-old has the least risk with a BMI of 27.3 (normal weight) and gynoid shape; the 42-year-old has BMI of 24.2 (normal weight) with one risk factor in the waist-hip ratio of 1.0, and the 68-year-old has BMI of 27.9 (overweight) with waist-hip ratio of 0.9, but risk is not as great as in the 56-year-old.

4. b. Rationale: A patient who is obese (BMI 32.2) but has a waist-hip ratio of less than 0.8, indicating a gynoid obesity, has an increased risk for osteoporosis. The other conditions are risks associated with android obesity.

5. a. Rationale: Motivation is essential. Focus on the reasons for wanting to lose weight.

6. a. Restrict dietary intake so that it is below energy requirements.
   b. A goal for weight loss must be set, and 1 to 2 pounds a week is realistic. A more rapid loss often causes skin and underlying tissue to lose elasticity and become flabby folds of tissue.
   c. May gain support from others trying to modify eating habits. Often provide education and dieting tips.
   d. Determine portion sizes. Portion sizes have increased over the years and are larger than they should be. Teach to weigh portions or learn equivalencies such as a serving of fruit is the size of a baseball.
   e. Alcohol should be limited or avoided because it increases caloric intake and has low nutritional value.
   f. Exercise increases energy expenditure, decreases appetite, and is important in maintaining weight loss.
   g. Programs de-emphasize diet and focus on how and when the person eats, help to modify eating habits, and may lead to more success in maintaining weight loss over time.

7. a. When reducing diets that severely restrict carbohydrates, the body's glycogen stores become depleted within a few days. The glycogen normally binds to water in fat cells, and it is this water loss that causes weight loss in the first few days. Fat is not burned until the glycogen-water pool is depleted.
   b. Daily weighing is not recommended because of the frequent fluctuation from retained water (including urine) and elimination of feces. A weekly weight is a more reliable indicator of weight loss.
   c. Men are able to lose weight more quickly than are women because women have a higher percentage of metabolically less-active fat.

8. a. Rationale: Plateau periods during which no weight is lost are normal occurrences during weight reduction and may last for several days to several weeks, but weight loss will resume if the prescribed weight-reduction plan is continued. Weight loss may stop if former eating habits are resumed, but this is not the most common cause of plateaus.

9. d. Rationale: A chicken breast the size of a deck of cards is about 3 oz, a normal portion size of meat. Other normal portions include a 3-inch bagel, 1/2 cup of chopped vegetables, and a piece of cheese the size of six dice.

10. b. Rationale: Medications are used only as adjuncts to diet and exercise programs in the treatment of obesity. Drugs do not cure obesity without changes in food intake and physical activity, and weight gain will occur when the medications are discontinued. The medications used work in a variety of ways to control appetite, but over-the-counter (OTC) drugs are probably the least effective and most abused of these drugs.

11. b. Rationale: Sibutramine (Meridia) has cardiovascular side effects and can increase both blood pressure (BP) and heart rate (HR). Valvular heart disease was seen with fenfluramine (Pondimin) and dexfenfluramine (Redux) use, and these drugs have been removed from the market. Some selective serotonin reuptake inhibitors that are approved for depression may have a short-term effect on weight loss.

12. d. Rationale: People who have undergone behavior therapy are more successful in maintaining weight losses over time because most programs deemphasize the diet and focus on how and when the person eats. Weighing daily is not recommended, and plateaus may not allow for consistent weight loss. Exercising more often depresses appetite and need not be limited.

13. a. 2; b. 1; c. 4; d. 3; e. 2; f. 4; g. 1; h. 3

14. c. Rationale: Special considerations are needed for the care of the morbidly obese patient because most hospital units are not prepared with beds, chairs, BP cuffs, and other equipment that will need to be used with the very obese patient. Consideration of all aspects of care should be made before implementing care for the patient, including extra time and perhaps assistance for positioning, physical assessment, and transferring the patient.

15. d. Rationale: Turning, coughing, and deep breathing are essential to prevent postoperative complications. Protecting the incision from strain is important since wound dehiscence is a problem for obese patients. If an NG tube that is present following gastric surgery for morbid obesity becomes blocked or needs repositioning, the health care provider should be notified. Ambulation is usually started in the evening of surgery, and additional help will be needed to support the patient. Respiratory function is promoted by keeping the head of the bed elevated at a 30-degree angle.

16. b. Rationale: Patients with histories of untreated depression or psychosis are not good candidates.

All other historical information includes medical complications of severe obesity that would help qualify the patient for the surgery.

17. a. Rationale: Fluids and foods high in carbohydrates tend to promote diarrhea and symptoms of the dumping syndrome in patients with gastric bypass surgery. The diet generally should be high in protein and low in carbohydrates, fat, and roughage, and consist of six small feedings a day because of the small stomach size. Liquid diets are likely to be used longer for the patient with a gastroplasty.

18. b, c, d. Rationale: Patients with metabolic syndrome need to lower risk factors by reducing and maintaining weight, increasing physical activity, and establishing healthy diet habits. Some patients with metabolic syndrome are diabetic and would need to monitor glucose levels frequently. When monitoring weight reduction, it is recommended to check weight weekly, not daily.

19. c. Rationale: The other factors are not specifically associated with metabolic syndrome.

Case Study

1. His BMI is about 45 kg/m^2: 296/4624 [68 × 68] × 703

2. L.C. has a risk for almost all health problems associated with obesity: type 2 diabetes, obesity hypoventilation syndrome, osteoarthritis, gout, lumbar disk disease, chronic low back pain, sudden cardiac death, heart failure, coronary artery disease (CAD), deep vein thrombosis (DVT), gallstones, nonalcoholic steatohepatitis, renal disease, and cancer. He already has hypertension, hyperlipidemia, sleep apnea, metabolic syndrome, impaired mobility, and depression.

3. L.C. would qualify for bariatric surgery; he has a BMI >40 kg/m^2: one or more obesity-related medical complication, is 18 years old or older, understands the risks and benefits of the surgery, has tried and failed other methods of weight loss, has no serious endocrine problems causing the obesity, is psychiatric and socially stable, and is able to follow up on a long-term basis. Surgery would lessen the risks of obesity complications.

4. Vertical banded surgery:
Pros: Stomach remains intact, small stoma size delays stomach emptying, successful weight loss
Cons: Possible intractable vomiting, distention of pouch wall, rupture of staple line, erosion of the band into the stomach
Roux-en-Y:
Pros: Excellent patient tolerance, sustained long-term weight loss, low complication rates, most commonly used procedure
Cons: absorption deficiencies of iron, cobalamin, folic acid, and calcium; mortality rates 2% in first month; dumping syndrome

5. L.C. needs to be instructed in proper coughing technique, deep breathing, and turning methods.

He should be taught to use an incentive spirometer and be informed about having an NG tube postoperatively. He will also need to take several showers per day for a few days before surgery. He should be told what to expect postoperatively: early ambulation, the use of antiembolism stockings or pneumatic compression devices, low-dose heparin administered subcutaneously, the need for pain medication, and initiation of oral liquids.

6. *Nursing diagnoses:*
   - Imbalanced nutrition: More than body requirements related to imbalance between energy expenditure and energy intake
   - Activity intolerance related to fatigue
   - Powerlessness related to lack of control of eating
   - Health-seeking behavior: Expressed desire for weight loss and health maintenance mechanisms
   Collaborative problems:
   Potential complications: CAD, renal failure, liver failure, musculoskeletal problems, type 2 diabetes, postoperative wound infection, respiratory complications, pain

CHAPTER 42

1. a. *F*, parasympathetic nervous system; b. *F*, labyrinthine stimulation; c. *F*, metabolic alkalosis, hydrochloric acid

2. c. Rationale: The loss of gastric hydrochloric acid causes metabolic alkalosis and an increase in pH; loss of potassium, sodium, and chloride; and loss of fluid, which increases the hematocrit.

3. d. Rationale: The patient with severe or persistent vomiting requires IV replacement of fluids and electrolytes until able to tolerate oral intake to prevent serious dehydration and electrolyte imbalances. Oral fluids are not given until vomiting has been relieved, and parenteral antiemetics are often not used until a cause of the vomiting can be established. NG intubation may be indicated in some cases, but fluid and electrolyte replacement is the first priority.

4. a. Rationale: Water is the fluid of choice for rehydration by mouth. Very hot or cold liquids are not usually well tolerated, and although broth and Gatorade have been used for the patient with severe vomiting, these substances are high in sodium and should be administered with caution.

5. d. Rationale: Ondansetron (Zofran) is one of several serotonin antagonists that act both centrally and peripherally to reduce vomiting—centrally on the vomiting center in the brainstem and peripherally by promoting gastric emptying. Dronabinol (Marinol) is an orally active cannabinoid that causes sedation and has a potential for abuse and is used when other therapies are ineffective. Antihistamines used as antiemetics also cause sedation.

6. Any three of the following are acceptable: monitor the patient's fluid and electrolyte status more closely

(lab, I&O); monitor vital signs along with breath sounds; assess mucous membranes, skin turgor, and color to assess for dehydration; assess level of consciousness closely; implement safety precautions (placement close to the nurses station, call bell in reach, hourly visual checks, use of sitters); check dosing of antiemetics; assess for weakness/fatigue.

7. a. 4; b. 6; c. 2; d. 3; e. 1; f. 5; g. 3; h. 7; i. 4; j. 6; k. 2

8. c. Rationale: A positive history of use of tobacco and alcohol is the most significant etiologic factor in oral cancer. Excessive exposure to ultraviolet radiation from the sun is a factor in the development of cancer of the lip. Herpes simplex infections have not been associated with oral cancer, and difficulty swallowing and ear pain are symptoms of advanced oral cancer, not risk factors.

9. b. Rationale: Because surgical treatment of oral cancers involves extensive excision, a tracheostomy is usually performed with the radical dissections. The first goal of care is that the patient will have a patent airway. The other goals are appropriate but of lesser priority.

10. b. Rationale: Measures to assess and treat withdrawal from alcohol should be implemented with patients who have heavy use of this substance because alcohol is a strong risk factor and withdrawal can be life threatening. Nutritional needs may need to be addressed with tube feedings postoperatively, and pain medications may need to be increased because of cross-tolerance. Counseling about lifestyle changes is not a priority in the early postoperative course.

11 a. fatty foods; b. chocolate; c. alcohol; d. tea, coffee
Also: peppermint and spearmint

12. c. Rationale: The use of blocks to elevate the head of the bed facilitates gastric emptying by gravity and is strongly recommended to prevent nighttime reflux. Small meals should be eaten frequently, but patients should not eat at bedtime or lie down for 2 to 3 hours after eating. Liquids should be taken between meals to prevent gastric distention with meals. Activities that involve increasing intraabdominal pressure, such as bending over, lifting, or wearing tight clothing, should be avoided.

13. c. Rationale: Dysphagia—occurring with meats, then soft foods, and eventually liquids—is the most common symptom of esophageal cancer and is often pronounced by the time the patient seeks medical attention. The patient frequently has poor nutritional status because of the inability to ingest adequate amounts of food before surgery. Fluid-volume deficit could occur, but this is a late finding in comparison with inadequate food intake.

14. b. Rationale: Following esophageal surgery, the patient should be positioned in semi-Fowler's or Fowler's position to prevent reflux and aspiration of gastric sections. NG drainage is expected to be bloody for 8 to 12 hours postoperatively. Abdominal distention is not a major concern following esophageal surgery, and even though the thorax may be opened during the surgery, clear breath sounds should be expected in all areas of the lungs.

15. a. 2; b. 5; c. 3; d. 1; e. 4

16. a. Arterial blood that has not been in contact with gastric secretions, as in esophageal or oral bleeding
 b. Blood that has been in the stomach for some time and has reacted with gastric secretions
 c. Slow bleeding from an upper GI source when blood passes through the GI tract and is digested
 d. Presence of guiaic-positive stools or NG aspirate

17. b. Rationale: Although all the interventions may be indicated when a patient has upper GI bleeding, the first nursing priority is to perform an assessment of the patient's condition, with emphasis on BP, pulse, and peripheral perfusion to determine the presence of hypovolemic shock.

18. d. Rationale: Octreotide is a somatostatin analog that has been shown to reduce upper GI bleeding and inhibit the release of GI hormones such as gastrin, thereby decreasing hydrochloric acid secretion. Ranitidine is a histamine H_2-receptor blocker that decreases acid secretion, and omeprazole inhibits the proton pump necessary for the secretion of hydrochloric acid. Vasopressin has a vasoconstriction action useful in controlling upper GI bleeding.

19. b. Rationale: All OTC drugs should be avoided because their contents may include drugs that are contraindicated because of the irritating effects on the gastric mucosa. Patients are taught to test suspicious vomitus or stools for occult blood, but all stools do not need to be tested. Antacids cannot be taken with all medications because they prevent the absorption of many drugs. Misoprostol is used to protect the gastric mucosa in patients who must take nonsteroidal antiinflammatory drugs (NSAIDs) for other conditions because it inhibits acid secretion stimulated by NSAIDs.

20. a. Rationale: The patient's BUN is usually elevated with a significant hemorrhage because blood proteins are subjected to bacterial breakdown in the GI tract. With control of bleeding, the BUN will return to normal. During the early stage of bleeding, the hematocrit is not always a reliable indicator of the amount of blood lost or the amount of blood replaced and may be falsely high or low. A urinary output of ≤ 20 mL/hr indicates impaired renal perfusion and hypovolemia, and a urine-specific gravity of 1.030 indicates concentrated urine typical of hypovolemia.

21. a. acute; b. autoimmune atrophic; c. endoscopy or biopsy; d. *Helicobacter pylori*; e. intrinsic factor; f. H_2R blocker, PPI

22. b. Rationale: A nonirritating diet with six small meals a day is recommended to help control the symptoms of gastritis. NSAIDs are often as irritating

to the stomach as aspirin and should not be used in the patient with gastritis. Antacids are often used for control of symptoms but have the best neutralizing effect if taken after meals, and alcohol and caffeine should be entirely eliminated because they may precipitate gastritis.

23. a. D; b. G; c. B; d. D; e. B; f. G; g. G; h. B; i. G; j. G; k. B; l. D
24. a. 2; b. 3; c. 1; d. 4
25. a. Rationale: The ultimate damage to the tissues of the stomach and duodenum, precipitating ulceration, is acid back-diffusion into the mucosa. The gastric mucosal barrier is protective of the mucosa, but without the acid environment and damage, ulceration does not occur. Ammonia formation by *H. pylori* and release of histamine impair the barrier but are not directly responsible for tissue injury.
26. b. Rationale: Back pain is a common manifestation of ulcers located on the posterior aspect of the duodenum and is important for nurses to keep in mind during assessment of the patient, because the more typical epigastric burning and pain may not be present. Duodenal ulcers are more often relieved by food than are gastric ulcers, and when epigastric discomfort occurs, it is lower than that of gastric ulcers. Eating stimulates gastric acid production, increasing discomfort for patients with gastric ulcers, whereas the pain of duodenal ulcers usually occurs several hours after eating.
27. c. Rationale: There is no specific diet used for the treatment of peptic ulcers, and patients are encouraged to eat as normally as possible, eliminating foods that cause discomfort or pain. Eating six meals a day prevents the stomach from being totally empty and is also recommended. Caffeine and alcohol should be eliminated from the diet because they are known to cause gastric irritation, and milk and milk products do not need to be avoided but they can add fat content to the diet.
28. a. Remove stimulation for HCl acid and pepsin secretion by keeping stomach empty
    b. Stop spillage of GI contents into the peritoneal cavity
    c. Remove excess fluids and undigested food from the stomach
29. a. 3; b. 6; c. 4; d. 2; e. 7; f. 3; g. 1; h. 5; i. 3; j. 7
30. c. Rationale: Increased vagal stimulation from emotional stress causes hypersecretion of hydrochloric acid, and stress reduction is an important part of the patient's management of peptic ulcers, especially duodenal ulcers. If side effects to medications develop, the patient should notify the health care provider before altering the drug regimen. Although effective treatment

will promote pain relief in several days, the treatment regimen should be continued until there is evidence that the ulcer has completely healed. Interchanging brands and preparations of antacids and H$_2$-receptor blockers without checking with health care providers may cause harmful side effects, and patients should take only prescribed medications.

31. c. Rationale: Perforation of an ulcer causes sudden, severe abdominal pain that is often referred to the shoulder, accompanied by a rigid, boardlike abdomen and other signs of peritonitis. Vomiting of blood indicates hemorrhage of an ulcer, and gastric outlet obstruction is characterized by projectile vomiting of undigested food, hyperactive stomach sounds, and upper abdominal swelling.
32. a. Rationale: If symptoms of gastric outlet obstruction, such as nausea, vomiting, and stomach distention, occur while the patient is on NPO status or has an NG tube, the patency of the NG tube should be suspected. A recumbent position should not be used in a patient with an outlet obstruction because it increases abdominal pressure on the stomach, and vital sign and circulatory status assessment are important if hemorrhage or perforation is suspected. Deep breathing and relaxation may help some patients with nausea but not when stomach contents are obstructed from flowing into the small intestine.
33. d. Rationale: Abdominal pain that causes the knees to be drawn up and shallow, grunting respirations in a patient with peptic ulcer disease are characteristic of perforation, and the nurse should assess the patient's vital signs and abdomen before notifying the health care provider. Irrigation of the NG tube should not be performed because the additional fluid may be spilled into the peritoneal cavity, and the patient should be placed in a position of comfort, usually on the side with the head slightly elevated.
34. a. 3; b. 4; c. 2; d. 1
35. d. Rationale: Because there is no sphincter control of food taken into the stomach following a Billroth procedure, concentrated food and fluid move rapidly into the small intestine, creating a hypertonic environment that pulls fluid from the bowel wall into the lumen of the intestine, reducing plasma volume and distending the bowel. Postprandial hypoglycemia occurs when the concentrated carbohydrate bolus in the small intestine results in hyperglycemia and the release of excessive amounts of insulin into the circulation, resulting in symptoms of hypoglycemia.
36. a. Rationale: Dietary control of dumping syndrome includes small, frequent meals with low carbohydrate content and elimination of fluids with meals. The patient should also lie down for 30 to

60 minutes after meals. These measures help delay stomach emptying, preventing the rapid movement of a high-carbohydrate food bolus into the small intestine.

37. d. Rationale: If the patient's NG tube becomes obstructed following a gastrectomy with an intestinal anastomosis, gastric secretions may put a strain on the sutured anastomosis and cause serious complications. Because of the danger of perforating the gastric mucosa or disrupting the suture line, the nurse should notify the health care provider if the tube needs to be repositioned or replaced.

38. b. Rationale: A total gastrectomy removes the parietal cells responsible for secreting intrinsic factor necessary for absorption of cobalamin, and lifelong administration of cobalamin is necessary to prevent the development of pernicious anemia. Wound healing is usually impaired in the patient with a total gastrectomy performed for gastric cancer because of impaired nutritional status before surgery. Following a total gastrectomy, the patient also requires diet modifications as a result of dumping syndrome and postprandial hypoglycemia. Peptic ulcers are not a common finding after total gastrectomy.

39. b. Rationale: Food poisoning caused by *Escherichia coli* is characterized by profuse diarrhea, abdominal cramping, and bloody stools and is most often associated with contaminated beef, especially ground beef. Salmonella contamination most often occurs with poultry, staphylococcal infections occur with milk and salad dressings, and botulism occurs with fish and low-acid canned products.

Case Study

1. Infiltration of the gastric wall by a tumor causes epigastric discomfort; growth of the tumor into the gastric lumen can cause anorexia and weight loss.

   Release of substances by cancer cells also contributes to anorexia, nausea, and vomiting. Nausea and vomiting may also be caused if the tumor obstructs the gastric outlet. Fatigue and other symptoms of anemia occur because of chronic blood loss as the lesion erodes through the mucosa.

2. Malnutrition is indicated in S.E. by weight loss, decreased hemoglobin and hematocrit, decreased serum albumin, skin changes and discoloration, and her emaciated appearance.

3. Other factors that may contribute to malnutrition in S.E. include the increased metabolic demands of tumor cells; responses to radiation therapy, such as vomiting, stomatitis, esophagitis, diarrhea, and decreased bone marrow function; and perhaps pernicious anemia resulting from the achlorhydria common with gastric cancer.

4. Malnourished patients do not respond well to radiation therapy, and normal cells do not recover from radiation damage when malnutrition is present. Depletion of protein stores also places S.E. at risk for impaired immune function.

5. A plan for S.E. and her family should include the following:
   - Increasing nutrition with bland, warm, high-calorie, high-protein foods; small, frequent feedings; and nutritional supplements as tolerated
   - Skin care for radiation therapy
   - Anticipatory planning for pain relief and continuing care as she becomes more impaired
   - Discussion of feelings and concerns of S.E. and her family, with explanations of realistic expectations of outcome of her condition

6. In responding to S.E., the nurse should provide accurate information in a way that will decrease her stress and promote her decision-making and coping skills. It is important to tell her that although it is unlikely she will recover from her cancer, the radiation treatment can help shrink the tumor mass, improve her nutritional status, and promote a feeling of well-being. She should be told that her family and health care providers will help her function effectively as long as possible.

7. *Nursing diagnoses:*
   - Imbalanced nutrition: Less than body requirements related to inability to ingest, digest, and absorb nutrients
   - Fatigue related to anemia and effects of radiation therapy
   - Activity intolerance related to generalized weakness
   - Impaired skin integrity related to malnutrition and radiation therapy
   - Ineffective self-health management related to lack of knowledge regarding disease progression
   Collaborative problems:
   Potential complications: Sepsis related to immunosuppression; negative nitrogen balance; organ failure

CHAPTER 43

1. d. Rationale: Antiperistaltic agents, such as loperamide and paregoric, should not be used in infectious diarrhea because of the potential of prolonging exposure to the infectious agent. Demulcent agents may be used to coat and protect mucous membranes in these cases. The other options are all appropriate measures to use in cases of infectious diarrhea.

2. d. Rationale: The first interventions to establish bowel regularity include promoting bowel evacuation at a regular time each day, preferably by placing the

patient on the bedpan, using a bedside commode, or walking the patient to the bathroom. To take advantage of the gastrocolic reflex, an appropriate time is 30 minutes after the first meal of the day or at the patient's usual individual timing. Perianal pouches are used to protect the skin only when regularity cannot be established, and evacuation suppositories are also used only if other techniques are not successful.

3. All the following factors indicate causes of constipation that are responsive to nursing intervention:
   a. Ignoring the urge to defecate causes the muscles and mucosa in the rectal area to become insensitive to the presence of feces, and drying of the stool occurs. The urge to defecate is decreased, and stool becomes more difficult to expel.
   b. Diverticulosis is seen in individuals with low fiber intake, small stool mass, and development of hard stool.
   c. A belief that one must have a daily bowel movement may lead to chronic laxative use and chronic dilation and loss of tone in the colon.
   d. Hemorrhoids are the most common complication of chronic constipation, caused by straining to pass hardened stool. The straining may cause problems in patients with hypertension.
   e. Increased fiber intake without increasing fluids may predispose the patient to impaction or obstruction.

4. c. Rationale: Of the foods listed, dried beans contain the highest amount of dietary fiber and are an excellent source of soluble fiber. Bran and berries also have large amounts of fiber.

5 a. Rationale: Enemas are fast-acting and beneficial in the immediate treatment of acute constipation but should be limited in their use. Bulk-forming medication stimulates peristalsis but take 24 hours to act; stool softeners have a prolonged action, taking up to 72 hours for an effect and fluids can help decrease the incidence of constipation.

6. a. Rationale: The patient with an acute abdomen may have significant fluid or blood loss into the abdomen, and evaluation of blood pressure (BP) and heart rate (HR) should be the first intervention, followed by assessment of the abdomen and the nature of the pain. Analgesics should be used cautiously until a diagnosis can be determined so that symptoms are not masked.

7. a, c, d, f

8. d. Rationale: Adequately functioning NG should prevent nausea and vomiting because stomach contents are continuously being removed. The first intervention in this case is to check the amount and character of the recent drainage and check the tube for patency. Decreased or absent bowel sounds are

expected after a laparotomy, and the Jackson-Pratt drains only fluid from the tissue of the surgical site. Antiemetics may be given if the NG tube is patent because anesthetic agents may cause nausea.

9. a. Rationale: The abdominal pain and distention that occur from the decreased motility of the bowel should be treated with increased ambulation and frequent position changes to increase peristalsis. If the pain is severe, cholinergic drugs, rectal tubes, or application of heat to the abdomen may be ordered. Assessment of bowel sounds is not an intervention to relieve the pain, and a high Fowler's position is not indicated. Opioids may still be necessary for pain control, and motility can be increased by other means.

10. d. Rationale: The patient is having symptoms of an acute abdomen and should be evaluated by a health care provider immediately. The patient's age, location of pain, and other symptoms are characteristic of appendicitis. Heat application and laxatives should not be used in patients with undiagnosed abdominal pain because they may cause perforation of the appendix or other inflammations. Fluids should not be taken until vomiting is controlled, nor should they be taken in the event that surgery may be performed.

11. b. Rationale: Because there is no definite treatment for irritable bowel syndrome (IBS) and patients become frustrated and discouraged with uncontrolled symptoms, it is important to develop a trusting relationship that will support the patient as different treatments are implemented and evaluated. High-fiber diets may help, but they might also increase the bloating and gas pains of IBS. Diagnosis of IBS can be established by Rome criteria and by elimination of other problems. Although IBS can be precipitated and aggravated by stress and emotions, it is not a psychogenic illness. Medications are available but usually used as a last resort because of side effects.

12. a. Rationale: It is likely that the patient could be developing a peritonitis, which could be life-threatening, and assessment of vital signs for hypovolemic shock should be done to report to the health care provider. If an IV line is not in place, it should be inserted, and pain may be eased by flexing the knees.

13. a. *T*; b. *F*, perforation with peritonitis; c. *F*, McBurney's point; d. *T*; e. *T*

14. a. B; b. UC; c. CD; d. B; e. UC; f. CD; g. UC; h. B; i. B; j. B; k. CD; l. B; m. B

15. a. decreased hemoglobin, hematocrit; b. increased BUN, hypernatremia; c. decreased Na, K, Mg, Cl, and bicarbonate; d. elevated WBC

16. c. Rationale: Ulcerative colitis and Crohn's disease have many of the same extraintestinal symptoms, including erythema nodosum and arthritis, as well

as uveitis, conjunctivitis, and gallstones; however, osteoporosis and peptic ulcer disease are specific to ulcerative colitis, and gluten intolerance is more commonly seen in Crohn's disease.

17. a. 2; b. 1, 4; c. 4; d. 6; e. 2; f. 1; g. 5; h. 2; i. 1; j. 4; k. 1

18. a. Rationale: The initial procedure for a total colectomy and ileal reservoir includes a colectomy, rectal mucosectomy, ileal reservoir construction, ileoanal anastomosis, and a temporary ileostomy. The ileostomy is closed in the second surgery after healing from the first surgery is complete. A loop ileostomy is the most common temporary ileostomy, and it is opened the first or second day postoperatively. A rectal tube to suction is not indicated in any of the surgical procedures for ulcerative colitis. A catheter placed in an ileostomy stoma would be expected following a total proctocolectomy with a continent ileostomy (Kock pouch), whereas a permanent ileostomy stoma would be expected following a total proctocolectomy with a permanent ileostomy.

19. a. Rationale: Initial output from a newly formed ileostomy may be as high as 1500 to 2000 mL daily, and intake and output must be accurately monitored for fluid and electrolyte imbalance. Ileostomy bags may need to be emptied every 3 to 4 hours, but the appliance should not be changed for several days unless there is leakage onto the skin. A terminal ileum stoma is permanent, and the entire colon has been removed. A return to a normal, presurgical diet is the goal for the patient with an ileostomy, with restrictions based only on the patient's individual tolerances.

20. a. Rationale: Signs of malnutrition include pallor from anemia, hair loss, bleeding, cracked gingivae, and muscle weakness, which support a nursing diagnosis that identifies impaired nutrition. Diarrhea may contribute to malnutrition but is not a defining characteristic. Anorectal excoriation and pain relate to problems with skin integrity, and the hypotension relates to problems with fluid deficit.

21. a. 3; b. 4; c. 5; d. 2; e. 6; f. 1

22. a. *F*, upper small bowel obstruction; b. *T*; c. *T*; d. *T*; e. *F*, strangulated; f. *F*, mechanical obstruction.

23. b. Rationale: Mouth care should be done very frequently for the patient with a small bowel obstruction who has an NG tube because of vomiting, fecal taste and odor, and mouth breathing. No ice chips are allowed with the NPO of a bowel obstruction. The NG tube should be checked for patency and irrigated as ordered. The position of the patient should be one of comfort.

24. c. Rationale: Although all polyps are abnormal growths, the most common type of polyps (hyperplastic) is non-neoplastic, as are several other types of polyps. However, adenomatous polyps are characterized by neoplastic changes in the epithelium, and most colorectal cancers appear to arise from these polyps. Only patients with a family history of familial adenomatous polyposis have close to a 100% lifetime risk of developing colorectal cancer.

25. a. Rationale: A diet that includes red meat is associated with development of colorectal cancer; smoking, alcohol, or other environmental agents are not known to be related to colorectal cancer.

26. An abdominal incision is made, and the proximal sigmoid colon is brought through the abdominal wall and formed into a colostomy. The patient is repositioned, a perineal incision is made, and the distal sigmoid colon, rectum, and anus are removed through the perineal incision.

27. b. Rationale: A normal new colostomy stoma should appear bright red, have mild to moderate edema, and have a small amount of bleeding or oozing of blood when touched. A purplish stoma indicates inadequate blood supply and should be reported. The colostomy will not have any fecal drainage for 2 to 4 days, but there may be some earlier mucus or serosanguineous drainage. Bowel sounds after extensive bowel surgery will be diminished or absent.

28. d, e. Rationale: The LPN can monitor and record observations related to the drainage and can measure and record the amount. The LPN could also monitor the skin around the stoma for breakdown. LPNs can irrigate a colostomy in a stable patient but this patient is only 2 days postop. The other actions are responsibilities of the RN (teaching, assessing stoma, and developing a care plan).

29. d. Rationale: Sexual dysfunction may result from an abdominal-perineal resection, but the nurse should discuss with the patient that different nerve pathways affect erection, ejaculation, and orgasm and that a dysfunction of one does not mean total sexual dysfunction and also that an alteration in sexual activity does not have to alter sexuality. Simple reassurance of desirability and ignoring concerns about sexual function do not help the patient regain positive feelings of sexuality.

30. a. liquid to semiliquid, constant, extremely irritating to skin, less odor than colostomy
    b. formed, may be able to be regulated with irrigation, least irritating
    c. semiformed, irregular, irritating to skin, foul odor

31. b. Rationale: A nursing diagnosis of disturbed body image is characterized by patients' comments that express shame or an altered image of themselves because of a change in appearance. Although this patient does not yet have the knowledge to care for the colostomy, the primary problem is that the patient cannot or will not yet learn because the colostomy is not acceptable to his image of himself.

32. b. Rationale: Following infusion of the fluid into the stoma, the solution and feces will take about 30 to 45 minutes to return, and the patient can plan to read or perform other quiet activities during the wait time. Between 500 and 1000 mL of warm tap water should be used; a cone tip on the end of the tubing prevents bowel damage that could occur if a stiff plastic catheter is used; and the fluid should be elevated about 18 to 24 inches above the stoma, or about shoulder level, to prevent too-rapid infusion of the solution.

33. c. Rationale: Formation of diverticula is common when decreased bulk of stool, combined with a more narrowed lumen in the sigmoid colon, causes high intraluminal pressures that result in saccular dilation or outpouching of the mucosa through the muscle of the intestinal wall. To prevent the high intraluminal pressure, fecal volume should be increased with use of high-fiber diets and bulk laxatives, such as psyllium hydrophilic mucilloid (Metamucil). Anticholinergic drugs are used only during an acute episode of diverticulitis, and the lesions are not premalignant.

34. a. Rationale: The inflammation and infection of diverticula cause small perforations with spread of the inflammation to the surrounding area in the intestines. Abscesses may form, or complete perforation with peritonitis may occur. Systemic antibiotic therapy is often used, but medicated enemas would increase intestinal motility and increase the possibility of perforation, as would the application of heat. Surgery is indicated when it is necessary to drain abscesses or to resect an obstructing inflammatory mass.

35. a. 6; b. 4; c. 1; d. 5; e. 2; f. 3

36. b. Rationale: Scrotal edema is a common and painful complication after an inguinal hernia repair and can be relieved in part by application of ice and elevation of the scrotum with a scrotal support. Heat would increase the edema and the discomfort, and a truss is used to keep unrepaired hernias from protruding. Coughing is discouraged postoperatively because it increases intraabdominal pressure and stress on the repair site.

37. b. Rationale: The most common type of malabsorption syndrome is lactose intolerance, and it is managed by restricting the intake of milk and milk products. Antibiotics are used in cases of bacterial infections that cause malabsorption, pancreatic enzyme supplementation is used for pancreatic insufficiency, and restriction of gluten is necessary for control of adult celiac disease (nontropical sprue, celiac sprue, gluten-induced enteropathy).

38. c. Rationale: The autoimmune process associated with celiac disease continues as long as the body is exposed to gluten, regardless of the symptoms that it produces, and a lifelong gluten-free diet is necessary. The other statements regarding celiac disease are all true.

39. c. Rationale: Short bowel syndrome results from extensive resection of portions of the small bowel and would occur if a patient had an extensive resection of the ileum. The other conditions primarily affect the large colon and result in fewer and less severe symptoms.

40. a. 5; b. 4; c. 2; d. 1; e. 3

41. d. Rationale: Warm sitz baths provide comfort, healing, and cleaning of the area following all anorectal surgery and may be done three or four times a day for 1 to 2 weeks. Stool softeners may be ordered for several days postoperatively to help keep stools soft for passage, but laxatives may cause irritation and trauma to the anorectal area and are not used postoperatively. Early passage of a bowel movement, although painful, is encouraged to prevent drying and hardening of stool resulting in an even more painful bowel movement.

Case Study

1. Changes in bowel patterns with alternating constipation and diarrhea; changes in stool caliber with ribbon or pencil stools; rectal bleeding; sensation of incomplete evacuation

2. Assess drains placed in the wound and the type and amount of drainage; assess the incision for suture integrity and signs and symptoms of wound infection; assess drainage from the wound for amount, color, and characteristics; warm sitz baths at 100.4° to 106° F for 10 to 20 minutes three to four times a day; pressure-reducing chair cushions for comfort

3. To be able to manage care independently; have normal skin integrity; adjust to altered body image

4. It appears that C.D. is depersonalizing the stoma and, to preserve his body image, is seeing it as something separate from himself with a name and personality of its own.

5. Anxiety, ineffective coping, and fear may influence his tolerance to pain

6. Care of the perineal wound; importance of fluids and diet; care for colostomy, including skin care, odor control, supplies needed, and where to obtain supplies; signs and symptoms of complications to report and when to seek medical care; name and contact for enterostomy nurse; name and address of ostomy association

7. *Nursing diagnoses:*
   • Disturbed body image related to presence of stoma
   • Acute pain related to surgical incisions and inadequate pain-control measures
   • Risk for impaired skin integrity related to stoma drainage and open perineal wound
   Collaborative problems:
   Potential complications: Perineal infection; stomal necrosis, retraction, prolapse, obstruction

CHAPTER 44

1. a. obstructive; both conjugated and unconjugated
   b. increased breakdown of red blood cells; unconjugated (indirect)
   c. hepatocellular; both conjugated and unconjugated
2. a. 3; b. 5; c. 4; d. 2; e. 3; f. 1; g. 2; h. 1; i. 5; j. 1
3. a. hepatitis B surface antigen (HBsAg), Anti-HBs;
   b. hepatitis B early antigen (HBeAg), Anti-HBe;
   c. hepatitis B core antigen (HBcAg), Anti-HBc IgM and Anti-HBc IgG
4. a. hepatitis B virus (HBV) DNA; b. anti-HBs; c. anti-HBc IgG; d. HbsAg; e. anti-hepatitis A virus (HAV) IgM, anti-HAV IgG; f. anti-HDV; g. anti-hepatitis C virus (HCV); h. HCV RNA; i. recombinant immunoblot assay (RIBA)
5. d. Rationale: The systemic manifestations of rash, angioedema, arthritis, fever, and malaise in viral hepatitis are caused by the activation of the complement system by circulating immune complexes. Liver manifestations include jaundice from hepatic cell damage and cholestasis as well as anorexia perhaps caused by toxins produced by the damaged liver. Impaired portal circulation usually does not occur in uncomplicated viral hepatitis but would be a liver manifestation.
6. c. Rationale: Incubation symptoms occur before the onset of jaundice and include a variety of gastrointestinal (GI) symptoms as well as discomfort and heaviness in the upper right quadrant of the abdomen. Pruritus, dark urine, and light-colored stools occur with the onset of jaundice in the acute phase.
7. d. Rationale: Although fulminant hepatitis can occur with hepatitis A and hepatitis C, it is more common in hepatitis B, especially in hepatitis B infection accompanied by infection with hepatitis D virus (HDV).
8. a. hepatitis B vaccine (Recombivax HB or Engerix-B)
   b. hepatitis B immune globulin (HBIG) and hepatitis B vaccine
9. d. Rationale: Individuals who have been exposed to hepatitis A through household contact or foodborne outbreaks should be given immune globulin within 1 to 2 weeks of exposure to prevent or modify the illness. Hepatitis A vaccine is used to provide preexposure immunity to the virus and is indicated for individuals at high risk for hepatitis A exposure. Although hepatitis A can be spread by sexual contact, the risk is higher for transmission with the oral-fecal route.
10. a. Rationale: No specific drugs are effective in treating acute viral hepatitis, although supportive drugs, such as antiemetics, sedatives, or antipruritics, may be used for symptom control. Antiviral agents, such as lamivudine or ribavirin, and α-interferon may be used for treating chronic hepatitis B or C.
11. b. Rationale: The patient with hepatitis B is infectious for 4 to 6 months, and precautions to prevent transmission through percutaneous and sexual contact should be maintained until tests for HbsAg are negative. Close contact does not have to be avoided, but close contacts of the patient should be vaccinated. Alcohol should not be used for at least a year, and rest with increasing activity during convalescence is recommended.
12. a. Rationale: Adequate nutrition is especially important in promoting regeneration of liver cells, but the anorexia of viral hepatitis is often severe, requiring creative and innovative nursing interventions. Strict bed rest is not usually required, and the patient usually has only minor discomfort with hepatitis. Diversional activities may be required to promote psychologic rest but not during periods of fatigue.
13. c. Rationale: Immunosuppressive agents are indicated in hepatitis associated with immune disorders to decrease liver damage caused by autoantibodies. Autoimmune hepatitis is similar to viral hepatitis in presenting signs and symptoms and may become chronic and lead to cirrhosis.
14. a. 5; b. 3; c. 6; d. 3; e. 7; f. 8; g. 2; h. 4; i. 3; j. 1
15. a. Scarring and nodular changes in liver lead to compression of the veins and sinusoids, causing resistance of blood flow through the liver from the portal vein.
    b. Development of collateral channels of circulation in inelastic, fragile esophageal veins as a result of portal hypertension.
16. a. decreased albumin production
    b. decreased, decreased, decreased
    c. decreased, aldosterone, antidiuretic hormone (ADH)
    d. peripheral edema
    e. aldosterone
    f. hypoalbuminemia, hypokalemia (from hyperaldosteronism)
17. b. Rationale: Serum bilirubin, both direct and indirect, would be expected to be increased in cirrhosis. Serum albumin and cholesterol are decreased, and liver enzymes, such as AST and ALT, are elevated.
18. a. Helps to promote diuresis and fluid excretion and may enable the liver to restore itself
    b. Increases plasma colloid osmotic pressure and maintains intravascular volume and kidney perfusion
    c. Increases fluid loss through the kidneys and mobilizes peritoneal fluid; spironolactone (Aldactone) blocks effects of the excess aldosterone
    d. Decreases intake of fluid-retaining sodium
    e. Is temporary measure to relieve impaired respiration or pain of severe ascites
    f. Shunts peritoneal fluid from the abdomen to the venous system, decreasing ascites and improving hemodynamic factors.

19. d. Rationale: Early signs of this neurologic condition include euphoria, depression, apathy, irritability, confusion, agitation, drowsiness, and lethargy. Loss of consciousness is usually preceded by asterixis, disorientation, hyperventilation, hypothermia, and alterations in reflexes. Increasing oliguria is a sign of hepatorenal syndrome.

20. a. Reduction of ammonia formation by decreasing absorption of ammonia from bowel
    b. Reduction of ammonia formation by reducing bacterial flora that produce ammonia
    c. Reduction of ammonia formation by removing red blood cells as a source of protein

21. b. Rationale: The patient with advanced, complicated cirrhosis requires a high-calorie, high-carbohydrate diet with moderate to low fat. Patients with cirrhosis are at risk for edema and ascites and their sodium intake should be limited. The tomato sandwich with salt-free butter best meets these requirements. Rough foods, such as popcorn, may irritate the esophagus and stomach and lead to bleeding. Peanut butter is high in sodium and fat, and canned chicken noodle soup is very high in sodium.

22. c. Rationale: Bleeding esophageal varices are a medical emergency. During an episode of bleeding, management of the airway and prevention of aspiration of blood are critical factors. Occult blood as well as fresh blood from the GI tract would be expected and is not tested. Vasopressin causes vasoconstriction, decreased heart rate, and decreased coronary blood flow; nitroglycerin is given with the vasopressin to counter these side effects. Portal shunting surgery is performed for esophageal varices but not during an acute hemorrhage.

23. d. Rationale: By shunting fluid sequestered in the peritoneum into the venous system, pressure on esophageal veins is decreased, and more volume is returned to the circulation, improving CO and renal perfusion. However, because ammonia is diverted past the liver, hepatic encephalopathy continues. These procedures do not prolong life or promote liver function.

24. c. Rationale: Abstinence from alcohol is very important in alcoholic cirrhosis and may result in improvement if started when liver damage is limited. Although further liver damage may be reduced by rest and nutrition, most changes in the liver cannot be reversed. Exercise does not promote portal circulation, and very moderate exercise is recommended. Acetaminophen should not be used by the patient with liver disease because it is potentially hepatotoxic.

25. c. Rationale: Because the prognosis for cancer of the liver is poor, and treatment is largely palliative, supportive nursing care is appropriate. The patient exhibits clinical manifestations of liver failure, as seen in any patient with advanced liver failure. Whether the cancer is primary or metastatic, there is usually a poor response to chemotherapy, and surgery is indicated only in the few patients that have localization of the tumor to one portion of the liver.

26. d. Rationale: Liver transplantation is indicated for patients with cirrhosis as well as for many adults and children with other irreversible liver diseases. Although health care providers make the decisions regarding the patient's qualifications for transplant, nurses should be knowledgeable about the indications for transplantation and be able to discuss the patient's questions and concerns related to transplantation. Rejection is less of a problem in liver transplants than in kidney or heart transplantation.

27. a. 2; b. 5; c. 3; d. 1; e. 4

28. c. Rationale: The predominant symptom of acute pancreatitis is severe, deep abdominal pain that is usually located in the left upper quadrant (LUQ) but may be in the midepigastrium. Bowel sounds are decreased or absent, temperature is elevated only slightly, and the patient has hypovolemia and may manifest symptoms of shock.

29. b. Rationale: Although serum lipase levels and urinary amylase levels are increased, an increased serum amylase level is the criterion most commonly used to diagnose acute pancreatitis. Serum calcium levels are decreased.

30. c. Rationale: Pancreatic rest and suppression of secretions are promoted by preventing any gastric contents from entering the duodenum, which would stimulate pancreatic activity. Surgery is not indicated for acute pancreatitis but may be used to drain abscesses or cysts. An ERCP pancreatic sphincterotomy may be performed when pancreatitis is related to gallstones. Pancreatic enzymes are necessary in chronic pancreatitis if a deficiency in secretion occurs.

31. c. Rationale: Positions that flex the trunk and draw the knees up to the abdomen help relieve the pain of acute pancreatitis, and positioning the patient on the side with the head elevated decreases abdominal tension. Diversional techniques are not as helpful as positioning in controlling the pain. The patient is usually NPO because food intake increases the pain and inflammation. Bed rest is indicated during the acute attack because of hypovolemia and pain.

32. c. Rationale: Sodium restriction is not indicated for patients recovering from acute pancreatitis, but the stools should be observed for steatorrhea, indicating that fat digestion is impaired, and glucose levels should also be monitored for indication of impaired β-cell function. Alcohol is a primary cause of pancreatitis and should not be used.

33. c. Rationale: Chronic damage to the pancreas causes pancreatic exocrine and endocrine insufficiency, resulting in a deficiency of digestive enzymes and insulin. Malabsorption and diabetes often result. Abstinence from alcohol is necessary in both types

of pancreatitis, as is a high-carbohydrate, high-protein, and low-fat diet. Although abdominal pain is a major manifestation of chronic pancreatitis, more commonly a heavy, gnawing feeling occurs.

34. a, b, c. Rationale: Measures to prevent attacks of pancreatitis are those that decrease the stimulation of the pancreas. Lower fat intake and foods that are less stimulating/irritating (bland) should be encouraged. Higher carbohydrates are less stimulating. Avoid alcohol and nicotine, since both stimulate the pancreas. Monitor for steatorrhea, since it may indicate worsening pancreatic function. Pancreatic enzymes should be taken with, not after, meals.

35. b. Rationale: Major risk factors for pancreatic cancer are believed to be cigarette smoking, high-fat diet, diabetes, and exposure to benzidine and cocaine. It is not associated with alcohol intake, as pancreatitis is.

36. a. duodenum; b. proximal pancreas; c. partial gastrectomy; d. distal segment common bile duct; e. pancreatic duct to jejunum; f. common bile duct to jejunum; g. stomach to jejunum

37. a. *T*; b. *F*, cholesterol; c. *T*; d. *T*

38. a, c, d, g, h

39. a. Obstruction of the common duct prevents bile drainage into the duodenum, with congestion of bile in the liver and subsequent absorption into the blood
    b. Absence of bile in the intestine
    c. Soluble bilirubin in the blood excreted into the urine
    d. Absence of bile salts in duodenum, preventing fat emulsion and digestion
    e. Contraction of the inflamed gallbladder and obstructed ducts, stimulated by cholecystokinin when fats enter the duodenum

40. a. Rationale: Ultrasonography is 90% to 95% accurate in detecting gallstones and is a noninvasive procedure. Liver-function tests will be elevated if liver damage has occurred but do not indicate gallbladder disease. An IV cholangiogram uses radiopaque dye to outline the gallbladder and the ducts.

41. a. Prevents gallbladder stimulation by food or fluids moving into the duodenum
    b. Inflammation of the gallbladder may be caused by bacterial infection or lead to bacterial colonization.
    c. Counteracts smooth muscle spasms of the bile ducts

42. a. 2; b. 1; c. 3; d. 4

43. c. Rationale: The laparoscopic cholecystectomy requires four small abdominal incisions to visualize and remove the gallbladder, and the patient has small dressings placed over these incisions. The patient with an incisional cholecystectomy is usually hospitalized 3 to 5 days, whereas the laparoscopic procedure allows same- or next-day discharge with return to work in 2 to 3 days. A T-tube is placed in the common bile duct after exploration of the duct during an incisional cholecystectomy.

44. c. Rationale: After removal of the gallbladder, bile drains directly from the liver into the duodenum, and a low-fat diet is recommended until adjustment to this change occurs. Most patients tolerate a regular diet with moderate fats but should avoid excessive fats, as large volumes of bile previously stored in the gallbladder are not available, and steatorrhea could occur with a large fat intake.

45. a. Rationale: The T-tube drains bile from the common bile duct until swelling from trauma has subsided and bile can freely enter the duodenum. The tube is placed to gravity drainage and should be kept open and free from kinks to prevent bile from backing up into the liver. The tube is not normally irrigated.

46. c. Rationale: Bile-colored drainage or pus from any incision may indicate an infection and should be reported to the health care provider immediately. The bandages on the puncture sites should be removed the day after surgery, followed by bathing or showering. Referred shoulder pain is a common and expected problem following laparoscopic procedures, when carbon dioxide used to inflate the abdominal cavity is not readily absorbed by the body. Nausea and vomiting are not expected postoperatively and may indicate damage to other abdominal organs and should be reported to the health care provider.

Case Study

1. Some etiologic factor causes injury to pancreatic cells or activation of the pancreatic enzymes in the pancreas rather than in the intestine, and the activated enzymes digest the pancreas itself, a process known as autodigestion. Activated trypsin can digest the protein of the pancreas and activate elastase and phospholipase. Elastase causes hemorrhage by dissolving the elastic fibers of blood vessels, and phospholipase A causes fat necrosis. The pancreas may be merely edematous, or it may become necrotic.

2. Alcohol abuse and gallbladder disease

3. The serum and urinary amylase levels are elevated, indicating release of these enzymes into the blood circulating through the pancreas. The white blood cell (WBC) count is high, indicating marked inflammation. The blood glucose level is elevated, indicating impairment of insulin production and release by the β cells. The decreased calcium indicates hypocalcemia, a sign of severe pancreatitis.

4. Hypocalcemia occurs in part because calcium combines with fatty acids released during fat necrosis of the pancreas. The nurse should observe for symptoms of tetany, such as jerking, irritability, muscular twitching, and positive Chvostek's and Trousseau's signs. Numbness or tingling around the lips and in the fingers is an early indicator of hypocalcemia.

5. The pain is usually located in the LUQ but may be in the midepigastric area and frequently radiates to the back.

It has a sudden onset and is described as severe, deep, piercing, and continuous. It is aggravated by eating and often begins when the patient is recumbent. It is not relieved by vomiting and may be accompanied by flushing, cyanosis, and dyspnea.

6. Hypovolemia, shock, and the local complications of pseudocysts and abscesses

7. Morphine, for pain relief; ranitidine, to decrease hydrochloric acid production by the stomach because the hydrochloric acid stimulates pancreatic activity

8. NPO status and suction with an NG tube prevent gastric contents from entering the duodenum and stimulating pancreatic secretion.

9. *Nursing diagnoses:*
   - Acute pain related to distention of the pancreas and peritoneal irritation
   - Deficient fluid volume related to nausea, vomiting, NG suction, restricted oral intake
   - Impaired oral mucous membrane related to NG tube and NPO status
   - Imbalanced nutrition: Less than body requirements related to dietary restrictions, nausea and vomiting, impaired digestion
   Collaborative problems:
   Potential complications: Hypovolemia/shock; hypocalcemia; hyperglycemia; fluid and electrolyte imbalance

CHAPTER 45

1. a. adrenal gland; b. right renal artery; c. right renal vein; d. vena cava; e. bladder; f. urethra; g. ureter; h. aorta; i. kidney; j. pyramid; k. papilla; l. renal pelvis; m. ureter; n. cortex; o. medulla; p. major calyx; q. minor calyx; r. fibrous capsule

2. a. 4; b. 1; c. 2, 5; d. 2, 3; e. 1; f. 5; g. 2; h. 2, 5; i. 5; j. 2; k. 5

3. a. *T*; b. *F*, regulate the volume and composition of extracellular fluid; c. *T*; d. *F*, high antidiuretic hormone (ADH) or renin or angiotensin II; e. *T*; f. *T*

4. a. Rationale: Renin is released in response to decreased arterial blood pressure (BP), renal ischemia, eosinophil chemotactic factor (ECF) depletion, and other factors affecting blood supply to the kidney. It is the catalyst of the renin-angiotensin-aldosterone system, which raises BP when stimulated. ADH is secreted by the posterior pituitary in response to serum hyperosmolality and low blood volume. Aldosterone is secreted within the renin-angiotensin system only after stimulation by angiotensin II, and kidney prostaglandins lower BP by causing vasodilation.

5. a. Rationale: Erythropoietin is released when the oxygen tension of the renal blood supply is low and stimulates production of red blood cells in the bone marrow. Hypotension causes activation of the renin-angiotensin-aldosterone system, as well as release of ADH. Hyperkalemia stimulates the release of

aldosterone from the adrenal cortex, and fluid overload does not directly stimulate factors affecting the kidney.

6. a. ureteropelvic junction and ureterovesical junction; b. ureterovesical junction; c. 200 to 250; d. 600, 1000; e. urothelium

7. a. Rationale: The short urethra of women allows easier ascension and colonization of bacteria in the bladder than occurs in men. Relaxation of pelvic floor muscles may contribute to stress and urge incontinence but is not associated with urinary tract infections (UTIs). The bladder capacity of men and women is the same, and the muscular support at the rhabdosphincter in men increases the risk for stricture at this point.

8. d. Rationale: The decreased ability to concentrate urine results in an increased volume of dilute urine, which does not maintain the usual diurnal elimination pattern. A decrease in bladder capacity also contributes to nocturia, but decreased bladder muscle tone results in urinary retention. Decreased renal mass decreases renal reserve, but function is generally adequate under normal circumstances.

9. a. Smoking history, history of exposure to carcinogenic and nephrotoxic chemicals, family history of kidney disease, geographic residence
   b. Low fluid intake or loss of fluids, high calcium and purine intake, coffee intake, weight gain resulting from fluid retention
   c. Change in appearance and amount of urine, change in urinary patterns, necessary assistance in emptying bladder
   d. Change in energy level, sedentary lifestyle, urine leakage during activity
   e. Sleep deprivation from nocturia
   f. Pain in flank, groin, suprapubic area; dysuria; absence of pain with other urinary symptoms; cognitive impairment affecting continence
   g. Decreased self-esteem and body image because of urinary problems
   h. Problems maintaining job and social relationships
   i. Change in sexual pleasure or performance
   j. Withdrawal or ineffective coping with incontinence or urinary problem
   k. Any treatment decisions that are affected by value system

10. c. Rationale: To assess for kidney tenderness, the nurse strikes the fist of one hand over the dorsum of the other hand at the posterior costovertebral angle. The upper abdominal quadrants and costovertebral angles are auscultated for vascular bruits in the renal vessels and aorta, and an empty bladder is not palpable. The kidneys are palpated through the abdomen, with the patient supine.

11. Word Search. a. Hematuria; b. Oliguria; c. Stress incontinence; d. Micturition; e. Pneumaturia; f. Enuresis; g. Dysuria; h. Anuria; i. Nocturia; j. Retention; k. Incontinence; l. Frequency; m. Polyuria; n. Hesitancy

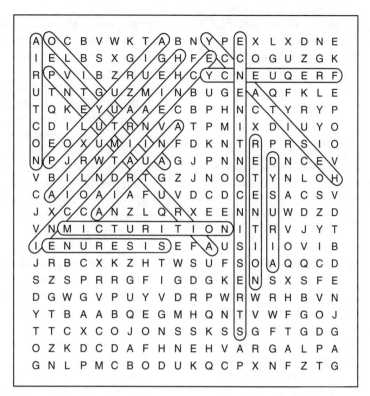

12. b. Rationale: Bacteria in warm urine specimens multiply rapidly, and false or unreliable bacterial counts may occur with old urine. Glucose, specific gravity, and WBCs do not change in urine specimens, but pH becomes more alkaline, RBCs are hemolyzed, and casts may disintegrate.

13. b. Rationale: Cloudiness from a fresh urine specimen, WBC count above 5/high-power field (hpf), and the presence of casts are all indicative of UTI, and pH is usually elevated because bacteria split the urea in urine into alkaline ammonia. Cloudy, brown urine usually indicates hematuria or the presence of bile, and colorless urine is usually very dilute. Option "a" is normal.

14. a. Rationale: A urine specific gravity of 1.002 is low, indicating dilute urine and the excretion of excess fluid. Fluid overload, diuretics, or lack of ADH can cause dilute urine. Normal urine specific gravity is 1.003 to 1.030. A high specific gravity indicates concentrated urine that would be seen in dehydration.

15. d. Rationale: During a renal arteriogram, a catheter is inserted, most commonly at the femoral artery, and following the procedure the patient is positioned with the affected leg extended with a pressure dressing applied. Peripheral pulse monitoring is essential to detect the development of thrombi around the insertion site, which may occlude blood supply to the leg. Gross bleeding in the urine is a complication of a renal biopsy. Allergy to the contrast medium should be established before the procedure, but the medium can be nephrotoxic, and renal function should be monitored after the procedure.

16. b. Rationale: The BUN is increased in renal problems but may also be increased when there is rapid or extensive tissue damage from other causes. Serum creatinine is more specific to renal function and does not vary with other tissue damage.

17. d. Rationale: The rate at which creatinine is cleared from the blood and eliminated in the urine approximates the glomerular filtration rate (GFR) and is the most specific test of renal function. The renal scan is useful in showing the location, size, and shape of the kidney and general blood perfusion.

18. a. Impaired conversion of inactive vitamin D to active vitamin D results in poor calcium absorption from the bowel, resulting in a hypocalcemia.
    b. Loss of cells that produce erythropoietin results in no stimulation of bone marrow to produce RBCs.
    c. This serum creatinine level is high, indicating the loss of tubular secretion (passage of substances from the blood into the tubule) by the kidney.

19. b. Rationale: Bleeding from the kidney following a biopsy is the most serious complication of the procedure, and urine must be examined for both gross and microscopic blood, in addition to vital signs and hematocrit levels being monitored. Following a cystoscopy, the patient may have

burning with urination, and warm sitz baths may be used. Urinary infections are a complication of any procedure requiring instrumentation of the bladder.

20. a. 5; b. 6; c. 8; d. 9; e. 7; f. 4; g. 3; h. 1; i. 6; j. 3; k. 2; l. 3; m. 7

CHAPTER 46

1. a. 4; b. 6; c. 3; d. 1; e. 2; f. 7; g. 5
2. c. Rationale: The usual classic symptoms of UTI are often absent in older adults, who tend to experience nonlocalized abdominal pain rather than dysuria and suprapubic pain. They may also experience cognitive impairment characterized by confusion or decreased level of consciousness.
3. d. Rationale: Unless a patient has a history of recurrent UTIs or a complicated UTI, TMP-SMX or nitrofurantoin (Macrodantin) is usually used to empirically treat an initial UTI without a culture and sensitivity or other testing. Asymptomatic bacteriuria does not justify treatment, but symptomatic UTIs should always be treated.
4. b. Rationale: The bladder should be emptied at least every 2 to 3 hours. Fluid intake should be increased to about 2000 mL/day without caffeine, alcohol, citrus juices, and chocolate drinks because they are potential bladder irritants. Cleaning the urinary meatus with an antiinfective agent after voiding will irritate the meatus, but the perineal area should be wiped from front to back after urination and defecation to prevent fecal contamination of the meatus.
5. c. Rationale: Ascending infections from the bladder to the kidney are prevented by the normal anatomy and physiology of the urinary tract unless a preexisting condition, such as bladder tumors, prostatic hyperplasia, strictures, or stones, is present. Resistance to antibiotics and failure to take a full prescription of antibiotics for a UTI usually result in relapse or reinfection of the lower urinary tract.
6. a. Rationale: Systemic symptoms of fever and chills with leukocytosis and nausea and vomiting are more common in pyelonephritis than in cystitis, and local symptoms of bladder involvement may or may not be present. Either patient may have a knowledge deficit regarding prevention of recurrence.
7. a. *F*, chronic; b. *T*; c. *T*; d. *F*, urine culture; e. *T*
8. d. Rationale: The symptoms of interstitial cystitis imitate those of an infection of the bladder, but the urine is free of infectious agents. Unlike a bladder infection, the pain with interstitial cystitis increases as urine collects in the bladder and is temporarily relieved by urination. Acidic urine is very irritating to the bladder in interstitial cystitis, and the bladder is small, but urinary retention is not common.
9. d. Rationale: Calcium glycerophosphate (Prelief) alkalinizes the urine and can help relieve the irritation from acidic foods. A diet low in acidic foods is recommended, and if a multivitamin is used,

high-potency vitamins should be avoided because these products may irritate the bladder. A voiding diary is useful in diagnosis but does not need to be kept indefinitely.

10. d. Rationale: Glomerulonephritis is not an infection but rather an antibody-induced injury to the glomerulus, where either autoantibodies against the glomerular basement membrane (GBM) directly damage the tissue, or antibodies reacting with nonglomerular antigens are randomly deposited as immune complexes along the GBM. Prior infection by bacteria or viruses may stimulate the antibody production but is not present or active at the time of glomerular damage.
11. d. Rationale: An elevated blood urea nitrogen (BUN) indicates that the kidneys are not clearing nitrogenous wastes from the blood, and protein may be restricted until the kidney recovers. Proteinuria indicates loss of protein from the blood and possibly a need for increased protein intake. Hypertension is treated with sodium and fluid restriction, diuretics, and antihypertensive drugs. The hematuria is not specifically treated.
12. a. Rationale: Most patients recover completely from acute poststreptococcal glomerulonephritis (APSGN) with supportive treatment. Chronic glomerulonephritis that progresses insidiously over years and rapidly progressive glomerulonephritis that results in renal failure within weeks or months occur in only a few patients with APSGN. In Goodpasture syndrome, antibodies are present against both the GBM and the alveolar basement membrane of the lungs, and dysfunction of both kidney and lung is present.
13. c. Rationale: The massive proteinuria that results from increased glomerular membrane permeability in nephrotic syndrome leaves the blood without adequate proteins (hypoalbuminemia) to create an oncotic colloidal pressure to hold fluid in the vessels. Without oncotic pressure, fluid moves into the interstitium, causing severe edema. Hypercoagulability occurs in nephrotic syndrome but is not a factor in edema formation, and GFR is not necessarily affected in nephrotic syndrome.
14. c. Rationale: Both humoral and cellular immune responses are altered in nephrotic syndrome, and infection is a serious complication. Skin integrity is at risk from massive edema, and hypercoagulability increases the risk for thrombosis. The elevated serum cholesterol level characteristic of nephrotic syndrome results from increased hepatic synthesis and not dietary intake.
15. a. 7; b. 4; c. 1; d. 5; e. 9; f. 2; g. 6; h. 3; i. 8
16. Crossword Puzzle
    Across: 7. Urethral diverticula; 10. Urosepsis
    Down: 1. Vesicoureteral reflux; 2. Goodpasture syndrome; 3. Pyelonephritis; 4. Urethritis; 5. Interstitial cystitis; 6. Glomerulonephritis; 8. Renal tuberculosis; 9. Cystitis

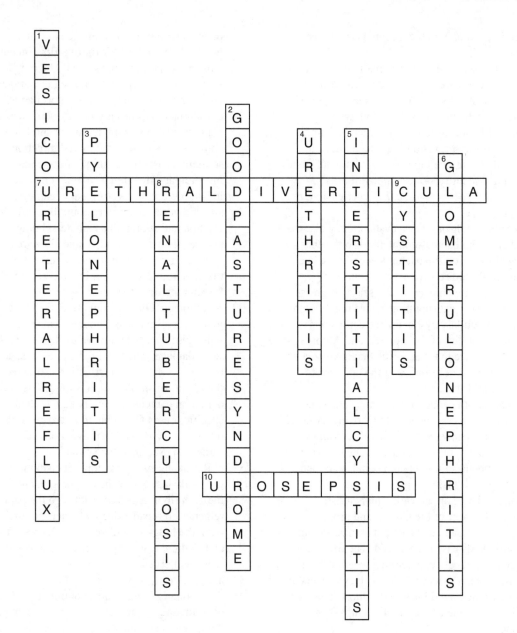

17. c. Rationale: Because crystallization of stone constituents can precipitate and unite to form a stone when in supersaturated concentrations, one of the best ways to prevent stones of any type is by drinking adequate fluids to keep the urine dilute and flowing, which is an output of about 2 L of urine a day. Sedentary lifestyle is a risk factor for renal stones, but exercise also causes fluid loss and a need for additional fluids. Protein foods high in purine should be restricted only for the small percentage of patients with uric acid stones, and although UTIs contribute to stone formation, prophylactic antibiotics are not indicated.

18. a. 3; b. 5; c. 2; d. 1; e. 3; f. 4; g. 5; h. 1; i. 3; j. 4; k. 2

19. c. Rationale: A classic sign of the passage of a calculus down the ureter is intense, colicky back pain that may radiate into the testicles, labia, or groin and may be accompanied by mild shock with cool, moist skin. Stones obstructing a calyx or at the ureteropelvic junction may produce dull costovertebral flank pain, and large bladder stones may cause bladder fullness and lower obstructive symptoms. Many patients with renal stones do not have a history of chronic UTIs.

20. d. Rationale: Currently it is believed that high dietary calcium intake may actually lower the risk for renal stones by reducing the urinary excretion of oxalate, and oxalate-rich foods should be limited to reduce oxalate excretion. Foods high in oxalate include spinach, rhubarb, asparagus, cabbage, and tomatoes, in addition to chocolate, coffee, and cocoa. Milk, milk products, dried beans, and dried fruits are high sources of calcium, and organ meats

are high in purine, which contributes to uric acid lithiasis.

21. b. Rationale: A high fluid intake maintains dilute urine, which decreases bacterial concentration in addition to washing stone fragments and expected blood through the urinary system following lithotripsy. Moist heat to the flank may be helpful to relieve muscle spasms during renal colic, and all urine should be strained in patients with renal stones to collect and identify stone composition.

22. a. *T*; b. *F*, antihypertensives; c. *F*, hypertension; d. *F*, anticoagulants; e. *T*

23. b. Rationale: Adult-onset polycystic kidney disease is an inherited autosomal-dominant disorder that often manifests after the patient has children, but the children should receive genetic counseling regarding their life choices. The disease progresses slowly, eventually causing progressive renal failure. Hereditary medullary cystic disease causes poor concentration ability of the kidneys, and Alport's syndrome is a hereditary nephritis that is associated with deafness and deformities of the optic lens.

24. a. 2; b. 3; c. 5; d. 1; e. 4

25. a. Rationale: Both cancer of the kidney and cancer of the bladder are associated with smoking. A family history of renal cancer is a risk factor for kidney cancer, and cancer of the bladder has been associated with use of phenacetin-containing analgesics and recurrent upper UTIs.

26. c. Rationale: There are no early characteristic symptoms of cancer of the kidney, and gross hematuria, flank pain, and a palpable mass do not occur until the disease is advanced. The treatment of choice is a radical nephrectomy, which can be successful in early disease. Many kidney cancers are diagnosed as incidental imaging findings. The most common sites of metastases are the lungs, liver, and long bones.

27. b. Rationale: Sitz baths following local bladder surgery promote muscle relaxation and reduce urinary retention. Fluids should be increased to dilute blood in the urine and prevent clots. Irritative bladder symptoms most commonly occur with local instillation of chemotherapeutic agents, and urinary catheterization is not usually necessary with laser photocoagulation.

28. a. 2; b. 1; c. 1; d. 4; e. 2; f. 1; g. 5; h. 3; i. 4; j. 2; k. 3; l. 1

29. a. Urge; relaxes bladder tone and increases sphincter tone, decreasing unwanted contractions
    b. Overflow; reduce urethral sphincter resistance to urine flow

30. c. Rationale: Pelvic floor exercises (Kegel exercises) increase the tone of the urethral sphincters and should be done in sets of 10 or more contractions four to five times a day (total of 40-50 per day). Frequent bladder emptying is recommended for patients with urge incontinence and an increase in pressure on the bladder for overflow incontinence. Absorptive perineal pads should be only a temporary measure because long-term use discourages continence and can lead to skin problems.

31. c. Rationale: All urinary catheters in hospitalized patients pose a very high risk for infection, especially antibiotic-resistant, nosocomial infections, and scrupulous aseptic technique is essential in the insertion and maintenance of all catheters. Routine irrigations are not performed. Cleaning the insertion site with soap and water should be performed for urethral and suprapubic catheters, but lotion or powder should be avoided, and site care for other catheters may require special interventions. Turning the patient to promote drainage is recommended only for suprapubic catheters.

32. b. Rationale: Output from ureteral catheters must be monitored every 1 to 2 hours because an obstruction will cause overdistention of the kidney pelvis and renal damage. The renal pelvis has a capacity of only 3 to 5 mL, and if irrigation is ordered, no more than 5 mL of sterile saline is used. The patient with a ureteral catheter is usually kept on bed rest until specific orders for ambulation are given. Suprapubic tubes may be milked to prevent obstruction of the catheter by sediment and clots.

33. b. Rationale: A nephrectomy incision is usually in the flank, just below the diaphragm, and occasionally the 12th rib is removed. Although the patient is reluctant to breathe deeply because of incisional pain, the lungs should be clear. Decreased sounds and shallow respirations are abnormal and would require intervention.

34. a. 2; b. 3; c. 1; d. 4

35. d. Rationale: Urine drains continuously from an ileal conduit, and the drainage bag must be emptied every 2 to 3 hours and measured to ensure adequate urinary output. With an ileal conduit, mucus is present in the urine because it is secreted by the ileal segment as a result of the irritating effect of the urine, but the surgery causes paralytic ileus, and the patient will be NPO for several days postoperatively. Fitting for a permanent appliance is not done until the stoma shrinks to its normal size in several weeks. Self-catheterization is performed when patients have formation of a continent Kock pouch.

36. b. Rationale: Because the stoma continuously drains urine, a wick formed of a rolled-up 4 × 4 gauze or a tampon is held against the stoma to absorb the urine while the skin is cleaned and a new appliance is attached. The skin is cleaned with warm water only because soap and other agents cause drying and irritation, and clean, not sterile, technique is used. The appliance should be left in place as long as possible before it loosens and allows leakage onto the skin, perhaps up to 14 days.

37. b, e, f. Rationale: An RN should perform the assessments, teaching, and determination of incontinence type. An LPN/LVN could perform the bladder scan or insert an indwelling catheter in an uncomplicated patient once taught the skill and known to be competent. In long-term care and rehabilitation facilities NAP may use bladder scans after they are trained.

Case Study

1. The Jewett-Strong-Marshall classification of bladder cancer identifies the tumor as superficial (CIS, O, A), invasive (B1, B2, C), or metastatic (D1-D4). The A classification for P.G. indicates that the tumor is superficial with submucosal involvement. The TNM grading system indicates the characteristics of the tumor (T), the nodal involvement (N), and the presence of distant metastasis (M). (See Chapter 16 for TNM classification.)

2. The drug will be instilled into the bladder and needs to be retained for about 2 hours. His position will be changed about every 15 minutes to ensure that the drug comes into maximum contact with all areas of the bladder, especially the dome. He may have irritative symptoms, such as frequency, urgency, and bladder spasms, in addition to hematuria during the weeks of treatment. BCG therapy may cause flulike symptoms or systemic infection, but the usual side effects of cancer chemotherapy are not experienced with BCG therapy or with intravesical chemotherapy. BCG stimulates the immune system rather than directly destroying cancer cells.

3. Stop smoking—it is the only significant risk factor in his history.

4. Follow-up is essential to evaluate the effectiveness of the treatment and detect any new tumors while they are in a superficial stage.

5. A cystectomy with urinary diversion would be indicated.

6. *Nursing diagnoses:*
   - Anxiety related to unknown outcome
   - Impaired urinary elimination related to effects of treatment
   - Acute pain related to effects of treatment
   - Risk for infection related to effects of treatment
   Collaborative problem:
   Potential complication: Bladder injury

CHAPTER 47

1. a. 1; b. 3; c. 1; d. 3; e. 2; f. 1; g. 3; h. 2; i. 3; j. 1; k. 2; l. 1
2. a. renal ischemia; nephrotoxic injury or sepsis
   b. basement membrane; tubular epithelium
   c. tubular epithelium; tubules
   d. basement membrane
3. **R**isk
   Injury
   Failure
   Loss
   End-stage kidney disease

4. d. Rationale: In prerenal oliguria, the oliguria is caused by a decrease in circulating blood volume, and there is no damage yet to the renal tissue. It can be reversed potentially by correcting the precipitating factor, such as fluid replacement for hypovolemia. Prerenal oliguria is characterized by urine with a high specific gravity and a low sodium concentration, whereas oliguria of intrarenal failure is characterized by urine with a low specific gravity and a high sodium concentration. Malignant hypertension causes damage to renal tissue and intrarenal oliguria.

5. b. Rationale: A urine-specific gravity that is consistently 1.010 and a urine osmolality of about 300 mOsm/kg is the same specific gravity and osmolality as plasma and indicates that tubules are damaged and unable to concentrate urine. Hematuria is more common with postrenal damage, and tubular damage is associated with a high sodium concentration (>40 mEq/L).

6. a. Rationale: Metabolic acidosis occurs in acute kidney injury (AKI) because the kidneys cannot synthesize ammonia needed to excrete H^+, resulting in an increased acid load. Sodium is lost in urine because the kidneys cannot conserve sodium, and impaired excretion of potassium results in hyperkalemia. Bicarbonate is normally generated and reabsorbed by the functioning kidney to maintain acid-base balance.

7. c. Rationale: The blood urea nitrogen (BUN) and creatinine levels remain high during the oliguric and diuretic phases of AKI. The recovery phase begins when the glomerular filtration returns to a rate at which BUN and creatinine stabilize and then decrease. Urinary output of 3 to 5 L/day, decreasing sodium and potassium levels, and fluid weight loss are characteristic of the diuretic phase of acute renal failure (ARF).

8. d. Rationale: Hyperkalemia is a potentially life-threatening complication of AKI in the oliguric phase. Muscle weakness and abdominal cramping are signs of the neuromuscular impairment that occurs with hyperkalemia, in addition to cardiac conduction abnormalities of peaked T wave, prolonged PR interval, prolonged QRS interval, and depressed ST segment. Urine output of 300 mL/day is expected during the oliguric phase, as is the development of peripheral edema.

9. a. *F*, infection; b. *T*; c. *F*, 600; d. *F*, sodium and potassium serum levels; e. *T*

10. a. Potassium above 6 mEq/L with cardiac changes; b. Bicarbonate level of 14 mEq/L, indicating metabolic acidosis; c. Change in mental status

11. a, b, c, d, e. High-risk patients include those exposed to nephrotoxic agents (a); prolonged hypovolemia or hypotension (possibly b and c); preexisting chronic kidney disease, advanced age (a); cardiac failure

(c), massive trauma (b); extensive burns, sepsis, or obstetric complications (d). Patients with prostate cancer may have obstruction of the outflow tract, which increases risk of postrenal AKI (e).

12. b. Rationale: Dysrhythmias may occur with an elevated potassium and they are potentially lethal. Monitor the rhythm while contacting the physician or calling the rapid response team. Vital signs should be checked. Depending on the patient history and cause of increased potassium, instruct the patient on diet sources of potassium but this would not help at this point. The nurse may want to recheck the value but until then, he or she should monitor the heart rhythm.

13. b. Rationale: During acidosis, potassium moves out of the cell in exchange for H^+ ions, increasing the serum potassium level. Correction of the acidosis with sodium bicarbonate will help lower the potassium levels. A decrease in pH and the bicarbonate and $PaCO_2$ levels would indicate worsening acidosis.

14. b. Rationale: Stages of chronic kidney disease are based on the glomerular filtration rate (GFR) or the presence of kidney damage over a period of 3 months. No specific markers of urinary output, azotemia, or urine output classify the degree of CKD.

15. See table below.

	Findings	Cause
a. Skin	Uremic frost	Urea crystallization on skin with very high BUN levels.
	Excoriations	Pruritus causes scratching from calcium-phosphate deposition in the skin.
b. Cardiovascular	Hypertension	Sodium retention and fluid overload, increased renin production.
	Pericardial friction rub	Uremic pericarditis.
	Peripheral edema	Sodium and fluid retention.
c. Respiratory	Kussmaul respiration	Respiratory compensation of metabolic acidosis.
	Dyspnea	Pulmonary edema of heart failure and fluid overload.
	Predisposed to respiratory infections	Decreased pulmonary macrophage activity.
	Pleural friction rub	Uremic pleuritis.
d. GI	Mucosal ulcerations	Increased ammonia from bacterial breakdown of urea.
	Anorexia, nausea, vomiting	Irritation of the GI tract from urea.
	Constipation	Iron salts/calcium–containing phosphate binders and limited fluid intake and limited activity.
	Urine odor of breath	High urea content of the blood.
e. Neurologic	General CNS depression	High nitrogenous waste products.
	Coma and convulsions	Rapidly increasing BUN, hypertensive encephalopathy.
	Peripheral neuropathy/restless leg syndrome	Increasing BUN, slowed nerve conduction.

BUN, Blood urea nitrogen.

16. a. increased BUN; b. increased creatinine; c. increased glucose; d. decreased red blood cell (RBC) count; e. increased very-low-density lipoprotein (VLDL); f. increased potassium, normal or decreased sodium; g. decreased high-density lipoprotein (HDL); h. increased magnesium; i. decreased fibrinogen; j. decreased factor VIII. Others: increased phosphorus; decreased calcium.

17. c. Rationale: The calcium-phosphorus imbalances that occur in CKD result in hypocalcemia, from a deficiency of active vitamin D and increased phosphorus levels. This leads to an increased rate of bone remodelling with a weakened bone matrix. Aluminum accumulation is also believed to contribute to the osteomalacia. Osteitis fibrosa involves replacement of calcium in the bone with fibrous tissue and is primarily a result of elevated levels of parathyroid hormone resulting from hypocalcemia.

18. d. Rationale: A patient with CKD may have unlimited intake of sugars and starches (unless the patient is diabetic), and hard candy is an appropriate snack and may help relieve the metallic and urine taste common in the mouth. Raisins are a high-potassium food, pickled foods have high sodium contents, and ice cream contains protein.

19. a. 3; b. 1; c. 4; d. 2; e. 1; f. 2; g. 4; h. 2; i. 1

20. a. *F*, folic acid; b. *F*, uremia; c. *T*; d. *F*, meperidine (Demerol)

21. c. Rationale: The most common causes of CKD in the United States are hypertension and diabetes mellitus. The nurse should obtain information on long-term health problems that are related to kidney disease. The other disorders are not closely associated with renal disease.

22. c. Rationale: A patient on hemodialysis will continue to have dietary and fluid restrictions for which the machine cannot compensate, and the patient needs additional teaching regarding her therapeutic regimen. The other nursing diagnoses are not supported with defining characteristics.

23 a. HD; b. PD; c. HD; d. PD; e. PD; f. PD; g. HD; h. HD; i. PD

24. d. Rationale: Dextrose is added to dialysate fluid to create an osmotic gradient across the membrane to remove excess fluid from the blood. The dialysate fluid has no potassium so that potassium will diffuse into the dialysate from the blood. Dialysate also usually contains higher calcium to promote its movement into the blood. Dialysate sodium is usually less than or equal to that of blood to prevent sodium and fluid retention.

25. a. fill or inflow, dwell, drain; b. 2; c. automated

26. b. Rationale: Peritonitis is a common complication of PD and may require catheter removal and termination of dialysis. Infection occurs from contamination of the dialysate or tubing or from progression of exit-site or tunnel infections, and strict sterile technique must be used by health professionals as well as the patient to prevent contamination. Too-rapid infusion may cause shoulder pain, and pain may be caused if the catheter tip touches the bowel. Difficulty breathing, atelectasis, and pneumonia may occur from pressure of the fluid on the diaphragm, which may be prevented by elevating the head of the bed and promoting repositioning and deep breathing.

27. a. 3; b. 2; c. 1; d. 3; e. 1; f. 2

28. d. Rationale: A more permanent, soft, flexible Silastic double-lumen catheter is being used for long-term access when other forms of vascular access have failed. Femoral vein catheters may only remain in place for up to 1 week and jugular catheters for 1 to 3 weeks.

29. a. Rationale: While patients are undergoing HD, they can perform quiet activities that do not require the limb that has the vascular access. BP is monitored frequently, and the dialyzer monitors dialysis function, but cardiac monitoring is not indicated. The HD machine continuously circulates both the blood and the dialysate past the semipermeable membrane in the machine. Graft and fistula access involve the insertion of two needles into the site to remove blood from and return blood to the dialyzer.

30. b. Rationale: A patent AV graft creates turbulent blood flow that can be assessed by listening for a bruit or palpated for a thrill as the blood passes through the graft. Assessment of neurovascular status in the extremity distal to the graft site is important to determine that the graft does not impair circulation to the extremity, but the neurovascular status does not indicate whether the graft is open.

31. d. Rationale: Continuous renal replacement therapy (CRRT) is indicated for the patient with AKI as an alternative or adjunct to HD to slowly remove solutes and fluid in the hemodynamically unstable patient. It is especially useful for treatment of fluid overload, but HD is indicated for treatment of hyperkalemia, pericarditis, or other serious effects of uremia.

32. d. Rationale: Extensive vascular disease is a contraindication of renal transplantation, primarily because adequate blood supply is essential to both the health of the new kidney and the circulation of immunosuppressive drugs. Other contraindications include disseminated malignancies, refractory or untreated cardiac disease, chronic respiratory failure, chronic infection, or unresolved psychosocial disorders. CAD may be treated with bypass surgery before transplantation, and transplantation can relieve hypertension. Hepatitis B or C infection is not a contraindication.

33. a. Rationale: Fluid and electrolyte balance is critical in the transplant-recipient patient, especially because diuresis often begins soon after surgery. Fluid replacement is adjusted hourly, based on kidney function and output. Urine-tinged drainage on the abdominal dressing may indicate leakage from the ureter implanted into the bladder, and the health care provider should be notified. The donor patient has a flank incision where the kidney was removed; the recipient patient has an abdominal incision where the kidney was placed in the iliac fossa. The urinary catheter is usually used for 2 to 3 days to monitor urine output and kidney function.

34. Suppression of body's normal defense mechanisms
    1. by surgery
    2. by immunosuppressive medications
    3. by the effects of end-stage renal disease

Case Study

1. T-cytotoxic lymphocytes recognize the kidney as foreign tissue and attack it, setting in process the inflammatory and complement systems. It usually occurs 4 days to 4 weeks after the transplant, but it may occur later, and it is not uncommon to have at least one rejection episode.

2. All laboratory results are abnormal, except potassium at high normal, and are typical of renal insufficiency that occurs during acute rejection:
   - Serum creatinine—decreased excretory function of tubules
   - BUN—decreased ability of the kidney to excrete urea
   - Glucose—insulin resistance occurs in chronic renal failure from unknown cause; may also be increased by corticosteroid therapy

- Potassium—decreased ability of the kidney to excrete potassium
- Bicarbonate—impaired generation and reabsorption by the kidney as it is being used to buffer acid load

Nursing care includes monitoring for CNS depression and skin and oral mucus breakdown from high urea; monitoring capillary blood glucose and administering insulin to keep glucose within normal range; and monitoring for increasing weakness and cardiac changes related to hyperkalemia and for symptoms of metabolic acidosis, such as Kussmaul respiration.

3. Immunosuppressive therapy: designed to reduce proliferation and action of T-cytotoxic lymphocytes that are responsible for acute rejection
   - Muromonab-CD3 (Orthoclone OKT3) is a monoclonal antibody that binds to CD3 receptors on lymphocytes and lyses the cells; is given IV to reverse acute rejection
   - Mycophenolate mofetil (CellCept) is an antimetabolite that inhibits purine synthesis and suppresses proliferation of T and B cells.
   - Methylprednisolone (Solu-Medrol) is a corticosteroid that inhibits cytokine production and T-cell activation.
   - Tacrolimus (Prograf) is a calcineurin inhibitor that prevents production and release of IL-2, IL-4, and α-interferon in addition to inhibiting production of T-cytotoxic lymphocytes.

   Supportive therapy: Designed to control the symptoms produced by renal insufficiency
   - Furosemide is a loop diuretic that is not influenced by GFR and is used to promote sodium, potassium, and fluid loss through the kidney; it helps to relieve hypervolemia and hypertension.
   - Nifedipine is a calcium channel blocker that reduces CO to control BP.
   - Sodium bicarbonate helps control the metabolic acidosis of renal insufficiency and replaces that which is not produced or reabsorbed by the kidney.
   - Insulin controls the hyperglycemia resulting from insulin resistance.

4. Many side effects may occur from immunosuppressive therapy, but the most common is decreased resistance to infection and increased incidence of cancer because of depression of T-cytotoxic lymphocytes.
   - Muromonab-CD3 causes fever, tachycardia, infections, headache, vomiting, chills, joint and muscle pain, and diarrhea.
   - Mycophenolate mofetil causes GI toxicity, leukopenia, and thrombocytopenia.
   - As a corticosteroid, methylprednisolone causes Cushing syndrome with sodium and water retention, redistribution of fat, muscle weakness

with protein wasting, hyperglycemia, and osteoporosis.
   - Tacrolimus is nephrotoxic and neurotoxic with headaches, seizures, and tremors; nausea and vomiting; hyperglycemia; hypertension; and hair loss.

5. Increased risk for infections, malignancies; chronic liver disease; increased risk for atherosclerosis with CAD a major cause of death; joint necrosis from chronic steroid therapy; psychologic adjustment—constant fear of rejection and wondering how long the transplant will last; depression if there is failure and a return to dialysis

6. *Nursing diagnoses:*
   - Excess fluid volume related to inability of kidney to excrete fluid
   - Grieving related to threat of loss of kidney
   - Risk for acute confusion related to CNS changes induced by uremic toxins and immunosuppressive drugs
   - Risk for infection related to suppressed immune system

   Collaborative problems:
   Potential complications: Hypertension; hyperkalemia with cardiac dysrhythmias; hyperglycemia; metabolic acidosis; infection

CHAPTER 48

1. a. hypothalamus; b. pituitary; c. parathyroids; d. thyroid; e. thymus; f. adrenals; g. pancreatic islets; h. ovaries; i. testes
2. a. 3; b. 8; c. 6; d. 1; e. 10; f. 1; g. 3; h. 1; i. 5; j. 1; k. 3; l. 1; m. 7; n. 9; o. 1; p. 2; q. 4
3. a. *T*; b. *F*, growth hormone, T3/T4 or cortisol; c. *T*; d. *F*, false-low; e. *F*, thyroid hormones; f. *T*; g. *F*, thyroid gland and adrenal cortex (also gonads); h. *T*; i. *F*, steroid hormones
4. a. 3, 2; b. 1, 4; c. 13, 14; d. 6, 5; e. 9, 10; f. 11, 12; g. 8, 7; h. 10, 9; i. 7, 8
5. b. Rationale: Antidiuretic hormone (ADH) release is controlled by the osmolality of the blood, and as the osmolality rises, ADH is released from the posterior pituitary gland and acts on the kidney to cause reabsorption of water from the kidney tubule, resulting in more dilute blood and more concentrated urine. Aldosterone, the major mineralocorticoid, causes sodium reabsorption from the kidney and potassium excretion. Calcium levels are not a factor in serum osmolality.
6. d. Rationale: Atrial natriuretic peptide (ANP) is secreted in response to high blood volume and high serum sodium levels and has an inhibiting effect on ADH and the renin-angiotensin-aldosterone system, the effects of which would make the blood volume even higher. Glucagon secretion inhibits insulin secretion, but insulin does not inhibit glucagon. The relationship between cortisol and insulin is

indirect—cortisol raises blood glucose levels, and insulin secretion is stimulated by the high glucose levels. Testosterone and estrogen have no reciprocal action, and both are secreted by the body in response to tropic hormones.

7. d. Rationale: Usually insulin and glucagon function in a reciprocal manner, except after a high-protein, carbohydrate-free meal, in which both hormones are secreted. Glucagon increases gluconeogenesis, and insulin causes target tissue to accept the amino acids for protein synthesis.

8. a. Rationale: Hypokalemia inhibits aldosterone release as well as insulin release; these are the major hormones affected by hypokalemia.

9. a. Decreased energy level in relation to the past; family history of similar problem
    b. Changes in appetite and weight, difficulty swallowing; changes in hair distribution, color, and texture; skin changes; hot and cold intolerances
    c. Increased thirst with frequent urination; kidney stones; frequent defecation or constipation; change in stool consistency or pattern
    d. Decrease in previous activity levels; fatigue, hyperactivity
    e. Sleep disturbances, nightmares, sweating, nocturia, insomnia, or excessive sleep
    f. Memory deficits, depression, inability to concentrate; visual disturbances or exophthalmos; apathy
    g. Changes in body appearance and self-perception
    h. Changes in ability to maintain usual roles
    i. Menstrual irregularity and infertility; history of delivering large babies; male sexual dysfunction; changes in secondary sex characteristics
    j. perception of stress in life and usefulness of previous coping mechanisms, changes in response to stress
    k. commitment to lifestyle changes, value of health

10. a. Rationale: The mineralocorticoid effects of cortisol causes sodium retention and potassium excretion from the kidney, resulting in hypokalemia. Because water is reabsorbed with the sodium, serum sodium remains normal. In its effect on glucose and fat metabolism, cortisol causes an elevation in blood glucose as well as increases in free fatty acids and triglycerides.

11. b. Rationale: Many symptoms of hypothyroidism, such as fatigue, mental impairment, dry skin, and constipation, that would be apparent in younger persons are attributed to general aging in the older adult, thus going unrecognized as a treatable condition.

12. c. Rationale: Assessment of the endocrine system is often difficult because hormones affect every body tissue and system, causing great diversity in the signs and symptoms of endocrine dysfunction. Weight loss, fatigue, and depression are signs that may occur with many different endocrine problems; but goiter,

exophthalmos, and the three "polys" are specific findings of endocrine dysfunction.

13. c. Rationale: In the patient with thyroid disease, palpation can cause the release of thyroid hormone into circulation, increasing the patient's symptoms and potentially causing a thyroid storm. Examination should be deferred to a more experienced clinician if possible. Pressure should not be so great as to damage the cricoid cartilage or laryngeal nerve, and if the thyroid is palpated correctly, the carotid arteries are not compressed.

14. a. parathyroid; b. adrenal; c. thyroid; d. excessive; e. thyroid; f. growth; g. adrenal; h. thyroid

15. a. Rationale: Endocrine disorders related to hormone secretion from glands that are stimulated by tropic hormones can be caused by a malsecretion of the tropic hormone or of the target gland. If the problem is in the target gland, it is known as a *primary endocrine disorder*, and a problem with tropic hormone secretion is known as a *secondary endocrine disorder*. Serum levels of tropic hormones can illustrate the status of the negative feedback system in relation to target-organ hormone levels. If a target organ produces low amounts of hormone, tropic hormones will be increased; if a target organ is overproducing hormones, tropic hormones will be low or undetectable.

16. b. Rationale: Normal secretion and action of insulin will usually result in fasting levels of glucose in 2 to 3 hours after carbohydrate ingestion, but to ensure that the level is a fasting level, a minimum of 4 hours should be allowed. Water may be taken, however, and does not affect the glucose level.

17. a. 4; b. 1; c. 5; d. 8; e. 3; f. 7; g. 6; h. 2

CHAPTER 49

1. d. Rationale: Insulin is an anabolic hormone, responsible for growth, repair, and storage, and it facilitates movement of amino acids into cells, synthesis of protein, storage of glucose as glycogen, and deposition of triglycerides and lipids as fat into adipose tissue. Glucagon is responsible for hepatic glycogenolysis and gluconeogenesis, and fat is used for energy when glucose levels are depleted.

2. a. skeletal muscle, adipose; b. pancreatic beta (β); c. cortisol, epinephrine, glucagon, growth hormone; d. type 1

3. a. 2; b. 2; c. 2; d. 1; e. 1; f. 2; g. 1; h. 2; i. 2; j. 1

4. a. High glucose levels cause loss of glucose in urine with osmotic diuresis; b. thirst caused by fluid loss of polyuria; c. cellular starvation from lack of glucose and use of fat and protein for energy

5. d. Rationale: Type 2 diabetes has a strong genetic influence, and offspring of parents who both have type 2 diabetes have an increased chance of

developing it. Whereas type 1 diabetes is associated with genetic susceptibility related to human leukocyte antigens (HLAs), offspring of parents who both have type 1 diabetes have only a 6% to 10% chance of developing the disease. Lower risk factors for type 2 diabetes include obesity; being a Native American, Hispanic, or African American; and being 55 years or older.

6. a. Rationale: Metabolic syndrome is a cluster of abnormalities that include elevated insulin levels, elevated triglycerides and low-density lipoproteins (LDL), and decreased high-density lipoproteins (HDL). These abnormalities greatly increase the risk for cardiovascular disease associated with diabetes that can be prevented or delayed with weight loss. Exercise is also important, but normal weight is most important.

7. b, c. Rationale: The patient has one prior test result that meets criteria for a diagnosis of diabetes, but on a subsequent day must again have results from one of the three tests that meet the criteria for diabetes diagnosis. These criteria include a fasting plasma glucose level ≥126 mg/dL (7.0 mmol/L), or A1C ≥6.5% or a 2-hour OGTT level ≥200 mg/dL (11.1 mmol/L). Both the fasting plasma glucose (FPG) and A1C would confirm a diagnosis of diabetes in this patient.

8. c. Rationale: Impaired glucose tolerance exists when a 2-hour plasma glucose level is higher than normal but lower than the level diagnostic for diabetes (i.e., 140-199 mg/dL). Impaired fasting glucose exists when fasting glucose levels are greater than the normal of 100 mg/dL but less than the 126 mg/dL diagnostic of diabetes. Both conditions represent a condition known as prediabetes.

9. c. Rationale: U100 insulin must be used with a U100 syringe, but for those using low doses of insulin, syringes are available that have increments of 1 unit instead of 2 units. Errors can be made in dosing if patients switch back and forth between different sizes of syringes. Aspiration before injection of the insulin is not recommended, nor is the use of alcohol to clean the skin. Because the rate of peak serum concentration varies with the site selected for injection, injections should be rotated within a particular area, such as the abdomen.

10. b. Rationale: A split-mixed dose of insulin requires that the patient adhere to a set meal pattern to provide glucose for the action of the insulins, and a bedtime snack is usually required when patients take a long-acting insulin late in the day to prevent nocturnal hypoglycemia. Hypoglycemia is most likely to occur with this dose late in the afternoon and during the night. When premixed formulas are used, flexible dosing based on glucose levels is not recommended.

11. d. Rationale: Lispro is a rapid-acting insulin that has an onset of action of 5 to 15 minutes and should be injected at the time of the meal to within 15 minutes of eating. Regular insulin is short acting with an onset of action in 30 to 60 minutes following administration and should be given 30 to 45 minutes before meals.

12. a. Rationale: When mixing regular with a longer-acting insulin, regular insulin should always be drawn into the syringe first to prevent contamination of the regular insulin vial with longer-acting insulin additives. Air is added to the neutral protamine Hagedorn (NPH) vial; then air is added to the regular vial, and the regular insulin is withdrawn, bubbles are removed, and the dose of NPH is withdrawn.

13. b. Rationale: Checking the temperature of the bath water is part of assisting with activities of daily living (ADLs) and within the scope of care for the nursing assistive personnel (NAP). Discussion of complications, teaching, and assessing learning are appropriate for RNs.

14. d. Rationale: Insulin glargine (Lantus), a long-acting insulin that is continuously released with no peak of action, cannot be diluted or mixed with any other insulin or solution. Mixed insulins should be stored needle-up in the refrigerator and warmed before administration. Currently used bottles of insulin can be kept at room temperature.

15. a. Rationale: Insulin pumps provide tight glycemic control by continuous subcutaneous insulin infusion based on the patient's basal profile, with bolus doses at mealtime at the patient's discretion. Errors in insulin dosing and complications of insulin therapy are still potential risks with insulin pumps.

16. c. Rationale: The patient's elevated glucose on arising may be the result of either dawn phenomenon or Somogyi effect, and the best way to determine whether the patient needs more or less insulin is by monitoring the glucose at bedtime, between 2:00 and 4:00 AM, and on arising. If predawn levels are below 60 mg/dL, the insulin dose should be reduced, but if the 2:00 to 4:00 AM blood glucose is high, the insulin should be increased.

17. a. 5; b. 2; c. 1; d. 1; e. 2; f. 4; g. 1; h. 3; i. 3; j. 4; k. 4; l. 5.

18. c. Rationale; rapid deep respirations are symptoms of diabetic ketoacidosis (DKA). Stage II ulcers and bilateral numbness are chronic complications of diabetes. The lumps and dents on the abdomen indicate a need to teach the patient about site rotation.

19. a. Rationale: The body requires food at regularly spaced intervals throughout the day, and omission or delay of meals can result in hypoglycemia, especially for the patient taking insulin or oral hypoglycemic agents.

Weight loss may be recommended in type 2 diabetes if the individual is overweight, but many patients with type 1 diabetes are thin and require an increase in caloric intake. Fewer than 7% of total calories should be from saturated fats, and simple sugar should be limited, but moderate amounts can be used if counted as a part of total carbohydrate intake.

20. b. Rationale: Maintenance of as near-normal blood glucose levels as possible and achievement of optimal serum lipid levels with dietary modification are believed to be the most important factors in preventing both short- and long-term complications of diabetes. There is no specific "diabetic diet," and use of dietetic foods is not necessary for diabetes control. Most diabetics eat three meals a day, and some require a bedtime snack for control of nighttime hypoglycemia. A reasonable weight, which may or may not be an ideal body weight, is also a goal of nutritional therapy.

21. b. Rationale: During exercise, a diabetic person needs both adequate glucose to prevent exercise-induced hypoglycemia and adequate insulin because counterregulatory hormones are produced during the stress of exercise and may cause hyperglycemia. Exercise after meals is best, but a 10- to 15-g carbohydrate snack may be taken if exercise is performed before meals or is prolonged. Blood glucose levels should be monitored before, during, and after exercise to determine the effect of exercise on the levels.

22. c. Rationale: Cleaning the puncture site with alcohol is not necessary and may interfere with test results and lead to drying and splitting of the fingertips. Washing the hands with warm water is adequate cleaning and promotes blood flow to the fingers. Blood flow is also increased by holding the hand down. Punctures on the side of the finger pad are less painful. Self-monitored blood glucose (SMBG) should be performed before and after exercise.

23. b. Rationale: The American Diabetes Association recommends that testing for type 2 diabetes with a FPG should be considered for all individuals at the age of 45 and above and, if normal, repeated every 3 years. Testing for immune markers of type 1 diabetes is not recommended. Testing at a younger age or more frequently should be done for members of a high-risk ethnic population, including African Americans, Hispanics, Native Americans, Asian Americans, and Pacific Islanders.

24. a. Rationale: During minor illnesses, the patient with diabetes should continue drug therapy and food intake. Insulin is important because counterregulatory hormones may raise blood glucose during the stress of illness, and food or a carbohydrate liquid substitution is important because

during illness the body requires extra energy to deal with the stress of the illness. Blood glucose monitoring should be done every 4 hours, and the health care provider should be notified if the level is >240 mg/dL (13.9 mmol/L) or if fever, ketonuria, or nausea and vomiting occur.

25. c. Rationale: When insulin is insufficient and glucose cannot be used for cellular energy, the body releases and breaks down stored fats and protein to meet energy needs. Free fatty acids from stored triglycerides are released and metabolized in the liver in such large quantities that ketones are formed. Ketones are acidic and alter the pH of the blood, causing acidosis. Osmotic diuresis occurs as a result of loss of both glucose and ketones in the urine.

26. a. Kussmaul's respirations; b. ketonuria; c. sweet, fruity odor to breath; d. decreased arterial pH (acidosis); e. ketonemia

27. c. Rationale: The management of DKA is similar to that of HHS except HHS requires greater fluid replacement because of the severe hyperosmolar state. Bicarbonate is not usually given in DKA to correct acidosis unless the pH is <7.0 because administration of insulin will reverse the abnormal fat metabolism. Total-body potassium deficit is high in both conditions, requiring potassium administration, and, in both conditions, glucose is added to IV fluids when blood glucose levels fall to 250 mg/dL (13.9 mmol/L).

28. a. 1; b. 3; c. 2; d. 1; e. 2; f. 1; g. 2; h. 3

29. d. Rationale: If a diabetic patient is unconscious, immediate treatment for hypoglycemia must be given to prevent brain damage, and IM or subcutaneous administration of 1 mg of glucagon should be done. If the unconsciousness has another cause, such as ketosis, the rise in glucose caused by the glucagon is not as dangerous as the low glucose level. Following administration of the glucagon, the patient should be transported to a medical facility for further treatment and evaluation. Insulin is contraindicated without knowledge of the patient's glucose level, and oral carbohydrate cannot be given when patients are unconscious.

30. a. Rationale: Blood glucose levels of 80 to 90 mg/dL (4.4-5 mmol/L) are within the normal range and are desired in the patient with diabetes, even following a recent hypoglycemic episode. Hypoglycemia is often caused by a single event, such as skipping a meal or taking too much insulin or vigorous exercise; once corrected, normal control should be maintained.

31. b. Rationale: The development of atherosclerotic vessel disease seems to be promoted by the altered lipid metabolism common to diabetes, and although tight glucose control may help delay the process,

it does not prevent it completely. Atherosclerosis in diabetic patients does respond somewhat to a reduction in general risk factors, as it does in nondiabetics, and reduction in fat intake, control of hypertension, abstention from smoking, maintenance of normal weight, and regular exercise should be carried out by diabetic patients.

32. a. 3; b. 1; c. 2; d. 1; e. 4; f. 1; g. 4; h. 2; i. 4; j. 3; k. 2; l. 3

33. d. Rationale: Complete or partial loss of sensitivity of the feet is common with peripheral neuropathy of diabetes, and diabetics may suffer foot injury and ulceration without ever having pain. Feet must be inspected during daily care for any cuts, blisters, swelling, or reddened areas.

34. a. Rationale: Because the clinical manifestations of long-term complications of diabetes take 10 to 20 years to develop, and because tight glucose control in the older patient is associated with an increased frequency of hypoglycemia, the goals for glycemic control are not as rigid as in the younger population. Treatment is indicated, and insulin may be used if the patient does not respond to oral agents. The patient's needs, rather than age, determine the responsibility of others in care.

Case Study

1. The hypoglycemia might have been prevented by the patient taking time to eat breakfast and perhaps increasing food intake in anticipation of strenuous exercise. She also should have checked her glucose level before exercising.

2. *Sympathetic response to hypoglycemia:*
   Weakness, nervousness, tremor
   Vasoconstriction with pallor, numbness, coldness, headache, tachycardia
   Brain neuroglycemia:
   Confusion, slurred speech, unsteady gait

3. The hypoglycemia should be treated with a fast-acting carbohydrate—120 to 180 mL of orange juice or regular soda, five or six hard candies, or 8 oz of low-fat milk.
   - Repeat the carbohydrate in 10 to 15 minutes if symptoms are still present or if blood glucose remains < 70 mg/dL (3.9 mmol/L).
   - When glucose is >70 mg/dL, a regularly scheduled meal or snack of complex carbohydrate and protein should be eaten.
   - The blood glucose should be checked again about 45 minutes after treatment to ensure that hypoglycemia does not recur.

4. How to recognize situations that lead to hypoglycemia; review the effects of exercise on glucose levels and the need for both adequate glucose and insulin

5. Monitor her blood glucose before, during, and after exercise; increase dietary intake before exercise;

maintain insulin doses; exercise 60 to 90 minutes after meals; carry simple carbohydrates to take at first symptoms

6. *Nursing diagnoses:*
   Ineffective self-health management related to noncompliance with recommended regimen
   Collaborative problems:
   Potential complications: Brain damage, coma, seizures, death

CHAPTER 50

1. d. Rationale: A normal response to growth hormone (GH) secretion is stimulation of the liver to produce somatomedin C, or insulin-like growth factor-1 (IGF-1), which stimulates growth of bones and soft tissues. The increased levels of somatomedin C normally inhibit GH, but in acromegaly, the pituitary gland secretes GH despite elevated IFG-1 levels. When both GH and IGF-1 levels are increased, overproduction of GH is confirmed. GH also causes elevation of blood glucose, and normally GH levels fall during an oral glucose challenge but not in acromegaly.

2. c. Rationale: The increased production of GH in acromegaly causes an increase in thickness and width of bones and enlargement of soft tissues, resulting in marked changes in facial features, oily and coarse skin, and speech difficulties. Height is not increased in adults with GH excess because the epiphyses of the bones are closed; infertility is not a common finding because GH is usually the only pituitary hormone involved in acromegaly.

3. a. Rationale: A transsphenoidal hypophysectomy involves entry into the sella turcica through an incision in the upper lip and gingiva into the floor of the nose and the sphenoid sinuses. Postoperative clear nasal drainage with glucose content indicates cerebrospinal fluid (CSF) leakage from an open connection to the brain, putting the patient at risk for meningitis. After surgery, the patient is positioned with the head elevated to avoid pressure on the sella turcica. Coughing and straining are avoided to prevent increased intracranial pressure and CSF leakage, and although mouth care is required every 4 hours, toothbrushing should not be performed because injury to the suture line may occur.

4. a. *F*, somatostatin analog, reduce levels; b. *F*, smaller; c. *T*; d. *T*

5. a. cortisol; b. thyroid; c. vasopressin/ADH analog; d. growth hormone; e. sex hormones: testosterone; follicle-stimulating hormone (FSH), and luteinizing hormone (LH) if fertility is desired; estrogen/progesterone if fertility is not an issue

6. See chart below.

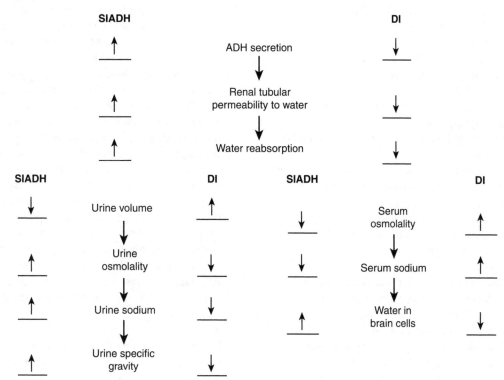

7. a. Rationale: The patient with syndrome of inappropriate secretion of antidiuretic hormone (SIADH) has marked dilutional hyponatremia and should be monitored for decreased neurologic function and convulsions every 2 hours. ADH release is reduced by keeping the head of the bed flat to increase left atrial filling pressure, and sodium intake is supplemented because of the hyponatremia and sodium loss caused by diuretics. A reduction in blood pressure (BP) indicates a reduction in total fluid volume and is an expected outcome of treatment.

8. b. Rationale: The patient with SIADH has water retention with hyponatremia, decreased urine output, and concentrated urine with high specific gravity. Improvement in the patient's condition is reflected by increased urine output, normalization of serum sodium, and more water in the urine, decreasing the specific gravity.

9. d. Rationale: A patient with diabetes insipidus has a deficiency of ADH with excessive loss of water from the kidney, hypovolemia, hypernatremia, and dilute urine with a low specific gravity. When vasopressin is administered, the symptoms are reversed, with water retention, decreased urinary output that increases urine osmolality, and an increase in BP.

10. c. Rationale: Normal urine specific gravity is 1.003 to 1.030, and urine with a specific gravity of 1.002 is very dilute, indicating that there continues to be excessive loss of water and that treatment of diabetes insipidus is inadequate. Headache,

weight gain, and oral intake greater than urinary output are signs of volume excess that occur with overmedication. Nasal irritation and nausea may also indicate overdosage.

11. b. Rationale: In nephrogenic diabetes insipidus, the kidney is unable to respond to ADH, so vasopressin or hormone analogs are not effective. Thiazide diuretics slow the glomerular filtration rate (GFR) in the kidney and produce a decrease in urine output. Low-sodium diets (<3 g/day) are also thought to decrease urine output. Fluids are not restricted because the patient could easily become dehydrated.

12. a. 4; b. 3; c. 1; d. 5; e. 6; f. 2

13. a. *T*; b. *F*, Graves' disease; c. *T*; d. *F*, decreased thyroid-stimulating hormone (TSH) level.

14. d. Rationale: In Graves' disease, antibodies to the TSH receptor are formed, attach to the receptors, and stimulate the thyroid gland to release triiodothyronine (T_3), thyroxine (T_4), or both, creating hyperthyroidism. The disease is not directly genetic, but individuals appear to have a genetic susceptibility to develop autoimmune antibodies. Goiter formation from insufficient iodine intake is usually associated with hypothyroidism.

15. c. Rationale: A hyperthyroid crisis results in marked manifestations of hyperthyroidism, with severe tachycardia, heart failure, shock, hyperthermia, agitation, nausea, vomiting, diarrhea, delirium, and coma. Although exophthalmos may be present in the patient with Graves' disease, it is not a significant factor in hyperthyroid crisis. Hoarseness

and laryngeal stridor are characteristic of the tetany of hypoparathyroidism, and lethargy progressing to coma is characteristic of myxedema coma, a complication of hypothyroidism.

16. a. 4; b. 2; c. 1; d. 2; e. 3; f. 1; g. 4; h. 4

17. a. Risk for injury: corneal ulceration related to inability to close eyelids

    b. Imbalanced nutrition: less than body requirements related to hypermetabolism

    c. Disturbed body image related to change in body appearance

    d. Activity intolerance related to fatigue and dyspnea

18. a. Rationale: To prevent strain on the suture line postoperatively, the patient's head must be manually supported while turning and moving in bed, but range-of-motion exercises for the head and neck are also taught preoperatively to be gradually implemented after surgery. There is no contraindication for coughing and deep breathing, and these should be carried out postoperatively. Tingling around the lips or fingers is a sign of hypocalcemia, which may occur if the parathyroid glands are inadvertently removed during surgery. This sign should be reported immediately.

19. a. To use in case airway obstruction occurs because of vocal cord paralysis from recurrent laryngeal nerve damage during surgery or laryngeal stridor occurs with tetany

    b. Needed in case hypocalcemia occurs from parathyroid gland removal or damage during surgery, resulting in tetany

    c. In case of airway obstruction, laryngeal stridor or edema around trachea

20. d. Rationale: With the decrease in thyroid hormone postoperatively, calories need to be reduced substantially to prevent weight gain. When a patient has had a subtotal thyroidectomy, thyroid replacement therapy is not given because exogenous hormone inhibits pituitary production of TSH and delays or prevents the restoration of thyroid tissue regeneration. Regular exercise stimulates the thyroid gland and is encouraged. Saltwater gargles are used for dryness and irritation of the mouth and throat following radioactive iodine therapy.

21. d. Rationale: Both Graves' disease and Hashimoto's thyroiditis are autoimmune disorders that eventually destroy the thyroid gland, leading to primary hypothyroidism. Thyroid tumors most often result in hyperthyroidism. Secondary hypothyroidism occurs as a result of pituitary failure, and iatrogenic hypothyroidism results from thyroidectomy or radiation of the thyroid gland.

22. a. depression and altered metabolism; as evidenced by excessive sleeping, no relief of somnolence, altered sleep stages

    b. calorie intake greater than need; as evidenced by weight gain, slow metabolism

    c. slowed metabolism; as evidenced by personality changes, forgetfulness, memory loss.

    d. decreased metabolic rate and mucin deposits in joints; as evidenced by fatigue, weakness, muscular aches, and pains

23. d. Rationale: All these manifestations may occur with treatment of hypothyroidism, but as a result of the effects of hypothyroidism on the cardiovascular system, when thyroid replacement therapy is started, myocardial oxygen consumption is increased, and the resultant oxygen demand may cause angina, cardiac dysrhythmias, and heart failure.

24. b. Rationale: Because of the mental sluggishness, inattentiveness, and memory loss that occur with hypothyroidism, it is important to provide written instructions and repeat information when teaching the patient. Replacement therapy must be taken for life, and alternate-day dosing is not therapeutic. Although most patients return to a normal state with treatment, cardiovascular conditions and psychoses may persist.

25. a. 1; b. 2; c. 1; d. 1; e. 2; f. 2; g. 2; h. 1; i. 2; j. 1, 2

26. b. Rationale: A high fluid intake is indicated in hyperparathyroidism to dilute the hypercalcemia and flush the kidneys so that calcium stone formation is reduced. Seizures are not associated with hyperparathyroidism, but impending tetany of hypoparathyroidism can be noted with Trousseau's phenomenon and Chvostek's sign. The patient with hyperparathyroidism is at risk for pathologic fractures resulting from decreased bone density, but mobility is encouraged to promote bone calcification.

27. b. Rationale: Rebreathing in a paper bag promotes carbon dioxide retention in the blood, which lowers pH and creates an acidosis. An acidemia enhances the solubility and ionization of calcium, increasing the proportion of total body calcium available in physiologically active form and relieving the symptoms of hypocalcemia. Saline promotes calcium excretion, as does furosemide. Phosphate levels in the blood are reciprocal to calcium, and an increase in phosphate promotes calcium excretion.

28. c. Rationale: The hypocalcemia that results from parathyroid hormone (PTH) deficiency is controlled with calcium and vitamin D supplementation and possibly oral phosphate binders. Replacement with PTH is not used because of antibody formation to PTH, the need for parenteral administration, and cost. Milk products, although good sources of calcium, also have high levels of phosphate, which reduce calcium absorption. Whole grains and foods containing oxalic acid also impair calcium absorption.

29. a. Rationale: The effects of glucocorticoid excess include weight gain from accumulation and redistribution of adipose tissue, sodium and water retention, glucose intolerance, protein wasting, loss

of bone structure, loss of collagen, and capillary fragility. Clinical manifestations of corticosteroid deficiency include hypotension, dehydration, weight loss, and hyperpigmentation of the skin.

30. c. Rationale: Although the patient with Cushing syndrome has excess corticosteroids, removal of the glands and the stress of surgery require that high doses of cortisone be administered postoperatively for several days before weaning the dose. The nurse should monitor the patient postoperatively to detect whether large amounts of hormones were released during surgical manipulation and to ensure that healing is satisfactory.

31. c. Rationale: Vomiting and diarrhea are early indicators of addisonian crisis, and fever indicates an infection, which is causing additional stress for the patient. Treatment of a crisis requires immediate glucocorticoid replacement, and IV hydrocortisone, fluids, sodium, and glucose are necessary for 24 hours. Addison's disease is a primary insufficiency of the adrenal gland, and adrenocorticotropic hormone (ACTH) is not effective, nor would vasopressors be effective with the fluid deficiency of Addison's disease. Potassium levels are increased in Addison's disease, and KCl would be contraindicated.

32. b. Rationale: A weight reduction in the patient with Addison's disease may indicate a fluid loss and a dose of replacement therapy that is too low rather than too high. Patients with Addison's disease are taught to take two to three times their usual dose of steroids if they become ill, have teeth extracted, or engage in rigorous physical activity and should always have injectable hydrocortisone available if oral doses cannot be taken. Because vomiting and diarrhea are early signs of crisis and because fluid and electrolytes must be replaced, patients should notify their health care provider if these symptoms occur.

33. a. Sodium and fluid retention because of mineralocorticoid effect; b. gastrointestinal (GI) irritation with an increase in secretion of pepsin and hydrochloric acid; c. corticosteroid-induced osteoporosis; d. glucose intolerance with hyperglycemia; e. hypokalemia because of mineralocorticoid effect

34. c. Rationale: Taking corticosteroids on an alternate-day schedule for pharmacologic purposes is less likely to suppress ACTH production from the pituitary and prevent adrenal atrophy. Normal adrenal hormone balance is not maintained during glucocorticoid therapy because excessive exogenous hormone is used.

35. a. Rationale: Hyperaldosteronism is an excess of aldosterone, which is manifested by sodium and water retention and potassium excretion. Furosemide is a potassium-wasting diuretic that would increase

the potassium deficiency. Aminoglutethimide blocks aldosterone synthesis; amiloride is a potassium-sparing diuretic; and spironolactone blocks mineralocorticoid receptors in the kidney, increasing the excretion of sodium and water but retaining potassium.

36. b. Rationale: A pheochromocytoma is a catecholamine-producing tumor of the adrenal medulla, which may cause severe, episodic hypertension; severe, pounding headache; and profuse sweating. Monitoring for a dangerously high BP before surgery is critical, as is monitoring for BP fluctuations during medical and surgical treatment.

Case Study

1. All the blood tests are altered because of the effect of glucocorticoids:
   - Elevated glucose—increased gluconeogenesis by liver and induced insulin resistance
   - Elevated white blood cell (WBC) count—granulocytosis
   - Decreased lymphocytes—lymphocytopenia
   - Increased red blood cell (RBC) count—polycythemia
   - Decreased K—increased mineralocorticoid effect causing sodium retention and potassium excretion

2. Cushing syndrome has several causes:
   - ACTH-secreting pituitary tumor is the most common cause of endogenous Cushing syndrome
   - Adrenal tumors
   - Ectopic ACTH production by tumors outside the hypothalamic-pituitary-adrenal axis
   - The pathophysiology of Cushing syndrome reflects an excess of normal glucocorticoid and mineralocorticoid activity, an exaggeration of normal functions.

3. ACTH levels: High or normal levels of ACTH indicate ACTH-dependent Cushing or a tumor of the pituitary gland; low or undetectable levels of ACTH indicate an adrenal or ectopic cause.

4. Pituitary cause—transsphenoidal hypophysectomy; adrenal cause—adrenalectomy; ectopic cause—removal if possible

5. A medical adrenalectomy involves treatment with mitotane (Lysodren), a drug that suppresses cortisol production, alters peripheral metabolism of steroids, and decreases plasma and urine steroid levels by actually killing adrenocortical cells.

6. Major nursing responsibilities are included in the following list:
   - Assessment of signs and symptoms of hormone toxicity:
     - Vital signs q4hr
     - Daily weights
     - Glucose monitoring
     - Changes in mental status

- Assessment for complications:
  - Signs and symptoms of infection, such as pain or purulent drainage, because fever and inflammation may be minimal or absent
  - Signs and symptoms of thromboembolic phenomena, such as chest pain, dyspnea, and tachypnea
  - Signs and symptoms of bone pain or limitations in motion, indicating pathologic fractures
  - Signs and symptoms of nephrolithiasis from increased calcium excretion
- Preoperative preparation:
  - Instruction about exercises, coughing, and deep breathing
  - Explanations about early monitoring for circulatory instability
  - Explanations about hormone replacement

7. *Nursing diagnoses:*
   - Risk for infection related to suppression of inflammation and immune function
   - Risk for injury related to loss of bone structure
   - Risk for impaired skin integrity related to edema and altered skin fragility
   - Disturbed body image related to altered physical appearance
   Collaborative problems:
   Potential complications: Thromboembolism, cardiac dysrhythmias, pathologic fractures, nephrolithiasis, diabetes mellitus, hypertensive crisis

CHAPTER 51

1. a. seminal vesicle; b. ejaculatory duct; c. prostate gland; d. rectum; e. Cowper's gland; f. anus; g. epididymis; h. testis; i. scrotum; j. glans; k. penis; l. urethra; m. ductus deferens; n. bladder; o. ureter; p. fallopian tube; q. ovary; r. body of uterus; s. fundus of uterus; t. round ligament; u. bladder; v. symphysis pubis; w. vagina; x. vaginal introitus; y. anus; z. rectum; aa. urethra; bb. cervix; cc. uterosacral ligament; dd. ureter
2. a. prepuce; b. labia minora; c. vaginal introitus; d. vestibule; e. perineum; f. anus; g. labia majora; h. urethra; i. clitoris; j. mons pubis; k. pectoralis major muscle; l. alveoli; m. areola; n. nipple
3. a. 3; b. 8; c. 2; d. 6; e. 1; f. 7; g. 4; h. 5
4. a. 4; b. 7; c. 5; d. 6; e. 3; f. 2; g. 1
5. a. *T*; b. *F*, fallopian tube; c. *F*, endocervix; d. *T*; e. *F*, 1 year
6. a. 2; b. 8; c. 6; d. 1; e. 1; f. 2, 7; g. 4; h. 3; i. 6; j. 8; k. 1; l. 1, 6; m. 5; n. 2
7. b. Rationale: Age-related changes in sexual function in men include a need for increased stimulation for an erection, a decreased need to ejaculate, and a possible decreased response to sexual stimuli. There is a decreased ability to attain an erection, but it is not related to prostatic changes. A negative social attitude toward sexuality in older adults also affects the sexual activity of people in this age group.

8. a. Potential congenital anomalies if rubella occurs during the first trimester of pregnancy
   b. Increased sterility in young men with mumps because of testicular atrophy resulting from orchitis
   c. Impotence and retrograde ejaculation in male diabetics, in addition to erectile problems from neuropathies
   d. Many may cause impotence in men
9. d. Rationale: The prostate is palpated through the wall of the rectum with a digital rectal examination. Inguinal hernias are detected by palpating the inguinal ring while the patient bears down, and scrotal palpation is done to detect testicular masses or tumors. No specific conditions are indicated by enlargement at the base of the penis.
10. a. Rationale: A decrease in the size of the penis is a normal finding in the older man. Loss of pubic hair is not normal, nor is any enlargement of the breasts. The normally darker color of the scrotum does not change with aging.
11. a. Lack of Pap testing, breast self-examination, prostate examinations, or testicular self-examination; smoking, alcohol, and caffeine use; family history of breast disease and reproductive cancers
    b. History of anorexia nervosa, decreased calcium intake
    c. Urge and stress incontinence; difficulty in urinating in male patients; vaginal and bladder infections
    d. Fatigue and activity intolerance related to menorrhagia
    e. Sleep interruption related to hot flashes and sweating; nocturia
    f. Pelvic pain; dyspareunia
    g. Changes in self-concept related to sexuality and aging
    h. Occupational hazards related to sexual functioning and reproductive capacity; dysfunctional or changing roles and relationships with others
    i. Recent changes in sexual practices; dissatisfaction with sexual expression; reproductive problems that affect sexual satisfactions; changes in menstrual patterns; multiple sexual partners; no protection against sexually transmitted diseases (STDs)
    j. Effect of STD on sex partners; stress of sexual problems or changes; infertility
    k. Conflict between value system and treatment; abortion issues; infertility issues
12. d. Rationale: The presence of dimpling or retractions can be observed by having the patient put her arms at her sides and over her head, lean forward, and press the hands on the hips. Lying down with the arm over the head flattens the breast for better palpation for lumps or thickness that can be felt with systematic palpation. Compressing the nipple is done to assess for drainage or galactorrhea.

13. d. Rationale: The vulva should be the color of the skin or slightly pink; redness indicates inflammation. A small amount of clear vaginal discharge is normal in females, as are episiotomy scars in a woman who has had children. Skene's ducts should be nonpalpable.

14. a. 6; b. 4; c. 9; d. 8; e. 3; f. 1; g. 5; h. 2; i. 7

15. b. Rationale: The risk for bleeding is increased following a D&C because the endometrial lining is scraped and injury to the uterus can occur. The nurse should closely assess the amount of bleeding with frequent pad checks the first 24 hours. Infection following D&C is uncommon, and the urinary system is not affected.

16. a. Rationale: A culdoscopy involves insertion of an endoscope through an incision made through the posterior fornix of the cul-de-sac and requires surgical anesthesia, as does the removal of cervical tissue during a conization. A D&C, laparoscopy, and breast biopsy are also operative procedures requiring surgical anesthesia; however, colposcopy, contrast mammography, and endometrial biopsies do not require surgical anesthesia.

17. a. Rationale: Huhner's (or Sims-Huhner's) test involves examination of a mucus sample of the cervix within 2 to 8 hours after intercourse to determine the number and mobility of sperm in the cervical mucus. A semen analysis is a simple examination of semen for the number, mobility, and structure of sperm. An endometrial biopsy provides a sample of endometrium to evaluate its changes under the influence of progesterone, and a hysterosalpingogram is a contrast x-ray of the uterine cavity and fallopian tubes.

CHAPTER 52

1. b. Rationale: The value of breast self-examination (BSE) in reducing mortality rates from breast cancer in women is currently controversial and is under review; however, it is still a useful tool in helping women become self-aware of how their breasts normally look and feel. None of the other options has been validated at this time.

2. a. Annual screening mammogram every year starting at the age of 40; b. clinical breast examination (CBE) every 3 years between the ages of 20 and 39 and every year for women beginning at age 40; c. optional monthly BSE starting at age 20; d. in women with increased risk, decisions for additional and more frequent testing to be determined with the health care provider.

3. a. Rationale: One of the major reasons women do not examine their breasts regularly is because of a lack of confidence in BSE skill, and a teaching program should include allowing time for women to use models to identify problems and perform a return demonstration of the examination on themselves.

Fear and denial often interfere with BSE even when women know the perceived risk for cancer is high, know the statistics, and know they should seek medical care if an abnormality is detected. Examinations in premenopausal women should be done right after the menstrual period, and specific dates are set for postmenopausal women or those who have had hysterectomies.

4. d. Rationale: A definitive diagnosis of breast cancer can be made only by a histologic examination of biopsied tissue. A stereotactic core biopsy is as reliable as an open surgical biopsy and has the advantages of decreased length of time for the procedure and recovery and reduced cost. A limitation of fine-needle aspiration is that if negative results are found, more definitive biopsy procedures are required.

5. d. Rationale: Most breast lesions are benign, and many mobile cystic lesions change in response to the menstrual cycle, whereas most malignant tumors do not. Caffeine has been associated with fibrocystic changes in some women, but research has not established caffeine as a cause of breast pain or cysts. Questions regarding a patient's last mammogram or family history are not closely related to the nurse's findings.

6. b. Rationale: Fibrocystic changes make breasts difficult to examine because of fibrotic changes and multiple lumps. A woman with this condition should be familiar with the characteristic changes in her breasts and monitor them closely for new lumps that do not respond in a cyclic manner over 1 to 2 weeks. Estrogen antagonizes the condition, and fibrocystic changes are not precancerous.

7. a. 3; b. 1; c. 2; d. 6; e. 5; f. 4; g. 2; h. 4; i. 6; j. 3; k. 1

8. b. Rationale: After the age of 60, the incidence of breast cancer increases dramatically, and advanced age is the highest risk factor for females. Obesity is a contributing factor for breast cancer, but fibrocystic breast changes are neither a precursor of cancer nor a known risk factor for cancer. Only about 5% to 10% of women with breast cancer have an alteration in the BRCA1 or BRCA2 gene, specific genetic abnormalities that contribute to the development of breast cancer.

9. b. Rationale: On palpation, malignant lesions are characteristically hard, irregularly shaped, poorly delineated, nontender, and nonmobile, and the most common site is the upper outer quadrant of the breast. A fibroademona is firm, defined, and mobile; fibrocystic lesions are usually large, tender, moveable masses found throughout the breast tissue. A painful, immobile mass under a reddened area of skin is most typical of a local abscess.

10. a. Rationale: Axillary lymph node status is one of the most important prognostic factors in primary breast cancer, and the more nodes involved, the higher the

risk for relapse or metastasis. Aneuploid DNA tumor content indicates that cells have abnormally high or low DNA content compared with normal cells and is associated with tumor aggressiveness. Cells in S-phase have a higher risk for recurrence and can produce earlier cancer death. Hormone receptor–negative tumors are usually poorly differentiated histologically, frequently recur, and are usually unresponsive to hormonal therapy.

11. d. Rationale: Even with negative axillary lymph nodes, recurrence occurs with breast cancer, illustrating that although most metastases occur through the lymphatic chains, metastasis can occur without invading the axillary nodes. Recurrence may be local or regional, with distant metastases most commonly to bone, lung, brain, and liver.

12. b. Rationale: Either treatment choice is indicated for women with early-stage breast cancer because the 10-year survival rate with lumpectomy with radiation is about the same as that with modified radical mastectomy. Each procedure has advantages and disadvantages that the patient must consider in making an informed choice, and the nurse should make that information available to the patient to assist in decision-making.

13. d. Rationale: Axillary lymph node dissection is almost always performed regardless of the treatment option selected because of its value in prognosis and decision-making regarding adjuvant therapy. A lumpectomy, or breast-conservation surgery, is followed by radiation therapy to the entire breast, and the use of chemotherapy or hormone therapy depends on the characteristics of the tumor and evidence of metastases.

14. c. Rationale: Lymphatic mapping with sentinel lymph node dissection (SLND) identifies one to four lymph nodes that drain first from the tumor site, and those nodes are examined for malignant cells. If any of the nodes have malignant cells, a complete axillary lymph node dissection is done. If the sentinel nodes are negative, no additional lymph nodes are removed.

15. a. adjuvant to surgery; b. palliative; c. high-dose brachytherapy; d. primary; e. high-dose brachytherapy

16. c. Rationale: Tamoxifen is an antiestrogen agent that blocks the estrogen-receptor sites of malignant cells and is the usual first choice of treatment in postmenopausal women with hormone receptor–positive tumors, with or without nodal involvement. Tamoxifen reduces the risk for recurrent breast cancer and also that for new primary tumors. The side effects of the drug are minimal and are those commonly associated with decreased estrogen.

17. c. Rationale: As early as in the recovery room following a modified radical mastectomy, the patient should start flexing and extending the fingers and wrist of the affected arm with daily increases

in activity. Postoperative mastectomy exercises, such as hair care, wall climbing with the fingers, and shoulder rotation and extension, are instituted gradually to prevent disruption of the wound.

18. b. Rationale: Removal of the axillary lymph nodes impairs lymph drainage from the affected arm and predisposes the patient to infection of the arm. The arm must be protected from even minor trauma, and blood pressure (BP), venipunctures, and injections should not be done on the arm. The arm should never be dependent, even during sleep, and should be elevated to promote lymph drainage.

19. c. Rationale: The Reach to Recovery program consists of volunteers, all women, who have had breast cancer and can answer questions about what to expect at home, how to tell people about the surgery, and what prosthetic devices are available. It is a valuable resource for patients who have breast cancer and should be used if available in the community. If a volunteer is not available, the nurse is responsible for assisting the patient in the same manner. Although the nurse should stress the importance of wearing a prosthesis, a permanent prosthesis cannot be used until healing is complete and inflammation is resolved.

20. b. Rationale: It is most important for the patient planning a mammoplasty that she have a realistic idea about what the surgery can accomplish and about possible complications. Currently surgery cannot restore nipple sensation or erectility, and the breast will not fully resemble its premastectomy appearance, but the outcome is usually more acceptable than the mastectomy scar. The woman's motives for breast reconstruction should not be questioned. There have been allegations of immune-related diseases associated with the use of silicone gel implants, but after further evaluation the Food and Drug Administration (FDA) has re-approved these implants for use.

21. a. Rationale: When an expander is used to stretch the skin and muscle at the mastectomy site, the expander is gradually increased in size by weekly injections of water or saline until the site is large enough to hold an implant. Placement of the expander can be at the time of mastectomy or at a later date. A musculocutaneous flap procedure is a type of reconstruction using the patient's own tissue. The nipple of the affected breast is removed at mastectomy, and a new nipple can be reconstructed after breast reconstruction from various normal tissues.

Case Study

1. It is likely that micrometastases to distant sites have occurred at the time of the diagnosis of breast cancer even in stage I disease and almost certainly in stage III disease, supporting indications for

systemic treatment of the cancer following local surgical treatment. Breast cancer is one of the solid tumors that is most responsive to chemotherapy, and destruction or control of tumor cells that have spread to distant sites is the goal of systemic chemotherapy.

2. a. cyclophosphamide [C]: alkylating agent, cell cycle–phase nonspecfic
   Side effects: Myelosuppression, nausea and vomiting, alopecia, hemorrhagic cystitis
   b. doxorubicin: Antitumor antibiotic, cell cycle–phase nonspecfic
   Side effects: Myelosuppression, mucositis, nausea and vomiting, alopecia, cardiotoxicity
   c. 5-fluorouracil: antimetabolite, cell cycle–phase specific
   Side effects: Myelosuppression, mucositis, nausea and vomiting, alopecia, photosensitivity

3. Teach P.T. to perform the following activities as necessary:
   • Myelosuppression:
     • Monitor her temperature every day.
     • Report any chilling; sore throat; cough; or rectal, urinary, or chest pain.
     • Keep the venous access catheter site clean and dry.
     • Avoid crowds and anyone with communicable diseases.
     • Wash the hands after toileting and before eating.
     • Report any bleeding, serious bruising, or persistent headaches.
     • Avoid using aspirin products.
     • Examine the mouth daily for blood-filled lesions.
     • Guard against bumping and other injury that might cause bleeding.
   • Mucositis:
     • Examine the mouth daily for bleeding, redness, or ulcers.
     • Use a mouthwash of baking soda or salt water every 2 hours as needed.
     • Use a soft-bristled toothbrush or sponge-tipped applicators for oral care.
     • Avoid hot, spicy, acidic foods and alcohol and tobacco.
     • Drink water frequently during the day.
   • Nausea and vomiting:
     • Use antiemetic medications as prescribed.
     • Use small, frequent meals that include bland, lukewarm, high-calorie, high-protein foods, and use liquid nutritional supplements if necessary.
     • Avoid strong odors and sights that increase nausea.
     • Eat and drink slowly.
     • Use gum, tea, or any food that stimulates salivation without causing nausea.
   • Alopecia:
     • Select a wig and begin to wear it before hair loss begins.
     • Wear a scarf or turban to conceal hair loss.

• Use a mild, protein-based shampoo and hair conditioner every 4 to 7 days to avoid drying remaining hair.
• Avoid excessive shampooing, brushing, and combing of hair.
• Avoid the use of curling irons, curlers, blow dryers, and hair spray.

4. An estrogen receptor–positive tumor is estrogen-dependent, and estrogen can promote growth of these breast cancer cells. Hormone receptor–positive cells usually are well differentiated, have low proliferative indices, and have a DNA content equal to that of normal cells. Drugs such as tamoxifen that block the estrogen receptor site of malignant cells can cause tumor regression and are widely used to treat recurrent or metastatic cancer that is estrogen-dependent.

5. The nurse should do the following:
   • Assist the patient to develop a positive but realistic attitude.
   • Help her identify sources of support and strength.
   • Encourage her to verbalize her guilt and anger and fears about her diagnosis and the impact it is having on her life.
   • Promote open communication between the patient and her husband.
   • Provide accurate and complete answers to her questions about her disease.
   • Offer information about community resources and local support groups.

6. Fear, denial, embarrassment, and being too busy are common reasons that women do not perform BSE or have a mammogram, and a lack of practice and skill at BSE undermines their confidence in performing the examination. Denial was probably a big factor for P.T. in view of the value of her breasts in her relationship with her husband.

7. Explain that some patients undergoing chemotherapy can have changes in maintaining focus/attention and memory and difficulties in concentration. We do not know currently why this happens, but research is being performed to determine the cause. This is called *chemobrain*, but that is not something that would need to be shared with the patient or the husband.

8. Teach P.T. that she will need follow-up for the rest of her life at regular intervals. She should expect to have a professional examination every 3 months for 2 years, every 6 months for the next 3 years, and then annually thereafter. She should be taught to perform BSE of both breasts every month and be informed that recurrence of breast cancer is likely to happen.

9. *Nursing diagnoses:*
   • Ineffective self-health management related to lack of compliance and information regarding breast cancer surveillance

- Ineffective coping related to reported feelings of guilt and perceived expectations of husband
- Impaired physical mobility related to decreased arm and shoulder mobility

Collaborative problems:

Potential complications: vascular access catheter displacement or infection; hyperuricemia; bleeding; septicemia; tumor recurrence

CHAPTER 53

1. c. Rationale: Although many factors relate to the current STD rates, one major factor is the widespread use of oral contraceptives, instead of condoms (both male and female), that provide a favorable environment for growth of STD organisms; in addition, condoms are the only contraceptive device that protects against STDs.

2. a. 3; b. 4; c. 1; d. 5; e. 2

3. d. Rationale: An established diagnosis of gonorrhea is treated with cefixime (Suprax) orally for one dose or a single dose of IM ceftriaxone (Rocephin). The doxycycline is often administered because of the high frequency of chlamydial infections coexisting with gonorrhea. Gram-stain smears are not useful in diagnosing gonorrhea in women because the female genitourinary tract normally harbors a large number of organisms that resemble *Neisseria gonorrhoeae*, and cultures must be performed to diagnose the disease in women. Penicillin G is used to treat syphilis, and although gonorrhea may lead to pelvic inflammatory disease (PID), its diagnosis would not necessarily indicate that the patient has PID.

4. a. Rationale: Upward extension of gonorrhea or chlamydia commonly causes PID, which can cause adhesions and fibrous scarring, leading to tubal pregnancies and infertility. Disseminated gonococcal infection is rare, and endocarditis and aneurysms are associated with syphilis.

5. d. Rationale: All sexual contacts of patients with gonorrhea must be notified, evaluated, and treated for STDs. The other information may be helpful in diagnosis and treatment, but the nurse must try to identify the patient's sexual partners.

6. a. S; b. T; c. T; d. P; e. T; f. S; g. L; h. T; i. S; j. T

7. d. Rationale: Many other diseases or conditions may cause false-positive test results on nontreponemal Venereal Disease Research Laboratory (VDRL) or rapid plasma reagent (RPR) tests, and additional testing is needed before a diagnosis is confirmed or treatment administered. Positive results on these tests should be confirmed by specific treponemal tests, such as the fluorescent treponemal antibody absorption (FTA-ABS) test or the TP-PA test, to rule out other causes. Analysis of cerebrospinal fluid (CSF) is used to diagnose asymptomatic neurosyphilis.

8. d. Rationale: The risk factors of drug abuse and sexual promiscuity are found in patients with both syphilis and HIV infection, and persons at highest risk for acquiring syphilis are also at high risk for acquiring HIV. Syphilitic lesions on the genitals enhance HIV transmission. Also, HIV-infected patients with syphilis appear to be at greatest risk for central nervous system (CNS) involvement and may require more intensive treatment with penicillin to prevent this complication of HIV.

9. b. Rationale: Although chlamydial infections may cause cervicitis and urethritis in women, it is more common for symptoms to be absent or minor in most infected women. The absence of symptoms necessitates screening of asymptomatic individuals at risk with nonculture tests, such as direct fluorescent antibody (DFA), or enzyme immunoassay (EIA) tests to identify and treat the disease.

10. b. Rationale: Notification and treatment of sex partners are necessary to prevent recurrence and the "ping-pong effect" of passing STDs between partners. Vibramycin is prescribed twice a day for 7 days, and although alcohol may cause more urinary irritation in the patient with chlamydia, it will not interfere with treatment.

11. c. Rationale: Gonorrhea and chlamydia have very similar symptoms in men, and chlamydial infections in men can be diagnosed by excluding gonorrhea. When Gram-stain smears and cultures for *N. gonorrhoeae* are negative, a diagnosis of NGU-chlamydia infection is made. Other testing for *N. gonorrhoeae* takes longer than a Gram stain.

12. a. *F*, oral or genital lesions; b. *T*; c. *F*, decrease recurrences of; d. *F*, sexual contact should be avoided; e. *T*

13. d. Rationale: The human papillomavirus (HPV) is responsible for causing genital warts, which manifest as discrete single or multiple white to gray warts that may coalesce to form large cauliflower-like masses on the vulva, vagina, cervix, and perianal area. Purulent vaginal discharge is associated with gonorrhea or chlamydia, painful perineal vesicles and ulcerations are characteristic of genital herpes, and a chancre of syphilis is a painless indurated lesion on the vulva, vagina, lips, or mouth.

14. a. Rationale: There is a strong association of genital warts to the development of dysplasia and neoplasia of the genital tract, especially when lesions involve the cervix, introitus, and perianal and intra-anal mucosa of women or the penis and perianal and anal mucosa of men. Regular Pap smears in women are critical in detecting early malignancies of the cervix. Oral acyclovir is used to treat herpes simplex virus-2 (HSV-2), but topical use has no value in treating viral STDs. Sexual partners of patients with HPV should be examined and treated, but because treatment does not destroy the virus, condoms should always be

used during sexual activity. Genital warts often grow more rapidly during pregnancy, but pregnancy is not contraindicated.

15. d. Rationale: Although gonorrhea and syphilis rank first and third, respectively, as the most common reportable communicable diseases in the United States, genital warts caused by HPV infection is not reportable in most states but is the most common STD in the United States today. An estimated 20 million people are currently infected with HPV, many of them young, sexually active adults.

16. a. Treatment with parenteral penicillin will cure both the mother and fetus. b. Erythromycin or silver nitrate required to be used in the eyes of all newborns. c. C-section if mother has active lesions. d. May be spread to the newborn by direct contact; cesarean section is not routine unless massive warts block the birth canal.

17. c. Rationale: Although sexual abstinence is the most certain method of avoiding all STDs, it is not usually a feasible alternative. A vaccine is available for HPV types 6, 11, 16, and 18 that protects against genital warts and cervical cancer. Conscientious hand washing and voiding after intercourse are positive hygienic measures that will help prevent secondary infections but will not prevent STDs.

18. a. Rationale: STDs that can be treated with a single dose or short course of antibiotic therapy often lead to a casual attitude about the outcome of the disease, which leads to noncompliance with instructions and delays in treatment. This is particularly true of diseases that initially show few distressing or uncomfortable symptoms, such as syphilis.

Case Study

1. The nurse should tell C.J. that he must tell his fiancée the truth about the sexual encounter and that it is most important for her to be evaluated for the disease. She may have the disease without symptoms and yet be at risk for development of pelvic inflammatory disease (PID) and infertility as a result of the gonorrhea. The nurse may offer a counseling referral, if necessary, for them to work through problems in their relationship.

2. Females often do not have any symptoms, but she could have a vaginal discharge, dysuria, urinary frequency, or changes in her menstrual patterns.

3. For C.J. the diagnosis can be confirmed by a positive Gram-stain smear of urethral drainage; in Ms. A., a positive culture of cervical secretions or of the urethra, anus, or oropharynx is necessary for confirmation of diagnosis.

4. Support and counseling may be needed from the nurse, and the couple should be assisted to verbalize their feelings and concerns. Active listening with a nonjudgmental attitude is important. Referral for professional counseling may be indicated.

5. Cefaxime (Suprax) orally in a single dose or ceftriaxone administered intramuscularly in a single dose and doxycycline twice daily is the recommended treatment for gonorrhea with a possible concurrent chlamydial infection. Because chlamydial infections are closely associated with gonococcal infections, both infections are usually treated concurrently even without diagnostic evidence.

6. Men: Prostatitis, urethral strictures, and sterility from orchitis or epididymitis
   Women: PID, Bartholin's abscess, ectopic pregnancy, infertility from tubal stricture
   Both men and women: Possible development of disseminated gonococcal infection

7. *Nursing diagnoses:*
   * Anxiety related to impact of condition on relationships and disease outcomes
   * Disturbed body image related to symptoms associated with gonorrhea
   * Risk for infection related to failure to practice precautionary measures
   Collaborative problems:
   Potential complication: Infertility

CHAPTER 54

1. a. Rationale: The initial visit of a couple seeking assistance with infertility includes a history and physical for both partners, testing for medical problems and sexually transmitted diseases (STDs), a cervical Pap test, possible semen analysis, and instruction for at-home ovulation testing. A discussion of possible future testing options and cost is also done. If the couple decides to continue with treatment, further visits will include more intensive evaluation, including postcoital testing, a hysterosalpingogram, pelvic ultrasound, and midluteal progesterone/prolactin levels.

2. b. Rationale: To determine the time of ovulation by body temperature, the woman must take and graph her temperature on awakening before any activity, noting any illness or variation in normal patterns. The increase in estrogen as ovulation approaches causes a temperature drop. When ovulation occurs, progesterone is produced and causes a sharp rise in temperature. Using basal body temperature to dictate the timing of sexual intercourse for conception is stressful and may decrease sexual performance and also the possibility of pregnancy. Anovulation can be detected but is treated primarily with hormone agents.

3. c. Rationale: In the presence of a confirmed pregnancy, uterine cramping with vaginal bleeding is the most important sign of spontaneous abortion. Other conditions causing vaginal bleeding, such as an incompetent cervix, do not usually cause cramping. There is no evidence that any medical treatment

improves the outcome for spontaneous abortion. Blood loss can be significant, and the loss of the pregnancy may cause long-term grieving. D&C is usually performed after the abortion to minimize blood loss and reduce the chance of infection.

4. d. Rationale: Mifepristone (RU 486) works by blocking progesterone, the hormone that supports pregnancy, and is effective within the first 49 days of pregnancy. Methotrexate is a chemotherapeutic agent that is toxic to trophoblastic tissue. Both agents are administered with misoprostol (Cytotec) to produce uterine contractions that expel the products of conception.

5. d. Rationale: Premenstrual syndrome (PMS) is diagnosed when other possible causes for symptoms have been eliminated and is based on a symptom diary that indicates the same symptoms during the luteal phase for two or three consecutive menstrual cycles. Oral contraceptives may be used to control the symptoms of PMS by suppressing ovulation, and although progesterone may also relieve the symptoms of PMS, its effectiveness is not associated with the diagnosis of PMS. There are no laboratory findings that account for the premenstrual symptoms.

6. c. Rationale: Limitation of salt, refined sugar, and caffeine in the diet has been shown to decrease the PMS symptoms of abdominal bloating, increased appetite, and irritability. Exercise is encouraged because it increases the release of endorphins, elevating the mood, and also has a tranquilizing effect on muscular tension. Estrogen is not used during the luteal phase, but progesterone may be tried. Vitamin B_6 and foods high in tryptophan may promote serotonin production, which improves symptoms.

7. c. Rationale: The release of excess prostaglandin F_2-α (PGF_2-α) from the endometrium at the time of menstruation or increased sensitivity to the prostaglandin is responsible for symptoms of primary dysmenorrhea, and drugs that inhibit prostaglandin production and release, such as nonsteroidal antiinflammatory drugs (NSAIDs), are effective in many patients with primary dysmenorrhea. Oral contraceptives are also used for primary dysmenorrhea to suppress ovulation and the associated production of prostaglandins.

8. a. 3; b. 1; c. 3; d. 3; e. 2; f. 3; g. 1

9. c. Rationale: When ovulation does not occur, estrogen continues to be unopposed by progesterone, and excessive buildup of the endometrium occurs. To prevent the risk of endometrial cancer by the buildup of the endometrium or to prevent menorrhagia from an unstable endometrium, progesterone or birth control pills are prescribed to ensure that the patient's endometrial lining will be shed at least four to six times a year. Balloon therapy to treat menorrhagia is contraindicated in women desiring future fertility.

10. b. Rationale: Ectopic pregnancy is a life-threatening condition; if the fallopian tube ruptures, profuse bleeding can lead to hypovolemic shock. All the interventions are indicated, but the priority should be monitoring the vital signs and pain for evidence of bleeding.

11. a. *F*, postmenopausal; b. *F*, estrogen (FSH levels rise); c. *T*; d. *T*; e. *T*

12. Benefits:
   • Control of vasomotor symptoms (hot flashes)
   • Relief of atrophic vaginal changes
   • Decreased risk of colorectal cancer
   • Decreased osteoporosis
   Risks:
   • Endometrial cancer
   • Breast cancer
   • Cardiovascular disease (myocardial infarction, stroke)
   • Venous thrombosis

13. a. 2; b. 1; c. 1; d. 4; e. 3; f. 1; g. 2; h. 1; i. 4

14. a. Rationale: *Gardnerella vaginalis* infection is a bacterial vaginosis that is sexually transmitted, and almost always both partners are infected. Successful treatment of the condition requires oral treatment with metronidazole (Flagyl) or clindamycin (Cleocin) for both partners. Minipads may be used to contain vaginal secretions, but they do not prevent reinfection.

15. b. Rationale: Sexual activity with multiple partners increases the risk for PID, and there is often a history of an acute infection of the lower genital tract caused by gonococcal or chlamydial microorganisms. The only significant contraceptive issue related to PID is that condom use will help prevent STDs that may lead to PID.

16. b. Rationale: Bed rest in semi-Fowler's position promotes drainage of the pelvic cavity by gravity and may prevent the development of abscesses high in the abdomen. Coitus, douching, and tampon use should be avoided to prevent spreading infection upward from the vagina, although frequent perineal care should be performed to remove infectious drainage.

17. b. Rationale: The risk for infertility following PID is high, and the nurse should allow time for the patient to express her feelings, clarify her concerns, and begin problem-solving with regard to the outcomes of the disease. Responses that do not allow for discussion of feelings and concerns or that tell the patient how she should feel or what she should worry about are not therapeutic.

18. a. *F*, endometriosis; b. *F*, endometriosis and uterine leiomyoma; c. *T*; d. *T*; e. *F*, pseudomenopause; f. *F*, metrorrhagia; g. *T*

19. b. Rationale: A stage 0 cervical cancer indicates cancer in situ that is confined to the epithelial layer of the cervix and requires treatment. Stage 0 is the

least invasive, and stage IVB indicates spread to distant organs.

20. c. Rationale: Conization (an excision of a cone-shaped section of the cervix) and laser treatment both are effective in locally removing or destroying malignant cells of the cervix and preserve fertility. Radiation treatments frequently impair ovarian and uterine function and lead to sterility. A subtotal hysterectomy would be contraindicated in treatment of cervical cancer because the cervix would be left intact in this procedure.

21. a. Rationale: Postmenopausal vaginal bleeding is the first sign of endometrial cancer; when it occurs, a sample of endometrial tissue must be taken to exclude cancer. An endometrial biopsy can be done as an office procedure and is indicated in this case. Abdominal x-rays and Pap smears are not reliable tests for endometrial cancer, and laser treatment of the cervix is indicated only for cervical dysplasia.

22. b. Rationale: Treatment of ovarian cancer is determined by staging from the results of laparoscopy with multiple biopsies of the ovaries and other tissue throughout the pelvis and lower abdomen. Although diagnosis of ovarian tumors may be made by ultrasound or computed tomography (CT) scan, the treatment of ovarian cancer depends on the staging of the tumor. The patient's desire for fertility is not a consideration because of the high mortality rate associated with ovarian cancer.

23. a. E; b. O; c. C; d. C; e. V; f. E; g. C; h. O; i. C; j. O

24. a. Rationale: Early signs of cancer of the vulva include pruritus, soreness of vulva, unusual odor, and discharge or bleeding of the vulva, with edema of the vulva and lymphadenopathy occurring as the disease progresses. Labial lesions and excoriation more commonly occur with infections, and nodules are more often cysts or lipomas.

25. c. Rationale: A total hysterectomy involves the removal of the uterus and the cervix, but the fallopian tubes and ovaries are left intact. Although menstruation is terminated, normal ovarian production of estrogen continues. A panhysterectomy is the procedure in which the uterus and cervix as well as the tubes and ovaries are removed.

26. c. Rationale: A pelvic exenteration is the most radical gynecologic surgery and results in removal of the uterus, ovaries, fallopian tubes, vagina, bladder, urethra, and pelvic lymph nodes and, in some situations, also the descending colon, rectum, and anal canal. There are urinary and fecal diversions on the abdominal wall, the absence of a vagina, and the onset of menopausal symptoms, all of which result in severe altered body structure.

27. d. Rationale: To prevent displacement of the intrauterine implant, the patient is maintained on absolute bed rest with turning from side to side. Bowel elimination is discouraged during the treatment by cleaning the colon before implantation, and urinary elimination is maintained by an indwelling catheter. Because the patient is radioactive, no individual nurse should spend more than 30 minutes daily with the patient, and visitors are restricted to less than 3 hours a day at a minimum of 6 ft from the patient.

28. a. Rationale: Kegel exercises help to strengthen muscular support of the perineum, pelvic floor, and bladder and are also beneficial for problems with pelvic support and stress incontinence. The muscles that should be exercised are those affected by trying to stop a flow of urine.

29. a. 5; b. 3; c. 2; d. 1; e. 4

30. a. Rationale: An anterior colporrhaphy involves repair of a cystocele, and an indwelling urinary catheter is left in place for several days postoperatively while healing occurs. Bowel function should not be altered and is maintained with a low-residue diet and a stool softener if necessary.

31. b. Rationale: Sexual assault is an act of violence, and the first priority of care for the patient should be assessment and treatment of serious injuries involving extragenital areas, such as fractures, subdural hematomas, cerebral concussions, and intra-abdominal injuries. All the other options are appropriate treatments, but treatment for shock and urgent medical injuries is the first priority.

32. b. Rationale: Specific informed consent must be obtained from the rape victim before any examination can be made or rape data collected. Following consent, the patient is advised not to wash, eat, drink, or urinate before the examination so that evidence can be collected for medicolegal use. Prophylaxis for STDs, hepatitis B, and tetanus is administered following examination, and follow-up testing for pregnancy and HIV is done in several weeks.

Case Study

1. The gonococcus spreads directly along the endometrium to the tubes and into the peritoneum, resulting in salpingitis, pelvic peritonitis, or tubo-ovarian abscesses.

2. Clinical manifestations include crampy or continuous bilateral lower abdominal pain that is increased with movement or ambulation; irregular menstrual bleeding and vaginal discharge that is yellow, green, or brownish with a foul odor; dyspareunia; fever; and chills, with possible nausea and vomiting.

3. Outpatient management would include oral antibiotics, increased fluid intake, good nutrition, restriction of activities, and rest with the head elevated. She should also be instructed to avoid intercourse, douching, and tampons.

4. Chronic PID is less acute, with increased cramps with menses, irregular bleeding, and moderate pain with intercourse.

5. Elevating the head of the bed promotes drainage of the pelvic cavity by gravity and may prevent the development of abscesses high in the abdomen. Application of heat with heating pads or sitz baths may help localize the infection.

6. Clarify the possible course and outcomes of the disease with the patient. Although early treatment may help prevent complications, it is realistic that sterility often results from PID because of adhesions and strictures of the fallopian tubes, and she is at increased risk for ectopic pregnancies. Discuss and listen to her concerns about her future childbearing ability.

7. *Nursing diagnoses:*
   - Ineffective health maintenance related to lack of protective measures against STDs
   - Anxiety related to outcome of disease on reproductive status
   - Risk for impaired skin integrity related to vaginal drainage

   Collaborative problems:

   Potential complications: Peritonitis, septic shock, thromboembolism

CHAPTER 55

1. d. Rationale: Hyperplasia is an increase in the number of cells, and in benign prostatic hyperplasia (BPH), it is thought that the enlargement caused by the increase in new cells results from endocrine changes associated with aging. Hypertrophy refers to an increase in the size of existing cells. The hyperplasia is not considered a tumor, nor does BPH predispose to cancer of the prostate.

2. c. Rationale: Classic symptoms of uncomplicated BPH are those associated with urinary obstruction and include diminished caliber and force of the urinary stream, hesitancy, difficulty initiating voiding, intermittent urination, dribbling at the end of urination, and a feeling of incomplete bladder emptying because of urinary retention. Irritative symptoms, including nocturia, frequency, dysuria, urgency, or hematuria, occur if infection results from urinary retention.

3. c. Rationale: Urinary flow meters are used to measure the urinary flow rate, which is decreased in vesicle neck obstruction. Cystourethroscopy may also evaluate the degree of obstruction, but a cystometrogram measures bladder tone, postvoiding catheterization measures residual urine, and a rectal ultrasound may determine the size and configuration of the prostate gland.

4. a. Rationale: Finasteride results in suppression of androgen formation by inhibiting the formation of the testosterone metabolite dihydroxytestosterone, the principal prostatic androgen, and results in a decrease in the size of the prostate gland.

Alpha-adrenergic blockers are used to cause smooth muscle relaxation in the treatment of BPH, but drugs affecting bladder tone are not indicated.

5. d. Rationale: Because of edema, urinary retention, and delayed sloughing of tissue that occurs with a laser prostatectomy, the patient will have postprocedure catheterization up to 7 days. The procedure is done under local anesthetic, and incontinence is not usually a problem.

6. d. Rationale: The prostate gland can be easily palpated by rectal examination, and enlargement of the gland is detected early if yearly examinations are performed. If symptoms of prostatic hyperplasia are present, further diagnostic testing, including a urinalysis, prostate-specific antigen (PSA), and cystoscopy, may be indicated.

7. a. 3; b. 5; c. 1; d. 6; e. 7; f. 1; g. 2; h. 1; i. 4; j. 7; k. 5; l. 3; m. 2, 7; n. 4

8. b. Rationale: Because of injury to the internal urinary sphincter, there is usually some degree of retrograde ejaculation following most transurethral surgeries, especially following a transurethral resection of the prostate (TURP). The semen is ejaculated into the bladder and is eliminated with the next voiding. Urinary incontinence, erectile dysfunction, and continued catheterization are rare following a TURP.

9. c. Rationale: Bleeding and blood clots from the bladder are expected after prostatectomy, and continuous irrigation is used to keep clots from obstructing the urinary tract. The rate of the irrigation may be increased to keep the clots from forming, if ordered, but the nurse should also check the vital signs because hemorrhage is the most common complication of prostatectomy. The traction on the catheter applies pressure to the operative site to control bleeding and should be relieved only if specific orders are given. The catheter does not need to be manually irrigated unless there are signs the catheter is obstructed, and clamping the drainage tube is contraindicated because it would cause distention of the bladder.

10. b. Rationale: Bladder spasms often occur after a TURP or suprapubic prostatectomy and are caused by bladder irritation, the presence of the catheter, or clots leading to obstruction of the catheter. The nurse should first check for the presence of clots obstructing the catheter or tubing and then may administer a belladonna and opium (B&O) suppository if one is ordered. The patient should not try to void around the catheter because this will increase the spasms. The flow rate on the irrigation fluid may be decreased if orders permit because fast-flowing, cold fluid may also contribute to spasms.

11. c. Rationale: Activities that increase intra-abdominal pressure should be avoided until the surgeon

approves these activities at a follow-up visit. Stool softeners and high-fiber diets may be used to promote bowel elimination, but enemas should not be used because they increase intra-abdominal pressure and may initiate bleeding. Because a TURP does not remove the entire prostate gland, the patient needs annual prostatic examinations to screen for cancer of the prostate. Fluid intake should be high, but caffeine and alcohol should not be used because they have a diuretic effect and increase bladder distention.

12. a. Hard, with asymmetric enlargement with areas of induration or nodules
    b. PSA higher than that usually seen in BPH; increased prostatic acid phosphatase (PAP), especially with metastasis; elevated alkaline phosphatase in advanced disease
    c. Pelvic or perineal pain, pain of metastasis, fatigue, malaise

13. c. Rationale: About the only modifiable risk factor for prostate cancer is its association with a high-fat diet. Age, ethnicity, and family history are risk factors for prostate cancer but are not modifiable. Simple enlargement or hyperplasia of the prostate is not a risk factor for prostate cancer.

14. b. Rationale: A prostatectomy performed with a perineal approach has a high risk for infection because of the proximity of the wound to the anus. Urinary retention and impaired bowel function may occur but do not necessarily lead to infection. Chemotherapy could lead to infection, but it is usually not the first choice of drug therapy following surgery.

15. a. *T*; b. *F*, luteinizing hormone-releasing hormone (LHRH) agonists (such as leuprolide [Lupron] or goserelin [Zoladex]) and androgen-receptor blockers; c. *F*, serum PSA measurements; d. *T*; e. *F*, African American; f. *F*, acute bacterial prostatitis; g. *T*

16. Word Search. a. Priapism; b. Hypospadias; c. Orchitis; d. Chordee; e. Testicular torsion; f. Circumcision; g. Phimosis; h. Spermatocele; i. Paraphimosis; j. Hydrocele; k. Epididymitis; l. Epispadias; m. Varicocele; n. Cryptorchidism

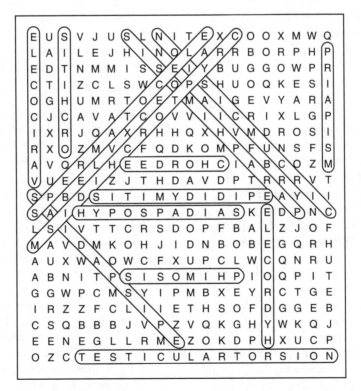

17. b. Rationale: Alpha-fetoprotein (AFP) and human chorionic gonadotropin (hCG) are glycoproteins that may be elevated in testicular cancer. If they are elevated before surgical treatment, the levels are noted, and if response to therapy is positive, the levels will decrease. PSA and PAP are used for screening of prostatic cancer; tumor necrosis factor (TNF) is a normal cytokine responsible for tumor surveillance and destruction; C-reactive protein (CRP) is found in inflammatory conditions and widespread malignancies; carcinoembryonic antigen (CEA) is a tumor marker for cancers of the GI system; and antinuclear antibody (ANA) is found most frequently in autoimmune disorders.

18. d. Rationale: Testicular tumors most often present on the testis as a lump or nodule that is very firm,

is nontender, and cannot be transilluminated. There may also be scrotal swelling and a feeling of heaviness. All the other options are normal findings.

19. c. Rationale: Until sperm distal to the anastomotic site is ejaculated or absorbed by the body, the semen will contain sperm, and alternative contraceptive methods must be used. When a postoperative semen examination reveals no sperm, the patient is considered sterile. Following vasectomy, there is rarely noticeable difference in the amount of ejaculate because ejaculate is primarily seminal fluid. Vasectomy does not affect testicular production of sperm or hormones, nor does it cause erectile dysfunction.

20. a. Rationale: Only a small percentage of erectile dysfunction is caused by psychologic factors, and before treatment for erectile dysfunction is initiated, the cause must be determined so that appropriate treatment can be planned. In the case of the 80% to 90% of erectile dysfunction that is of physiologic causes, interventions are directed at correcting or eliminating the cause or restoring function by medical means. New invasive or experimental treatments are not widely used and should be limited to research centers, and patients with systemic diseases can be treated medically if the cause cannot be eliminated.

21. a. 3; b. 1; c. 5; d. 2; e. 4; f. 5

Case Study

1. Testicular tumors develop either from the cellular components of the testis (very rare and usually benign) or from the embryonal precursors (germinal tumors that are almost always malignant). Risk factors include age between 15 and 35, a history of cryptorchidism, family history of testicular cancer, orchitis, HIV infection, maternal exposure to DES, and testicular cancer in the contralateral testis.

2. The primary difference on testicular examination between a spermatocele and a testicular cancer is that spermatocele will transilluminate, whereas cancer cannot be transilluminated.

3. About 95% of patients with testicular cancer that is found in early stages obtain a complete remission. C.E. has no back pain or gynecomastia, which would indicate metastatic disease. His prognosis is positive,

but he will need careful monitoring to detect any relapse early.

4. AFP and hCG are frequently elevated in testicular cancer and should be noted before treatment. If these markers are elevated before treatment and then decrease after treatment, a positive response to treatment is indicated. The levels of AFP and hCG are monitored during long-term follow-up to detect any relapse of the tumor.

5. Initiate conversation with him about his concerns, and allow him to talk about them. It is important to discuss the option of sperm banking before his surgery in case he later wants to have children.

6. The orchiectomy and lymph node resection will most likely be followed with radiation of the remaining lymph nodes and/or a single or multiple chemotherapy regimen. Germ-cell tumors are very sensitive to systemic chemotherapy, and its use is recommended. All these processes will cause sterility, but the surgery and additional treatment should not alter his sexual function.

7. *Nursing diagnoses:*
   • Anxiety related to effects of surgery
   • Fear related to outcome of disease process and prognosis
   Collaborative problems:
   No preoperative collaborative problems

CHAPTER 56

1. a. Golgi apparatus; b. mitochondrion; c. nucleolus; d. nucleus; e. Nissl bodies; f. axon hillock; g. axon; h. Schwann cell; i. myelin sheath; j. collateral axon; k. node of Ranvier; l. telodendria; m. synaptic knobs; n. neuron cell body; o. dendrites

2. a. dura mater; b. arachnoid; c. pia mater; d. ventral root; e. dorsal root; f. central canal; g. substansia gelatinosa; h. spinal cord; i. dorsal horn; j. lateral horn; k. ventral horn; l. spinal ganglia; m. spinal nerves; n. transverse process of vertebra; o. sympathetic ganglion; p. body of vertebra

3. Crossword Puzzle
   Across: 3. clefts; 6. synapse; 9. oligodendroglia; 11. myelin; 12. nucleus; 14. potential; 15. pia; 16. pons; 17. LOC; 18. neuron
   Down: 1. node of Ranvier; 2. astrocyte; 3. CSF; 4. LE; 5. Schwann cell; 7. axon; 8. regeneration; 10. dendrite; 13. limbic; 14. pain; 15. PO; 16. PO

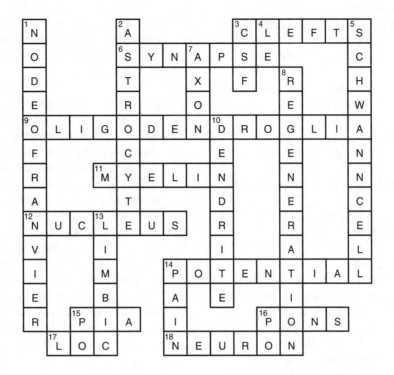

4. a. *F*, ependymal cells; b. *T*; c. *F*, faster; d. *F*, astrocytes; e. *T*

5. b. Rationale: The fasciculus gracilis and fasciculus cuneatus tracts carry information and transmit impulses concerned with touch, deep pressure, vibration, position sense, and kinesthesia. Spinothalamic tracts carry pain and temperature sensations; the spinocerebellar tracts carry subconscious information about muscle tension and body position; and descending corticobulbar tracts carry impulses responsible for voluntary impulses from the cortex to the cranial nerves.

6. a. Rationale: The cell bodies of lower motor neurons that send impulses to skeletal muscles in the arms, legs, and trunk are located in the anterior horn of the spinal cord, and lesions generally cause weakness or paralysis and decreased muscle tone. Upper motor neurons include the brainstem and cerebral cortex motor neurons that influence skeletal muscle movement, and lesions at this point cause weakness and paralysis with hyperreflexia and spasticity.

7. a. 8; b. 10; c. 7; d. 1; e. 11; f. 2; g. 12; h. 4; i. 3; j. 5; k. 9; l. 6

8. d. Rationale: Some cranial nerves are only efferent motor nerves (e.g., III, IV, VI, VII, XI, XII), some are only afferent sensory nerves (e.g., I, II, VIII), and some have both motor and sensory functions (e.g., V, IX, X), but spinal nerves always have both sensory and motor fibers. Both cranial and spinal nerves occur in pairs, and whereas most cell bodies of cranial nerves are located in the brain, the primary cell bodies of CN I, II, and XI are located outside of the brain.

9. a. S; b. S; c. P; d. P; e. S; f. P; g. S; h. P; i. P; j. P; k. P

10. b. Rationale: The circle of Willis is a vascular circle formed by the basilar artery and the internal carotid arteries and may act as an anastomotic pathway when occlusion of a major artery on one side of the brain occurs. The middle cerebral arteries supply the outer portions of the frontal, parietal, and superior temporal lobes, but the circle of Willis may accommodate for plaque in this artery.

11. a. 6; b. 4; c. 9; d. 7; e. 1; f. 8; g. 2; h. 5; i. 3

12. c. Rationale: A decrease in sensory receptors caused by degenerative changes leads to a diminished sense of touch, temperature, and peripheral vibrations in the older adult. Reflexes are decreased but not normally absent, and intelligence does not decrease, although there may be some loss of memory. Hypothalamic modifications lead to increased frequency of spontaneous awakening with interrupted sleep and insomnia.

13. a. Avoid suggesting symptoms.
    b. The onset, cause, and course of illness are especially important aspects of the nursing history.
    c. The mental status must be accurately assessed to ensure that the reported history is factual.

14. a. Uncontrolled hypertension, lack of appropriate helmet use, family history of neurologic problems, substance abuse, malnutrition
    b. Difficulty chewing and swallowing, B-vitamin deficiency
    c. Bowel or bladder incontinence, constipation
    d. Problems in mobility, strength, and coordination; history of falling

e. Sleep disturbances from pain or immobility; insomnia, frequently awakening

f. Sensory changes, dizziness; cognitive changes; language difficulties

g. Decreased self-worth and body image; unkempt physical appearance and hygiene

h. Changes in roles at work or in family from neurologic problems

i. Decreased sexual desire, stimulation, function, or response

j. Sense of being overwhelmed, inadequate coping patterns

k. Religious or cultural beliefs that interfere or assist with planned treatment

15. a. 7; b. 4; c. 8, 9; d. 9; e. 3, 6; f. 9, 12; g. 2, 6, 10; h. 13; i. 11; j. 11; k. 1; l. 5

16. c. Rationale: The primary purposes of the nursing neurologic examination are to determine the effects of neurologic dysfunction on daily living and the patient's and the family's ability to cope with neurologic deficits. The examination should be viewed in terms of functional disabilities, rather than dysfunction, of component parts of the nervous system, and findings of the examination should be used to plan appropriate care for deficits in self-care and in activities of daily living.

17. a. 6; b. 8; c. 5; d. 9; e. 10; f. 1; g. 4; h. 7; i. 2; j. 3

18. b. Rationale: The normal response of the triceps reflex is extension of the arm or visible contraction of the triceps. The normal response of the biceps reflex is flexion of the arm at the elbow, whereas the presence of the brachioradialis reflex is seen with flexion and supination at the elbow.

19. b. Rationale: Deep-tendon grading is as follows: 0/5 = absent; 1/5 = weak response; 2/5 = normal response; 3/5 = exaggerated response; 4/5 = hyperreflexia with clonus.

20. d. Rationale: To facilitate insertion of the spinal needle between the third and fourth lumbar vertebrae, the patient should round the spine by flexing the knees, hips, and neck while in a lateral position. Sitting on the edge of the bed and bending only the spine does not separate the vertebrae as efficiently. Stimulants are withheld for 8 hours before an electroencephalogram (EEG), and sedation is used for more invasive tests, such as myelograms and angiography.

21. a. Rationale: A spinal headache, which may be caused by loss of CSF at the puncture site, is common following a lumbar puncture or a myelogram, and nuchal rigidity may also occur as a result of meningeal irritation. The patient is not in danger of paralysis with a lumbar puncture, nor does hemorrhage from the site occur. Contrast media are not used with a lumbar puncture.

22. b. Rationale: Following a myelogram (and a lumbar puncture), the patient is positioned flat in bed for several hours to avoid a spinal headache, and fluids are encouraged to help in the excretion of the contrast medium. Pain at the insertion site is rare, and the most common complaint after a myelogram is a headache.

23. b. Rationale: Cerebral angiography involves the injection of contrast media through a catheter inserted into the femoral or brachial artery and passed into the base of a carotid or vertebral artery and is performed when vascular lesions or tumors are suspected. Allergic reactions to the contrast medium may occur, and vascular spasms or dislodgement of plaques is possible. Neurologic and vital signs must be monitored every 15 to 30 minutes for 2 hours, every hour for the next 6 hours, and then every 2 hours for 24 hours following the test. EEGs and transcranial Doppler sonography are not invasive studies.

24. d. Rationale: Normal glucose levels in CSF are 40 to 70 mg/dL. All types of organisms consume glucose, and decreased glucose level reflects bacterial activity. Increased levels are associated with diabetes. The other values are all normal.

CHAPTER 57

1. a. Increased absorption, decreased production, displacement into spinal canal; b. Herniation, lesion, edema, collapse of veins and dural sinuses, increased venous outflow and decreased blood flow; c. Distention of dura, slight compression of tissue

2. a. 5 to 15
   b. 50, ischemic; 150, constricted
   c. 60-100; 56 mm Hg: MAP = DBP + 1/3 (SBP – DBP) = 52 + 18 = 70
   CPP = MAP – ICP = 70 – 14 = 56
   d. 45: MAP = DBP + 1/3 (SBP – DBP) = 64 + 15 = 79
   CPP = MAP – ICP = 79 – 34 = 45
   e. 50; 30

3. a. D; b. I; c. D; d. D; e. I

4. a. 2; b. 1; c. 2; d. 1; e. 3

5. a. CO; b. CO; c. CB; d. CO; e. CB

6. c. Rationale: One of the most sensitive signs of increased intracranial pressure (ICP) is a decreasing level of consciousness (LOC). A decrease in LOC will occur before changes in vital signs, ocular signs, or projectile vomiting occur.

7. b. Rationale: Cushing's triad consists of three vital sign measures that reflect ICP and its effect on the medulla, the hypothalamus, the pons, and the thalamus. Because these structures are very deep, Cushing's triad is usually a late sign of ICP. The signs include an increasing systolic BP with a widening pulse pressure, a bradycardia with a full and bounding pulse, and irregular respirations.

8. c. Rationale: The dural structures that separate the two hemispheres and the cerebral hemispheres from the cerebellum influence the patterns of cerebral herniation. A cingulated herniation occurs where

there is lateral displacement of brain tissue beneath the falx cerebri.

9. a. Rationale: An intraventricular catheter is a fluid-coupled system that can provide direct access for microorganisms to enter the ventricles of the brain, and aseptic technique is a very high nursing priority to decrease the risk for infection. Constant monitoring of ICP waveforms is not usually necessary, and removal of CSF for sampling or to maintain normal ICP is done only when specifically ordered.

10. a. *T*; b. *F*, tragus of the ear; c. *T*; d. *T*; e. *F*, Licox brain tissue oxygenation catheter; f. *T*

11. a. 2; b. 4; c. 3; d. 5; e. 1

12. d. Rationale: A patient with increased ICP is in a hypermetabolic and hypercatabolic state and needs adequate glucose to maintain fuel for the brain and other nutrients to meet metabolic needs. Malnutrition promotes cerebral edema, and if a patient cannot take oral nutrition, other means of providing nutrition should be used, such as tube feedings or parenteral nutrition. Glucose alone is not adequate to meet nutritional requirements, and 5% dextrose solutions may increase cerebral edema by lowering serum osmolarity. Patients should remain in a normovolemic fluid state with close monitoring of clinical factors such as urine output, fluid intake, serum and urine osmolality, serum electrolytes, and insensible losses.

13. a. eyes open; b. best verbal response; c. best motor response

14. b. Rationale: No opening of eyes = 1; incomprehensible words = 2; flexion withdrawal = 4. Total = 7

15. d. Rationale: Of the body functions that should be assessed in an unconscious patient, cardiopulmonary status is the most vital function and gives priorities to the ABCs (airway, breathing, and circulation).

16. c. Rationale: One of the functions of CN III, the oculomotor nerve, is pupillary constriction, and testing for pupillary constriction is important to identify patients at risk for brainstem herniation caused by increased ICP. The corneal reflex is used to assess the functions of CN V and VII, and the oculocephalic reflex tests all cranial nerves involved with eye movement. Nystagmus is commonly associated with specific lesions or chemical toxicities and is not a definitive sign of ICP.

17. a. Rationale: Nursing care activities that increase ICP include hip and neck flexion, suctioning, clustering care activities, and noxious stimuli; they should be avoided or performed as little as possible in the patient with increased ICP. Lowering the $PaCO_2$ below 20 mm Hg can cause ischemia and worsening of ICP; the $PaCO_2$ should be maintained at 30 to 35 mm Hg.

18. c. Rationale: A PaO_2 of 50 mm Hg reflects a hypoxemia that may lead to further decreased cerebral perfusion and hypoxia and must be corrected. The pH and SaO_2 are within normal range, and a $PaCO_2$ of 30 mm Hg reflects an acceptable value for the patient with increased ICP.

19. a, b, d, e. The first sign of increased ICP is a change in LOC. Other manifestations are dilated ipsilateral pupil, changes in motor response such as posturing, and fever, which may indicate pressure on the hypothalamus. Changes in vital signs would be an increased systolic BP with widened pulse pressure and bradycardia.

20. c. Rationale: If reflex posturing occurs during range of motion (ROM) or positioning of the patient, these activities should be done less frequently until the patient's condition stabilizes, because posturing can cause increases in ICP. Neither restraints nor CNS depressants would be indicated.

21. a. 4; b. 9; c. 1; d. 7; e. 6; f. 10; g. 3; h. 8; i. 12; j. 11; k. 2; l. 5

22. b. Rationale: Testing clear drainage for CSF in nasal or ear drainage may be done with a Dextrostik or Tes-Tape strip, but if blood is present, the glucose in the blood will produce an unreliable result. To test bloody drainage, the nurse should test the fluid for a "halo" or "ring" that occurs when a yellowish ring encircles blood dripped onto a white pad or towel.

23. d. Rationale: An arterial epidural hematoma is the most acute neurologic emergency, and typical symptoms include unconsciousness at the scene, with a brief lucid interval followed by a decrease in LOC. An acute subdural hematoma manifests signs within 48 hours of an injury; a chronic subdural hematoma develops over weeks or months.

24. d. Rationale: When there is a depressed fracture and fractures with loose fragments, a craniotomy is indicated to elevate the depressed bone and remove free fragments. A craniotomy is also indicated in cases of acute subdural and epidural hematomas to remove the blood and control the bleeding. Burr holes may be used in an extreme emergency for rapid decompression, but with a depressed fracture, surgery would be the treatment of choice.

25. a. Rationale: In addition to monitoring for a patent airway during emergency care of the patient with a head injury, the nurse must always assume that a patient with a head injury may have a cervical spine injury. Maintaining cervical spine precautions in all assessment and treatment activities with the patient is essential to prevent additional neurologic damage.

26. c. Rationale: Residual mental and emotional changes of brain trauma with personality changes are often the most incapacitating problems following head injury and are common in patients who have been comatose longer than 6 hours. Families must be prepared for changes in the patient's behavior to avoid family-patient friction and maintain family functioning, and professional assistance may be

required. There is no indication he will be dependent on others for care, but he likely will not return to pretrauma status.

27. a. *F*, all; b. *F*, occipital; c. *F*, a glioblastoma multiforme; d. *T*; e. *T*

28. b. Rationale: Frontal lobe tumors often lead to loss of emotional control, confusion, memory loss, disorientation, and personality changes that are very disturbing and frightening to the family. Physical symptoms, such as blindness, disturbances in sensation and perception, and even seizures, that occur with other tumors are more likely to be understood and accepted by the family.

29. a. 4; b. 6; c. 1; d. 5; e. 2; f. 3

30. a. Rationale: To prevent undue concern and anxiety about hair loss and postoperative self-esteem disturbances, a patient undergoing cranial surgery should be informed preoperatively that the head is usually shaved in surgery while the patient is anesthetized and that methods can be used after the dressings are removed postoperatively to disguise the hair loss. In the immediate postoperative period, the patient is very ill, and the focus is on maintaining neurologic function, but preoperatively the nurse should anticipate the patient's postoperative need for self-esteem and maintenance of appearance.

31. d. Rationale: The primary goal after cranial surgery is prevention of increased ICP, and interventions to prevent ICP and infection postoperatively are nursing priorities. The residual deficits, rehabilitation potential, and ultimate function of the patient depend on the reason for surgery, the postoperative course, and the patient's general state of health.

32. a. M; b. E; c. E; d. M; e. E; f. M; g. M; h. E; i. M

33. d. Rationale: Meningitis is often a result of an upper respiratory infection or middle-ear infection, where organisms gain entry to the CNS. Epidemic encephalitis is transmitted by ticks and mosquitoes, and nonepidemic encephalitis may occur as a complication of measles, chickenpox, or mumps. Encephalitis caused by the herpes simplex virus carries a high fatality rate.

34. b. Rationale: High fever, severe headache, nuchal rigidity, and positive Brudzinski's and Kernig's signs are such classic symptoms of meningitis that they are usually considered diagnostic for meningitis. Other symptoms, such as papilledema, generalized seizures, hemiparesis, and decreased LOC, may occur as complications of increased ICP and cranial nerve dysfunction.

35. a. increased seizures; b. increased ICP; c. dehydration; d. direct neurologic damage

36. c. Rationale: The symptoms of brain abscess closely resemble those of meningitis and encephalitis, including fever, headache, and increased ICP, except the patient also usually has some focal symptoms that reflect the local area of the abscess.

Case Study

1. The temperature elevation and nuchal rigidity in the presence of increased ICP and decreasing LOC indicate that J.K. has developed a meningeal infection.

2. The risks for meningitis after head injury and surgery include penetrations into the intracranial cavity with the compound fracture that involves a depressed skull fracture with scalp lacerations with a communicating pathway to the intracranial cavity and the incisions necessary for craniotomy for hematoma evacuation. Postoperative drains, invasive monitoring, environmental pathogens, as well as impaired immune response, also contribute to the development of meningitis.

3. Acute inflammation and infection of the pia mater and the arachnoid membrane cause nuchal rigidity, a sign of meningeal irritation, and fever. The inflammatory response increases CSF production with an increase in pressure, and as the purulent secretion produced by microbial infection spreads to other areas of the brain, cerebral edema and increased ICP occur. Increased ICP is thought to be a result of swelling around the dura, increased CSF volume, and endotoxins produced by the bacteria.

4. Priority interventions include reduction of fever, reduction of ICP, maintaining antibiotic schedule to keep therapeutic levels, maintaining fluid balance, protection from injury if seizures occur, and minimizing environmental stimuli.

5. Access to the meninges could have occurred from facial and cranial fractures and the surgical incisions.

6. *Nursing diagnoses:*
   - Risk for ineffective cerebral tissue perfusion related to cerebral tissue swelling
   - Hyperthermia related to infection and abnormal temperature regulation
   - Ineffective breathing pattern related to decreased LOC and immobility
   - Risk for injury related to potential for seizures
   - Imbalanced nutrition: less than body requirements related to hypermetabolism and inability to ingest food and fluids
   - Risk for impaired skin integrity related to immobility

   Collaborative problems:

   Potential complications: Increased ICP; seizures; hydrocephalus; disseminated intravascular coagulation; brain herniation

CHAPTER 58

1. c. Rationale: The highest risk factors for thrombotic stroke are hypertension and diabetes. African Americans have a higher risk for stroke than do white persons but probably because they have a greater incidence of hypertension. Factors such as

obesity, diet high in saturated fats and cholesterol, cigarette smoking, and excessive alcohol use are also risk factors but carry less risk than hypertension.

2. c. Rationale: The communication between cerebral arteries in the circle of Willis provides a collateral circulation, which may maintain circulation to an area of the brain if its original blood supply is obstructed. All areas of the brain require constant blood supply, and atherosclerotic plaques are not readily reversed. Neurologic deficits can result from ischemia caused by many factors.

3. d. Rationale: A transient ischemic attack (TIA) is a temporary focal loss of neurologic function caused by ischemia of an area of the brain, usually lasting only about 3 hours. TIAs may be due to microemboli from heart disease or carotid or cerebral thrombi and are a warning of progressive disease. Evaluation is necessary to determine the cause of the neurologic deficit and provide prophylactic treatment if possible.

4. a. 2; b. 3; c. 3; d. 1; e. 4; f. 3; g. 4; h. 1; i. 2; j. 4; k. 1; l. 4; m. 2

5. c. Rationale: Clinical manifestations of altered neurologic function differ, depending primarily on the specific cerebral artery involved and the area of the brain that is perfused by the artery. The degree of impairment depends on rapidity of onset, the size of the lesion, and the presence of collateral circulation.

6. a. L; b. R; c. R; d. R; e. L; f. R

7. a. *T*; b. *F*, expressive aphasia; c. *T*; d. *F*, fluent dysphasia; e. *F*, spasticity

8. a. Rationale: A CT scan is the most commonly used diagnostic test to determine the size and location of the lesion and to differentiate a thrombotic stroke from a hemorrhagic stroke. Positron emission tomography (PET) will show the metabolic activity of the brain and provide a depiction of the extent of tissue damage after a stroke. Lumbar punctures are not performed routinely because of the chance of increased intracranial pressure causing herniation. Cerebral arteriograms are invasive and may dislodge an embolism or cause further hemorrhage; they are performed only when no other test can provide the needed information.

9. c. Rationale: An endarterectomy is a removal of an atherosclerotic plaque, and a plaque in the carotid artery may impair circulation enough to cause a stroke. A carotid endarterectomy is performed to prevent a cerebrovascular accident (CVA), as are most other surgical procedures. An extracranial-intracranial bypass involves cranial surgery to bypass a sclerotic intracranial artery. Percutaneous transluminal angioplasty uses a balloon to compress stenotic areas in the carotid and vertebrobasilar arteries and often includes inserting a stent to hold the artery open.

10. c. Rationale: The administration of antiplatelet agents, such as aspirin, dipyridamole (Persantine),

and ticlopidine (Ticlid), reduces the incidence of stroke in those at risk. Anticoagulants are also used for prevention of embolic strokes but increase the risk for hemorrhage. Diuretics are not indicated for stroke prevention other than for their role in controlling blood pressure (BP), and antilipemic agents have not been found to have a significant effect on stroke prevention. The calcium-channel blocker nimodipine is used in patients with subarachnoid hemorrhage to decrease the effects of vasospasm and minimize tissue damage.

11. d. Rationale: The first priority in acute management of the patient with a stroke is preservation of life. Because the patient with a stroke may be unconscious or have a reduced gag reflex, it is most important to maintain a patent airway for the patient and provide oxygen if respiratory effort is impaired. IV fluid replacement, treatment with osmotic diuretics, and perhaps hypothermia may be used for further treatment.

12. b. Rationale: Surgical management with clipping of an aneurysm to decrease rebleeding and vasospasm is an option for a stroke caused by rupture of a cerebral aneurysm. Placement of coils into the lumens of the aneurysm by interventional radiologists is increasing in popularity. Hyperventilation therapy would increase vasodilation and the potential for hemorrhage. Thrombolytic therapy would be absolutely contraindicated, and if a vessel is patent, osmotic diuretics may leak into tissue, pulling fluid out of the vessel and increasing edema.

13. a. Rationale: The body responds to the vasospasm and decreased circulation to the brain that occurs with a stroke by increasing the BP, frequently resulting in hypertension. The other options are important cardiovascular factors to assess, but they do not result from impaired cerebral blood flow.

14. a. self-care deficit; b. unilateral neglect; c. impaired swallowing; d. risk for aspiration
Also: Impaired urinary elimination; risk for impaired skin integrity; ineffective airway clearance; impaired physical mobility; impaired verbal communication; situational low self-esteem.

15. d. Rationale: Active ROM should be initiated on the unaffected side as soon as possible, and passive ROM of the affected side should be started on the first day. Having the patient actively exercise the unaffected side provides the patient with active and passive ROM as needed. Use of footboards is controversial because they stimulate plantar flexion. The unaffected arm should be supported, but immobilization may precipitate a painful shoulder-hand syndrome. The patient should be positioned with each joint higher than the joint proximal to it to prevent dependent edema.

16. a. Rationale: The presence of homonymous hemianopia in a patient with right-hemisphere brain

damage causes a loss of vision in the left field. Early in the care of the patient, objects should be placed on the right side of the patient in the field of vision, and the nurse should approach the patient from the right side. Later in treatment, patients should be taught to turn the head and scan the environment and should be approached from the affected side to encourage head turning. Eye patches are used if patients have diplopia (double vision).

17. a. Rationale: The first step in providing oral feedings for a patient with a stroke is ensuring that the patient has an intact gag reflex because oral feedings will not be provided if the gag reflex is impaired. The nurse should then evaluate the patient's ability to swallow ice chips or ice water after placing the patient in an upright position.

18. c. Rationale: Soft foods that provide enough texture, flavor, and bulk to stimulate swallowing should be used for the patient with dysphasia. Thin liquids are difficult to swallow, and patients may not be able to control them in the mouth. Pureed foods are often too bland and too smooth, and milk products should be avoided because they tend to increase the viscosity of mucus and increase salivation.

19. d. Rationale: tPA dissolves clots and increases the risk for bleeding. It is not used with hemorrhagic strokes. If the patient had a thrombotic/embolic stroke the time frame would be important as well as a history of surgery. The nurse should answer the question as accurately as possible and then encourage the individual to talk with the primary care physician if he or she has further questions.

20. b. Rationale: During rehabilitation, the patient with aphasia needs frequent, meaningful verbal stimulation that has relevance for him. Conversation by the nurse and family should address activities of daily living (ADLs) that are familiar to the patient. Gestures, pictures, and simple statements are more appropriate in the acute phase, when patients may be overwhelmed by verbal stimuli. Flashcards are often perceived by the patient as childish and meaningless.

21. c. Rationale: Unilateral neglect, or neglect syndrome, occurs when the patient with a stroke is unaware of the affected side of the body, which puts the patient at risk for injury. During the acute phase, the affected side is cared for by the nurse with positioning and support, but during rehabilitation the patient is taught to care consciously for and attend to the affected side of the body to protect it from injury. Patients may be positioned on the affected side for up to 30 minutes.

22. c. Rationale: Patients with left-brain damage from stroke often experience emotional lability, inappropriate emotional responses, mood swings, and uncontrolled tears or laughter disproportionate or out of context with the situation. The behavior is upsetting and embarrassing to both the patient and the family, and the patient should be distracted to minimize its presence. Patients with right-brain damage often have impulsive, rapid behavior that requires supervision and direction.

23. d. Rationale: The patient and family need accurate and complete information about the effects of the stroke to problem-solve and make plans for chronic care of the patient. It is uncommon for patients with major strokes to return completely to prestroke function, behaviors, and role, and both the patient and family will mourn these losses. The patient's specific needs for care must be identified, and rehabilitation efforts should be continued at home. Family therapy and support groups may be helpful for some patients and families.

24. c. Rationale: Medication administration is within the scope of practice for an LPN. Assessment and teaching are within the scope of practice for the RN.

Case Study

1. A CT or magnetic resonance imaging (MRI) scan would be able to determine the size and location of a lesion and to differentiate between an infarction and a hemorrhage. A lumbar puncture would not be indicated because of the chance that hemorrhage had increased ICP. Other tests that might be used when hemorrhage is evident include intraarterial angiography, digital subtraction angiography, and transcranial Doppler sonography.

2. Unconsciousness, Glasgow Coma Scale (GCS) score of 5, and wide pulse pressure with a decrease in pulse and respiration all indicate increased intracranial pressure (ICP).

3. The loss of consciousness is associated with a poor prognosis for recovery, and the family should be told that her condition is very guarded.

4. The highest priorities for interventions are those that support her life processes: airway and respiratory function with oxygen administration, fluid management without overloading the vascular system, and measures that decrease ICP.

5. Anything that impairs clotting is contraindicated in a hemorrhagic stroke: anticoagulants, antiplatelet agents, and thrombolytic therapy. Hyperosmolar diuretics are also contraindicated because they may escape from an injured vessel, causing increased edema in brain tissue.

6. Hypothermia and barbiturate therapy may be used, but these treatments have not proved effective. Surgery is the only other option, and clipping of an aneurysm may be performed, or the aneurysm may be wrapped or reinforced with muscle.

7. *Nursing diagnoses:*
   - Risk for ineffective cerebral tissue perfusion related to hemorrhage
   - Ineffective airway clearance related to unconsciousness
   - Self-care deficit related to altered mental state

- Risk for injury related to inability to monitor personal safety
- Risk for infection related to immobility
Collaborative problems:
Potential complications: increased ICP; brain herniation; seizures

CHAPTER 59

1. a. 3; b. 1; c. 2; d. 1; e. 3; f. 1; g. 3; h. 3; i. 2; j. 3; k. 2; l. 2

2. d. Rationale: The primary way to diagnose and differentiate between headaches is with a careful history of the headaches, requiring assessment of specific details related to the headache. Electromyelography (EMG) may reveal contraction of the neck, scalp, or facial muscles in tension-type headaches, but this is not seen in all patients. CT scans and cerebral angiography are used to rule out organic causes of the headaches.

3. d. Rationale: Both migraine headaches and cluster headaches appear to be related to vasodilation of cranial vessels, and drugs that cause vasoconstriction, like sumatriptan, are useful in treatment of migraine and cluster headaches. Methysergide is an ergot alkaloid that blocks serotonin receptors in the central and peripheral nervous systems and is used for treatment of migraine headaches and prevention of cluster headaches. Beta-blockers and tricyclic antidepressants are used prophylactically for migraine headaches but are not effective for cluster headaches.

4. a. Rationale: When the anxiety is related to a lack of knowledge about the etiology and treatment of a headache, helping the patient to identify stressful lifestyles and other precipitating factors and ways of avoiding them are appropriate nursing interventions for the anxiety. Interventions that teach alternative therapies to supplement drug therapy also give the patient some control over pain and are appropriate teaching regarding treatment of the headache. The other interventions may help reduce anxiety generally, but they do not address the etiologic factor of the anxiety.

5. c. Rationale: The NAP is able to obtain equipment from the supply cabinet or department. The RN may need to provide a list of necessary equipment and should set up the equipment and ensure proper functioning. The RN is responsible for the initial history and assessment as well as teaching the patient about the room's call system. Padded tongue blades are no longer used, and no effort should be made to place anything in the patient's mouth during a seizure.

6. d. Rationale: Generalized seizures have bilateral synchronous epileptic discharge affecting the entire brain at onset of the seizure, preventing any warning. Loss of consciousness (LOC) is also characteristic,

but many partial seizures also include an LOC. Partial seizures begin in one side of the brain but may spread to involve the entire brain. Partial seizures that start with a local focus and spread to the entire brain, causing a secondary generalized seizure, are associated with a transient residual neurologic deficit postictally known as Todd's paralysis.

7. a. 2; b. 4; c. 7; d. 1; e. 3; f. 6; g. 1; h. 5; i. 2; j. 7; k. 7; l. 1; m. 7; n. 4

8. a. *T*; b. *T*; c. *F*, patient history and description of seizure; d. *F*, first time or status; e. *T*

9. c. Rationale: A seizure is a paroxysmal, uncontrolled discharge of neurons in the brain, which interrupts normal function, but the factor that causes the abnormal firing is not clear. Seizures may be precipitated by many factors, and although scar tissue may stimulate seizures, it is not the usual cause of seizures. Epilepsy is established only by a pattern of spontaneous, recurring seizures.

10. b. Rationale: Most patients with seizure disorders maintain seizure control with medications, but if surgery is considered, three requirements must be met: The diagnosis of epilepsy must be confirmed, there must have been an adequate trial with drug therapy without satisfactory results, and the electroclinical syndrome must be defined. The focal point must be localized, but the presence of scar tissue is not required.

11. d. Rationale: Serum levels of antiseizure drugs are monitored regularly to maintain therapeutic levels of the drug, above which patients are likely to experience toxic effects and below which seizures are likely to occur. EEGs have limited value in diagnosis of seizures and even less in monitoring seizure control.

12. c. Rationale: If antiseizure drugs are discontinued abruptly, seizures can be precipitated, and patients should never stop their medication. Missed doses should be made up if the omission is remembered within 24 hours, and patients should not adjust medications without professional guidance because this, too, can increase seizure frequency and may cause status epilepticus. If side effects occur, the physician should be notified and drug regimens evaluated. Antiseizure drugs have numerous interactions with other drugs, and the use of other medications should be evaluated by health professionals.

13. a, b, c. The focus is on maintaining a patent airway and preventing patient injury.

14. b. Rationale: In the postictal phase of generalized tonic-clonic seizures, patients are usually very tired and may sleep for several hours, and the nurse should allow the patient to sleep as long as necessary. Suctioning is performed only if needed, and decreased LOC is not a problem postictally

unless a head injury has occurred during the seizure.

15. b. Rationale: One of the most common complications of a seizure disorder is the effect it has on the patient's lifestyle. This is because of the social stigma attached to seizures, causing patients to hide their diagnosis and to prefer not to be identified as having epilepsy. Job discrimination against the handicapped is prevented by federal and state laws, and patients need to identify their disease in case of medical emergencies. Medication regimens usually require only once- or twice-daily dosing, and the major restrictions of lifestyle usually involve driving and high-risk environments.

16. a. 3; b. 5; c. 4; d. 2; e. 1

17. b. Rationale: Most patients with MS have remissions and exacerbations of neurologic dysfunction that eventually cause progressive loss of motor, sensory, and cerebellar functions. Intellectual function generally remains intact, but patients may experience anger, depression, or euphoria. A few people have chronic progressive deterioration, and some may experience only occasional and mild symptoms for several years after onset.

18. c. Rationale: Motor and sensory dysfunctions, including paresthesias as well as patchy blindness, blurred vision, and hearing loss, are the most common manifestations of multiple sclerosis (MS). Bowel and bladder dysfunctions and ataxia also occur, but excessive involuntary movements, tremors, and memory loss are not seen in MS.

19. c. Rationale: There is no specific diagnostic test for MS, and a diagnosis is made primarily by history and clinical manifestations. In later MS, CT and MRI may detect sclerotic plaques. Some patients have elevations of oligoclonal immunoglobulin G, lymphocytes, and monocytes in CSF, but these findings do not establish a diagnosis of MS.

20. b. Rationale: Mitoxantrone (Novantrone) is an immunosuppressant drug that reduces both B and T lymphocytes and impairs antigen presentation. It is similar to other immunosuppressants in that it increases the risk for infection, but it cannot be used for more than 2 to 3 years because it causes cardiac toxicity. It is administered intravenously monthly.

21. d. Rationale: The main goal in care of the patient with MS is to keep the patient active and maximally functional, promoting self-care as much as possible to maintain independence. Assistive devices encourage independence while preserving the patient's energy. No care activity that the patient can do for himself or herself should be performed by others. Involvement of the family in the patient's care and maintenance of social interactions are also important but are not the priority in care.

22. b. Rationale: Corticosteroids used in treating acute exacerbations should not be abruptly stopped by the patient because adrenal insufficiency may result, and prescribed tapering doses should be followed. Infections may exacerbate symptoms and should be avoided, and high-protein diets with vitamin supplements are advocated. Long-term planning for increasing disability is also important.

23. a. Tremor: Impaired handwriting and hand activities
    b. Rigidity: Muscle soreness and pain; slowness of movement
    c. Bradykinesia: Lack of blinking, arm swinging while walking, and facial expression; shuffling gait; difficulty initiating movement

24. b. Rationale: Although clinical manifestations are characteristic in Parkinson's disease, no laboratory or diagnostic tests are specific for the condition. A diagnosis is made when at least two of the three signs of the classic triad are present and it is confirmed with a positive response to antiparkinsonian medication. Essential tremors increase during voluntary movement, whereas the tremors of Parkinson's disease are more prominent at rest.

25. c. Rationale: The bradykinesia of Parkinson's disease prevents automatic movements, and activities such as beginning to walk, rising from a chair, or even swallowing saliva cannot be executed unless they are consciously willed. Handwriting is affected by the tremor and results in the writing trailing off at the end of words. Specific limb weakness and muscle spasms are not characteristic of Parkinson's disease.

26. c. Rationale: Peripheral dopamine does not cross the blood-brain barrier, but its precursor, levodopa, is able to enter the brain, where it is converted to dopamine, increasing the supply that is deficient in Parkinson's disease. Other drugs used to treat Parkinson's disease include bromocriptine, which stimulates dopamine receptors in the basal ganglia, and amantadine, which is believed to promote the release of dopamine from brain neurons. Carbidopa is an agent that is usually administered with levodopa to prevent the levodopa from being metabolized in peripheral tissues before it can reach the brain.

27. c. Rationale: The shuffling gait of Parkinson's disease causes the patient to be off balance and at risk for falling. Teaching the patient to use a wide stance with the feet apart, to lift the toes when walking, and to look ahead helps promote a more balanced gait. Use of an elevated toilet seat and rocking from side to side will enable a patient to initiate movement. Canes and walkers are difficult for patients with Parkinson's disease to maneuver and may make the patient more prone to injury.

28. b. Rationale: The reduction of acetylcholine (ACh) effect in myasthenia gravis (MG) is treated with anticholinesterase drugs, which prolong the action of ACh at the neuromuscular synapse, but too much of these drugs will cause a cholinergic crisis with symptoms very similar to those of MG. To determine

whether the patient's manifestations are due to a deficiency of ACh or to too much anticholinesterase drug, the anticholinesterase drug edrophonium chloride (Tensilon) is administered. If the patient is in cholinergic crisis, the patient's symptoms will worsen, but if the patient is in a myasthenic crisis, the patient will improve.

29. c. Rationale: The patient in myasthenic crisis has severe weakness and fatigability of all skeletal muscles, affecting the patient's ability to swallow, talk, move, and breathe. However, the priority of nursing care is monitoring and maintaining adequate ventilation.

30. c. Rationale: Restless legs syndrome that is not related to other pathologic processes, such as diabetes mellitus or rheumatic disorders, may be caused by an alteration in dopaminergic transmission in the basal ganglia because dopaminergic agents, such as those used for parkinsonism, are effective in managing sensory and motor symptoms. Polysomnography studies during sleep are the only tests that have diagnostic value, and although exercise should be encouraged, excessive leg exercise does not have an effect on the symptoms.

31. b. Rationale: In acute amyotrophic lateral sclerosis (ALS), there is gradual degeneration of motor neurons with extreme muscle wasting from lack of stimulation and use. However, cognitive function is not impaired, and patients feel trapped in a dying body. Chorea manifested by writhing, involuntary movements is characteristic of Huntington's disease. As an autosomal-dominant genetic disease, Huntington's disease also has a 50% chance of being passed to each offspring.

32. c. Rationale: Many chronic neurologic diseases involve progressive deterioration in physical or mental capabilities and have no cure, with devastating results for patients and families. Health care providers can only attempt to alleviate physical symptoms, prevent complications, and assist patients in maximizing function and self-care abilities as long as possible.

Case Study

1. The cause of MS is unknown, although research findings suggest MS is related to infectious (viral), immunologic, and genetic factors. T cells are activated by some unknown factor, and these T cells migrate to the CNS and cause a disruption in the blood-brain barrier. Subsequent antigen-antibody reaction within the CNS results in activation of the inflammatory response, and through multiple mechanisms, destruction of the myelin of axons occurs. There is loss of myelin, disappearance of oligodendrocytes, and proliferation of astrocytes. These changes result in characteristic plaque formation, or sclerosis, scattered through the CNS and loss of nerve impulse transmission.

2. The role of precipitating factors, such as exposure to pathogenic agents, in the etiology of MS is controversial. It is possible that their association with MS is random and that there is no cause-and-effect relationship. Possible precipitating factors include emotional stress, excessive fatigue, pregnancy, and a poorer state of health. In D.S.'s case, it is possible that the viral neuritis was a precipitating factor.

3. Because there is no definitive diagnostic test for MS, diagnosis is based primarily on history and clinical manifestations. Although MRI can detect sclerotic plaques, D.S.'s initial symptoms were so nonspecific and transient that often a "wait-and-see" approach is taken.

4. Patient education should focus on preventing exacerbations or worsening of the disease. Building general resistance to illness, including avoiding fatigue, stress, extremes of heat and cold, and exposure to infection, is an important measure in maintaining general health. Vigorous and early treatment of infection is critical if it does occur. It is important to teach the patient to (1) achieve a good balance of exercise and rest, (2) eat nutritious and well-balanced meals, and (3) avoid the hazards of immobility (contractures and pressure sores). Patients should know their treatment regimens, the side effects of medications and how to watch for them, and drug interactions with over-the-counter medications. The patient should consult a health care provider before taking nonprescription medications.

5. Because there is no cure for MS, treatment is aimed at slowing the disease process and providing symptomatic relief. The disease process is treated with drugs, and the symptoms are controlled with a variety of medications and other forms of therapy. Corticosteroids are helpful in treating acute exacerbations of the disease, probably by reducing edema and acute inflammation at the site of demyelination. Immunosuppressive drugs, such as azathioprine (Imuran), cyclosporine (Sandimmune), and cyclophosphamide (Cytoxan), have been shown to produce some beneficial effects in patients with severe and relapsing MS. A new immunosuppressant drug, mitoxantrone (Novantrone), reduces both B and T lymphocytes. However, the potential benefits of these drugs in patients with MS need to be counterbalanced against the potentially serious side effects. Immunomodulator drugs, such as interferon β-1b (Betaseron), interferon β-1a (Avonex), and glatiramer acetate (Copaxone), have been effective in reducing frequency and severity of exacerbations, but all these agents must be administered parenterally. Physical therapy and speech therapy may also help improve neurologic function.

6. *Nursing diagnoses:*
   - Ineffective role performance
   - Anxiety
   - Disturbed sensory perception: visual
   - Risk for impaired parenting
   Collaborative problems:
   Potential complication: blindness

CHAPTER 60

1. a. DL; b. DM; c. DL; d. DL; e. DM; f. DL; g. DM; h. DM; i. DL; j. DM
2. a. *T*; b. *F*, vascular; c. *T*; d. *T*; e. *F*, beta-amyloid protein
3. a. Rationale: Depression is often associated with Alzheimer's disease (AD), especially early in the disease when the patient has awareness of the diagnosis and the progression of the disease. When dementia and depression occur together, intellectual deterioration may be more extreme. Depression is treatable, and use of antidepressants often improves cognitive function.
4. c. Rationale: The Mini-Mental State Examination is a tool to document the degree of cognitive impairment, and it can be used to determine a baseline from which changes over time can be evaluated. It does not evaluate mood or thought processes but can detect dementia and delirium and differentiate these from psychiatric mental illness. It cannot help to determine etiology.
5. d. Rationale: Hypothyroidism can cause dementia but is a treatable condition if it has not been long standing. The other conditions are causes of irreversible dementia.
6. c. Rationale: The only definitive diagnosis of AD can be made on examination of brain tissue on autopsy, but a clinical diagnosis is made when all other possible causes of dementia have been eliminated. Patients with AD may have β-amyloid proteins in the blood, brain atrophy, or isoprostanes in the urine, but these findings are not exclusive to those with AD.
7. b. Rationale: Because there is no cure for AD, collaborative management is aimed at improving or controlling the decline in cognition and controlling the undesirable manifestations that the patient may exhibit. Anticholinesterase agents help increase acetylcholine (ACh) in the brain, but a variety of other drugs are also used to control behavior. Memory-enhancement techniques have little or no effect in patients with AD, especially as the disease progresses. Patients with AD have limited ability to communicate health symptoms and problems, leading to a lack of professional attention for acute and other chronic illnesses.
8. a. 3, 10; b. 4, 9; c. 1, 8; d. 6, 9; e. 5, 9; f. 7, 8; g. 3, 10; h. 2, 10; i. 5, 9; j. 1, 8; k. 2, 10
9. b. Rationale: Patients with late AD frequently become agitated, but because their short-term memory is so pronounced, distraction is a very good way to calm them. "Why" questions are upsetting to them because they don't know the answer, and they cannot respond to normal relaxation techniques.
10. a, b, d, e
11. c. Rationale: Adhering to a regular, consistent daily schedule helps the patient avoid confusion and anxiety and is important both during hospitalization and at home. Clocks and calendars may be useful in early AD, but they have little meaning to a patient as the disease progresses. Questioning the patient about activities and events they cannot remember is threatening and may cause severe anxiety. Maintaining a safe environment for the patient is important but does not change the disturbed thought processes.
12. b. Rationale: Caregiver-role strain is characterized by such symptoms of stress as inability to sleep, make decisions, or concentrate and is frequently seen in family members who are responsible for the care of the patient with AD. Assessment of the caregiver may reveal a need for assistance to increase coping skills, effectively use community resources, or maintain social relationships. Eventually the demands on a caregiver exceed the resources, and the person with AD may be placed in an institutional setting.
13. a. Rationale: Adult day care is an option to provide respite for caregivers and a protective environment for the patient during the early and middle stages of AD. The respite from the demands of care allows the caregiver to maintain social contacts and perform normal tasks of living and be more responsive to the patient's needs. Visits by home care nurses involve the caregiver and cannot provide adequate respite. Institutional placement is not always an acceptable option at earlier stages of AD, nor is hospitalization an acceptable form of respite care.
14. a. Rationale: Conditions that decrease the CNS production of ACh are believed to be a critical factor in the development of delirium. Patients with Parkinson's disease are treated with anticholinergics that decrease ACh in the brain, increasing the risk for delirium. It is true that delirium and Parkinson's disease are seen in older people, but the relationship is more specific than just age.
15. a, b, d. All caregivers are responsible for the patient's safety. Basic care activities, such as those associated with personal hygiene, and ADLs can be delegated to an NAP. The RN will perform ongoing assessments and develop/revise the plan of care, as needed. The RN will assess the patient's safety risk factors, provide education and make referrals. The LPN could check the patient's environment for safety hazards.

16. a. age; b. infection (cytokines); c. hypoxemia (lung disease); d. intensive care unit (ICU) hospitalization (change in environment, sensory overload); e. preexisting dementia; f. dehydration. Also: hyperthermia

17. d. Rationale: Delirium is an acute problem that usually has a rapid onset in response to a precipitating event, especially when the patient has underlying health problems, such as heart disease and sensory limitations. In the absence of prior cognitive impairment, a sudden onset of confusion, disorientation, and agitation is usually delirium. Delirium may manifest with both hyporeactive and hyperactive symptoms.

18. c. Rationale: Care of the patient with delirium is focused on identifying and eliminating precipitating factors if possible. Treatment of underlying medical conditions, changing environmental conditions, and discontinuing medications that induce delirium are important. Drug therapy is reserved for those patients with severe agitation, because the drugs themselves may worsen delirium.

Case Study

1. The pathophysiology of AD includes cellular changes with neurofibrillary tangles with altered tau proteins and neuritic plaques containing β-amyloid protein in the cerebral cortex and hippocampus. There is also a loss of the connections between neurons.

2. AD is diagnosed by exclusion. When all other possible causes of mental impairment and persistence of dementia are ruled out, the diagnosis of Alzheimer's remains. Brain atrophy and enlarged ventricles seen in some patients with AD are also seen in normal people and in other conditions. Newer techniques such as SPECT, MRS and PET detect changes earlier in the disease and can be used to monitor response to therapy. Only on autopsy can AD be confirmed by the presence of neurofibrillary tangles in brain tissue.

3. All functions of mental capacity and ability to care for oneself are lost as the disease progresses. There will be deterioration of personal hygiene and all activities of daily living, progression of psychotic symptoms now evidenced by his hallucinations, loss of long-term memory and recognition of his family, and loss of communication.

4. Assess what she is doing now to manage his care. Teach her about the expected progression of the disease, and assist her in planning respite care or arranging for home health assistants. Help her identify problem areas. Encourage her to keep G.D. awake and busy during the day so that he will sleep better at night, and so will she.

5. Community resources may include Alzheimer's support groups, adult day care, home health assistants and home nursing, and various forms of assisted living and long-term care facilities.

6. *Nursing diagnoses:*
   - Risk for injury related to impaired judgment, nighttime wandering
   - Risk for other-directed violence related to misinterpretation of environmental stimuli
   - Impaired memory related to effects of dementia
   - Wandering related to cognitive impairment
   - Disturbed sleep pattern related to circadian asynchrony
   Collaborative problems:
   Potential complication: Psychosis

7. *Nursing diagnoses:*
   - Anxiety related to erratic behavioral patterns and cognitive decline of husband
   - Ineffective health maintenance related to fatigue and chronic stress
   - Caregiver role strain related to grieving over the family member's illness
   - Risk for other-directed violence (patient abuse) related to ineffective coping
   Collaborative problems:
   Potential complication: Depression

CHAPTER 61

1. a. *T*; b. *F*, Bell's palsy; c. *F*, corticosteroids; d. *F*, Bell's palsy; e. *T*; f. *T*

2. a. Rationale: The pain of trigeminal neuralgia is excruciating, and it may occur in clusters that continue for hours. The condition is considered benign with no major effects except the pain. Corneal exposure is a problem in Bell's palsy, or it may occur following surgery for the treatment of trigeminal neuralgia. Maintenance of nutrition is important but not urgent because chewing may trigger trigeminal neuralgia and patients then avoid eating. Except during an attack, there is no change in facial appearance in a patient with trigeminal neuralgia, and body image is more disturbed in response to the paralysis typical of Bell's palsy.

3. a. Rationale: Although percutaneous radiofrequency rhizotomy and microvascular decompression provide the greatest relief of pain, glycerol rhizotomy causes less sensory loss and fewer sensory aberrations with comparable or better pain relief. Gamma knife radiosurgery provides precise radiation useful for persistent pain after other surgery.

4. c. Rationale: Because attacks of trigeminal neuralgia may be precipitated by hot or cold air movement on the face, jarring movements, or talking, the environment should be of moderate temperature and free of drafts, and patients should not be expected to converse during the acute period. Patients often prefer to carry out their own care because they are afraid someone else may inadvertently injure them or precipitate an attack. The nurse should stress that

oral hygiene be performed because patients often avoid it, but residual food in the mouth after eating occurs more frequently with Bell's palsy.

5. a. Rationale: The most serious complication of Guillain-Barré syndrome is respiratory failure, and it is essential that respiratory rate, depth, and vital capacity are monitored to detect involvement of the nerves that affect respiration. Corticosteroids may be used in treatment but do not appear to have an effect on the prognosis or duration of the disease. Rather, plasmapheresis or administration of high-dose immunoglobulin does result in shortening recovery time. The peripheral nerves of both the sympathetic and parasympathetic nervous systems are involved in the disease and may lead to orthostatic hypotension, hypertension, and abnormal vagal responses affecting the heart. Guillain-Barré syndrome may affect the lower brainstem and CNs VII, VI, III, XII, V, and X, affecting facial, eye, and swallowing functions.

6. c. Rationale: As nerve involvement ascends, it is very frightening for the patient, but most patients with Guillain-Barré syndrome recover completely with care. Patients also recover if ventilatory support is provided during respiratory failure. Guillain-Barré syndrome affects only peripheral nerves and does not affect the brain.

7. a. 3; b. 1; c. 2; d. 1; e. 2; f. 3; g. 2; h. 1; i. 2; j. 3; k. 1

8. d. Rationale: Spinal cord injuries are highest in young adult men between the ages of 15 and 30 and those who are impulsive or risk takers in daily living. Other risk factors include alcohol and drug abuse as well as participation in sports and occupational exposure to trauma or violence.

9. b. Rationale: At the C7 level, spinal shock is manifested by tetraplegia and sensory loss. The neurologic loss may be temporary or permanent. Paraplegia with sensory loss would occur at the level of T1. A hemiplegia occurs with central (brain) lesions affecting motor neurons and spastic tetraplegia occurs when spinal shock resolves.

10. a. 5; b. 4; c. 1; d. 3; e. 2

11. c. Rationale: The primary injury of the spinal cord rarely affects the entire cord, but the pathophysiology of secondary injury may result in damage that is the same as mechanical severance of the cord. Complete cord dissolution occurs through autodestruction of the cord by hemorrhage, edema, and the presence of metabolites and norepinephrine, resulting in anoxia and infarction of the cord. Edema resulting from the inflammatory response may increase the damage as it extends above and below the injury site.

12. c. Rationale: Spinal shock occurs in about half of all people with acute spinal cord injury. In spinal shock, the entire cord below the level of the lesion fails to function, resulting in a flaccid paralysis and hypomotility of most processes without any reflex activity. Return of reflex activity signals the end of spinal shock. Sympathetic function is impaired below the level of the injury because sympathetic nerves leave the spinal cord at the thoracic and lumbar areas, and cranial parasympathetic nerves predominate in control over respirations, heart, and all vessels and organs below the injury. Neurogenic shock results from loss of vascular tone caused by the injury and is manifested by hypotension, peripheral vasodilation, and decreased CO. Rehabilitation activities are not contraindicated during spinal shock and should be instituted if the patient's cardiopulmonary status is stable.

13. b. Rationale: Until the edema and necrosis at the site of the injury are resolved in 72 hours to 1 week after the injury, it is not possible to determine how much cord damage is present from the initial injury, how much secondary injury occurred, or how much the cord was damaged by edema that extended above the level of the original injury. The return of reflexes signals only the end of spinal shock, and the reflexes may be inappropriate and excessive, causing spasms that complicate rehabilitation.

14. a. above T5; b. above C4; c. below C4; d. above T6

15. b. Neurogenic shock associated with cord injuries above the level of T6 greatly decrease the effect of the sympathetic nervous system, and bradycardia and hypotension occur. A heart rate of 42 is not adequate to meet oxygen needs of the body, and while low, the blood pressure is not at a critical point. The oxygen saturation is satisfactory, and the motor and sensory loss are expected.

16. a. 7; b. 3; c. 9; d. 7; e. 1; f. 6

17. d. Rationale: Although surgical treatment of spinal cord injuries often depends on the preference of the health care provider, surgery is usually indicated when there is continued compression of the cord by extrinsic forces or when there is evidence of cord compression. Other indications may include progressive neurologic deficit, compound fracture of the vertebra, bony fragments, and penetrating wounds of the cord.

18. a. Rationale: The need for a patent airway is the first priority for any injured patient, and a high cervical injury may decrease the gag reflex and ability to maintain an airway, as well as the ability to breathe. Maintaining cervical stability is then a consideration, along with assessing for other injuries and the patient's neurologic status.

19. c. Rationale: Cervical injuries usually require skeletal traction with the use of Crutchfield, Vinke, or other types of skull tongs to immobilize the cervical vertebrae, even if fracture has not occurred. Hard cervical collars are used for minor injuries or for stabilization during emergency transport of the patient. Sandbags are also used temporarily

to stabilize the neck during insertion of tongs or during diagnostic testing immediately following the injury. Special turning or kinetic beds may be used to turn and mobilize patients who are in cervical traction.

20. c. Rationale: Dopamine is a vasopressor that is used to maintain blood pressure during states of hypotension that occur during neurogenic shock associated with spinal cord injury. Atropine would be used to treat a bradycardia. The temperature reflects some degree of poikilothermism, but this is not treated with medications.

21. c. Rationale: Because pneumonia and atelectasis are potential problems related to ineffective coughing and the loss of intercostal and abdominal muscle function, the nurse should assess the patient's breath sounds and respiratory function to determine whether secretions are being retained or whether there is progression of respiratory impairment. Suctioning is not indicated unless lung sounds indicate retained secretions; position changes will help mobilize secretions. Intubation and mechanical ventilation are used if the patient becomes exhausted from labored breathing or if ABGs deteriorate.

22. d. Rationale: During the first 2 to 3 days after a spinal cord injury, paralytic ileus may occur, and nasogastric suction must be used to remove secretions and gas from the GI tract until peristalsis resumes. IV fluids are used to maintain fluid balance but do not specifically relate to paralytic ileus. Tube feedings would be used only for patients who had difficulty swallowing and not until peristalsis returned; parenteral nutrition would be used only if the paralytic ileus was unusually prolonged.

23. a. Rationale: During the acute phase of spinal cord injury, the bladder is hypotonic, causing urinary retention with the risk for reflux into the kidney or rupture of the bladder. An indwelling catheter is used to keep the bladder empty and closely monitor urinary output. Intermittent catheterization or other urinary drainage methods may be used in long-term bladder management. Use of incontinent pads is inappropriate because the bladder fails to empty.

24. b. Rationale: In 1 week following a spinal cord injury, there may be a resolution of the edema of the injury and an end to spinal shock. When spinal shock ends, reflex movement and spasms will occur, which may be mistaken for return of function, but with the resolution of edema, some normal function may also occur. It is important when movement occurs to determine whether the movement is voluntary and can be consciously controlled, which would indicate some return of function.

25. 5, 2, 6, 3, 1, 4. Rationale: Initial response by the nurse should be to elevate the head of bed (HOB) to decrease BP and to remove noxious stimulation.

Frequently the trigger is bladder distention, which can be dealt with quickly. The physician needs to be notified as soon as possible and, depending on the communication system available to the nurse, he/she should get the call placed. Meanwhile, stay with the patient and loosen any restrictive clothing. The physician may order an antihypertensive and documentation should be an accurate and thorough description of the entire episode.

26. b. Rationale: Intermittent self-catheterization five to six times a day is the recommended method of bladder management for the patient with a spinal cord injury because it more closely mimics normal emptying and has less potential for infection. The patient and family should be taught the procedure using clean technique, and if the patient has use of the arms, self-catheterization should be performed. Indwelling catheterization is used during the acute phase to prevent overdistention of the bladder, and surgical urinary diversions are used if urinary complications occur.

27. d. Rationale: Most patients with a complete lower motor neuron lesion are unable to have either psychogenic or reflexogenic erections, and alternative methods of obtaining sexual satisfaction may be suggested. Patients with incomplete lower motor neuron lesions have the highest possibility of successful psychogenic erections with ejaculation, whereas patients with incomplete upper motor neuron lesions are more likely to experience reflexogenic erections with ejaculation. Patients with complete upper motor neuron lesions usually only have reflex sexual function with rare ejaculation.

28. a. Rationale: Working through the grief process is a lifelong process that is triggered by new experiences, such as marriage, child rearing, employment, or illness, which the patient must adjust to throughout life within the context of his or her disability. The goal of recovery is related to adjustment, rather than acceptance, and many patients do not experience all components of the grief process. During the anger phase, patients should be allowed outbursts, and the nurse should use humor to displace some of the patient's anger.

29. b. Rationale: Most metastatic tumors are extradural lesions that may be removed successfully with surgery. Most tumors of the spinal cord are slow-growing, do not cause autodestruction, and, with the exception of intradural-intramedullary tumors, can be removed with complete functional restoration. Radiation is used to treat metastatic tumors that are sensitive to radiation and that have caused only minor neurologic deficits in the patient; radiation is also used as adjuvant therapy to surgery for intramedullary tumors.

Case Study

1. S.M. is experiencing central cord syndrome of the cervical cord, in which there is compression on anterior horn cells. It usually occurs as a result of hyperextension.
2. The cell bodies of lower motor neurons, which send axons to innervate the skeletal muscles of arms, trunk, and legs, are located in the anterior horn of the spinal cord. The cervical segments of the spinal cord contain the lower motor neurons for the arms, and a cervical injury that affects the anterior horn will affect the arms to a greater extent than it affects the legs.
3. Injury to the cord may occur without fracture of the vertebrae, with traumatic twisting or stretching of the cord. The response to the trauma includes secondary injury leading to edema, hemorrhage, and ischemia of the cord, impairing function.
4. Methylprednisolone has been found to improve blood flow and reduce edema in the spinal cord, with the effects of reduction of posttraumatic spinal cord ischemia, improvement of energy balance, restoration of extracellular calcium, improvement of nerve impulse condition, and repression of the release of free fatty acids from spinal cord tissues.
5. Shock and denial are common first reactions to the loss of function with spinal cord injuries, followed by anger and depression. During the acute phase, S.H. will probably have unrealistic expectations concerning her recovery, sleep a lot, and withdraw. As she progresses, she will become angry and refuse to discuss her limitations. Altered body image will be a big problem because she will see herself as different from her peers, an important developmental issue during adolescence.

6. Intensive rehabilitation that focuses on refined retraining physiologic function of her limbs should be planned and will involve much physical therapy over time. She should be mobilized as quickly as appropriate to prevent hazards of immobility and to encourage her in her progress.
7. *Nursing diagnoses:*
   - Impaired physical mobility related to spinal cord injury and prescribed bed rest
   - Risk for disuse syndrome related to immobilization
   - Self-care deficit: Feeding, bathing, and grooming related to upper extremity weakness
   - Risk for injury related to sensory deficit and lack of self-protective abilities

   Collaborative problems:
   Potential complications: Progression of lesion; hypoventilation; spinal shock

CHAPTER 62

1. a. epiphysis; b. diaphysis; c. articular cartilage; d. spongy bone; e. epiphyseal line; f. red marrow cavities; g. compact bone; h. medullary cavity; i. endosteum; j. yellow marrow; k. periosteum
2. a. periosteum; b. canaliculi; c. blood vessels; d. osteon
3. a. joint cavity; b. bursa; c. articular cartilage; d. periosteum; e. joint capsule; f. nerve; g. blood vessel; h. synovial membrane; i. bone
4. Word Search. a. haversian; b. sarcomere; c. epiphysis; d. osteocyte; e. tendon; f. periosteum; g. synovium; h. isometric; i. calcium; j. canaliculi; k. osteoclast; l. atrophy; m. actin; n. bursae; o. osteoblast; p. cartilage; q. ligament; r. fascia; s. hyaline; t. striated

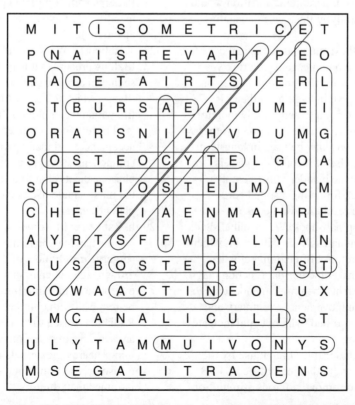

5. a. 1; b. 1, 2, 3; c. 1, 2, 3; d. 4; e. 1, 2, 3; f. 1; g. 1, 2, 3
6. d. Rationale: Loss of water from disks between vertebrae, vertebral disk compression, and narrowing of intervertebral spaces all contribute to a loss of height in the older adult. Although bone density decreases and cartilage is lost from joints, these do not affect the long bones or the height of the person.
7. b. Rationale: Loss of muscle mass and strength, decreased motor neurons, limited movement because of joint changes, and less flexible tendons and ligaments all contribute to the older adult's risk for falls. Self-care deficits are not widespread, and fatigue and a high risk for impaired skin integrity are not directly related to changes in the musculoskeletal system that are associated with aging.
8. a. Rationale: Corticosteroids cause protein catabolism with skeletal muscle wasting and increased osteoclast activity with loss of bone mass, which can have a marked detrimental effect on mobility and activity. Potassium-depleting diuretics may cause hypokalemia, which is associated with muscle weakness and cramps. Oral hypoglycemic drugs and NSAIDs are not known to affect the musculoskeletal system.
9. a. History of musculoskeletal injuries, poor use of body mechanics or excessive muscular or joint stress, family history of joint and bone disease
   b. Presence of obesity, inadequate calcium, vitamin D or C, or protein intake
   c. Inability to physically access toilet; constipation
   d. Limitation of movement; pain, weakness, crepitus; extremes of occupational activity and recreational activities—sedentary or heavy use of body
   e. Pain interfering with sleep; frequent position changes
   f. Musculoskeletal pain; pain-management measures
   g. Loss of body image or self-worth, caused by musculoskeletal deformity
   h. Change in work and family roles and responsibilities caused by immobility or pain
   i. Decreased sexual activity and satisfaction because of pain, deformity
   j. Decreased coping ability related to effect of musculoskeletal problems
10. c. Rationale: Muscle strength is graded on a scale of 0 to 5, with 0 = no detection of muscle strength and 5 = active movement against full resistance (normal). Active movement against gravity and some resistance = 4.
11. b. Rationale: There is no indication to measure the length of limbs during assessment unless a gait disturbance or limb-length discrepancy is noted, and then the limb should be measured between two bony prominences and compared with the measurement of the opposite extremity. Muscle mass measurement and joint movement may affect gait, but differences in limb length will always affect gait. Palpating for crepitus will identify friction between bones, usually at joints.
12. c. Rationale: A goniometer is a protractor device that measures the angle of joints and can be used to determine specific degrees of joint range of motion. It is used when a specific musculoskeletal problem has been identified that affects ROM.
13. a. 13; b. 6; c. 3; d. 12; e. 1; f. 7; g. 11; h. 10; i. 9; j. 5; k. 2; l. 8; m. 4
14. a. standard x-ray; b. arthrocentesis; c. diskogram; d. dual-energy x-ray absorptiometry (DEXA); e. electromyogram; f. creatine kinase
15. a. rheumatoid factor (RF); b. erythrocyte sedimentation rate (ESR); c. antinuclear antibody (ANA)

CHAPTER 63

1. d. Rationale: Musculoskeletal problems in the older adult can be prevented with appropriate strategies, especially exercise. Almost all older adults have some degree of decreased muscle strength, joint stiffness, and pain with motion. The use of mild antiinflammatory agents decreases inflammation and pain and can help the patient maintain activity and prevent further deconditioning. Stair walking can create enough stress on fragile bones to cause a hip fracture, and use of ramps may help prevent falls. Walkers and canes should be used as necessary to decrease stress on joints so that activity can be maintained.
2. c. Rationale: Warm-up exercises "prelengthen" potentially strained tissues by avoiding the quick stretch often encountered in sports and also increase the temperature of muscle, resulting in increased speed of cell metabolism, increased speed of nerve impulses, and improved oxygenation of muscle fibers. Stretching is also thought to improve kinesthetic awareness, lessening the chance of uncoordinated movement. Taping or wrapping joints may actually predispose a person to injury, and muscle strength is not a key factor in soft-tissue injuries.
3. Word Search. a. Bursitis; b. Subluxation; c. Carpal tunnel syndrome; d. Rotator cuff injury; e. Dislocation; f. Meniscus injury; g. Sprain; h. Repetitive strain injury; i. Strain; j. Greenstick; k. Spiral; l. Open; m. Oblique; n. Comminuted; o. Pathologic; p. Transverse; q. Avulsion fracture

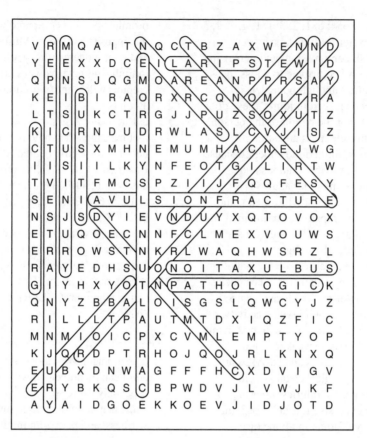

4. b. Rationale: Application of cold, compression, and elevation is indicated to prevent edema resulting from sprain and strain injury. Muscle spasms are usually treated with heat applications and massage, and repetitive strain injuries require cessation of the precipitating activity and physical therapy. Dislocations or subluxations require immediate reduction and immobilization to prevent vascular impairment and bone cell death.

5. a, b, c, e. Rationale: Consider the principle of RICE. Rest: movement should be restricted. Ice: cold should be used to promote vasoconstriction and to reduce edema. C: compression helps to decrease swelling. E: elevate the extremity above the level of the heart. Mild nonsteroidal antiinflammatory drugs (NSAIDs) may be needed to manage pain.

6. a. 3; b. 5; c. 1; d. 6; e. 2; f. 6; g. 2; h. 5, 6; i. 4; j. 6; k. 3; l. 2; m. 5; n. 4

7. b. Rationale: Deformity is the cardinal sign of fracture but may not be apparent in all fractures. Other supporting signs include edema and swelling, localized pain and tenderness, muscle spasm, ecchymosis, loss of function, crepitation, and an inability to bear weight.

8. a. Rationale: A malunion occurs when the bone heals in the expected time but in an unsatisfactory position, possibly resulting in deformity or dysfunction. Nonunion occurs when the fracture fails to heal properly despite treatment, and delayed union is healing of the fracture at a slower rate than expected. The loss of bone substances as a result of immobilization occurs in posttraumatic osteoporosis.

9. a. *F*, reduction; b. *T*; c. *F*, infection; d. *F*, skin; e. *T*

10. d. Rationale: Complaints of abdominal pain or pressure, nausea, and vomiting are signs of cast syndrome that occur when body casts are applied too tightly, causing compression of the superior mesenteric artery against the duodenum. The cast may need to be split or removed, and the health care provider should be notified. Elevation is not indicated for a spica cast, and the patient with a spica cast should not be placed in the prone position during the initial drying stage, because the cast is so large and heavy it may break. A cast should never be covered with a blanket because heat builds up in the cast and may increase edema.

11. b. Rationale: Infection is the greatest risk with an open fracture, and all open fractures are considered contaminated. Tetanus prevention is always indicated if the patient has not been immunized or does not have current boosters. Prophylactic antibiotics are often used in management of open fractures, but recent antibiotic therapy is not relevant, nor are previous injuries to the site.

12. d. Rationale: Pulses distal to the injury should be checked before and after splinting to assess for nerve or vascular damage and documented to avoid doubts about whether a problem discovered later was missed during the original examination or was caused by the

treatment. Elevation of the limb and application of ice should be instituted after the extremity is splinted.

13. b. Rationale: Neurologic assessment includes evaluation of motor and sensory function and, in the upper extremity, includes abduction and adduction of the fingers, opposition of the fingers, and supination and pronation of the hands. It would also include sensory perception in the fingers. Evaluation of the feet would occur in lower-extremity injuries. Assessment of color, temperature, capillary refill, peripheral pulses, and edema evaluates vascular status.

14. b. Rationale: A patient with any type of cast should exercise the joints above and below the cast frequently, and moving the fingers frequently will improve circulation and help prevent edema. Unlike plaster casts, thermoplastic resin or fiberglass casts are relatively waterproof and, if they become wet, can be dried with a hair dryer on low setting. Tape petals are used on plaster casts to protect the edges from breaking and crumbling but are not necessary for synthetic casts. After the cast is applied, the extremity should be elevated at about the level of the heart to promote venous return, and ice may be used to prevent edema.

15. a. Rationale: A swing-to gait is a three-point gait in which the patient places the crutches ahead of the unaffected leg and swings up to the level of the crutches, keeping weight off the affected leg. It is safer than a swing-through gait because it provides better balance and stability. Two- and four-point gaits are used when at least partial weight-bearing is allowed on the limb.

16. c. Rationale: Progressive pain that is distal to the injury and is unrelieved by usual analgesics is the earliest sign of compartment syndrome. Paralysis and absence of peripheral pulses will eventually occur if it is not treated, but these are late signs that often appear after permanent damage has occurred. The overlying skin may appear normal because the surface vessels are not occluded.

17. a. paresthesia; b. pain; c. pressure; d. pallor; e. paralysis; f. pulselessness

18. a. Rationale: Soft-tissue edema in the area of the injury may cause an increase of pressure within the closed spaces of the tissue compartments formed by the nonelastic fascia, creating a compartment syndrome. If symptoms occur, it may be necessary to incise the fascia surgically, a procedure known as a fasciotomy. Amputation is usually necessary only if the limb becomes septic because of untreated compartment syndrome.

19. a. 2; b. 3; c. 1; d. 7; e. 4; f. 2; g. 1, 4, 6; h. 5; i. 7; j. 1; k. 6; l. 3; m. 5; n. 4, 5; o. 6

20. a. Rationale: Initial manifestations of fat embolism usually occur 24 to 48 hours after injury and are associated with fractures of long bones and multiple fractures related to pelvic injuries, including fractures of the femur, tibia, ribs, and pelvis.

21. d. Rationale: Patients with fractures are at risk for both fat embolism and pulmonary embolism from venous thromboembolism, but there is a difference in the time of occurrence, with fat embolism occurring shortly after the injury and thrombotic embolism occurring several days after immobilization. They both may cause pulmonary symptoms of chest pain, tachypnea, dyspnea, apprehension, tachycardia, and cyanosis, but fat embolism may cause petechiae located around the neck, anterior chest wall, axilla, buccal membrane of the mouth, and conjunctiva of the eye, which differentiate it from thrombotic embolism.

22. a. *F*, intracapsular; b. *T*; c. *F*, femoral neck; d. *T*; e. *T*

23. d. Rationale: The classic signs of a hip fracture are shortening of the leg and external rotation accompanied by severe pain at the fracture site, and additional injury could be caused by weight bearing on the extremity. The patient may not be able to move the hip or the knee, but movement in the ankle and toes is not affected.

24. c. Rationale: Although surgical repair is the preferred method of managing intracapsular and extracapsular hip fractures, initially patients frequently may be treated with skin traction, such as Buck's extension or Russell's traction, to immobilize the limb temporarily and to relieve the painful muscle spasms before surgery is performed. Prolonged traction would be required to reduce the fracture or immobilize it for healing, creating a very high risk for complications of immobility.

25. a. Rationale: Because the fracture site is internally fixed with pins or plates, the fracture site is stable, and the patient is moved from the bed to the chair on the first postoperative day, with ambulation beginning on the first or second postoperative day, without weight bearing on the affected leg. Weight bearing on the affected extremity is usually restricted for 6 to 12 weeks until adequate healing is evident on x-ray. The patient may be positioned on the operative side following internal fixation, and abductor pillows are used for patients who have total hip replacements.

26. d. Rationale: Patients with hip prostheses must avoid extreme flexion, adduction, or internal rotation for at least 6 weeks to prevent dislocation of the prosthesis. Gradual weight bearing on the limb is allowed, and ambulation should be encouraged.

27. c. Rationale: The low-bulk, high-carbohydrate liquid diet and intake of air through a straw required during mandibular fixation often lead to constipation and flatus, which may be relieved with bulk-forming laxatives, prune juice, or ambulation. Wires or rubber bands should be cut only in the case of cardiac or respiratory arrest, and patients should be taught to clear their mouth of vomitus or secretions. The mouth should be thoroughly cleaned with water,

saline, or alkaline mouthwashes or using a Water Pik as necessary to remove food debris. Hard candy should not be held in the mouth.

28. c. Rationale; The compression dressing/bandage supports the soft tissues, reduces edema, hastens healing, minimizes pain, and promotes residual limb shrinkage. If the dressing is left off, edema will form quickly and may delay rehabilitation. Elevation and ice will not be as effective at preventing the edema that will form. Dressing the incision with dry gauze will not provide the benefits of a compression dressing.

29. b. Rationale: The disruption in body image caused by an amputation often causes a patient to go through psychologic stages of grieving, and the patient should be allowed to go through a period of depression as a normal consequence of the amputation. The grieving process is not ineffective coping or impaired adjustment but a normal process of adjusting to loss.

30. b. Rationale: Phantom sensation or phantom pain may occur following amputation, especially if pain was present in the affected limb preoperatively. The pain is a real sensation to the patient and should be treated with analgesics and other pain interventions. As recovery and ambulation progress, phantom limb sensation usually subsides.

31. b. Rationale: Because the device covers the residual limb, the surgical site cannot be directly seen, and postoperative hemorrhage is not apparent on dressings, requiring vigilant assessment of vital signs for signs of bleeding. Elevation of the residual limb with an immediate prosthetic fitting is not necessary because the device itself prevents edema formation. Exercises to the leg are not performed in the immediate postoperative period so as to avoid disruption of ligatures and the suture line.

32. a. Rationale: Flexion contractures, especially of the hip, may be debilitating and delay rehabilitation of the patient with a leg amputation. To prevent hip flexion, the patient should avoid sitting in a chair with the hips flexed or having pillows under the surgical extremity for prolonged periods, and the patient should lie on the abdomen for 30 minutes three to four times a day to extend the hip.

33. a. Rationale: Skin breakdown on the residual limb can prevent the use of a prosthesis, and the limb should be inspected every day for signs of irritation or pressure areas. No substances except water and mild soap should be used on the residual limb, and ROM exercises are not necessary when the patient is using a prosthesis. A residual limb shrinker is an elastic stocking that is used to mold the limb in preparation for prosthesis use, but a cotton residual limb sock is worn with the prosthesis.

34. a. 3; b. 4; c. 5; d. 1; e. 2

35. d. Rationale: Physical therapy is initiated 1 day postoperatively with ambulation and weight bearing using a walker for a patient with a cemented prosthesis and non–weight bearing on the operative side for an uncemented prosthesis. In addition, the patient is turned to both sides and back with support of the operative leg and sits in the chair at least twice a day.

36. b. Rationale: Following a total hip arthroplasty, extremes of internal rotation, adduction, and 90-degree flexion of the hip must be avoided for 4 to 6 weeks postoperatively to prevent dislocation of the prosthesis. During hospitalization an abduction pillow is placed between the legs to maintain abduction, and the leg is extended.

37. b. Rationale: Continuous passive motion machines are frequently used following knee surgery to promote earlier joint mobility. Because joint dislocation is not a problem with knee replacements, early exercise with straight leg raises and gentle ROM is also encouraged postoperatively.

38. b. Rationale: Neurovascular checks of the fingers following surgery of the hands are essential to detect compromised vascular and neurologic function caused by trauma or edema. Postoperatively the hands are elevated with a bulky dressing in place, and when the dressing is removed, a guided splinting program is started. Exercises are performed three to four times a day when the splints are removed and the patient is discharged. Before surgery, it must be made clear to the patient that the goal of the surgery is to restore function related to grasp, pinch, stability, and strength, and the hands will not necessarily have good cosmetic appearance.

39. d. Rationale: The patient with a tight cast may be at risk for neurovascular compromise (impaired circulation and peripheral nerve damage) and should be assessed first. The other patients should be seen as soon as possible. Providing analgesia for the patient with phantom pain would be the next priority. The patient in skeletal traction needs explanation of the purpose and functioning of the traction. She may need analgesia or muscle relaxants to help tolerate the traction.

Case Study

1. The knee and ankle should be immobilized with the splint. Unless the joints above and below the site are immobilized, the affected area is unstable.

2. The 6 Ps should be assessed—pulses, paresthesias, pallor, pressure, paralysis, and pain—especially unrelieved pain, which may indicate compartment syndrome.

3. The wound should be cleaned with extensive irrigation using normal saline, and if the wound is highly contaminated, surgical debridement may be necessary. Tetanus immunization is required if a dose of tetanus toxoid has not been given in the past 5 years, or if the patient has had fewer than three doses of toxoid, tetanus immunoglobulin should be administered. Bleeding should be controlled with sterile dressings.

4. Measures to relieve pain include elevating the limb and applying ice to decrease swelling, administering analgesics, and keeping the limb immobilized.

5. It can take up to one year for complete healing of the fracture, but ossification should take place in 3 weeks to 6 months. At that time the limb can be casted, and he can be mobile with crutches with no weight bearing on the affected limb. Weight bearing will be restricted for 6 to 12 weeks, depending on the rate of healing. His return to work will depend on how he is able to perform his responsibilities on crutches.

6. Mrs. A. should be called and informed of her husband's accident, and she should be told that H.A. is alert and oriented but has a fractured leg and will require hospitalization. Care should be taken not to panic her and to reassure her that his condition is stable.

7. *Nursing diagnoses:*
   • Acute pain related to edema and muscle spasms
   • Risk for peripheral neurovascular dysfunction related to edema
   • Risk for infection related to disruption of skin integrity and presence of environmental pathogens
   • Anxiety related to unknown outcome and restrictions
   Collaborative problems:
   Potential complications: Fat embolism; compartment syndrome; infection; malunion or nonunion

CHAPTER 64

1. b. Rationale: Chronic infection of the bone leads to formation of scar tissue from the granulation tissue. This avascular scar tissue provides an ideal site for continued microorganism growth and is impenetrable to antibiotics. Surgical debridement is often necessary to remove the poorly vascularized tissue and dead bone and to instill antibiotics directly to the area. Involucrum is new bone laid down at the infection site, which seals off areas of sequestra. Antibiotics can be effective during acute osteomyelitis, and prevention of chronic osteomyelitis requires early antibiotic treatment. Bone and skin grafting may be necessary following surgical removal of infection if destruction is extensive.

2. c. Rationale: The patient with osteomyelitis is at risk for pathologic fractures at the site of the infection because of weakened, devitalized bone, and careful handling of the extremity is necessary. ROM exercises should be limited because of the possibility of spreading infection, and edema is not a common finding in osteomyelitis. Careful handling of dressings is necessary to prevent the spread of infection to others.

3. c. Rationale: Because large doses of appropriate antibiotics are necessary in the treatment of acute osteomyelitis, it is important to identify the causative

microorganism. The definitive way to determine the causative agent is by bone biopsy or biopsy of the soft tissue surrounding the site. The other tests may help to establish the diagnosis but do not identify the causative agent.

4. c. Rationale: Activities such as exercise or heat application, which increase circulation and serve as stimuli for the spread of infection, should be avoided by patients with acute osteomyelitis. Oral or IV antibiotic therapy is continued at home for 4 to 6 weeks, and weight bearing is contraindicated to prevent pathologic fractures.

5. b. Rationale: One of the most common adverse effects of prolonged and high-dose antibiotic therapy is overgrowth of *Candida albicans* in the oral cavity and genitourinary tract. These infections are manifested by whitish-yellow, curdlike lesions of the mucosa. A dry, cracked, furrowed tongue is characteristic of severe dehydration; vesicles are characteristic of herpes simplex infections; and mouth and lip ulcers are characteristic of aphthous somatitis, or canker sores.

6. a. 1; b. 3; c. 1; d. 2; e. 2; f. 3

7. b. Rationale: Promotion of muscle activity is important in any patient with muscular dystrophy, but when the disease has progressed to cardiomyopathy or respiratory failure, activity must be balanced with oxygen supply. At this stage of the disease, care should be taken to prevent skin or respiratory complications. The patient should be encouraged to perform as much self-care and exercise as energy allows, but this will be limited.

8. a. *T*; b. *F*, mechanical strain and spasms of paravertebral muscles; c. *T*; d. *F*, herniated intervertebral disk; e. *T*

9. a. Rationale: Proper daily exercise is an important part of the prevention of back injury, with the goal of maintaining mobility and strength in the back. Patients should sit with the knees higher than the hips and should sleep in a side-lying position, with knees and hips bent, or on the back, with a device to flex the hips and knees. Good body mechanics with proper transfer and turning techniques are necessary in all jobs and activities.

10. b. Rationale: Urinary incontinence following spinal surgery may indicate nerve damage and should be reported to the health care provider. Paralytic ileus is common following surgery and is expected. Pain at the graft site, usually the iliac crest or the fibula, often is more severe than pain from the fused area, and although movement and sensation of the arms and legs should not be more impaired than before surgery, they often are not relieved immediately after surgery.

11. c. Rationale: After spinal surgery, patients are logrolled to maintain straight alignment of the spine at all times, requiring the patient to be turned with

a pillow between the legs and moving the body as a unit. The head of the bed is usually kept flat, and the legs are extended.

12. a. 4; b. 7; c. 5; d. 2; e. 3; f. 1; g. 4; h. 5; i. 1; j. 6

13. c. Rationale: Poorly fitted shoes selected for fashion rather than comfort are the primary factor in the development of foot problems. A few congenital problems predispose to foot problems, and poor hygiene in patients with peripheral vascular disease may lead to foot infections, but these factors are in the minority compared with the effect of ill-fitting shoes.

14. a. 3; b. 1; c. 2; d. 1; e. 3; f. 2, 3; g. 2

15. b, c, e. Rationale: Risk factors for osteoporosis include age >65, white or Asian ethnicity, cigarette smoking, inactive lifestyle, low body weight, and being postmenopausal including premature menopause. Other factors include family history, excessive alcohol use, long-term use of medications such as corticosteroids, thyroid replacement, heparin, long-acting sedatives or antiseizure drugs.

16. a. increased calcium intake and vitamin D;
b. weight-bearing exercise; c. postmenopausal estrogen replacement therapy
Also: bisphosphonates (e.g., etidronate [Didronel], alendronate [Fosamax])

17. a. Rationale: The bisphosphonates, such as alendronate, must be taken at least 30 minutes before food or other medications to promote their absorption, and, because they are very irritating to the stomach and esophagus, the patient must remain upright for at least 30 minutes after taking the medication to prevent reflux into the esophagus. These drugs will increase bone density, and calcium is still needed for bone formation.

Case Study

1. Risk factors for back pain in G.B. include excess body weight, cigarette smoking, and a job that requires heavy lifting and prolonged periods of sitting.

2. Preoperative preparation includes teaching about the restrictions on positioning and movement required following surgery, measures for pain control, and assessments that will be carried out postoperatively. The nurse should ensure that G.B. has received information about the procedure from the surgeon and understands the benefits and risks of the surgery.

3. G.B. will probably be restricted to flat bed rest for at least the first 24 hours to avoid straining the surgical area. Pillows may be used under the thigh of each leg to prevent strain on the back muscles. When turning is allowed, he must be turned with the help of several personnel to avoid changing the alignment of the spine, or he must be logrolled. Depending on the surgeon's preference, ambulation will usually begin by the second postoperative day, again keeping the spine in alignment.

4. These postoperative assessments should be carried out by the nurse q2-4hr during the first 24-48 hours:
   - Sensation: In all extremities in all appropriate dermatomes
   - Circulation and vital signs
   - Movement: Of all extremities
   - Muscle strength: Note any weakness of the extremities
   - Wound: Assess dressing for drainage and note amount, color, characteristics; clear or light yellow drainage should be tested for the presence of glucose, which would indicate spinal fluid leakage
   - Pain: Document location and intensity of pain; evaluate pain after administration of analgesia
   - Bowel activity: Assess bowel sounds, passage of flatus, and abdomen; paralytic ileus is common for several days
   - Urinary function: Incontinence or retention may indicate nerve damage and should be reported. Intermittent catheterization may be required for bladder emptying, especially until G.B. is allowed to stand to void.

5. Discharge instructions include teaching G.B. to report any persistent limb weakness, abnormal sensations, or pain to the health care provider. He should be instructed to avoid standing or sitting for prolonged periods. Walking, lying down, and shifting weight from one foot to another should be encouraged. Twisting of the spine is harmful, and he should be taught to think through any activity before bending, lifting, or stooping. A firm mattress or bed board should be used at home. To prevent further back problems, weight loss and smoking cessation should be encouraged. He should be taught correct body mechanics and to do strengthening back exercises after recovery from the surgery.

6. *Nursing diagnoses:*
   - Acute pain related to nerve root compression, muscle spasms, and surgical incision
   - Impaired physical mobility related to pain
   - Ineffective self-health management related to lack of knowledge regarding posture, exercises, body mechanics, and weight reduction
   Collaborative problems:
   Potential complication: Paralysis

CHAPTER 65

1. d. Rationale: Cartilage destruction in the joints affects 90% of people by the age of 40, and when the destruction becomes symptomatic, osteoarthritis (OA) is said to be present. Because degenerative changes cause symptoms in only about 60% of those over the age of 65, joint pain and functional disability should not be considered a normal finding in aging persons. OA is not a systemic disease, and although degenerative changes can be accelerated

by excessive use of or stress on a joint, many people with joint pain have no history of previous joint stress or injury.

2. a. 3; b. 5; c. 6; d. 1; e. 4; f. 2
3. a. *F*, Heberden's; b. *F*, bone surfaces rubbing together; c. *T*; d. *F*, acetaminophen; e. *T*
4. b. Rationale: Principles of joint protection and energy conservation are critical in being able to maintain functional mobility in the patient with osteoarthritis, and patients should be helped to find ways to perform activities and tasks with less stress. ROM, isotonic, and isometric exercises of the affected joints should be balanced with joint rest and protection, but during an acute flare of joint inflammation, the joints should be rested. If a joint is painful, it should be used only to the point of pain, and masking the pain with analgesics may lead to greater joint injury.
5. c. Rationale: Common side effects of NSAIDs include GI irritation and bleeding, dizziness, rash, headache, and tinnitus. Oral lesions and blood dyscrasias are common in patients receiving immunosuppressive agents and disease-modifying agents. Fluid retention, hypertension, and bruising from capillary fragility are frequently seen in patients using systemic corticosteroids.
6. a. Rationale: Some strong results from the use of over-the-counter glucosamine and chondroitin sulfate in the treatment of arthritis have been validated, and overall, these substances have few side effects.
7. a. Rationale: Misoprostol (Cytotec) is used to prevent nonsteroid antiinflammatory drug (NSAID)–induced gastric ulcers and gastritis and would increase the patient's tolerance of any of the NSAIDs. The use of naproxen would cause the same gastric effects as ibuprofen. The daily dose of acetaminophen should not exceed 4 g/day to prevent liver damage, and antacids interfere with the absorption of NSAIDs.
8. d. Rationale: In rheumatoid arthritis (RA), autoantibodies known as rheumatoid factors are formed against abnormal IgG, which is stimulated by an unknown factor. When the autoantibodies and the abnormal IgG combine, they form immune complexes that are deposited in the joints, blood vessels, and pleura and cause activation of complement with a resulting inflammatory response. The joint and systemic manifestations of RA are a result of the action of inflammatory mediators and cells. Some patients with RA have a prevalence of the HLA-DR4 antigen, but it does not directly cause damage.
9. a. RA; b. OA; c. OA; d. B; e. RA; f. RA; g. RA; h. OA; i. RA; j. O; k. RA
10. c. Rationale: A patient with moderate RA has no joint deformities but may have limited joint mobility, adjacent muscle atrophy, and inflammation of the joints. Synovial hypertrophy and thickening of the joint capsule may cause spindle-shaped fingers.

Splenomegaly may be found with RA, and crepitus on movement and Heberden's nodes are associated with osteoarthritis.

11. d. Rationale: The inflammatory reactions of RA cause an elevation in C-reactive protein (CRP), a finding that is useful in monitoring the response to therapy. The WBC count may be increased in response to inflammation and is also elevated in synovial fluid. Anemia, rather than polycythemia, is common, and normal IgG levels are not affected.
12. a. Rheumatoid nodules: Firm, nontender, subcutaneous masses occurring over the extensor surfaces of joints, such as fingers and elbows
    b. Sjögren's syndrome: Diminished lacrimal and salivary gland secretions
    c. Felty's syndrome: Inflammatory eye disorders, splenomegaly, lymphadenopathy, pulmonary disease, and blood dyscrasias
13. a. 7; b. 6; c. 5; d. 1; e. 9; f. 2; g. 3; h. 1; i. 7; j. 2; k. 5; l. 4; m. 2, 8; n. 2; o. 10
14. c. Rationale: Because older adults are more likely to take many drugs, the use of multidrug therapy in RA is particularly problematic because of the increased likelihood of adverse drug interactions and toxicity. Rheumatic disorders do occur in older adults but usually in milder form. Interpretation of laboratory values in older adults is more difficult in diagnosing RA because of age-related serologic changes, but the disease can be diagnosed. Older adults are not less compliant with drug regimens but may need help with complex regimens.
15. b. Rationale: Most patients with RA experience morning stiffness, and morning activities should be scheduled later in the day after the stiffness subsides. A warm shower in the morning and time to become more mobile before activity are advised. Management of RA includes daily exercises for the affected joints and protection of joints with devices and movements that prevent joint stress. Splinting should be done during an acute flare to rest the joint and prevent further damage.
16. b. Rationale: Pacing activities and alternating rest with activity are important in maintaining self-care and independence of the patient with RA, in addition to preventing deconditioning and a negative attitude. The nurse should not carry out activities for patients that they can do for themselves but instead should support and assist patients as necessary.
17. d. Rationale: Cold therapy is indicated to relieve pain during an acute inflammation, can be applied with frozen packages of vegetables, and should only last 10 to 15 minutes at a time. Heat in the form of heating pads, moist warm packs, paraffin baths, or warm baths or showers is indicated to relieve stiffness and muscle spasm. Heat should not be applied for more than 20 minutes at a time.

18. c. Rationale: Aquatic exercises in warm water allow easier joint movement because of the buoyancy of the water, and water produces more resistance and can strengthen the muscles. Tai chi is also a good form of gentle, stretching exercise that would be appropriate. Dancing and even walking impact the joints of the feet, and even low-impact aerobics could be damaging. Exercises for patients with RA should be gentle.

19. d. Rationale: An unusually high frequency of HLA-B27 is found in patients with ankylosing spondylitis, psoriatic arthritis, and reactive arthritis, and these diseases have a predilection for involvement of the spine, peripheral joints, and periarticular structures as well as an absence of rheumatoid factor and autoantibodies.

20. d. Rationale: Kyphosis and involvement of costovertebral joints in ankylosing spondylitis lead to a bent-over posture and a decrease in chest expansion, manifestations that are managed with chest expansion and deep-breathing exercises. Postural training emphasizes avoiding forward flexion during any activities, and the patient should sleep on the back without the use of pillows.

21. a. 6; b. 4; c. 1; d. 2; e. 3; f. 5; g. 6; h. 1; i. 3; j. 5; k. 4; l. 2

22. d. Rationale: The diagnosis of gout is established by finding monosodium urate monohydrate crystals in the synovial fluid of an inflamed joint or tophus. Hyperuricemia and elevated urine uric acid are not diagnostic for gout because they may be related to a variety of drugs or may exist as a totally asymptomatic abnormality in the general population. Although there is a familial predisposition to hyperuricemia, both environmental and genetic factors contribute to gout.

23. b. Rationale: Colchicine has an antiinflammatory action specific for gout and is the treatment of choice during an acute attack, often producing dramatic pain relief in 24 to 48 hours. It may also be used prophylactically to reduce the frequency of attacks. Probenecid is a uricosuric drug that is used to control hyperuricemia by increasing the excretion of uric acid through the kidney, and allopurinol is also used to control hyperuricemia by blocking production of uric acid. Aspirin inactivates the effect of uricosuric drugs and should not be used when patients are taking probenecid and other uricosuric drugs.

24. b. Rationale: During therapy with probenecid or allopurinol, the patient must have periodic determination of blood uric acid levels to evaluate the effectiveness of the therapy and to ensure that levels are kept low enough to prevent future attacks of gout. Patients should not alter their doses of medications without medical direction, and the drugs used for control of gout are not useful in the treatment of an acute attack. With the use of medications, strict dietary restrictions on alcohol and high-purine foods are usually not necessary. When the patient is taking probenecid, urine output should be maintained at 2 to 3 L to prevent urate from precipitating in the urinary tract and causing kidney stones.

25. a. Rationale: In systemic lupus erythematosus (SLE), autoantibodies are produced to nucleic acids, erythrocytes, coagulation proteins, lymphocytes, platelets, and many other self proteins. Overproduction of collagen is characteristic of systemic sclerosis, and abnormal IgG reactions with autoantibodies are characteristic of RA.

26. a. cutaneous vascular lesions on sun-exposed skin with classic butterfly rash on face; b. polyarthralgia and polyarthritis; c. pericarditis and dysrhythmias; d. restrictive lung disease with cough, tachypnea, and pleurisy; e. proteinuria resulting from nephritis; f. seizures, peripheral neuropathy, cognitive dysfunction; g. anemia, leukopenia, and thrombocytopenia

27. b. Rationale: Patients with SLE often find that one of the most difficult facets of the disease is its extreme variability in severity and progression. There is no characteristic pattern of progressive organ involvement, nor is it predictable as to which systems may become affected. SLE is now associated with a normal life span, but patients must be helped to adjust to the unknown course of the disease.

28. c. Rationale: Efficacy of treatment with corticosteroids or immunosuppressive drugs is best monitored by serial serum complement levels and anti-DNA titers, both of which will decrease as the drugs have an effect. A reduction in ESR is not as specific, and the patient with SLE often has a chronic anemia that is not affected by drug therapy.

29. a. Rationale: Acute exacerbations of SLE may be precipitated by overexposure to ultraviolet light, physical and emotional stress, fatigue, and infection or surgery. The major concern in planning a pregnancy is that exacerbations are also common following delivery, and there are increased risks for the mother and fetus during pregnancy. Although SLE has an identified genetic association with HLA-DR2 and HLA-DR3, genetic counseling is not usually recommended. Dietary recommendations include small, frequent meals and adequate iron intake. Although nonpharmacologic methods of pain control are encouraged, the use of NSAIDs is often necessary to help control inflammation and pain.

30. a. Rationale: Systemic sclerosis is a disorder of connective tissue that causes skin thickening and tightening, resulting in expressionless facial features, puckering of the mouth, and a small oral orifice. It also causes symmetric, painless swelling or thickening of the skin of the fingers and hands. It does not cause the swan-neck or ulnar drift deformities seen in RA or SLE, and low back pain and spinal stiffness are associated with ankylosing spondylitis.

31. d. Rationale: One of the most common and early manifestations of CREST syndrome is Raynaud's phenomenon, which causes paroxysmal vasospasms of the digits with diminished blood flow to the fingers and toes on exposure to cold, followed by cyanosis and then erythema on rewarming. The hands and feet must be protected from cold exposure and possible burns or cuts that might heal slowly, and smoking is contraindicated. Sensitivity to ultraviolet light is not a factor in systemic sclerosis, nor is fluid intake. Cardiovascular involvement may occur, but it does not require patient monitoring.

32. b. Rationale: Dermatomyositis produces symmetric weakness of striated muscle, and weak neck and pharyngeal muscles may produce dysphagia. Weakened pharyngeal muscles lead to a poor cough, difficulty swallowing and increased aspiration risk. Muscle tenderness or pain is uncommon, as is joint involvement. During an acute attack the patient is so weak that bed rest is needed, and passive ROM is usually required.

33. b. Rationale: People with fibromyalgia syndrome (FMS) typically experience nonrestorative sleep, morning stiffness, irritable bowel syndrome, and anxiety in addition to the widespread, nonarticular musculoskeletal pain and fatigue. FMS is nondegenerative, nonprogressive, and noninflammatory. Neither muscle weakness nor muscle spasms are associated with the disease, although there may be tics in the muscle at the tender points.

34. d. Rationale: Two criteria for the diagnosis of FMS are that (1) pain is experienced in 11 of the 18 tender points on palpation and (2) the patient has a history of widespread pain for at least 3 months. The other findings may also be present but are not diagnostic for FMS.

35. d. Rationale: The pain and related symptoms of FMS cause significant stress, and anxiety is a common finding. Stress management is an important part of the treatment and may include any of the commonly used relaxation strategies as well as psychologic counseling.

36. a. Unexplained, persistent, or relapsing chronic fatigue that is of new and definite onset
b. Fatigue is not due to ongoing exertion.
c. Fatigue is not substantially alleviated by rest.
d. Fatigue results in substantial reduction in occupational, educational, social, or personal activities.

Case Study

1. N.M. should be told that RA is a disease that affects all of her body, even though her joints are primarily affected at this time. She needs to know that it is not known what causes RA but that antibodies are formed that react with substances causing inflammation and damage to a variety of organs. Joint changes include inflammation of the lining of the joints and eventual filling of the joint with bone, completely immobilizing the joint and causing deformities similar to those she is developing in her hands. She should be told that the fatigue and low-grade fever she has are part of the disease and that with disease control these symptoms will improve.

2. The painful, stiff hands and feet; the fatigue; the low-grade fever; and the ulnar drift deviation are all manifestations of RA.

3. Methotrexate is a chemotherapeutic agent that has an antiinflammatory effect but causes bone marrow suppression and hepatotoxicity. Its dosage in RA is much smaller than that used for cancer therapy, and side effects are not as common. When used in RA, it frequently reduces clinical symptoms in days to weeks with few, if any, adverse effects. Teaching N.M. about methotrexate is an important nursing responsibility. Periodic blood chemistry and hematology tests must be done, the patient should take a daily supplement of folic acid, and the patient should report signs of anemia or any infection. Methotrexate is teratogenic, and N.M. should be informed that contraception must be used during and 3 months after treatment.

4. Protection of her joints will be enhanced if she can maintain a normal weight, avoid tasks that cause pain, use assistive devices to prevent joint stress, and avoid forceful, repetitive movements. She should plan regularly scheduled rest periods alternated with activity throughout the day and should develop organizing and pacing techniques that spread tasks through the day or the week. Suggesting that she take a warm shower or bath in the morning to relieve her morning stiffness might be helpful. Exercise regimens will be prescribed for N.M., and she should be encouraged to follow the regimens daily.

5. Because of the chronicity and disability associated with arthritis, patients are often vulnerable to claims of unproven remedies. The nurse should recognize that the copper bracelet will do no harm but may be a waste of money for N.M. It is important to encourage her to recognize that regular, proven methods of treatment used on a consistent basis are the best way to control her condition. The more she is taught about the disease and its management, the more compliant she will be with treatment regimens.

6. Additional sources of information and sharing are available from the Arthritis Foundation and should be suggested to N.M.

7. *Nursing diagnoses:*
   • Acute and chronic pain related to joint inflammation
   • Impaired physical mobility related to joint pain, stiffness, and deformity
   • Fatigue related to disease activity

- Ineffective self-health management related to use of unproven remedies
- Risk for infection related to altered immune function

Collaborative problems:

Potential complication: Bone marrow suppression

CHAPTER 66

1. d. Rationale: One of the primary characteristics of critical care nurses that is different from those of generalist medical-surgical nurses is the use of advanced technology to measure physiologic parameters accurately to manage life-threatening complications. All nursing addresses human responses to health problems and requires knowledge of physiology, pathophysiology, pharmacology, and psychologic support to the patient and family. Diagnosis and treatment of life-threatening diseases are roles of medicine.

2. a. physiologically unstable; b. risk for serious complications; c. risk for serious complications; d. intensive nursing support

3. b. Rationale: When anxiety in the ICU patient is related to the environment, which has unfamiliar equipment, high noise and light levels, and an intense pace of activity, which leads to sensory overload, the nurse should eliminate as much of this source of stress as possible by muting phones, limiting overhead paging, setting alarms appropriate to the patient's condition, and eliminating unnecessary alarms. Offering flexible visiting schedules for family members and providing as much autonomy in decisions about care as possible are indicated when impaired communication and loss of control contribute to the anxiety. Use of sedation to reduce anxiety should be carefully evaluated and implemented when nursing measures are not effective.

4. c. Rationale: The caregivers of the critically ill patient are very important in the recovery and well-being of the patient, and the extent to which the family is involved and supported affects the patient's clinical course. Although the cost of planning and providing critical care is a concern to caregivers, it is not the major reason caregivers are included in the patient's care. Caregivers may be responsible for making decisions about the patient's care only when the patient is unable to make personal decisions. Most caregivers have questions regarding the patient's quality of care because of anxiety and lack of information about the patient's condition.

5. a. decreased; b. increased; c. decrease; d. increase; e. increased; f. increases

6. d. Rationale: Cardiac output (CO) is dependent on heart rate and stroke volume, and stroke volume is determined by preload, afterload, and contractility. If CO is decreased and heart rate is unchanged, stroke volume is the variable factor. If the preload determined by pulmonary artery wedge pressure (PAWP) and the afterload determined by SVR are unchanged, the factor that is changed is the contractility of the myocardium.

7. b. Rationale: Referencing hemodynamic monitoring equipment means positioning the monitoring equipment so that the zero reference point is at the vertical level of the left atrium of the heart. The port of the stopcock nearest the transducer is placed at the phlebostatic axis, the external landmark of the left atrium. The phlebostatic axis is the intersection of two planes: a horizontal line midchest, halfway between the outermost anterior and posterior surfaces, transecting a vertical line through the fourth intercostal space at the sternum.

8. a. *T*; b. *F*, pulmonary artery; c. *F*, left ventricle; d. *T*; e. *T*

9. c. Rationale: During insertion of a pulmonary artery catheter, it is necessary to monitor the ECG continuously because of the risk for dysrhythmias, particularly when the catheter reaches the right ventricle. It is the health care provider's responsibility to obtain informed consent regarding the catheter insertion. During the catheter insertion, the patient is placed supine with the head of the bed flat. An Allen test to confirm adequate ulnar artery perfusion is performed before insertion of an arterial catheter in the radial artery for arterial pressure monitoring.

10. a. Slowly inflate the pulmonary artery catheter balloon with 1.0 to 1.5 mL of air while observing the pressure tracing, and measure the PAWP at the end of expiration, limiting the balloon inflation to fewer than four respiratory cycles.
    b. Rapidly inject the prescribed amount and temperature of solution into the right atrial lumen of the pulmonary artery catheter, and read the computer display of the CO.

11. a. MAP: 75 mm Hg (90 + 136)/3
    PAMP: 26 mm Hg (38 + 40)/3
    SV: 25.8 mL/beat (3.2 × 1000)/124
    SVR: 1525 dyne sec/cm^5 (75 − 14 × 80/3.2)
    b. All the changes in the hemodynamic parameters are characteristic findings in the patient with heart failure: increased pulmonary congestion and pressures; increased pressure in the left atrium and ventricle; increased SVR; and decreased stroke volume, CO, and systemic BP.

12. b. Rationale: The normal mixed venous oxygen saturation of 60% to 80% becomes decreased with decreased arterial oxygenation, low CO, low hemoglobin, or increased oxygen consumption. With normal CO, arterial oxygenation, and hemoglobin, the factor that is responsible for decreased SvO_2 is increased oxygen consumption, which can result from increased metabolic rate, pain, movement, or fever.

13. d. Rationale: When a pulmonary artery pressure tracing indicates a wedged waveform when the balloon is deflated, this indicates that the catheter has advanced and has become spontaneously wedged. If the catheter is not repositioned immediately, a pulmonary infarction or a rupture of a pulmonary artery may occur. If the catheter is becoming occluded, the pressure tracing becomes blunted, and pulmonary edema and increased pulmonary congestion increase the pulmonary artery waveform. Balloon leaks found when injected air does not flow back into the syringe do not alter waveforms.

14. d. Rationale: The counterpulsation of the intraaortic balloon pump (IABP) increases diastolic arterial pressure, forcing blood back into the coronary arteries and main branches of the aortic arch, increasing coronary artery perfusion pressure and blood flow to the myocardium. The balloon pump also causes a drop in aortic pressure just before systole, decreasing afterload and myocardial oxygen consumption. These effects make the IABP valuable in treating unstable angina, acute myocardial infarction with heart failure, cardiogenic shock, and a variety of surgical heart situations. Its use is contraindicated in incompetent aortic valves, dissecting aortic aneurysms, and generalized peripheral vascular disease.

15. a. *F*, afterload; b. *T*; c. *F*, diastolic

16. c. Rationale: Because the IABP is inserted into the femoral artery and advanced to the descending thoracic aorta, compromised distal extremity circulation is common and requires that the cannulated extremity be extended at all times. Repositioning the patient is limited to side-lying or supine positions with the head of the bed elevated no more than 30 to 45 degrees. Assessment for bleeding is important because the IABP may cause platelet destruction, and occlusive dressings are used to prevent site infection.

17. d. Rationale: Weaning from the IABP involves reducing the pumping to every second or third heartbeat until the IABP catheter is removed. The pumping and infusion flow are continued to reduce the risk for thrombus formation around the catheter until it is removed.

18. b. Rationale: Ventricular assist devices are temporary devices that can partially or totally support circulation until the heart recovers and can be weaned from cardiopulmonary bypass or when a donor heart can be obtained. The devices currently available do not permanently support circulation.

19. c. Rationale: A nasal endotracheal (ET) tube is longer and smaller in diameter than an oral ET tube, creating more airway resistance and increasing the

work of breathing. Suctioning and secretion removal are also more difficult with nasal ET tubes, and they are more subject to kinking than are oral tubes. Oral tubes require a bite block to stop the patient from biting the tube and may cause more laryngeal damage because of their larger size.

20. a. Rationale: The patient is positioned with the mouth, pharynx, and trachea in direct alignment, with the head extended in the "sniffing position," but the head must not hang over the edge of the bed. The patient may be asked to extrude the tongue during nasal intubation. Speaking is not possible during intubation or while the tube is in place because the tube splits the vocal cords.

21. c. Rationale: The first action of the nurse is to use an end-tidal CO_2 detector. If no CO_2 is detected, the tube is in the esophagus. The second action by the nurse following ET intubation is to auscultate the chest to confirm bilateral breath sounds and observe to confirm bilateral chest expansion. If this evidence is present, the tube is secured and connected to an O_2 source. Then the placement is confirmed immediately with x-ray, and the tube is marked where it exits the mouth. Then the patient should be suctioned as needed.

22. c. Rationale: The minimal occluding volume (MOV) involves adding air to the ET tube cuff until no leak is heard at peak inspiratory pressure but ensures that minimal pressure is applied to the tracheal wall to prevent pressure necrosis of the trachea. The minimal occluding volume should apply between 20 to 25 mm Hg of pressure on the trachea to prevent injury. The cuff does not secure the tube in place but rather prevents escape of ventilating gases through the upper airway.

23. a. 8, between 20 and 25 mm Hg; b. suctioning, bag-valve mask (BVM); c. half; d. 100 to 120 mm Hg; e. 10; f. hyperoxygenates

24. c. Rationale: Suctioning an ET tube is performed when adventitious sounds over the trachea or bronchi confirm the presence of secretions that can be removed by suctioning. Visible secretions in the ET tube, respiratory distress, suspected aspiration, increase in peak airway pressures, and changes in oxygen status are other indications. Peripheral crackles are not an indication for suctioning, and suctioning as a means of inducing a cough is not recommended because of the complications associated with suctioning.

25. d. Rationale: If serious dysrhythmias occur during suctioning, the suctioning should be stopped, and the patient should be slowly ventilated via BVM with 100% oxygen until the dysrhythmia subsides. Patients with bradycardia should not be suctioned excessively. Ventilation of the patient with slow, small-volume breaths using the BVM is performed when severe coughing results from suctioning.

26. a. Use two nurses: one to hold the tube while it is untaped or the holder is loosened, and another to perform care.
    b. After completion of care, confirm the presence of bilateral breath sounds to ensure that the position of the tube was not changed and reconfirm cuff pressure.

27. b, c, d. Rationale: Because the patient with an ET tube cannot protect the airway from aspiration and cannot swallow, the cuff should always be inflated and the head of the bed (HOB) elevated while the patient is receiving tube feedings or mouth care is being performed. The HOB elevated 30 to 45 degrees helps reduce risk. The mouth and oropharynx should be suctioned with Yankauer or tonsil suction to remove accumulated secretions that cannot be swallowed. Clearing the ventilatory tubing of condensed water is important to prevent respiratory infection.

28. c. Rationale: Sedation may be appropriate as well as having someone the patient knows at the bedside talking to him; reassuring him may decrease his anxiety and calm him. The other methods may need to be used. Restraints will need ongoing and frequent assessment of need. Reminding the patient may help, but it may not be enough to prevent the patient from pulling the tube if the patient becomes extremely anxious.

29. 1. Apnea or impending inability to breathe
    2. Acute respiratory failure
    3. Severe hypoxia
    4. Respiratory muscle fatigue

30. a. N; b. P; c. B; d. N; e. N; f. P; g. N

31. a. 2; b. 1; c. 2; d. 2; e. 1

32. a. CPAP—continuous positive airway pressure; b. SIMV—synchronized intermittent mandatory ventilation; c. PSV—pressure support ventilation; d. ACV—assist-control ventilation; e. PEEP—positive end-expiratory pressure; f. HFV—high-frequency ventilation; g. PC/IRV—pressure-controlled/inverse-ratio ventilation

33. a. Rationale: Positive-pressure ventilation, especially with end-expiratory pressure, increases intrathoracic pressure with compression of thoracic vessels, resulting in decreased venous return to the heart, decreased left ventricular end-diastolic volume (preload), decreased CO, and lowered BP. None of the other factors is related to increased intrathoracic pressure.

34. d. Rationale: Decreased CO associated with positive-pressure ventilation and positive end-expiratory pressure (PEEP) results in decreased renal perfusion, release of renin, and increased aldosterone secretion, which causes sodium and water retention. ADH may be released because of stress, but ADH is responsible only for water retention, and increased intrathoracic pressure decreases, not increases, the release of atrial natriuretic factor, causing sodium retention. There is decreased, not increased, insensible water loss via the airway during mechanical ventilation.

35. a. LPN; b. RN; c. LPN; d. NAP; e. RN; f. LPN; g. RN; h. NAP; i. RN; j. NAP

36. c. Rationale: Neuromuscular blocking agents produce a paralysis that facilitates ventilation, but they do not sedate the patient. It is important for the nurse to remember that the patient can hear, see, think, and feel and should be addressed and given explanations accordingly. Communication with the patient is possible, especially from the nurse, but visitors for an anxious and agitated patient should provide a calming, restful effect on the patient.

37. a. anemia resulting in poor O_2 transport; b. decreased respiratory strength; c. delayed weaning; d. decreased resistance to infection; e. prolonged recovery

38. b. Rationale: A leaking cuff can lower tidal volume or respiratory rates. An SIMV rate that is too low, the presence of lung secretions, or obstruction can decrease tidal volume. A decreased $PaCO_2$ and increased pH indicate a respiratory alkalosis from hyperventilation, and cardiac dysrhythmias can occur with either hyperventilation or hypoventilation.

39. b. Rationale: A variety of ventilator weaning methods is used, but all should provide weaning trials with adequate rest between weaning trials to prevent respiratory muscle fatigue. Weaning is usually carried out during the day, with the patient ventilated at night until there is sufficient spontaneous ventilation without excess fatigue. In all methods, patients usually require a 10% increase in fraction of inspired oxygen (FiO_2) to maintain arterial oxygen tension. If the patient becomes hypoxemic, ventilator support is indicated.

40. a. Rationale: Care of a ventilator-dependent patient in the home requires that the caregiver know how to manage the ventilator and take care of the patient on it. The nurse should ensure that caregivers understand the potential sacrifices they may have to make and the impact that home mechanical ventilation will have over time, before final decisions and arrangements are made. Placement in long-term care facilities is not usually necessary unless the caregiver can no longer manage the care or the patient's condition deteriorates.

Case Study

1. The best indicators to use to monitor D.V.'s hemodynamic status are the values determined from the pulmonary artery catheter, the urinary output, and the BP because infectious processes are altering his LOC, skin temperature, and other vital signs that may commonly be used to monitor hemodynamic status. Of the hemodynamic parameters, it is most important to monitor CO, SVR, and SvO_2 because

these parameters are the most out of range and suggest septic shock.

2. PEEP is used for D.V. to increase his oxygenation because his PaO_2 is decreased, but it can increase intrathoracic pressure, suppressing venous return and increasing ICP.

3. D.V.'s MAP is 64 mm Hg (100 + (46 × 2)/3). The MAP necessary to promote tissue and cerebral perfusion and yet not increase ICP would be a MAP that maintains a CPP of 70 mm Hg. With an ICP of 22 mm Hg, MAP needs to be 92 mm Hg to maintain cerebral perfusion and yet not increase ICP (CPP = MAP – ICP, or 70 = 92 – 22). His current MAP results in a cerebral perfusion pressure of 42, which is inadequate to maintain cerebral perfusion.

4. Fluid therapy would include rapid administration of 0.9% sodium chloride, colloids, or both to expand vascular volume and maintain tissue perfusion, with monitoring of PAP, PAWP, and CO to evaluate fluid replacement. Lactated Ringer's is contraindicated because of the patient's elevated lactate levels. Antibiotics specific for cryptococcal infections, such as fluconazole (Diflucan), should be initiated immediately, and a broad-spectrum antibiotic, such as an aminoglycoside, is indicated for bacterial prophylaxis. Vasopressor agents, such as norepinephrine (Levophed), dopamine (Intropin), or phenylephrine (Neo-Synephrine), are indicated to promote vasoconstriction and increase SVR. After fluid therapy has been initiated, an osmotic diuretic, such as mannitol, may be used to pull water out of the brain tissue and decrease ICP. Aspirin or other antipyretics should be given to control his temperature because increased temperature increases the metabolic rate and oxygen need. Sodium bicarbonate is not indicated to correct the patient's acidosis unless the pH is below 7.20.

5. Gastrointestinal ischemia may cause translocation of bowel bacteria into the systemic circulation, creating a source of further infection and sepsis. Early institution of enteral tube feedings may help promote GI function and prevent bacterial translocation.

6. Subjective assessment findings:
Seizures reflect the cerebral irritation caused by the inflammation of the meninges and the increased ICP.
Objective assessment findings:
- Increased ICP is responsible for the GCS score of 6 and is reflected by the ICP of 22 mm Hg.
- The infectious process of the meningitis is reflected by the increased body temperature and the WBC count of 18,500/μL.
- The response of the sympathetic nervous system to the inflammation and sepsis is seen in the elevated blood glucose level.
- Most of the other findings reflect the development of septic shock, systemic inflammatory response

syndrome (SIRS), and possible development of multiple-organ dysfunction syndrome (MODS).
- Shock is evident from the lowered BP, metabolic acidosis, markedly reduced SVR, and decreased urinary output resulting from poor renal perfusion.
- Septic shock is characterized by activation of mediators that cause widespread vasodilation and increased capillary permeability, resulting in decreased SVR and high CO because of the decreased peripheral resistance. The vasodilation causes the skin to be warm and dry. Septic shock also results in poor oxygen utilization, resulting in elevated mixed venous oxygen saturation (SvO_2). All these processes are reflected in the assessment findings in this patient.
- The ABGs and increased lactate indicate the metabolic acidosis resulting from anaerobic metabolism of cells. The $PaCO_2$ and HCO_3^- are low, and the respiratory rate is increased, indicating the body's attempt to compensate for the metabolic acidosis by using bicarbonate to buffer lactic acid and by hyperventilation to blow off extra carbon dioxide.
- The decreased urinary output and decreased arterial oxygenation may reflect not only poor perfusion to the kidneys and lungs but also initial organ damage and development of MODS.

7. *Nursing diagnoses:*
- Risk for ineffective cerebral tissue perfusion related to cerebral tissue swelling
- Ineffective peripheral tissue perfusion related to deficit in capillary blood supply
- Ineffective protection related to neurosensory alterations
- Hyperthermia related to inflammatory process
- Ineffective airway clearance related to unconsciousness and presence of artificial airway
- Risk for injury related to endotracheal intubation, mechanical ventilation, seizure activity, and environmental hazards
- Risk for aspiration related to presence of artificial airway
- Imbalanced nutrition: less than body requirements related to increased caloric demands and inability to take nourishment orally
- Risk for decreased CO related to impeded venous return by PEEP

Collaborative problems:
Potential complications: ARDS; DIC; organ ischemia—neurologic, renal, GI, respiratory; pneumothorax or pneumomediastinum; MODS

CHAPTER 67

1. d. Rationale: Although all the factors may be present, regardless of the cause, the end result is inadequate supply of oxygen and nutrients to body cells from inadequate tissue perfusion.

2. a. 2; b. 3; c. 5; d. 1; e. 2; f. 6; g. 5; h. 4; i. 1; j. 5; k. 4; l. 5; m. 5; n. 6; o. 1; p. 3
3. a. *F*, hypovolemic; b. *T*; c. *T*; d. *T*; e. *F*, absolute; f. *T*
4. a. decreased capillary hydrostatic pressure; b. α-Adrenergic stimulation; c. β-Adrenergic stimulation, increased cardiac output; d. renin release; e. aldosterone secretion; f. increased venous return to heart, increased BP; g. Increased serum osmolality, release of ADH; h. renal water reabsorption
5. a. increased heart rate (β-adrenergic stimulation); b. cool, pale skin (α-adrenergic stimulation); c. thirst (with fluid shift to intravascular space); d. decreased urinary output (ADH and aldosterone); e. fluctuating BP; f. decreased bowel sounds (α-adrenergic stimulation)
   Others: abdominal distention, edema (sodium retention)
6. c. Rationale: When sepsis is the cause of shock, the endotoxins stimulate a cascade of inflammatory responses that start with release of TNF and interleukin-1 (IL-1), which stimulate other inflammatory mediators that increase neutrophil and platelet aggregation and adhesion to the endothelium. There is an increase in coagulation and inflammation and fibrinolysis, and platelet-activating factor causes formation of microthrombi and vessel obstruction. The process does not occur in other types of shock until late stages.
7. a. Renin-angiotensin activation causes arteriolar constriction, decreasing perfusion.
   b. Vasoconstriction of the pulmonary arterioles decreases the blood flow to pulmonary capillaries, and a ventilation-perfusion mismatch occurs. Areas of the lung that are oxygenated are not perfused by blood because of the decreased blood flow, resulting in additional hypoxemia and decreased oxygen for cells.
   c. Increased capillary permeability and profound vasoconstriction cause increased hydrostatic pressure with shift of fluid to interstitial spaces and decreased circulating blood volume.
   d. Decreased myocardial perfusion occurs as the heart fails, leading to dysrhythmias and myocardial ischemia, further decreasing CO and oxygen delivery to cells.
8. b. Rationale: During both the compensated and progressive stages of shock, the sympathetic nervous system is activated in an attempt to maintain CO and SVR. In the irreversible stage of shock, the sympathetic nervous system can no longer compensate to maintain homeostasis, and a loss of vasomotor tone leading to profound hypotension affects perfusion to all vital organs, causing increasing cellular hypoxia, metabolic acidosis, and cellular death.
9. d. Rationale: In every type of shock there is a deficiency of oxygen to the cells, and high-flow oxygen therapy is indicated. Fluids could be started next, blood cultures done before any antibiotic therapy, and lab specimens then could be drawn.
10. b. Rationale: In early compensated shock, activation of the renin-angiotensin system stimulates the release of aldosterone, which causes sodium reabsorption and potassium excretion by the kidney, elevating serum sodium levels, and decreasing serum potassium levels. Blood glucose levels are elevated during the compensated stage of shock in response to catecholamine stimulation of the liver, which releases its glycogen stores in the form of glucose. Metabolic acidosis does not occur until the progressive stage of shock, when compensatory mechanisms become ineffective and anaerobic cellular metabolism causes lactic acid production.
11. d. Rationale: In late irreversible shock, progressive cellular destruction causes changes in lab findings that indicate organ damage. Increasing ammonia levels indicate impaired liver function. Metabolic acidosis is usually severe as cells continue anaerobic metabolism, and the respiratory alkalosis that may occur in the progressive stage has failed to compensate for the acidosis. Potassium levels increase and blood glucose decreases.
12. a. Rationale: Lactated Ringer's solution may increase lactate levels, which a damaged liver cannot convert to bicarbonate, and may intensify the metabolic lactic acidosis that occurs in progressive shock, necessitating careful attention to the patient's acid-base balance. Sodium and potassium levels as well as hemoglobin and hematocrit levels should be monitored in all patients receiving fluid replacement therapy.
13. b. Rationale: The endpoint of fluid resuscitation in septic and hypovolemic shock is a CVP of 15 mm Hg or a PAWP of 10-12 mm Hg. The CO is too low, and the heart rate is too high, to indicate adequate fluid replacement.
14. a. Rationale: A decreased mixed venous oxygen saturation (SvO_2) indicates that the patient has used the venous oxygen reserve and is at greater risk for anaerobic metabolism. The SvO_2 decreases when more oxygen is used by the cells, as in activity or hypermetabolism. All the other values indicate an improvement in the patient's condition.
15. d. Rationale: As a vasopressor, norepinephrine may cause severe vasoconstriction, which would further decrease tissue perfusion, especially if fluid replacement is inadequate. Vasopressors generally cause hypertension, reflex bradycardia, and decreased urine output because of decreased renal blood flow; they do not directly affect acid-base balance.
16. c. Rationale: Vasoactive drugs are those that can either dilate or constrict blood vessels, and both are used in various stages of shock treatment. When

using either vasodilators or vasoconstrictors, it is important to maintain a MAP of at least 60 mm Hg so that adequate perfusion is maintained.

17. a. Restore coronary artery blood flow with thrombolytic therapy, angioplasty, emergency revascularization; increase CO with inotropic agents; reduce workload by dilating coronary arteries, decreasing preload and afterload; use circulatory assist devices, such as an intraaortic balloon pump
    b. Fluid and blood replacement, control of bleeding with pressure, surgery
    c. Fluid resuscitation, antimicrobial agents, inotropic agents with vasopressors
    d. Epinephrine, inhaled bronchodilators, colloidal fluid replacement, diphenhydramine, corticosteroids
18. a. Diuretics (e.g., furosemide [Lasix] to decrease the workload of the heart by decreasing fluid volume and reducing preload.
    b. Milrinone (Primacor) increases cardiac contractility and output and decreases preload and afterload by directly relaxing vascular smooth muscles.
    c. Nitroglycerin (Nitrol, Tridil) primarily dilates veins, reducing preload.
    d. Nitroprusside (Nipride) acts as a potent vasodilator of veins and arteries and may increase

or decrease CO, depending on the extent of preload and afterload reduction.
Others: Diuretics, ACE inhibitors, β-adrenergic blockers

19. c. Rationale: Prevention of shock necessitates identification of persons who are at risk and a thorough baseline nursing assessment with frequent ongoing assessments to monitor and detect changes in patients at risk. Frequent monitoring of all patients' vital signs is not necessary. Aseptic technique for all invasive procedures should always be implemented but will not prevent all types of shock. Health-promotion activities that reduce the risk for precipitating conditions, such as coronary artery disease or anaphylaxis, may help prevent shock in some selected cases.
20. Vital signs, including pulse oximetry; level of consciousness; skin (color, temperature, moisture); urine output; peripheral pulses with capillary refill
21. a. 3; b. 1; c. 3; d. 5; e. 2; f. 1; g. 3, 4; h. 1; i. 2; j. 5
22. c. Rationale: If the metabolic acidosis is compensated, the pH will be within the normal range, and if the patient is hyperventilating to blow off carbon dioxide to reduce the acid load of the blood, $PaCO_2$ will be decreased.
23. See table below.

	O_2 Supplement	Volume Expansion—Crystalloid	Volume Expansion—Colloid	Circulatory Assist Device	Anti-biotics	Anti-histamine	Vaso-dilator	Vaso-pressor	Inotropes	Anti-inflammatory
Anaphylactic	X		X			X				
Cardiogenic	X			X			X		X	
Hypovolemic	X	X	X					X		
Neurogenic	X	X cautious						X		
Obstructive	X	X temporary								
Septic	X	X	X		X			X		X (Xigris)

24. d. Rationale: Although some patients in shock may be treated with antianxiety and sedative drugs to control anxiety and apprehension, the nurse should always acknowledge the patient's feelings, explain procedures before they are carried out, and inform the patient of the plan of care and its rationale. Members of the clergy should be called only if the patient requests or agrees to a visit, and whereas visits by family may have a therapeutic effect on some patients, family visits may increase stress in others.
25. a. *T*; b. *F*, results; c. *F*, SIRS; d. *T*; e. *T*
26. a. 1; b. 4; c. 5; d. 3; e. 3; f. 2; g. 1; h. 4

27. a. Rationale: Early enteral feedings in the patient in shock are believed to increase the blood supply to the GI tract and help to prevent translocation of GI bacteria and endotoxins into the blood, preventing initial or additional infection in patients in shock. Surgical removal of necrotic tissue, especially from burns, eliminates a source of infection in critically ill patients, as does the use of strict aseptic technique in all patient procedures. Known infections are treated with specific agents, and broad-spectrum agents are used only until organisms are identified.

28. b. Rationale: Generally, the first organ system affected by mediator-induced injury in MODS is the respiratory system. Adventitious sounds and areas absent of breath sounds will be present. Other organ damage also occurs, but lungs are usually first.

29. d. Rationale: The presence of MODS is confirmed when there is defined clinical evidence of failure of more than one organ. Elevated serum lipase and amylase levels indicate pancreatic failure, a serum creatinine of 3.8 mg/dL indicates kidney failure, and a platelet count of 15,000/μL indicates hematologic failure. Other criteria include urine output less than 0.5 mL/kg/hr, BUN 100 mg/dL or greater, WBC count 1000/μL, upper or lower GI bleeding, GCS score 6 or less, and hematocrit 20% or less. A respiratory rate of 45/min, $PaCO_2$ of 60, and a chest x-ray with bilateral diffuse, patchy infiltrates indicate respiratory failure but not other organ damage.

Case Study

1. Indwelling catheter leading to UTI; compromised patient—elderly, chronic illnesses of diabetes, myocardial infarction, and heart failure

2. Aseptic technique in catheter placement; increased fluid intake to flush catheter; consult with health care provider regarding prophylactic antimicrobials; early detection of changes in urine, temperature

3. Release of endotoxins by gram-negative bacteria that cause inflammatory responses is the initial insult. The endotoxins bind to monocytes and lymphocytes, stimulating the release of TNF and IL-1, which in turn cause release or activation of platelet-activating factor, prostaglandins, leukotrienes, thromboxane A-2, kinins, and complement. The result is widespread vasodilation and increased capillary permeability. Histamine is also released, which causes increased capillary permeability. The end result is decreased SVR and normal or increased CO as a result of the decreased SVR. Myocardial function is also suppressed by myocardial depressant factor. Death is associated with persistent increase in heart rate and CO, with low SVR and refractory hypotension with progression to MODS.

4. The widespread vasodilation caused by the inflammatory processes and increased capillary permeability causing fluid loss to the interstitium cause hypotension.

5. Decreased LOC—decreased tissue perfusion to the brain and hypoxia of brain cells
Warm, dry, and flushed skin—massive vasodilation
Tachycardia—activation of sympathetic nervous system with β-adrenergic stimulation increasing heart rate
Tachypnea—compensation for tissue hypoxia and metabolic acidosis
Fever—bacterial infection
Decreased SVR—profound vasodilation

Increased CO—occurs as a result of decreased vascular resistance
Oliguria—inadequate renal perfusion and possible renal failure
Hyperglycemia—sympathetic nervous system stimulation causes glycogenolysis by the liver

6. To monitor fluid replacement and cardiac function because of multiple system involvement

7. Blood gases:
   - pH—indicates an acidosis, typical of the metabolic acidosis of anaerobic metabolism of shock
   - PaO_2—very low, indicating a marked hypoxemia
   - $PaCO_2$—also low as a result of hyperventilation to compensate for the metabolic acidosis
   - HCO_3^-—the bicarbonate is low because it is used to neutralize the acids of anaerobic metabolism.
   - SaO_2—a very low oxygen saturation. Normal should be 96% to 100%, and the patient's level indicates severe hypoxemia.

8. Hemodynamic pressures:
   - Right atrial pressure (RAP)—normal is 2 to 8 mm Hg. Marked vasodilation would decrease venous return to the heart, and it would be expected to be decreased.
   - PAP—normal is 10 to 20 mm Hg and is an indicator of afterload or systemic vascular resistance. The patient's PAP would be expected to be decreased in septic shock, where there is profound vasodilation.
   - PAWP—normal is 6 to 12 mm Hg and is an indicator of afterload or systemic vascular resistance. The patient's PAWP would be expected to be low.
   - CO—normal is 4 to 8 L/min. Initially, the patient's CO would be expected to be elevated, illustrating the high CO typical of septic shock.
   - SVR—normal is 900 to 1400 dynes/sec/cm^{-5}. Vasodilation would produce a decreased SVR.

9. Fluid therapy is used to increase vascular volume and BP to increase tissue perfusion. Dopamine is used to increase vasoconstriction and strengthen myocardial contractions to elevate systemic vascular resistance.

10. *Nursing diagnoses:*
    - Ineffective peripheral tissue perfusion related to deficit in capillary blood supply
    - Altered protection related to neurosensory alterations
    - Hyperthermia related to inflammatory process
    - Risk for disuse syndrome related to perceptual-cognitive impairment
    Collaborative problems:
    Potential complications: Heart failure; acute respiratory disease (ARDS); disseminated intravascular coagulopathy (DIC); organ ischemia—neurologic, renal, GI; MODS

CHAPTER 68

1. c. Rationale: Respiratory failure results when the transfer of oxygen or carbon dioxide function of the respiratory system is impaired, and although the

definition is determined by PaO_2 and $PaCO_2$ levels, the major factor in respiratory failure is inadequate gas exchange to meet tissue O_2 needs. Absence of ventilation is respiratory arrest, and partial airway obstruction may not necessarily cause respiratory failure. Acute hypoxemia may be caused by factors other than pulmonary dysfunction.

2. a. HO; b. HO; c. HC; d. HO; e. HO; f. HC; g. HC; h. HO; i. HC

3. a. *T*; b. *F*, 1 or less; c. *T*; d. *F*, air in the lung from passing into the blood; e. *F*, V/Q mismatch; f. *F*, diffusion limitation

4. a. 3; b. 4; c. 2; d. 5; e. 1

5. a. 3; b. 1; c. 2; d. 4

6. b. Rationale: Hypercapnic respiratory failure is associated with alveolar hypoventilation with increases in alveolar and arterial CO_2 and often is caused by problems outside the lungs. A patient with slow, shallow respirations is not exchanging enough gas volume to eliminate CO_2. Deep, rapid respirations reflect hyperventilation and often accompany lung problems that cause hypoxemic respiratory failure. Pulmonary edema and large airway resistance cause obstruction of oxygenation and result in a V/Q mismatch or shunt typical of hypoxemic respiratory failure.

7. d. Rationale: In a patient with normal lung function, respiratory failure is commonly defined as a PaO_2 ≤60 mm Hg or a $PaCO_2$ >45 mm Hg or both, but because the patient with chronic pulmonary disease normally maintains low PaO_2 and high $PaCO_2$, acute respiratory failure in these patients can be defined as an acute decrease in PaO_2 or increase in $PaCO_2$ from the patient's baseline parameters, accompanied by an acid pH. The pH of 7.28 reflects an acidemia and a loss of compensation in the patient with chronic lung disease.

8. a. HO; b. HC; c. HC; d. HO; e. HO; f. HC; g. HC

9. a. Rationale: Because the brain is very sensitive to a decrease in oxygen delivery, restlessness, agitation, disorientation, and confusion are early signs of hypoxemia, for which the nurse should be alert. Mild hypertension is also an early sign, accompanied by tachycardia. Central cyanosis is an unreliable, late sign of hypoxemia, and cardiac dysrhythmias also occur later.

10. d. Rationale: The increase in respiratory rate required to blow off accumulated CO_2 predisposes to respiratory muscle fatigue, and the slowing of a rapid rate in a patient in acute distress indicates tiring and the possibility of respiratory arrest unless ventilatory assistance is provided. A decreased I/E ratio, orthopnea, and accessory muscle use are common findings in respiratory distress but do not necessarily signal respiratory fatigue or arrest.

11. a. Rationale: Patients with a shunt are usually more hypoxemic than are patients with a V/Q mismatch because the alveoli are filled with fluid, which prevents gas exchange. Hypoxemia resulting from an intrapulmonary shunt is usually not responsive to high O_2 concentrations, and the patient will usually require positive pressure ventilation. Hypoxemia associated with a V/Q mismatch usually responds favorably to oxygen administration at 1 to 3 L/min by nasal cannula. Removal of secretions with coughing and suctioning is not generally effective in reversing an acute hypoxemia resulting from a shunt.

12. a. Rationale: When there is impaired function of the one lung, the patient should be positioned with the unaffected lung in the dependent position to promote perfusion to the functioning tissue. If the diseased lung is positioned dependently, more V/Q mismatch would occur. The head of the bed may be elevated, or a reclining chair may be used, with the patient positioned on the unaffected side, to maximize thoracic expansion if the patient has increased work of breathing.

13. b. Rationale: Augmented coughing by applying pressure on the thorax or abdominal muscles at the beginning of expiration helps to produce muscle movement, increases pleural pressure and expiratory flows, and assists the cough to remove secretions in the patient who is exhausted. An oral airway is used only if there is a possibility that the tongue will obstruct the airway. Huff coughing is indicated for patients with problems with ET tubes in place, which prevent glottal closure, and slow, pursed-lip breathing is used to prevent air trapping and give the patient a sense of control over breathing.

14. a. Rationale: Although sedation, analgesia, and neuromuscular blockade are often used to control agitation and pain, these treatments may contribute to prolonged ventilator days. It is most important to assess the patient for the cause of the restlessness and agitation (e.g., pain, hypoxemia, electrolyte imbalances), and treat the underlying cause before sedating the patient more.

15. d. Rationale: Hemodynamic monitoring with a pulmonary artery catheter is instituted in severe respiratory failure to determine the amount of blood flow to tissues and the response of the lung and heart to hypoxemia. Continuous BP monitoring may be performed, but BP is a reflection of cardiac activity, which can be determined by the pulmonary artery catheter findings. ABGs are important to evaluate oxygenation and ventilation status and V/Q mismatches.

16. a. inhaled albuterol, metaproterenol; b. IV corticosteroids; c. IV furosemide (Lasix), nitroglycerine (Tridil); d. vancomycin (Vancocin), ceftriaxone (Rocephin).

17. d. Rationale: Noninvasive positive-pressure ventilation (NIPPV) involves the application of a face mask and delivery of a volume of air under inspiratory pressure. Because the device is worn externally, the patient must be able to cooperate in its use, and frequent access to the airway for suctioning

or inhaled medications must not be necessary. It is not indicated when high levels of oxygen are needed or respirations are absent.

18. a. Rationale: Although ARDS may occur in the patient who has virtually any severe illness or trauma and may be both a cause and result of SIRS, the most common precipitating insults of ARDS are septic shock and gastric aspiration.

19. a. Interstitial and alveolar edema from damage to vascular endothelium and increased capillary permeability
    b. Atelectasis from destruction of type II cells, resulting in inactivation of surfactant
    c. Hyaline membrane formation from exudation of high-molecular-weight substances in the edema fluid

20. c. Rationale: In the fibrotic phase of ARDS, diffuse scarring and fibrosis of the lungs occur, resulting in decreased surface area for gas exchange and continued hypoxemia caused by diffusion limitation. Although edema is resolved, lung compliance is decreased because of interstitial fibrosis, and long-term mechanical ventilation is required with a poor prognosis for survival.

21. b. Rationale: Hypoxemia that does not respond to oxygenation by any route is a hallmark of ARDS and is always present. $PaCO_2$ levels may be normal until the patient is no longer able to compensate in response to the hypoxemia. Bronchial breath sounds may be associated with the progression of ARDS. Pulmonary capillary wedge pressures that are normally elevated in cardiogenic pulmonary edema are normal in the pulmonary edema of ARDS.

22. c. Rationale: Early signs of ARDS are insidious and difficult to detect, but the nurse should be alert for any early signs of hypoxemia, such as restlessness, dyspnea, and decreased mentation, in patients at risk for ARDS. Abnormal findings on physical examination or diagnostic studies, such as adventitious lung sounds, signs of respiratory distress, respiratory alkalosis, or decreasing PaO_2, are usually indications that ARDS has progressed beyond the initial stages.

23. b. Rationale: Hospital-acquired pneumonia is one of the most common complications of ARDS, and early detection requires frequent monitoring of sputum smears and cultures and assessment of the quality, quantity, and consistency of sputum. Blood in gastric aspirate may indicate a stress ulcer, and subcutaneous emphysema of the face, neck, and chest occurs with barotrauma during mechanical ventilation. Oral infections may result from prophylactic antibiotics and impaired host defenses but are not common.

24. a. Rationale: Because ARDS is precipitated by a physiologic insult, a critical factor in its prevention and early management is treatment of the underlying condition. Prophylactic antibiotics,

treatment with diuretics and fluid restriction, and mechanical ventilation are also used as ARDS progresses.

25. a. Rationale: PEEP used with mechanical ventilation applies positive pressure to the airway and lungs at the end of exhalation, keeping the lung partially expanded and preventing collapse of the alveoli and helping to open up collapsed alveoli. Permissive hypercapnia is allowed when the patient with ARDS is ventilated with smaller tidal volumes to prevent barotrauma. Extracorporeal membrane oxygenation and extracorporeal CO_2 removal involve passing blood across a gas-exchanging membrane outside the body and then returning oxygenated blood back to the body.

26. c. Rationale: PEEP increases intrathoracic and intrapulmonic pressures, compresses the pulmonary capillary bed, and reduces blood return to both the right and left side of the heart. Preload (CVP) and CO are decreased, often with a dramatic decrease in blood pressure.

27. d. Rationale: When a patient with ARDS is supine, alveoli in the posterior areas of the lung are dependent and fluid-filled, and the heart and mediastinal contents place more pressure on the lungs, predisposing to atelectasis. If the patient is turned prone, air filled, nonatelectatic alveoli in the anterior portion of the lung receive more blood, and perfusion may be better matched to ventilation, causing less V/Q mismatch. Lateral rotation therapy is used to stimulate postural drainage and help mobilize pulmonary secretions.

Case Study

1. The patient is experiencing hypercapnic respiratory failure, reflected by the elevated $PaCO_2$ and pH of 7.3. In this case, severe COPD, with destruction of alveoli and terminal respiratory units, has led to hypoventilation, with less removal of CO_2 and less space for O_2 in the alveoli. The patient with severe COPD always has some degree of decompensation resulting in chronic respiratory failure, but an acute exacerbation or infection may cause an acute decompensation, thus producing an acute or chronic respiratory failure.

2. The primary contributing factor to the onset of the acute failure is the pneumonia, but other factors include the presence of chronic lung disease, her age, and immunosuppression with steroids.

3. The primary pathophysiologic effects of hypercapnia are a respiratory acidosis resulting from retained CO_2 and a hypoxemia resulting from alveolar retention of CO_2. Clinical manifestations of hypercapnic respiratory failure that P.C. is experiencing include the dyspnea, shortness of breath, sitting in a tripod position, and using pursed-lip breathing, in addition to her ABG values. Other manifestations

of hypercapnia that the nurse should assess P.C. for include morning headache, somnolence, confusion, dysrhythmias, and muscle weakness. Because she is also hypoxemic, she should be assessed for mild hypertension, tachycardia, prolonged expiration, and accessory respiratory muscle use.

4. The tripod position helps decrease the work of breathing, because propping the arms up increases the anterior-posterior diameter of the chest and changes pressures in the thorax. Pursed-lip breathing causes an increase in SaO_2 because it slows respiration, allows more time for expiration, and prevents the small bronchioles from collapsing.

5. Noninvasive positive pressure ventilation (NIPPV) is delivered by placing a mask over the patient's nose or nose and mouth, and the patient breathes spontaneously while positive pressure is delivered. It may be used as a treatment for patients with acute or chronic respiratory failure and helps decrease the work of breathing, without the need for endotracheal intubation. It is not appropriate for the patient who has absent respirations, excessive secretions, a decreased LOC, high O_2 requirements, facial trauma, or hemodynamic instability.

6. Treatment of acute respiratory failure is directed toward reversing the disease process that resulted in the failure. P.C.'s COPD is chronic and irreversible, but the IV antibiotics are critical in treating the pneumonia that precipitated the acute or chronic respiratory failure. The bronchodilators and corticosteroids will help with airway inflammation and spasm, but it cannot be expected that she will recover without treatment of the infection.

7. *Nursing diagnoses:*
   - Ineffective breathing pattern related to expiratory obstruction to airflow
   - Ineffective airway clearance related to increased airway resistance
   - Impaired gas exchange related to alveolar hypoventilation
   - Risk for impaired skin integrity related to NIPPV mask

   Collaborative problems:
   Potential complications: hypoxia; hypercapnia; respiratory and metabolic acidosis; dysrhythmias

CHAPTER 69

1. a. 3; b. 1; c. 2; d. 4; e. 1; f. 5; g. 2; h. 3
2. d. Rationale: During the primary survey of emergency care, assessment and immediate interventions are made for life-threatening problems affecting airway, breathing, circulation, disability, and exposure/environmental control. The triage system is used initially to determine the priority of care for patients, and history of the illness or accident is part of the secondary survey. Any emergency department should be able to stabilize and initially treat a patient who requires specialized care unavailable at the admitting facility.

3. *Airway with Cervical Spine Stabilization and/ or Immobilization:* Inhalation injury, airway obstruction, upper airway wounds or trauma, seizures, near-drowning
   Interventions: Jaw-thrust maneuver, application of cervical immobilization device, artificial airway, suctioning
   Breathing: Anaphylaxis, flail chest, hemothorax, open or tension pneumothorax
   Interventions: Supplemental oxygen or ventilation with BVM at 100% oxygen, chest tube insertion or needle thoracostomy, ET intubation
   Circulation: Cardiac injury, pericardial tamponade, shock, uncontrolled external hemorrhage
   Interventions: CPR and ALS if no pulse, two large-bore IVs with infusions of fluids or blood, direct pressure to bleeding; obtain blood samples; assist with pelvic splints
   Disability: Head injury, stroke
   Interventions: Monitor LOC, elevate the head of bed 30 degrees, if permitted; two large-bore IVs if possible candidate for thrombolytic

4. a. Rationale: Specific injuries are associated with specific types of accidents and events surrounding an incident, and details of the incident and the trajectory of penetrating injuries are important in identifying and treating injury. Alcohol use is assessed with blood testing, and although information may be used for regulatory agencies, the primary use of the information is for treatment of the patient.

5. a. Continuous cardiac monitoring; b. obtain full set of vital signs, including oxygen saturation; c. CXR; d. insert indwelling urinary catheter; e. insert orogastric or nasogastric tube. Others: facilitate laboratory and diagnostic studies, continuous pulse oximetry monitoring, determine need for tetanus prophylaxis, facilitate family presence

6. b. Rationale: A nasally placed tube is contraindicated if the patient has facial fractures or a possible basilar skull fracture because the tube could enter the brain. It would not be contraindicated in the other conditions.

7. a. allergies; b. medications; c. past health history, pregnancy status; d. last meal; e. events/environment leading to the illness or injury

8. b. Rationale: Tetanus immunoglobulin provides passive immunity for tetanus and is used in treatment of a tetanus-prone wound if the patient has not had at least three doses of active tetanus toxoid. The patient would also receive tetanus toxoid to initiate active immunity in the case of tetanus-prone wounds. If the patient has fewer than three doses of tetanus toxoid and a non–tetanus-prone wound, only tetanus toxoid would be administered to initiate active immunity. In the actively immunized patient, tetanus toxoid is

administered for tetanus-prone wounds if it has been more than 5 years since the last dose, and it is also administered for non–tetanus-prone wounds if it has been more than 10 years since the last dose.

9. b. Rationale: Therapeutic hypothermia after resuscitation improves mortality and neurologic outcomes. This patient might benefit from this therapy. Patient "a" will need airway maintenance and evaluation of cause for unconsciousness. Patient "c" should have ABCs monitored and begin the cooling process. Watch for dysrhythmias. Provide fluid and electrolyte replacement. Patient "d" will need mechanical ventilation and diuretics.

10. b. Rationale: Organ procurement agencies are now called to talk with families as they are trained to screen and counsel families.

11. a. 3; b. 4; c. 2; d. 4; e. 3; f. 4; g. 4; h. 3; i. 1

12. c. Rationale: Rewarming of frostbitten tissue is extremely painful, and analgesia should be administered during the process. The affected part is submerged in a warm water bath at approximately 104°–108° F (40°–42° C), and massage or scrubbing of the tissue should be avoided because of the potential for tissue damage. Blisters form in hours to days following the injury and are not an immediate concern.

13. a. Rationale: Rigidness, bradycardia, and slowed respiratory rate are signs of moderate hypothermia. The ABCs are the initial priority. Active core rewarming is indicated for moderate to severe hypothermia. Axillary temperatures are inadequate to monitor core temperature, so esophageal, rectal, or indwelling urinary catheter thermometers are used. The patient should be assessed for other injuries but should not be exposed in order to prevent further loss of heat.

14. b. Rationale: Patients with profound hypothermia appear dead on presentation and exhibit fixed, dilated pupils; difficult to detect vital signs;

unconsciousness; and apnea. Shivering is seen in mild hypothermia, and moderate hypothermia is characterized by slowed respirations, BP obtainable only by Doppler, and rigidity.

15. a. F; b. B; c. B; d. S; e. B

16. a. Rationale: The most important life-threatening consequence of near-drowning of any type is hypoxia from fluid-filled and poorly ventilated alveoli—airway and oxygenation are first priorities. Correction of metabolic (anaerobic) acidosis occurs with effective ventilation and oxygenation; lactated Ringer's or normal saline solution is started to manage fluid balance; and mannitol or furosemide may be used to treat free water and cerebral edema.

17. a. Rationale: Wood ticks or dog ticks release a neurotoxin as long as the tick head is attached to the body, and tick removal is essential for effective treatment. Tick removal leads to return of muscle movement, usually within 48 to 72 hours. There is no antidote, and hemodialysis is not known to remove the neurotoxin. Antibiotics are used to treat Lyme disease and Rocky Mountain spotted fever, infections spread by tick bites.

18. a. *F, Pasteurella* species; b. *T*; c. *F*, washing with large amounts of water; d. *F*, water or milk; e. *F*, hemodialysis

19. a, b, c, d. Rationale: Patients who ingest caustic agents, co-ingest sharp objects, or ingest nontoxic substances should not receive lavage.

20. d. Rationale: Activated charcoal will absorb any of the medication left in the stomach. Cathartics are usually given with activated charcoal to increase elimination of the toxins absorbed by the charcoal. Gastric lavage may be indicated to remove any drug that is not already absorbed from the stomach for some patients; however, there is a risk of aspiration and esophageal perforation. Vomiting should never be induced in a patient who is unconscious.

21. See table below.

Agent	Bacterial	Viral	Person-to-Person Spread	Antibiotic Treatment	Vaccine
Botulism	X				X
Anthrax	X			X	X
Plague	X		X	X, immediately	In development
Hemorrhagic fever		X	X		
Tularemia	X			X	In development
Smallpox		X	X		X

22. a. 6; b. 4; c. 2; d. 1; e. 4; f. 6; g. 3; h. 2; i. 5; j. 3; k. 1
23. b. Rationale: Ionizing radiation exposure in a sublethal dose will cause nausea and vomiting within 2 to 4 hours of exposure, hair loss in 2 days to 2 weeks, and coagulopathies in 2 days to 2 weeks.
24. d. Rationale: Disaster medical assistance teams are composed of members with health or medical skills and directly provide medical care in disaster situations. Triage is performed by first responders such as police and designated emergency medical personnel. The hospital's emergency response plan is a specific plan that addresses how personnel and resources will be used in case of a disaster, and community emergency response teams provide training to communities in general to respond to disasters.

Case Study

1. Advanced age and prolonged exposure to heat over several days are risk factors for M.M.'s development of heat stroke.
2. ABGs—decreased PaO_2; electrolytes—decreased serum sodium, chloride, potassium; CBC—hemoconcentration with elevated hemoglobin and hematocrit; BUN and creatinine—elevated; serum glucose—decreased; coagulation studies—decreased prothrombin time, decreased bleeding times; liver function tests—elevated enzymes; UA—elevated specific gravity, protein, possible microscopic hematuria
3. Clothing would be removed and the patient covered with wet sheets and placed in front of a fan; consider immersion in a cool water bath. If the temperature is not reduced by these methods, administer cool fluids intravenously or lavage with cool fluids.
4. 100% oxygen to compensate for the hypermetabolic state, with intubation and mechanical ventilation if necessary; IV crystalloid salt solution with CVP or PA pressure monitoring to evaluate fluid status; cooling methods with monitoring of core temperature; indwelling catheter and I&O; administration of chlorpromazine (Thorazine) to control shivering during cooling process
5. Mrs. M. should be told that M.M. is seriously ill and that there is a chance he might not recover because heat stroke has a very high morbidity and mortality rate. She should be kept informed of the treatment he is receiving and his response to treatment, and she should be provided with emotional support and an opportunity to be at her husband's bedside during invasive procedures.
6. *Nursing diagnoses:*
   - Hyperthermia related to environmental exposure
   - Decreased CO related to hypermetabolic process
   - Deficient fluid volume related to fluid loss greater than intake
   - Altered protection related to altered mental state
   - Risk for impaired skin integrity related to immobility
   Collaborative problems:
   Potential complications: Hypovolemic shock; cerebral edema; seizures; hypoxia; electrolyte imbalance; renal failure